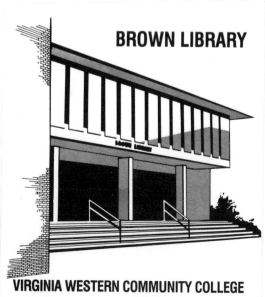

Periodontology *for the* Dental Hygienist

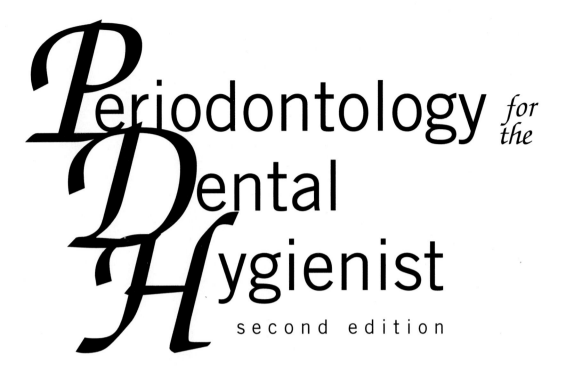

Periodontology *for the* Dental Hygienist

second edition

Dorothy A. Perry, RDH, PhD
Associate Professor and Vice Chair
Department of Preventive and Restorative Dental Sciences
Chair, Division of Dental Hygiene
School of Dentistry
University of California, San Francisco
San Francisco, California

Phyllis Beemsterboer, RDH, EdD
Associate Professor of Periodontology
Associate Dean for Academic Affairs
School of Dentistry
Oregon Health Sciences University
Portland, Oregon

Edward J. Taggart, Jr, DDS, MS
Clinical Professor
Division of Periodontology
Department of Stomatology
School of Dentistry
University of California, San Francisco
San Francisco, California

W.B. SAUNDERS COMPANY
A Harcourt Health Sciences Company
Philadelphia London New York St. Louis Sydney Toronto

087692

W.B. SAUNDERS COMPANY
A Harcourt Health Sciences Company

The Curtis Center
Independence Square West
Philadelphia, Pennsylvania 19106

Library of Congress Cataloging-in-Publication Data

Perry, Dorothy A.
Periodontology for the dental hygienist / Dorothy A. Perry, Phyllis Beemsterboer,
Edward J. Taggart, Jr.–2nd ed.

p.   cm.

Includes bibliographical references and index.

ISBN 0–7216–8559–5

1. Periodontics.   2. Dental hygienists.   I. Beemsterboer, Phyllis.
II. Taggart, Edward J. III. Title.
[DNLM: 1.   Periodontal   Diseases.   2. Periodontics.   WU   240   P462p
2001]

RK361.P4679 2001   617.6′32–dc21

DNLM/DLC   00-057416

Editor-in-Chief: Andrew Allen
Acquisitions Editor: Shirley A. Kuhn
Developmental Editor: Katherine A. Macciocca
Production Manager: Peter Faber
Illustration Specialist: Peg Shaw
Book Designer: Kevin O'Malley
Indexer: Angela Holt

PERIODONTOLOGY FOR THE DENTAL HYGIENIST   ISBN 0-7216-8559-5

Printed in the United States of America.

Last digit is the print number: 9   8   7   6   5   4   3   2   1

Dedication

To memories of our parents:
Louis G. Beemsterboer (1922-1995), Claire
Berkhemer (1908-1960), Robert W. Berkhemer
(1917-2000), Edward J. Taggart, Sr. (1916-1991),
and Margaret C. Taggart (1916-1993)

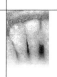

Contributors

GARY C. ARMITAGE, DDS, MS
Professor and Chairman, Division of Periodontology, School of Dentistry, University of California, San Francisco, California
Chapter 17 / Systemic Factors Influencing Periodontal Diseases

PHYLLIS L. BEEMSTERBOER, RDH, EdD
Associate Professor of Periodontology, Associate Dean for Academic Affairs, School of Dentistry, Oregon Health Sciences University, Portland, Oregon
Chapter 2 / Periodontium: Anatomic Characteristics and Host Response
Chapter 8 / Occlusion and Temporomandibular Disorders
Chapter 10 / Treatment Planning for the Periodontal Patient
Chapter 11 / Plaque Control for the Periodontal Patient
Chapter 12 / Nonsurgical Periodontal Therapy
Chapter 16 / Periodontal Emergencies

CHERYL A. CAMERON, RDH, PhD, JD
Professor, Department of Dental Public Health Sciences, School of Dentistry, University of Washington, Seattle, Washington
Chapter 9 / Clinical Assessment

GINA D. EVANS, RDH, BS
Private Practice of Dental Hygiene, Seattle, Washington
Chapter 9 / Clinical Assessment

MARTHA H. FALES, PhD
Professor Emeritus, School of Dentistry, University of Washington, Seattle, Washington
Chapter 1 / Historical Perspectives on Dental Hygiene and Periodontology

MARI-ANNE L. LOW, RDH, MS
Manager, Product Development–Clinical Operations, Oral-B Laboratories Inc., Belmont, California
Chapter 15 / Periodontal Maintenance and Prevention

DOROTHY A. PERRY, RDH, PhD
Associate Professor and Vice Chair, Department of Preventive and Restorative Dental Sciences, Chair, Division of Dental Hygiene, School of Dentistry, University of California, San Francisco, California
Chapter 2 / Periodontium: Anatomic Characteristics and Host Response
Chapter 3 / Epidemiology of Periodontal Disease
Chapter 5 / Calculus and Other Disease-Associated Factors
Chapter 9 / Clinical Assessment
Chapter 11 / Plaque Control for the Periodontal Patient
Chapter 12 / Nonsurgical Periodontal Therapy
Chapter 13 / Periodontal Surgery
Chapter 14 / Dental Implants
Chapter 16 / Periodontal Emergencies

DOROTHY J. ROWE, RDH, MS, PhD
Associate Professor, Department of Preventive and Restorative Dental Sciences, School of Dentistry, University of California, San Francisco, California
Chapter 4 / Microbiology of Periodontal Diseases

EDWARD J. TAGGART, JR, DDS, MS
Clinical Professor, Division of Periodontology, Department of Stomatology, School of Dentistry, University of California, San Francisco, California
Chapter 6 / Gingival Diseases
Chapter 7 / Periodontal Diseases
Chapter 13 / Periodontal Surgery

Preface to the Second Edition

The goal of the dental hygienist is to educate and treat the patient to preserve oral health. The purpose of the second edition of *Periodontology for the Dental Hygienist* is the same as the first edition—to provide foundation knowledge in the discipline of dental hygiene, ultimately strengthening the ability to analyze patients' needs and to treat appropriately. We wish to share a few thoughts with you on the terminology and education that are relevant to this revised edition. First, the word patient is used throughout the book in preference to the word client. Second, differences in opinion exist about the use of the educational terms competency and objective. And third is the place of *Periodontology for the Dental Hygienist* in the context of information available on the World Wide Web.

Patients

Some dental hygiene educators and other health care professionals have stopped calling those we treat patients and now call them clients. Although this change is far from universal, it is of concern to some as to which word is preferred. We continue to use the term patient in this book when referring to human beings in need of periodontal care. The reason lies in the Latin origins of the two words. Patient is derived from the Latin *patiens,* meaning to suffer or bear. Client is derived from *cliens,* meaning to seek the protection or influence of someone powerful. The ability to help someone who is suffering is far more appropriate usage than to exert power over someone in need. Members of the health care community may disagree on the use of these terms, but it is a great reward to help those who are suffering. For

that reason, we are treating *patients* with periodontal diseases.

Educational Terms

Some dental hygiene educators have asked us to define competencies at the beginning of each chapter rather than refer to individual chapter objectives. We continue to believe, however, that the term objective is more appropriate because competency has a much broader application than the specific knowledge we artificially divide into chapters for study. Dental hygiene students in beginning classes and laboratories strive to achieve foundation knowledge and novice-level skills. Students must have this foundation to be able to begin their journey toward competency.

Competency describes the expected behavior of entry-level dental hygienists, including psychomotor skills, and knowledge and values that permit synthesis and application in the practice setting without an instructor for support and guidance. Competency is a journey that continues throughout the life of a professional person. Competency is a continuum and is expressed in five learning stages: novice, beginner, competent, proficient, and expert. Once a student graduates from the dental hygiene education program, he or she is competent and continues to build on the experiences gained from patient care interactions in order to move toward proficiency. True proficiency is achieved only after years of practice.

Proficiency is the ability to be accurate, handle complicated problems, and work comfortably under any circumstances. Expert is the highest level in the continuum and is the result of years of practice, experience and increased levels of expertise in treating patients with difficult and complex problems. The practice of dental hygiene is a professional journey. The objectives in this book form part of the foundation on which a student will build, working toward competency and eventually proficiency and expertise.

World Wide Web

Periodontology for the Dental Hygienist, second edition, is published during changing times for both colleges and universities and publishers. Enormous quantities of material on the subject of periodontology, and every other subject imaginable, are available on the World Wide Web. Photographs, cases, and descriptions of every sort can be downloaded and printed, providing access to a library too vast to even comprehend. In this atmosphere, we hope to provide a useful tool in the discipline that will be valued by both those who visit the Web regularly and those who do not.

This textbook is meant to include state-of-the-art analyses of all aspects of periodontology pertinent to dental hygienists in 2001 and shortly thereafter. Information and research are exploding, and one small book can give the reader only a high quality "snapshot" in time. We recommend augmenting this text with the resources on the Web. For example, by using one search engine and the term periodontitis, 2550 sites appear. By scrolling through them, the user can link to an array of resources, from Web pages by noted periodontal researchers such as Walter Loesche, to a noted lesson page such as the *Dental Hygiene Guide to the Internet.*

We suggest starting with professional organizations and moving to links from there. The American Dental Hygienists' Association provides an extremely valuable resource, available at http://www.adha.org. This site links you to state and local dental hygiene societies plus many more high quality locations. Information on oral health can also be gleaned from WebMD, federal government organizations such as the National Institute for Dental and Craniofacial Research, and university libraries such as UC Digital Library. Almost every college and university has digital access. The Journal of Dental Hygiene, JDH, is available electronically. To access it remotely, each person needs a password. Passwords are readily available to students and alumni at individual colleges and universities.

Many links are of high quality and are well-maintained resources. In fact, several dental hygiene educators requested that we list links at the end of each chapter. We believe it is more valuable to encourage you to seek resources on the World Wide Web, starting with these few locations and building from that foundation.

We wish you well in your career as a dental hygienist. We hope and expect you to augment the basic resources we provide you in this book through your teachers, mentors, libraries, and Web. We offer you one advantage with this book over the Web—you may sit more comfortably in your easy chair to read it. All the best to you.

Dorothy A. Perry
Phyllis L. Beemsterboer
Edward J. Taggart, Jr.

Preface to the First Edition

Periodontology is an integral part of the practice of dental hygiene. A foundation in science plus knowledge in the discipline permits the clinician to synthesize and apply treatment techniques with the goal of preserving teeth in comfort and function. This goal and level of achievement are essential to the dental hygiene professional.

The purpose of this book, *Periodontology for the Dental Hygienist,* is to prepare the dental hygienist to meet this goal. The book defines the scope of periodontal education for students of dental hygiene, places it in the context of clinical practice, and continues to be a resource of periodontal information. The material covers both the historical and scientific background of dental hygiene periodontal practice, pathogenesis of periodontal diseases, rationale for therapy, critical analysis of patient assessments, current theories of treatment, and specific rationales for techniques. The information is integrated in a logical order to provide the learner with a thoroughly readable text and a complete understanding of periodontology.

Mastery of this information facilitates both the dental hygiene student and the practicing dental hygienist to become periodontal therapists. The dental hygienist acting in this role is an essential member of the periodontal treatment team.

Acknowledgments

Many people provided expertise, resources, illustrations, and understanding during the genesis of this book. Without their support, this text could not have been written.

Our families sacrificed weekend time and pleasant evenings at home, and paid long-distance telephone bills. Those particularly to be thanked are Anne Perry, Carolyn Koster Taggart, and Joe Jedrychowski. Without their help and distraction this book and the first edition would have been finished in half the time but without their caring and concern.

Our contributors provided wonderful richness and expertise to both editions. Each of their chapters is a tribute to their academic interests and expertise. Special thanks to Martha Fales, Ken Fales, Dorothy Rowe, Cheryl Cameron, Gina Evans, Mari-Anne Low, and Gary Armitage for their help with the first edition and second edition, including galleys, and page proofs. Thanks for their friendship.

The outstanding illustrations and interesting cases presented on these pages are the collective work of many friends over many years. A special note of appreciation goes to Phil Melnick for giving us free access to his beautiful slide collection and for taking the best intraoral radiographs. Gary Armitage provided the unique and outstanding histologic illustrations, plus unlimited access to the slide library at the University of California, San Francisco. Others who shared were Dean Charles Bertolami, Carol Bibb, Tom Bramanti, Paulo Camargo, Glenn Clark, Jim Coggan, Greg Conti, Dennis Davis, Debbie Del Carlo, Fritz Finzen, Ron Fujitaki, Walter Fuller, Valerie Godfrey, Ed Green, Deborah Greenspan, Lisa Grosso, Paul Johnson, Sasha Jovanovic, Barry Kinney, Wilma Motley, Rick Nagy, Joe Regezi, Robbie Robinson, Randy Rowland, Jay Seibert, John Sottosanti, Bob Wirthlin, Larry Wolinsky, and Craig Yonemura.

No textbook is written by one or even three people. *Periodontology for the Dental Hygienist,* second edition, represents a state-of-the-art presentation of many of the achievements of all those mentioned here plus the discourse of generations of scientists who have advanced this field. We stand in awe of their many accomplishments. Thank you.

NOTICE

Periodontology is an ever-changing field. Standard safety precautions must be followed, but as new research and clinical experience broaden our knowledge, changes in treatment and drug therapy may become necessary or appropriate. Readers are advised to check the most current product information provided by the manufacturer of each drug to be administered to verify the recommended dose, the method and duration of administration, and the contraindications. It is the responsibility of the treating physician, relying on experience and knowledge of the patient, to determine the dosages and the best treatment for each individual patient. Neither the publisher nor the editor assume any liability for any injury and/or damage to persons or property arising from this publication.

THE PUBLISHER

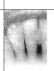

Contents

1

Martha H. Fales

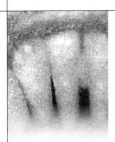

Historical Perspectives on Dental Hygiene and Periodontology

Chapter Objectives

1. Discuss the preventive oral health procedures of early civilizations.
2. Describe the factors that led to the establishment of the profession of dental hygiene.
3. Comment on the differences in the basic orientation of restorative dentists and periodontists.
4. Recognize the major contributions of anthropology to the knowledge of historical events in early dentistry.
5. Recognize the technological progress in periodontal care from magical cures to the use of ultrasonic instruments.
6. Understand the lag between oral health research findings and their application to dental practice.

Key Terms

Anthropology
Apprentice
Barber-surgeons
Gingivitis
Oral prophylaxis

Periodontitis
Periodontoclasia
Preceptor
Pyorrhea alveolaris

Study of the past shows that history unites objective actions with subjective interpretations. In this way, comprehension is combined with narration of what has happened. This chapter provides a brief review of historical events that have brought together the professions of dentistry and dental hygiene with the science of periodontology. These groups of clinicians provide oral health services today based on our history of education, research, and practice experiences. This panoramic view illustrates the need for dental hygienists to embrace an historical perspective and pursue lifelong learning to direct, modify, and expand their professional actions.

ANCIENT DOCUMENTATION OF DENTAL CONCERNS: 3000 B.C. TO 1800 A.D.

The dental profession owes a great deal to **anthropology** (the study of humans) for the knowledge of dental diseases that existed before there were written records. In a text published in 1948, Weinberger[1] described Arthur Keith's findings from a study of prehistoric skulls. These skulls showed an extreme form of true dental caries, evidence of alveolar bone resorption, periapical abscesses, supernumerary teeth, and impacted teeth. This research suggests that dental and periodontal diseases have plagued humans since the beginning of time.

Ancient Evidence of Periodontal Disease and Its Treatment

Anthropologic expeditions to Mesopotamian sites in Iraq found gold vanity sets and cases, including ear scoops, tweezers, and toothpicks. One set found in the Nigel Temple at Ur is estimated to have been used about 3000 B.C.

The oldest written documents related to teeth were found in the Sumerian civilization located in the geographic region between the Tigris and Euphrates Rivers in Asia. The documents included pictographic and cuneiform tablets. These tablets provide evidence of early concern for personal oral hygiene. An Assyrian medical text from approximately 3000 B.C. contained the following treatment:

> If a man's mouth has mouth trouble, thou shalt bray Lelium in well water, introduce salt, alum and vinegar therein, thou shalt leave it under the stars, in the morning, thou shalt wind a linen (strip) around his forefinger, without a meal thou shalt clean his mouth.[2]

A thousand years later, during the Greek and Roman periods, medical and dental knowledge progressed from a mixture of religion and magic to a true separation of religion and medicine. Cicero wrote that Aesculapius (1193–1164 B.C.), the ancient god of medicine and healing, was the first to recommend cleansing the mouth and teeth. Thus, Weinberger cited this reference as the origin of dental hygiene.[1]

Hippocrates (460–377 B.C.), a Greek physician, was the first to prescribe a dentifrice. He wrote:

> When a woman's mouth smells and her gums are black and unhealthy, one burns, separately, the head of a hare, and three mice, after having taken out the intestines of two of them (not however the liver or kidneys): one pounds in a stone mortar some marble and whitstone, and passes it through a sieve; one then mixes equal parts of these ingredients and with this mixture one rubs the teeth and the interior of the mouth; afterward one rubs them again with greasy wool and one washes the mouth with water. One soaks the dirty wool in honey and with it rubs the gums inside and outside. One pounds dill and anise seeds, 2 aboles [1 abole = ¾ gram] of myrrh; one immerses these substances in half a cotyle [1 cotyle = ¼ liter] of pure white wine; one then rinses the mouth with it, holding it in the mouth for some time; this is to be done frequently and the mouth to be rinsed with said preparation fasting, and after each meal. The medicament described above cleans the teeth and gives them a sweet smell.[3]

The whitstone mentioned by Hippocrates indicates the origin of chalk used in a dentifrice. Chalk is still a major ingredient in toothpaste and tooth powders.

In 1940, Leonard wrote an historical background of **periodontoclasia**, defining it as any destructive or degenerative disease of the periodontium. He stated the flashes of understanding, that started with Hippocrates, could have served as a basis for effective periodontal treatment many hundreds of years before such treatment became generally available.[4]

Aristotle (348–322 B.C.) was the first to mention instruments associated with teeth when he described "scrapers." Existing examples show that these instruments were similar to current scalers. However, Aristotle had a curious misperception: he wrote women did not have as many teeth as men.[1]

A fiber stick probably served as the first toothbrush. It was approximately the size of a pencil and was hammered on one end to separate the bristles. Such sticks were recorded in Babylonian, Chinese, Greek, and Roman literature. The stick was always taken from a tree or bush that contained, in its bark, a cleansing powder plus aromatic fumes that acted as an astringent. In this way, the stick provided a dentifrice and mouthwash combined. The Mohammedans called their sticks "siwaks." They were made of arrak (*Salvadora persica:* the toothbrush tree).[5] In Greece and Italy, sticks came from the mastic tree (*Pistacia lentiscus:* the toothpick tree). In Saudi Arabia, the sticks are called "miswaks" (Figure 1-1).

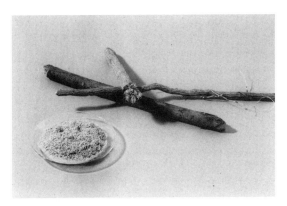

FIGURE 1-1. A chew stick made from a tree branch. (Courtesy of Dr. Lawrence Wolinsky.)

The Middle Ages

Little dental literature existed or survived during the Middle Ages, approximately 500 A.D. to 1500 A.D. The next reference to dental history came later, during the period of the Arab conquests. Albucasis (936-1013 A.D.) was a great Moorish surgeon in Spain and a very religious man. He was the first author to consider the formation of dental calculus or tartar. He recommended thorough cleansing of the teeth with a set of 14 scrapers he devised.

In the famous Latin treatise, *De Chirurgia,* Albucasis wrote:

On Scraping the Teeth

Sometimes on the surface of the teeth, both inside and outside, as well as under the gums, are deposited rough scales of ugly appearance and black, green or yellowish in color; thus corruption is communicated to the gums and so the teeth are in process of time denuded. It is necessary for thee to lay the patient's head upon thy lap and scrape the teeth and molars, on which are observed either true encrustations of something similar to sand, and do this until nothing more remains of such substances; and until the dirty color of the teeth disappears, be it black, green, or yellowish, or of any other color. If a first scraping is sufficient, so much the better; if not, thou shalt repeat it on the following day, or even on the third and fourth day, until the desired purpose is obtained. Thou must know, however, that the teeth need scrapers of various shapes and figure, on account of the various nature of the operation. In fact, the scalpel with which the teeth must be scraped on the inside is unlike that with which thou shalt scrape the outside; and that with which thou shalt scrape the interstices between the teeth shall likewise have another shape. Therefore, thou must have all the series of scalpels ready, if it so pleases God.[6]

Written in the 900s, this description shows an understanding of the character of dental calculus and periodontal therapy. Similar rules are found in periodontal instructions of more recent vintage.

The next mention of oral hygiene occurred in the writing of Johannes Aranculus (1412-1484) when he listed 10 rules of oral hygiene. These showed an early concern for diet in relation to oral diseases. He wrote:

Therefore it is essential to guard against corruption of food and drink in the stomach: (a) such food as milk and salt fish must not be eaten; shortly after meals, exercise, bathing, etc., should be avoided; (b) meat and other foods that might cause vomiting, and (c) desserts and sweets such as honey should not be eaten. (d) One should not bite hard things. (e) One should avoid all substances that can set the teeth on edge. (f) All things that are too hot or too cold should be avoided, and especially taken in rapid succession, hot or cold, or cold or hot drinks. (g) Onions should not be eaten as they are injurious to the teeth. (h) Teeth should be cleansed after each meal, using a thin piece of a certain wood, but care must be taken not to injure the gums. (i) After each meal it is necessary to rinse the mouth with a good strong wine, or mixture of various herbs. (j) The teeth must be rubbed before going to bed, or in the morning with a suitable dentifrice.[1]

The Development of Modern Dentistry

Europe must be given credit for beginning the era of modern dentistry. Dentists were trained by apprenticeship, learning by watching and assisting an established dentist. Ambroise Paré (1517-1590) was the first **apprentice** who was allowed to take the examination to become a member of the College of Surgeons in Paris. He extracted teeth, opened dental abscesses, and set fractured jaws. Pare performed these tasks not in the crude manner of members of the College, but with skill and good judgment, as though gained through educational experiences.[7]

Andreas Vesalius (1514-1564), a Flemish anatomist, and Bartolommeo Eustachio (1520-1574), an Italian anatomist, were responsible for early anatomic studies of the teeth. Then followed the discoveries of Anton van Leeuwenhoek (1632-1723), a Dutch naturalist and microscopist who discovered dental tubuli. Van Leeuwenhoek described them as being so fine that 600 to 700 of them were no thicker than a hair from a beard. He also examined tartar scrapings from teeth and saw microorganisms of the mouth.

Historians agree that no individual exerted a more powerful influence on dental progress than Pierre Fauchard (1678-1761). He is often regarded as the father of dentistry. Fauchard was self-educated in dentistry and through his long career, developed a systematic method for dental practice. His classic text, *Le Chiurgien Dentiste,* was first published in 1728. Fauchard described home care remedies:

It is without reason that I advise a discontinuance of this practice (brushing) and to wash out the mouth after having cleaned the teeth in this way every morning with tepid water, rubbing the teeth from below upwards and from above downwards outside and inside with a little sponge of the finest quality dipped in water. It is still better to mix it with a fourth part of brandy to strengthen the gums better and to fasten the teeth . . . It is good to use a half round toothpick to remove the fur which collects on the teeth in the night, sometimes it gets between the gums and the teeth.[8]

John Hunter (1728-1793), a surgeon and anatomist at St. Georges Hospital in London, England, published *The Natural History of the Teeth* in 1771. This book classified dentistry as an important part of surgical practice. He concluded that dental caries are initiated on the outside of the tooth on susceptible surfaces where food collects.[7]

In 1638, the Pilgrims brought to the American colonies some physicians, an apothecary, and three **barber-surgeons**, perhaps the first American dentists. However, history is not clear about the first dentist to practice in America. Woofendale, Mills, Baker, Flagg, Paul Revere, and the Greenwoods—all of the colonial era—were among the American pioneers in the dental arts. Their methods and products were only slightly removed from those of the barber-surgeons, but the new country offered great promise for education and advancement in all fields, including dentistry.

ESTABLISHING FORMAL DENTAL EDUCATION: 1800 TO 1900

During the early 1800s, dental leaders became convinced that dentistry required knowledge of anatomy, pathology, and physiology. They further believed that the apprentice method (working and learning in the office of a **preceptor**, a clinician-teacher), was no longer adequate because no one person was competent to teach all scientific subjects and, at the same time, instruct students in the mechanical requirements of dentistry. This opinion led to the establishment of dental educational programs.

The new dental educational programs had two main problems to overcome before they could be accepted: (1) the antagonism of dentists trained as apprentices, who expected to profit from being dentists and preceptors, and (2) the low regard with which dentistry was viewed by medicine. Medicine was firmly established as a healing profession, and many believed that dentistry should be a branch of medicine. Most of the dentists of the era had learned their trade by apprenticeship and were considered more artisans than healers, so they chose to establish a separate profession.[9]

In 1939, Stillman reflected on the conflicts of professionalism and provided insight into this discontinuity between dentistry and medicine. He described three conflicts that must be resolved in favor of a profession: (1) Was it a trade or a profession? (2) Was it technologic art or pathology and physiology? (3) Was it prosthesis or healing? When the first dental school was established, the leaders had a smattering of medical education and began to combine the dental trade with a healing profession. The restorative dentist dealing with nonregenerative enamel and dentin tended to define the trade of dentistry differently than the periodontist focused on diseased living periodontal tissue, whose work more nearly characterized a healing profession.[10]

The first dental school was officially opened in 1840 as the Baltimore College of Dental Surgery. There were five students in the first class. The lack of respect for dentistry among the medical profession started to be overcome in 1867, when Harvard University established a dental department in close association with its medical department. Between 1840 and 1867, 13 dental schools were established, some short-lived, but others eventually affiliated with universities and are still in existence. At Harvard's first dental school graduation in 1890, its president, Oliver Wendell Holmes, referred to dentistry as:

a branch of the medical profession to which this graduating class has devoted itself . . . yours is now an accepted province of this great and beneficent calling . . . medicine.[7]

INTERRELATIONSHIP OF EARLY PERIODONTICS TO DENTAL HYGIENE

Periodontal diseases are as old as human civilization. Descriptions of early attempts at treating them were recorded, but in general, periodontal diseases were assumed to be incurable. In 1845, John M. Riggs first publicly called attention to the disease in America. He asserted that it was a curable disease and that, with proper surgical treatment (cleaning of the pockets), 90 percent of the cases could be cured. He was respected in his time and was quoted at home and abroad as an authority on the subject. Periodontal disease became known as Riggs' disease, and curettage beyond the pocket to "stir up a healing reaction" was his original contribution to therapy.[11]

Leonard Koecker, a 19th century surgeon dentist of London, was acknowledged by H. J. Leonard to have recorded successful treatment of advanced cases of periodontal disease with conservative techniques. He is considered the first modern periodontist.[4] He was not widely recognized because Horace Hayden, the senior faculty member of the new Baltimore School of Dental Medicine, had branded Koecker a charlatan. In contrast to Koecker, Riggs could not be ignored or ridiculed because he demonstrated his technique in clinics. Riggs cured periodontoclasia, as periodontal disease was called at the time, and dentists saw the results. Hayden continued to disagree, believing that he had seen periodontal disease in all its forms and that a radical cure was beyond the reach of medical skill.[4]

F. H. Rehwinkel renamed periodontoclasia **pyorrhea alveolaris** in a report he presented to the American Dental Association in 1877. This name was never totally acceptable because it was descriptive of only one phase of pathology, bone loss. However, pyorrhea became a commonly used term that is still heard today.[4]

DEVELOPMENT OF THE PROFESSION OF DENTAL HYGIENE

Late in the 1800s, dental journals began to include articles about disease prevention and teaching prophylactic methods to patients. D. D. Smith of Philadelphia impressed many in the field with his arguments and demonstrations of these techniques. He emphasized systematic change in the environment of the teeth to prevent disease. Smith probably had the most profound influence on Alfred C. Fones, who originated the role of the dental hygienist. Fones attended a meeting of the Northeastern Dental Society in 1898 at which Smith described his system of periodic **oral prophylaxis** (cleaning of the teeth). The treatment required patients to return at intervals of a few weeks for office treatment and to perform daily home care as they were instructed. Fones visited Smith's office three times to observe the practice. Fones implemented this system in his own office for 5 years. During this time, he learned that the procedures took an inordinate amount of practice time. Smith believed that prophylaxis was too important to be delegated, but Fones disagreed.

First Dental Hygienist

In 1906, Fones taught his dental assistant, Irene Newman, to instruct and treat his patients to maintain their mouths in a clean state. His educational program for her was described at a presentation to the National Dental Association Meeting in Cleveland, Ohio, in July 1911. First, he gave her drawings and books so that she could study the anatomy of the teeth. Later, he mounted extracted teeth in modeling compound in the normal position, placed indelible pencil stain on all of the surfaces, and instructed her to remove the stain with an orangewood stick and wet pumice. This procedure was repeated many times until she could remove all the stain in 1 hour. Next, he used her as a patient and rehearsed each step as he cleaned her teeth and she watched in the hand mirror. Later, Fones became the patient and instructed Newman as he observed in the hand mirror. Her first patients were children whose teeth she polished. Later, scaling instruments were introduced. For some time, she removed only the gross deposits, but Fones found that even this assistance saved him a great deal of chair time. Eventually, her skills improved so that she could accomplish more for his patients.[12]

First Dental Hygiene Schools

Fones went on to establish the first school for dental hygienists in Bridgeport, Connecticut, in

1913. His school graduated hygienists for 3 years before colleges and universities began to train dental hygienists (Figure 1-2).

Robin Adair of Atlanta, Georgia, an oral surgeon with both MD and DDS degrees, read an article before the Florida State Dental Society in June 1911, entitled "The Introduction of Oral Prophylaxis into Dental Practice." He described the introduction of a system of regular cleanings in his practice. He performed all of the treatment originally, but later used a "dental nurse." He interviewed 150 applicants before selecting a middle-aged nurse to train. He asked her to help him at the chair, read everything published on the subject, and practice on her family and friends before treating office patients. Adair performed the initial treatment and had the dental nurse finish. He reported that his patients were delighted. He even sent out cards notifying his patients of the dental nurse and her skills.

Adair opened the fourth dental hygiene program in 1917 in Atlanta, but graduated only 17 students. His untimely death in an automobile accident resulted in closure of the school and was a great loss to development in dental hygiene.[13]

Licensure and Regulation

Early demonstration programs and the success of Fones' school in Bridgeport, followed by other dental hygiene education programs, led to regulation and licensure for dental hygienists. Professional dental practitioners were first granted licenses in 1841. By 1889, all states had adopted dental practice acts and eliminated the preceptorship method of training for dentists. Connecticut was the first state to regulate dental hygiene practice. The law was enacted in 1915. New York, Massachusetts, and Maine adopted laws regulating dental hygiene practice in 1917. The pattern of extending the laws in the United States followed the establishment and location of the dental hygiene educational programs.[13]

School Programs for Children

It was the general consensus during the period 1900 to 1930 that a clean tooth would not decay. Because of this philosophy, many school dental health education programs were established to teach tooth brushing and promote prevention. Some of these community programs had benefactors who financed clinics for the dental treatment of children. Three of these programs also educated dental hygienists in their clinics: Guggenhiem and Eastman, in New York state, and Forsyth, in Boston, Massachusetts (Figure 1-3). Graduate dental hygienists from these programs had little experience with adult patients. However, Fones' original educational program and textbook covered the peri-

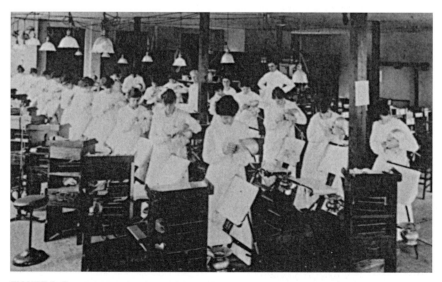

FIGURE 1-2. Dr. Fones' first class of dental hygiene students appears here as they worked on manikins in 1913. (Courtesy of Wilma E. Motley, RDH. Originally published by the American Dental Hygienists' Association in *History of the American Dental Hygienists' Association 1923—1982*. Chicago; 1986)

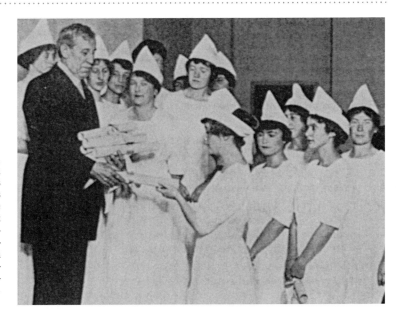

FIGURE 1–3. Mr. Thomas Forsyth, one of the founders of the Forsyth Dental Infirmary, delivered diplomas to the Forsyth dental hygiene class of 1918. The class members were reported to be wearing the latest fashion in professional caps. (Courtesy of Wilma E. Motley, RDH. Originally published by the American Dental Hygienists' Association in *History of the American Dental Hygienists' Association 1923-1982*. Chicago; 1986)

odontal membrane and its arrangement in relation to the alveolus and roots of the permanent teeth. It also had a chapter on pyorrhea alveolaris. Interestingly, Fones' book listed pyorrhea as a curable disease whose treatment required exacting and painstaking technique.[11]

Many public elementary school dental hygiene programs were initiated in the first half of the 20th century because the greatest cause of student absence at the time was toothaches. New York state had the most highly developed programs, which used dental hygiene teachers who had teaching credentials in the public schools. Boston also had an extensive number of school dental clinics located throughout the city. Flint, Michigan, had many dental clinics located within the school buildings. It was well into the 1930s before techniques for restoring primary teeth were generally taught and practiced, so these school clinics, staffed by dentists, mostly extracted primary teeth and restored 6-year molars. They operated in association with preventive dental hygiene programs in the schools.

Recognition of Periodontics as a Specialty

Only a small percentage of the dentists of the early 1900s believed in the philosophy of prevention of periodontal diseases. Most accepted the theory of their inability to cure or control periodontal disease and believed that areas of purulent discharge were foci of infection. Willa Yuretsky, in her historical review of oral prophylaxis, stated that it was often the tendency of the dental profession in the early part of the 20th century to regard pyorrhea alveolaris as a constitutional disease that should be treated by physicians.[14]

However, a small group of dental specialists interested in retaining the teeth persevered. In 1914, Grace Rogers Spaulding of Detroit, Michigan, and Gillette Hayden of Columbus, Ohio, formed the American Academy of Periodontology. This new group adopted the name of "periodontoclasia" for this ancient disease. There was considerable resistance to acceptance of the name, but these women dentists were accustomed to not being readily accepted. Some historians suggested that these women became periodontists to establish their place in dentistry in the face of the education of dental hygienists.

Early periodontists were dentists with particular interest in treating periodontal disease. The first periodontal specialty programs were established in the 1940s. References to the treatment of periodontal problems started to appear in the literature in the 1920s. The first periodontal textbook, published in 1922, was entitled *A Textbook of Clinical Periodontia.* It was written by Paul Stillman and John Oppie McCall of New York City.

Because of the theory of exquisitely clean teeth, many of the early periodontists developed their own scalers, as had the early dental and medical practitioners.[15] However, except for Riggs and his followers in 1845, the first choice of most dentists for treating periodontal diseases was surgical extraction. This method remained the treatment of choice until the 1920s.

Instruments for Evaluating and Treating Periodontal Diseases

The most important instrument introduced for use by dental hygienists and dentists is the periodontal probe. It first permitted the quantification of periodontal destruction. It came into use for measuring pocket depth in the post-World War II era, from 1948 to 1958. Periodontal probes varied in design and usually bore the name of the designer or school—the Marquis probe, Michigan probe, Goldman-Fox probe, and World Health Organization (WHO) probe, to name a few. The WHO probe is associated with an international system for evaluating periodontal treatment needs, known as the Community Index of Periodontal Treatment Needs (CIPTN).[16] Periodontal probes permit the accurate evaluation and recording of periodontal status, as described in Chapter 9. Unfortunately, in the last 20 years, it has taken several legal suits over untreated periodontal disease for the importance of identifying pocket depth and maintaining records of gingival condition to be emphasized in general dental practices.

The development of a broad range of curette and scaler designs, along with emphasis on thorough evaluation using periodontal probes has led to better understanding and techniques for preserving teeth. In the early 1960s, powered scalers using sonic or ultrasonic frequencies for calculus removal became available for periodontal treatment. These instruments have been proven through extensive research to remove calculus, subgingival plaque, and endotoxins as effectively as scalers and curettes.[17] For additional information on the development of the periodontal instruments, see Chapter 12, Development of Modern Periodontal Instruments.

DEVELOPMENTS IN THE TREATMENT OF PERIODONTAL DISEASES

The systematic treatment of diseased gums was initiated in 1845 by Riggs in his office in Hart-

ford, Connecticut. He frequently gave clinics demonstrating his methods for scaling and cleaning teeth. His contemporaries credited him with originating and publicly describing treatment for the cure of inflammation of the gums, now called **gingivitis**, and absorption of the alveolar process, known as "scurvy of the gums," now called **periodontitis**. This therapy restored loose teeth to comparative firmness. Riggs' treatment emphasized calculus removal and subgingival curettage. He believed that the cause of treatment failure was lack of thoroughness.[18]

Understanding the Etiology of Periodontal Diseases

Several reports that appeared in the 1880s presented bacteriologic theories of the etiology of periodontal diseases. In 1894, G. V. Black published an article on diseases of the periodontal membrane and uric acid diathesis, which he called "phagadenic pericementitis." Based on information available at the time, he concluded that the disease process was a "purely local affectation of an infectious character" related to the "glands of the periodontal membrane." Interestingly, G. V. Black is always listed among the early leaders in the science of dentistry, even though he was not educated beyond attendance at a country school. During his lifetime, he was awarded four honorary degrees, MD, DDS, ScD, and LLD.[18]

T.B. Hartzell, the author of many articles on periodontal disease and its treatment, considered streptococcal infection as one of its etiologic factors. In 1935, he expressed certainty that dentists should use the microbial principles of Pasteur and Dulaux. If so, periodontoclasia, or pyorrhea alveolaris, would be accepted as a "germ ferment disease" in which the destruction of the periodontal membrane and surrounding bone and tissues was the result of pus-making bacterial ferment. This idea led to enormous progress for dentistry as a learned profession and elevated it in the minds of medical colleagues, who tended to view dentistry as largely mechanical.[19]

OCCLUSION AND PERIODONTAL DISEASES

The issue of occlusion and its contribution to the etiology of periodontal disease has been controversial and widely discussed. In 1917,

P. R. Stillman wrote about possible damage to supporting tissues as a result of inharmonious relationships and stresses.[10] In many articles, Harold K. Box of Toronto pointed out the effects of excessive stress on the periodontal membrane and the alveolus. He also described a method of removing epithelium with soft tissue curettes designed specifically for the purpose. He offered histologic proof of reattachment in his booklet, *Studies in Periodontal Pathology.*[4] Currently, occlusion is thought to be a contributor to the periodontal disease process and is described in Chapter 8.

SYSTEMIC INFLUENCES ON PERIODONTAL DISEASES

After 1918, dentistry became concerned with the relationship of nutrition to periodontal disease. Percy Howe, whose major research related to dental caries, provided much valuable information about the effects of dietary deficiencies on the condition of the tissues that support the teeth.[19] A. W. Bryan, the author of a 1939 history of progress in the recognition of the causes of periodontal diseases, cautioned dental practitioners to look for the original causative factors, beyond the treatment of symptoms. He stated:

> It seems to the writer that drug treatment, unless directed at specific infection, and the surgical removal of unattached tissue are both essentially the treatment of symptoms. Unless the deep conditions that caused the unattached tissue to be formed or allowed the infection to become virulent are corrected, we have not treated our case scientifically.[19]

Developments in Treatment

Arthur D. Black, the son of G. V. Black and a renowned dental educator at Northwestern Dental School in Chicago, Illinois, advocated surgical resection of diseased gingival and alveolar tissue. A. W. Ward, a dentist, developed surgical instruments and also devised an adherent antiseptic and sedative cement to cover the cut tissues during healing. This bandage eliminated an objectionable feature of gum surgery, the painful and unsightly wound. Ward's periodontal pack is still used today.[19]

Electrosection, pocket packing with gutta percha or cotton dipped in wax or resin, the use of drugs to cause gum shrinking, and the use of ammonium hydrogen fluoride to remove calculus were all tried, but yielded poor results. Trichloracetic acid, silver nitrate, oxyphosphate of copper cement, and other cauterizing agents have also been tried and discarded. Dental researchers are still looking for the magic potion to dissolve calculus. Likewise, the search for vaccines or serums has been pursued for decades, with disappointing results.

PERIODONTAL EDUCATION IN SCHOOLS OF DENTISTRY

Much of the delay in the acceptance of new beliefs and theories in treating periodontal diseases was the result of their slow adoption in dental schools. Because most of the deans and educators were restorative dentists, the bulk of the curriculum covered restorative courses. In his survey of dental curricula for the American Dental Association in 1935, L. E. Blaugh stated that the treatment of periodontoclasia was unsatisfactory. Dental diagnosis and periodontal treatment were not adequately taught in dental schools.[20]

An analysis of dental school curricula in the 1947 Horner Report on Dentistry showed the historical distribution of curricular time devoted to periodontics. The report stated that periodontal instruction was first included under operative dentistry, as recommended in 1934 by the American Dental Association Curriculum Survey Committee. During 1941-1942, periodontics had a separate listing in the curriculum and accounted for 2.1 percent of the curricular time. Twelve years later, in the 1950s, the periodontal curriculum had doubled to 4.25 percent of the curricular time[20] (Table 1-1).

Specialty Programs in Periodontology

Specialty programs in periodontics arose in dental schools that had faculty members who were

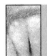

TABLE 1-1. Percentage of Dental School Curriculum Assigned to Periodontics 1934-1987	
Year	**% Periodontics Education**
1934*	
1941	2.10%
1950	4.25%
1976	6.00%
1987	7.10%

*Listed in Operative Dentistry. Solomon ES, Brown WE. Dental school curriculum: a 50 year update. J Dent Educ 1988;52:149–151.

conducting research in the specialty: McCall, Prichard, and Schluger at Columbia University; Miller, Bunting, Jay, and Hard at the University of Michigan; and Glickman at Tufts University. The first graduate programs in periodontics started in the late 1940s at those institutions. The American Dental Association recognized periodontics as a specialty in 1947, and a specialty board was created in 1950. Unfortunately, the creation of periodontics as a graduate specialty provided dental school curriculum committees additional reasons not to include more time for it in the undergraduate curriculum. Basic prevention teaching was also neglected. As a consequence, a large group of dental school graduates of the era had little knowledge of how to prevent, treat, and control periodontal diseases.[20]

Growth of Research

Research in the 1960s verified that periodontal diseases were infectious (see Chapter 4). Current research goals include identifying the pathogenic bacteria, clarifying host–bacterial interactions, understanding the pathologic process more fully, and determining the role of genetic and environmental factors in the natural history of periodontal disease.[21]

In 1984, teacher and researcher Sigurd Ramfjord reacted to the slow pace at which periodontal research was incorporated into dental practice. He stated:

> One problem in dentistry is the lag that often exists between publication of research findings and their application in clinical practice if there is no inherent economic reward in the new procedure. Crown margins are still routinely placed subgingivally by dentists although it has been known for more than 20 years that this is a periodontal hazard.[22]

Curriculum Development

The development of curriculum guidelines was initiated in 1985 by the joint efforts of the American Dental Association, the Council on Dental Education, and the American Association of Dental Schools, renamed the American Dental Education Association, ADEA, in 2000. These guidelines may have contributed to the increase in curriculum time allotted to periodontics. Solomon and Brown,[23] in their study of 50 years of dental school curricula, reported that periodontics accounted for 7.1 percent of the clinical science hours in 1987. This number

was an increase from 2.1 percent in 1941 and 6 percent in 1976. However, time allotted for the entire clinical science group increased 5.3 percent during that period, suggesting that any increase in periodontics teaching time was of little consequence in increasing the emphasis on periodontal diseases.

A simple comparison of the curriculum guidelines for periodontics, published in the *Journal of Dental Education* in 1985 and 1992, highlights changes in the treatment of periodontal diseases and the recognition of the role of the dental hygienist. For the first time, in 1992, behavioral objectives recommended that the dental students be taught to "consult with and refer to dental hygienists those patients needing nonsurgical periodontal therapy and supportive periodontal treatment."[24, 25]

Likewise, the 1992 article notes that dental hygienists may "be used in appropriate areas of the training program."[25] An example of the usefulness of dental hygienists in teaching about and treating periodontal disease is a recent advertisement for a tenured position in a dental school department of periodontics. A dental hygienist instructor with experience in a periodontal practice was being sought to teach clinical periodontics in a 1994 publication of the American Association of Dental Schools.[26] This advertisement supports the increased didactic and clinical instruction in periodontics currently mandated in the dental hygiene curriculum.

The success of the fluoridation regimen in the prevention of caries also has helped to increase the curriculum time devoted to periodontal diseases. National reports on the decline in decay rates in the pediatric population show that 50 percent of American schoolchildren now have no tooth decay and that interproximal caries are approaching eradication in fluoridated areas. In this light, dental school administrators recognized the need for greater emphasis on periodontics.[21]

The practice community now requires general dentists and periodontists to maintain detailed periodontal records to protect against malpractice suits and to provide evidence of evaluation and treatment of periodontal disease. A complete periodontal evaluation of every patient must be performed to meet the expectations of consumers. Much of the confusion surrounding periodontal diseases comes from the difficulties involved in measuring active disease. Research will eventually solve this problem, but until then, clinical attachment loss, probing depth, radiographic bone loss, and gingival bleeding continue to serve as measures of periodontal diseases, even though they may be cumbersome or inappropriate.[16] For further explanation of the assessments required for periodontal diseases, see Chapter 9.

Microbiologists have sought to identify the principal pathogenic organisms associated with periodontal diseases for some time. The research is complicated, but presumptive evidence shows that there are identifiable pathogenic organisms associated with a variety of periodontal diseases. However, it is increasingly clear that the host response to infection is a major determinant in the development of clinical disease. Host response is described in Chapter 2 and its role in disease development in Chapters 6 and 7. Control and prevention of periodontal diseases remain challenges for the future.[16]

ROLE OF DENTAL HYGIENISTS IN PERIODONTICS: 1913 AND BEYOND

Testimonies of the leading proponents of dental hygienists in the early 1900s indicate the attributes of the dentists who promoted the new profession. These individuals had great concern for the oral health of their patients, and they recognized the limitations of periodontal care at the time. They also realized that there was a cost-effective way to maintain the oral health of their patients. They recognized early on that individual preventive care was time consuming. Many also had a strong belief in social causes, particularly promoting oral health among children. This belief led to the employment of dental hygienists in education programs in the public schools, along with the introduction of dental hygiene services to private dental practices. Figure 1-4 shows an example of a school-based dental health program.

From 1913 to 1923, the first 10 years of the existence of dental hygiene, 11 programs were initiated to teach dental hygienists. A professional society, The American Dental Hygienists' Association was established, and a professional journal was published, the *Journal of the American Dental Hygienists' Association.* By 1923, the new dental hygiene schools had graduated 969 students, and 24 states had established licensure systems for dental hygienists.[13]

From 1924 to 1935, much emphasis was placed on dental hygiene care in children's programs because of rampant dental caries and extensive poverty in the United States during the Great Depression of the 1930s. The Children's Bureau, housed in the United States De-

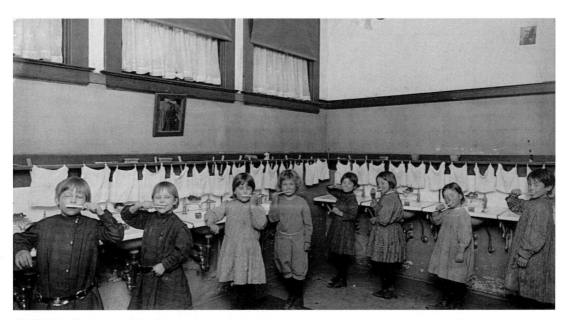

FIGURE 1–4. Toothbrushing drill in early 1900s. (Courtesy of Pemco, Webster, and Stevens Collection. Museum of History and Industry, Seattle, WA)

partment of Labor in Washington, DC, made sizable grants to the Bureaus of Maternal and Child Health in many states. The development of Child Health Conferences was one of the major goals of these grants (Figure 1-5). These conferences were held in all sections of the United States to educate mothers about child care. In addition, they provided local physicians and dentists with information about the needs of children who were seen in their offices. Many of these programs employed dental hygienists, as did more than 100 city health departments. The Social Security Act of 1935 provided traineeships in public health for many of these dental hygienists. Numerous public health dental hygienists went on to chair new dental hygiene programs as they earned advanced degrees through the support of Maternal and Child Health programs.[13]

Changes in Dental Hygiene Practice

The literature provides little information about the activities of the early dental hygienists in private practice. Many were appreciated by

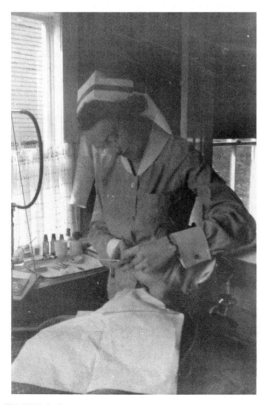

FIGURE 1-5. Dr. Martha Fales examining a clinic patient in 1941.

their patients and employers. However, they had minimal job security, earned low wages, and were required to perform many service functions, such as housework in dental offices, which could be demeaning. Many women left the profession when they married and established families.

An early report on dental hygiene graduates, licensure, and practice was authored by Walter J. Pelton, Chief of the Division of Dental Resources of the United States Public Health Service. His survey reported that by 1956, the cumulative number of graduate dental hygienists was 15,649. These dental hygienists were an average of 35.9 years old, and 78.2 percent practiced full time. Of those working at the time of the study, 68.6 percent were employed by private dentists and 26.5 percent were employed by government agencies. An additional 4.9 percent were employed by other sources, including 2 percent who worked in dental and dental hygiene schools. The remuneration as reported in this survey could explain why many women chose not to make dental hygiene a career at that time. Gross annual earnings for 1953-1954 were $3658 in private practice, $3484 in public health positions, and $4400 in education positions.[27]

A similar report by the Survey Research Laboratory of the University of Illinois for the American Dental Hygienists' Association in 1981-1982 summarized a sample as representative of the demographic and socioeconomic base of the dental hygiene profession. Their composite showed that the average dental hygienist in the early 1980s was 29 years old, possessed an Associate of Arts degree, had 10 years of experience in private practice, was married, shared a joint income, and lived in a small urban or suburban community. This dental hygienist treated between six and 10 patients a day, allowed 30 to 35 minutes for each visit, worked between 30 and 40 hours per week, and was paid on a daily basis totaling approximately $15,000 per year.[28]

Care Delivery Techniques Improve

These surveys highlight the statistical changes that have occurred in dental hygiene, but the physical changes have been even more radical. The early graduates followed the nursing education pattern because many people considered teaching and nursing the only acceptable career patterns for women. Thus, early dental hygiene graduates wore starched white uniforms, white stockings, and caps. Dental hygiene and dentistry were practiced standing up by the side of the dental chair (Figure 1-6).

It was not until the advent of four-handed dentistry, the dentist and dental assistant working while seated at the head of the reclined patient, in the early 1960s, that operating stools for dentists and dental assistants were introduced. This development necessitated dramatic changes in dental school clinic and operatory arrangements. The more relaxed and comfortable physical advantages of sit-down dentistry were quickly recognized by dental hygienists. They, too, learned to practice sitting down, both in training programs and in private practice (Figure 1-7). The next major physical change in practice patterns was the introduction of the fully reclining (contoured) dental chair. This type of chair permitted dentists and dental hygienists to work while seated and promoted the use of the reclined Trendelenburg position for the patient. This position kept the patient's brain lower than the heart, which precluded fainting while providing good access, light, and visibility (Figure 1-8).[29]

EXPANDING ROLE OF THE DENTAL HYGIENIST

The late 1960s and early 1970s was a time of concern about the growing population and the availability of health care for all. Dentists were concerned about how to meet the anticipated increased demands for care. One result was a significant increase in the number of dental hygiene programs in the United States, from 35 in 1956, to 61 in 1966, and 173 in 1976.[13] There was a smaller increase in the number of dental schools, but enrollments were substantially increased in the late 1960s. At that time, there was also movement toward increasing the duties of both dental hygienists and dental assistants. Both start-up grants and sizable supportive grants to evaluate these activities were available from the United States government. Some grant money supported experimental programs that were designed to provide additional skills for dental hygienists to treat periodontally involved patients. Specific duties varied across the country, but these skills became known generally as expanded-duty dental hygiene skills.

The University of Pennsylvania, the University of Iowa, Howard University, and Forsyth School for Dental Hygienists were among the institutions that received federal grants for research on expanded-duty dental hygiene functions. Because of a 1970 change in the laws permitting local anesthetic administration and restorative procedures to be taught to dental hygienists, the University of Washington received grants to teach the expanded duties to teachers in auxiliary education programs nationwide.[13] This change had an enormous effect on spreading expanded-duty education throughout the country.

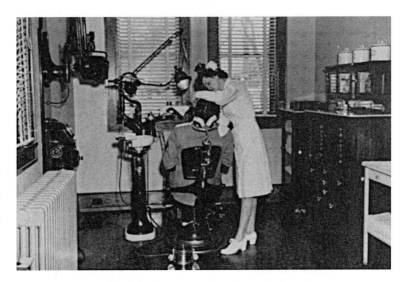

FIGURE 1–6. This photograph shows the typical appearance of a dental hygiene operatory from the 1940's. Dental hygienists routinely worked standing at the side of the patient who was seated but not reclined. (Courtesy of Wilma E. Motley, RDH. Originally published by the American Dental Hygienists' Association in *History of the American Dental Hygienists' Association 1923-1982.* Chicago; 1986)

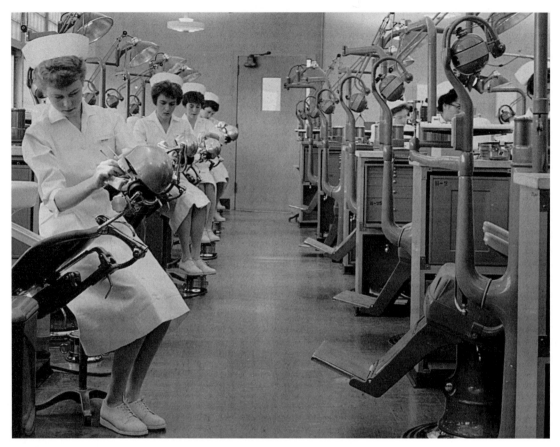

FIGURE 1–7. A dental hygiene school clinic in the 1960s.

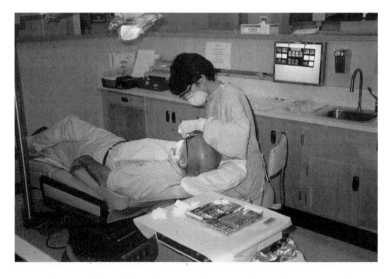

FIGURE 1–8. A dental hygienist providing dental hygiene care in a modern clinic setting.

The program at the University of Pennsylvania particularly focused on the expanded duties of dental hygienists in the area of local anesthesia administration and periodontal care. This program started in 1970 with several objectives: investigating the feasibility of teaching licensed dental hygienists to perform expanded duties in periodontics; developing and evaluating a training program course package designed to prepare dental hygienists to perform expanded duties in periodontics; evaluating the quality of work produced and the level of performance; and involving regional dental schools in evaluating the feasibility of incorporating this type of program into standard dental hygiene curricula. The expanded functions included in this experimental program were administration of local anesthetics; subgingival scaling, root planing, and curettage; gingivoplasty and gingivectomy; and intraoral photography.[13]

The Howard University Dental School and the Forsyth programs expanded into restorative functions. Interestingly, the Forsyth program evaluated educational costs. It determined that in the mid-1970s, educating a dentist cost $68,000 and educating an expanded-duty dental hygienist cost $10,400.[13]

The next federal attempt to help dentistry to function more efficiently and at less cost to consumers was the Teaching Expanded Auxiliary Management (TEAM) grant program. This federal grant program to dental schools was intended to develop behavioral relation skills for dental students who use auxiliaries in clinical practice. The cadre of dental graduates who benefited from the TEAM programs, from 1972 to 1978, are probably among the best employers of dental auxiliaries today. In many dental schools, the program terminated with the end of the grant funding period. Some practice management courses were continued as a result of these grants. These programs had limited involvement with periodontics because they focused on increased clinical production of restorative dental procedures.

Dental Hygiene Practices

In 1986, Colorado passed a law allowing dental hygienists to provide most of their services without the supervision of dentists. Reports describe many responsible dental hygienists who operated their own practices and devised innovative systems to provide quality dental hygiene care. The Colorado law does not permit radiographs to be taken or local anesthetics to be administered without supervision. These restrictions can limit the provision of periodontal treatment. Many independently practicing dental hygienists treat their periodontal patients in the offices of referring dentists. In this way, local anesthetics can be administered under supervision so that maximum comfort and therapeutic results for their patients can be achieved.[30]

Approaches to modify the practice acts for dental hygienists have been undertaken in several states and Canadian provinces since 1990. These proposals have attempted both to provide more independent practice opportunities for dental hygienists as well as to lower the educational standards of dental hygiene and allow dental assistants to assume more responsibilities without additional formal education. The experience in California has been an exception. Between 1987 and 1990 a research demonstration project in California tested the possibility of specially trained dental hygienists practicing independent of dentist supervision.[31] The project encountered many roadblocks but carefully documented educational requirements and practice experiences resulted in 1998 legislative approval for the graduates of the dental hygiene manpower project (HMPP) to become Registered Dental Hygienists in Alternative Practice (RDHAP).[32]

RESPONSIBILITIES OF THE PROFESSION OF DENTAL HYGIENE

Political changes in 1979 and 1980 gave national health care a lesser priority than in previous decades. Therefore, accelerated programs remained unchanged or were eliminated. The private practice of dentistry with specialty practices, such as periodontics, is currently available to approximately 50 percent of the population who have insurance coverage or sufficient income to afford care. An economic slump from 1981 to 1983, when dental appointment books were not full, led to concern about job security among some dental hygienists. Once the economy recovered, dental hygienists tended to have full employment. The fact that this full employment results in care for only approximately half of the total population is a source of concern to many health care providers and social-minded persons. For the other half of the population, periodontal and preventive care is almost nonexistent. Public health department dental clinics are operating on reduced budgets, and their coverage for periodontal needs has never been adequate. Most hospital emergency room dental care is only for relief of pain through the extraction of teeth.

Currently, many dental hygienists are contributing to the improved periodontal health of patients in general dental practices, specialty dental practices, public health practices, nursing homes, and a variety of educational programs—dental and dental hygiene, continuing education courses, and research. Many re-

port tremendous job satisfaction. They enjoy recognition of their skills; adequate compensation; respect from the community, patients, coworkers, and employers; and personal challenges in treating patients. Dental hygiene provides a wide range of practice options.

Now, more than 80 years after the first dental hygiene graduates started to maintain the oral health of patients in dental practices, the profession faces a new momentum amid the challenge of providing health care for all. It is hoped that dental care will soon include not only therapy for all, but also the application of all known preventive techniques. This approach could result in the prevention of oral diseases for the entire population.

STUDY QUESTIONS

MULTIPLE CHOICE

1. Periodontal diseases are as old as human civilization.
   Periodontal diseases in the early 1800s were considered incurable and beyond the reach of medical skill.

   a. Both statements are TRUE.
   b. Both statements are FALSE.
   c. The first statement is TRUE, the second statement is FALSE.
   d. The first statement is FALSE, the second statement is TRUE.

2. Dentists in the early 1900's developed an individual who would specialize in the cleaning of teeth BECAUSE that skill was too time consuming, difficult to perform, and limited the time for other dental procedures.

   a. Both the statement and the reason are correct and related.
   b. Both the statement and the reason are correct but NOT related.
   c. The statement is correct, but the reason is NOT.
   d. The statement is NOT correct, but the reason is correct.
   e. NEITHER the statement NOR the reason is correct.

3. Who erroneously believed that women did not have as many teeth as men?

   a. Aristotle
   b. Hippocrates
   c. Leonard
   d. Albucasis
   e. Aranculus

4. The first dental hygiene educational program was established in:

   a. Boston
   b. Bridgeport
   c. Atlanta
   d. New York
   e. Chicago

5. Some primitive groups in undeveloped countries chew fiber sticks to clean the teeth. The sticks are called:

   a. chewers
   b. arraks
   c. siwaks
   d. mastics
   e. tooth sticks

6. Dr. Alfred Fones' first office dental hygienist had been trained in what profession?

   a. nurse
   b. schoolteacher
   c. homemaker
   d. dental assistant
   e. secretary

7. The first state to pass a dental practice act that included licensure for dental hygienists was:

   a. Connecticut
   b. Georgia
   c. New York
   d. Massachusetts
   e. Michigan

8. There was a growing concern about the increase in population and the need for health care for all in the 1960s and 1970s. This resulted in the decrease in the number of dental hygiene programs in the United States.

   a. Both statements are TRUE.
   b. Both statements are FALSE.
   c. The first statement is TRUE, the second statement is FALSE.
   d. The first statement is FALSE, the second statement is TRUE.

9. The first dental school affiliated with a university was located in:

   a. New York
   b. Washington
   c. Baltimore
   d. Boston
   e. Hartford

10. The first dentist to practice in colonial America was:

   a. Revere
   b. Greenwood
   c. Woofendale
   d. Mills
   e. Never determined

SHORT ANSWER

11. Why does studying the history of periodontology lead to a better understanding of dentistry and dental hygiene?

   _____

   _____

12. What changes in periodontal thinking and treatment followed the introduction of the microscope? How rapidly was this knowledge assimilated into dental education and practice?

_____

_____

13. With the rapid transmission of scientific findings today, in addition to the explosion of knowledge, describe how the professional can evaluate what is important to know. How is this decision based on historical events and precedent?

_____

_____

14. Trace the role of mouth cleanliness from ancient times to today.

_____

_____

REFERENCES

1. Weinberger BW. An Introduction to the History of Dentistry in America, Vol. I. St. Louis: CV Mosby, 1948:14, 215.
2. Guerini V. A History of Dentistry from the Ancient Times Until the End of the Eighteenth Century. Philadelphia: Lea & Febiger, 1909.
3. Hippocrates. De Morbis Mulerum, Lib II, 606.
4. Leonard HJ. The historical background of periodontology. J Periodontol 1940;11:67, 70, 73.
5. Ring ME. Dentistry: An Illustrated History. St. Louis: Avery/CV Mosby, 1985:71, 303.
6. Albucasis A. De Chirurgia (translated from Latin by Channing S). Oxford, 1778:181-183.
7. Bremmer MDK. The Story of Dentistry, 2nd ed. New York: Dental Items of Interest Publishing Company, 1946:52, 68, 85.
8. Fauchard P. The Surgeon Dentist or Treatise on the Teeth (translated by Lindsay L from 2nd ed, 1746). New York: Milford House, 1969:28.
9. Hollingshead BS. The Survey of Dentistry. Washington, DC: American Council on Education, 1961:240.
10. Stillman PR. The past and future of periodontia. J Periodontol 1939;10:31-36.
11. Fones AC. Mouth Hygiene, 2nd ed, Philadelphia: Lea & Febiger, 1921:166-172, 276.
12. Fones AC. The origin and the history of the dental hygiene movement. J Am Dent Assoc 1920;13:1816.
13. Fales MJH. History of Dental Hygiene Education in the United States, 1913-1975 (dissertation). Ann Arbor, MI: University of Michigan, 1975.
14. Yuretskyy W. An historical review of oral prophylaxis. J Periodontol 1939;10:81-87.
15. McCall JO. The evolution of the scaler and its influence on the development of periodontia. J Periodontol 1939;10:69-81.
16. Burt BA, Eklund SA. Dentistry, Dental Practice and the Community. Philadelphia: WB Saunders, 1992:66-67, 114, 125.
17. Woodall IR, Dafoe BR, Young NS, Weed-Fonner L, Yankell SL. Comprehensive Dental Hygiene Care, 2nd ed. St. Louis: CV Mosby, 1985:407.
18. Merritt AH. The historical background of periodontology. J Periodontol 1939;10:7-25.
19. Bryan AW. Progress in the recognition of etiologic factors of periodontal diseases. J Periodontol 1939;10:25-30.
20. Commission on the Survey of Dentistry in the US. The Survey of Dentistry. Washington, DC: American Council on Education, 1960:246, 247, 315.
21. US Department of Health and Human Services. Dental science: dental health NIDR at 40. Bethesda, MD: Public Health Service, National Institutes for Health, 1988: Publication no. 88-1868:19, 30, 41.
22. Ramfjord SP. Changing concepts in periodontics. J Prosthet Dent 1984;52:781-786.
23. Solomon ES, Brown WE. Dental school curriculum: a 50 year update. J Dent Educ 1988;52:149-151.
24. Curriculum guidelines for periodontics. J Dent Educ 1985;49:611-615.
25. Curriculum guidelines for periodontics. J Dent Educ 1992;56:773-778.
26. Bulletin of Dental Education. Washington, DC: American Association of Dental Schools, 1994;27:7.
27. Pelton WJ, Pennell E, Vavra H. Section 8: Dental Hygienists. Health Manpower Sourcebook. Bethesda MD: Public Health Service, US Dept of Health Education and Welfare, Division of Public Health Resources, 1957: Publication no 263-1957.
28. American Dental Hygienists' Association. Who we are: a report on the survey of dental hygiene issues. Attitudes, perceptions and preferences. Dent Hyg 1982;56:13-19.
29. Wilkins EM. Clinical Practice of the Dental Hygienist, 6th ed. Philadelphia: Lea & Febiger, 1989:65.
30. Thomas RD. On their own. RDH 1994;14:14-26.
31. Perry DA, Freed JR, Kushman JE. The California demonstration project in independent practice. J Dent Hyg 1994;68:137-142.
32. Stateline: Congratulations to California RDHAPs. Access 1999;13:41.

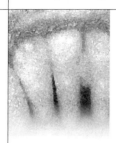

2

Dorothy A. Perry / Phyllis L. Beemsterboer

Periodontium: Anatomic Characteristics and Host Response

Chapter Objectives

1. Name and describe the anatomy and clinical characteristics of the tissues of the periodontium.
2. Differentiate among the three types of oral epithelial surfaces: keratinized, parakeratinized, and nonkeratinized.
3. Name the principal fiber bundles of the gingiva.
4. List the functions of the periodontal ligament.
5. Describe clinically normal gingiva in terms of color, size, contour, texture, and consistency.
6. Describe the interactions of the major elements in the host response.
7. Define the protective roles of gingival fluid and saliva.

Key Terms

Alveolar bone
Antibody
Antigen
Attachment apparatus
Cementum
Chemotaxis
Complement
Cytokine
Dehiscence
Effector molecule
Fenestration

Gingiva
Gingival fluid
Hypersensitivity reactions
Immunoglobulin
Junctional epithelium
Lysis
Mucogingival junction
Oral epithelium
Periodontal ligament
Phagocytize
Sulcular epithelium

Gingival and periodontal diseases are infectious diseases by nature. Their effects can best be understood with a basic background in the unique anatomy of the periodontium and knowledge of the response the human body undertakes to protect itself from infection. As will be further explained in Chapters 4, on microbial plaque, and Chapters 6 and 7, devoted to gingival and periodontal diseases, the effects and damages caused by these microbe-induced diseases are complex. They can result in irreversible changes to the normal architecture, loss of teeth, loss of function, and changes in appearance.

This chapter is divided into two parts. The first part presents a basic description of the normal periodontium. This description provides the reader with a basic understanding of the environment affected by gingival and periodontal diseases. The second part is an introduction into the rapidly growing area of host response, immunology. A basic understanding of these processes will inform the reader why tissue destruction occurs. Part two closes with a brief description of the protective influences that exist in the periodontium.

ANATOMIC CHARACTERISTICS OF THE PERIODONTIUM

The periodontium is defined simply as the tissues that surround, support, and are attached to the teeth. These include the **gingiva, periodontal ligament, cementum,** and **alveolar bone.**[1] These tissues support the teeth and oral structures. Maintaining the health and function of the periodontium is the most significant factor in the longevity of the dentition.

Gingiva

The gingiva includes the **oral epithelium, sulcular epithelium,** and **junctional epithelium.** Underlying the gingiva is the lamina propria, the connective tissue component.

The gingiva is the visible component of the periodontium inside the mouth. It is described as pink,[2] pale pink,[3] or coral pink.[4] In some cases, it has normal variation and melanin pigmentation. The gingiva is distinguished from the oral mucosa at the **mucogingival junction.** This line indicates the transition from the loosely attached and movable oral mucosa to the attached gingiva, which is more firmly attached to the bone by collagen fibers. The attached gingiva is the portion that extends coronally from the mucogingival junction. The width of the attached gingiva varies from individual to individual and from tooth to tooth in the same mouth. It has been suggested that 1 to 9 mm is the range of widths.[5] However, there is no absolute minimum width required for periodontal health.[6] Frenum and muscle attach-

ments are present in the gingiva, and those located coronally in the attached gingiva are associated with narrower widths of attached gingiva. Gingiva is keratinized or parakeratinized tissue on the oral surface and it is commonly stippled. Nonstippled gingiva is also seen in healthy mouths.[6] The degree of keratinization varies throughout the epithelium in the mouth, with the palatal gingiva being the most keratinized and the cheek the least. The tongue is also covered with keratinized epithelium.[4] The location of the gingival margin in fully erupted, healthy teeth is 0.5 to 2 mm coronal to the cementoenamel junction of the teeth (Figure 2–1).[3]

The free marginal gingiva surrounds the tooth and creates a cuff or collar of gingiva extending about 1.5 mm coronally. The surface of the free marginal gingiva next to the tooth forms the gingival wall of the sulcus.[6] The free gingiva may be distinguished from the attached gingiva by a free gingival groove, a slight depression on the gingiva corresponding to the depth of the sulcus. This groove varies from tooth to tooth, occurring 24 percent to 43 percent of the time, most commonly in the mandibular anterior and bicuspid areas.[2] The free gingiva on buccal and lingual surfaces rarely ends in a true knife-edged tip next to the tooth surface; the coronal termination of the

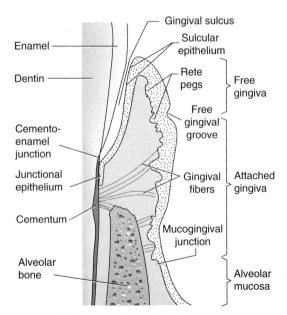

FIGURE 2–1. Cross-section of the gingiva and supporting structures.

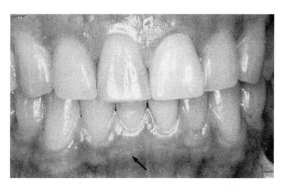

FIGURE 2–2. Clinical presentation of normal gingiva showing interdental papillae and free gingival margin. The arrow indicates the mucogingival junction on the mandible.

free gingiva is typically more rounded (Figure 2-2).

The papillae are gingiva that fill the embrasure (spaces). They are also referred to as interdental gingiva. The papillae between anterior teeth are commonly described as pyramidal.[2] When the papilla is broad, as is often the case between posterior teeth, there is a nonkeratinized area called the col. This area is a slight depression of tissue between the buccal and lingual interdental papillae. It indicates a fusion of two papillae to cover a wide space. The col is not usually present between anterior teeth. When adjacent teeth do not contact each other, whether they are anterior or posterior teeth, attached gingiva forms between the teeth, and the papillae and col are absent.[6]

The gingival epithelium is joined to the underlying connective tissue by a basal lamina, 300 to 400 angstroms thick. The basal lamina is joined to the connective tissue by fibrils. The connection between the free and attached gingiva and the underlying connective tissue occurs in ridges of epithelium called rete pegs.[4]

ORAL EPITHELIUM

The oral epithelium is also called the outer gingival epithelium.[3] It is composed of the attached gingiva, the papillae, and the outer surface of the free gingiva. Its function is protective, and the epithelium is typically keratinized. Epithelium becomes keratinized when the surface cells form scales of keratin and lose their nuclei. Keratohyaline granules are found in the subsurface, or granular layer. In some cases, epithelium shows signs of being keratinized, yet the cells of the superficial layers retain their nuclei. This surface condition is called

parakeratinization. If no signs of keratinization are present, the epithelial surface is considered nonkeratinized.[4]

SULCULAR EPITHELIUM

The sulcular epithelium is the nonkeratinized, or parakeratinized, extension of the oral epithelium into the gingival sulcus. It extends from the height of the gingiva apically to the junctional epithelium and forms the gingival wall of the sulcus (Figure 2-3). In health, the epithelium lining the sulcus is smooth and intact; there are no rete pegs projecting into the connective tissue.

The healthy sulcus is generally 1 to 3 mm deep. However, the sulcus depth determined clinically by measurement with a periodontal probe may be considerably different than the histologic sulcus depth. Probe measurements are subject to variation as a result of several influences: probe insertion pressure, accuracy of probe reading, and ability of the probe tip

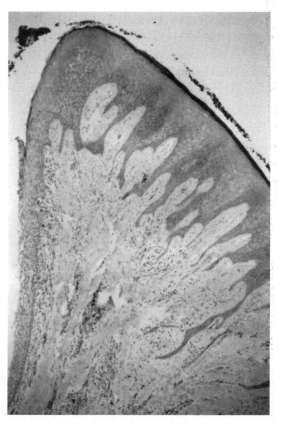

FIGURE 2–3. Histologic appearance of the normal free gingiva and sulcus. Rete pegs are seen subjacent to the oral epithelium but not the sulcular epithelium. (Courtesy of Dr. Gary Armitage.)

to penetrate tissue.[7] For this reason, Löe and colleagues suggested that the use of the term "sulcus depth" in reference to probe readings is misleading. A more accurate term would be "probing depth" or "probeable depth" of the gingival sulcus.[2]

SULCULAR OR GINGIVAL FLUID

A sulcular or **gingival fluid** flows from the underlying connective tissue into the sulcus. This fluid is also known as gingival or crevicular fluid. The flow is related to the permeability of the connective tissue capillaries. The fluid seeps out between the epithelial cells into the sulcus. The amount of fluid flow is small, considered to be minimal to none in the healthy state.[3] Gingival fluid is believed to perform several functions: cleansing the sulcus, improving epithelial cell adherence to the tooth surface, and possessing antimicrobial and immune properties.[4]

JUNCTIONAL EPITHELIUM

The junctional epithelium separates the periodontal ligament from the oral environment. It is composed of specialized epithelial cells that adhere organically to tooth structure, and its function is considered to be protection for the attachment of the tooth to the surrounding tissues. It forms a layer that is 15 or 20 cells thick at the coronal end and narrows to a few cells thick at the apical termination. Its length in the healthy state ranges from 0.25 to 1.35 mm.[3, 4] This epithelium continually renews itself, and its most coronal portion determines the histologic base of the gingival sulcus.[6]

The attachment of the junctional epithelium to the root surface is enhanced by fibers from the connective tissue. This attachment supports the free marginal gingival, and it is considered a functional unit called the dentogingival unit.[4]

GINGIVAL CONNECTIVE TISSUE

The connective tissue beneath the gingiva is called the lamina propria. The lamina propria is made up of two layers: the papillary layer that is immediately beneath the epithelium and consists of papillary projections between the rete pegs; and the reticular layer that extends to the periosteum.[4] Approximately 60 percent of the lamina propria is made up of connective tissue that is composed of collagen fibrils that form discrete fiber bundles.[6] Other elements

include cells such as fibroblasts, undifferentiated mesenchymal cells, mast cells, and macrophages as well as blood vessels and nerves.[2]

The fiber bundles are known as the gingival ligament.[6] These are not individual fibers, but fiber bundles, although they are commonly referred to as fibers. Their functions include protecting and supporting the junctional epithelium, maintaining the tone of the attached gingiva, and protecting the periodontal ligament. There are five principal fiber groups and six minor groups. All bundles are discrete, although some fibrils intertwine so that the gingival ligament supports its components. The bundles are best described by their orientation and attachment. These characteristics suggest the function of the specific bundle. All are interdependent and provide the most coronal connective tissue attachment for the teeth. The principal and secondary fiber bundles have been described. See Gingival Fiber Groups.

Principal Fiber Bundles of the Gingiva

1. Dentogingival fiber bundles radiate from the cementum into the free gingiva and attached gingiva. They probably support the gingiva.
2. Alveologingival fiber bundles radiate from the periosteum into the attached gingiva. They probably attach the gingiva to the bone.
3. Dentoperiosteal fiber bundles course from the cementum, near the cementoenamel junction, across to the alveolar crest. They may anchor the tooth to the bone and protect the periodontal ligament.

 GINGIVAL FIBER GROUPS

Principal Gingival Fiber Group
Dentogingival
Alveologingival
Dentoperiosteal
Circular
Transseptal

Secondary Gingival Fiber Group
Periostogingival
Interpapillary
Transgingival
Intercircular
Semicircular
Intergingival

4. Circular fiber bundles encircle the entire tooth coronal to the alveolar crest. These bundles probably support the free gingiva.
5. Transseptal fiber bundles span the interdental space, with the ends inserted into the cementum of the teeth. They probably help maintain the relationships between teeth.

Secondary Fiber Groups of the Gingiva

1. Periostogingival fiber bundles course from the periosteum of the alveolar bone and spread into the connective tissue, probably to attach the gingiva to the bone.
2. Interpapillary fiber bundles are found in the papillae, coronal to the transseptal fiber bundles. They probably support the papillary gingiva.
3. Transgingival fiber bundles are formed between the teeth, coronal to the cementoenamel junction. They probably support the marginal gingiva.
4. Intercircular fiber bundles run from the distal, facial and lingual surfaces of one tooth, around the adjacent tooth, and insert on the mesial surface of the tooth beyond the adjacent tooth. They may help to maintain arch form.
5. Semicircular fiber bundles course from the mesial surface to the distal surface of the same tooth. They may help to support the free gingiva.
6. Intergingival fiber bundles run mesiodistally in the connective tissue immediately beneath the gingival epithelium. They probably support the attached gingiva.

Periodontal Ligament

Teeth are not attached rigidly to the bone in humans and other mammals. The periodontal ligament provides a suspensory cushion in the 0.4 to 1.5 mm space between the surface of the tooth and the bone. The periodontal ligament is a connective tissue complex primarily filled with fiber bundles and cells.[6] The cells in the ligament perform an important formative function for the tissues: they generate a pericementum for the cemental surface of the root and a periosteum for the bone.[8] Unusual formations of cementum called cementicles can also occur in the periodontal ligament (Figure 2–4). Spe-

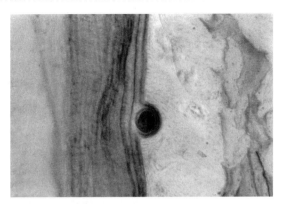

FIGURE 2–4. Histologic appearance of the dentin, cementum, periodontal ligament, and alveolar bone. The round structure in the cementum is a cementicle. (Courtesy of Dr. Gary Armitage.)

cific functions of the periodontal ligament include [6]:

1. Tooth anchorage.
2. Fibrous tissue development and maintenance.
3. Calcified tissue development and maintenance.
4. Nutritive and metabolite transport.
5. Sensory functions, including touch, pressure, pain, and proprioception (displacement sensitivity).

FIBER BUNDLES

The fiber bundles in the periodontal ligament are made of collagen, arranged in bundles, and are spread throughout the periodontal ligament with the other cellular, vascular, and nerve tissues. In addition to attaching the tooth to the bone, they are believed to transmit occlusal forces to the bone, resist occlusal forces (the "shock absorber" effect), and protect the vessels and nerves from injury.[9]

There are five principal fiber bundles in the periodontal ligament of all teeth. The principal fiber bundles are attached to the cementum with brush-like fibers called Sharpey's fibers, course from the cementum across the periodontal ligament, and terminate in the alveolar bone as Sharpey's fibers.[6, 9] The principal fiber bundles include:

1. Alveolar crest group. These run from the cementum, just apical to the cementoenamel junction, to crestal bone. They are thought to oppose lateral forces, and retain the tooth in the socket.

2. Horizontal fiber bundles. These attach the root surface to the alveolar bone directly across the periodontal ligament space.
3. Oblique group. These bundles course in an oblique direction across the periodontal ligament space and into the alveolar bone. They are the largest group of fiber bundles and are believed to transform occlusal stresses on to the alveolar bone.
4. Apical fiber bundles. These run from the apex of the root into the alveolar bone, both apical and lateral to the root apex. They do not occur in partially erupted teeth.
5. Interradicular fiber bundles. These are only present in multirooted teeth. They spread apically into the bone, from the furcation (See Periodontal Ligament Fiber Bundles and Figure 2-5).

In addition to the principal fiber bundles, small collagen fibers have been identified that run in all directions in the periodontal ligament. These are referred to as the indifferent fiber plexus and their function is unknown. Less well formed collagen bundles and immature forms of elastin are also observed in the periodontal ligament, mostly in association with blood vessels.[6]

PHYSIOLOGIC DRIFT

Gradual tooth movement occurs throughout life, in both mesial and occlusal directions. This movement is probably the result of wear of proximal and occlusal tooth surfaces. The movement is gradual, totaling no more than 1 cm during lifetime. Physiologic drift is considered an adjustment process that allows the dentition to retain balance among its complex structures. The cells of the periodontal ligament probably mediate the changes needed in the bone and the cementum to permit movement and maintain balance.[6]

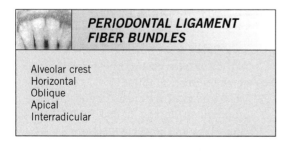

PERIODONTAL LIGAMENT FIBER BUNDLES
Alveolar crest
Horizontal
Oblique
Apical
Interradicular

Cementum

The cementum covering the root surfaces of the teeth is a calcified structure varying in thickness from 20 to 50 µm near the cementoenamel junction to 50 to 200 µm at the apex.[8] It contains Sharpey's fibers and attaches the fiber bundles to the root. There are no vascular or nerve connections, so the cementum cannot transmit pain sensations. This is why the cementum is not sensitive to scaling procedures.

The cementum anchors the teeth, maintains occlusal relationships,[6] and provides a seal for the dentinal tubules.[3]

Hassell[6] described four types of cementum: type I acellular, afibrillar; type II acellular, fibrillar; type III cellular, containing intrinsic fibers; and type IV cellular, containing intrinsic and extrinsic fibers. Type I cementum is located near the cementoenamel junction. It contains no fibers or cementocytes. Type II cementum is present on the coronal third of the root. It contains Sharpey's fibers but no cementocytes. Type III cementum consists of intrinsic fibers secreted by cementoblasts and contains lacunae with encased cementocytes. It is considered secondary, or repair, cementum. Type IV cementum contains intrinsic fibers, Sharpey's fibers, and cellular elements. Incremental lines are readily seen in cementum, suggesting the dynamic nature of cementum, with alternating periods of apposition and periods of rest (Figure 2-6).

Alveolar Process

The alveolar process is the support system for the teeth. The alveolar process is similar to bone elsewhere in the body,[8] and it is an extension of the bone from the body of the mandible and the body of the maxilla. The alveolar bone lines the sockets of the teeth and provides bony support for the sockets. The walls of the sockets are called the lamina dura when viewed on radiographs. They may also be referred to as the cribiform plate based on histologic appearance[3] (Figure 2-7).[8] The term cribiform plate simply means a plate of bone with many perforations to permit the passage of blood vessels and nerves. The tooth sockets are called the alveoli.[9] The alveolar process is composed of three components: (1) the alveolar bone, the bone comprising the cribiform plate encompassing

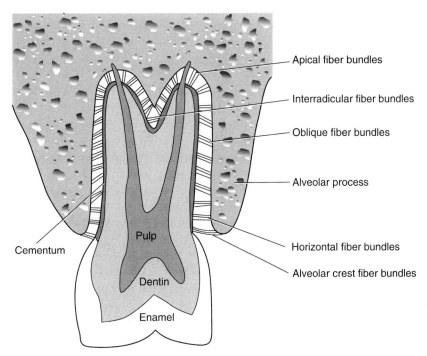

Apical fiber bundles

Interradicular fiber bundles

Oblique fiber bundles

Alveolar process

Horizontal fiber bundles

Alveolar crest fiber bundles

Cementum

Pulp

Dentin

Enamel

FIGURE 2–5. Cross-section of a maxillary first premolar showing the five principal fiber bundles of the periodontal ligament. Horizontal and oblique fiber are present throughout the periodontal ligament, not limited to the lateral portions of the root.

the alveoli, and adjacent cancellous bone; (2) the compact bone, which makes up the facial and lingual cortical plates of bone; and (3) the trabecular and cancellous bone between the cortical plates and surrounding the alveoli.[6] The alveolar process functions as a unit, as indicated by its gradual resorption when teeth are lost.[9]

The alveolar process is dependent on the teeth: the crest of the alveolar process follows the cementoenamel junction of the teeth. It is actually 2 to 3 mm apical to the cementoenamel junction, and 0.5 to 1.5 mm apical to the epithelial attachment to the tooth, in the state of periodontal health. The alveolar process is in a constant state of remodeling. This remodeling accommodates the physiologic tooth migration,

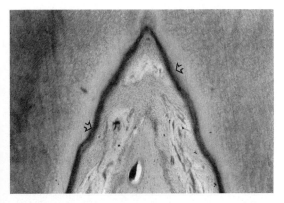

FIGURE 2–6. Histologic appearance of a maxillary first premolar furcation area. Note the orientation of the periodontal ligament to the cementum (dark line with arrows). The interradicular alveolar bone appears as a triangular structure at the bottom of the illustration. The round lumen in the alveolar bone is a channel filled with a blood vessel. (Courtesy of Dr. Gary Armitage.)

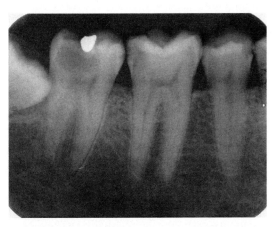

FIGURE 2–7. Radiographic appearance of normal alveolar bone showing the lamina dura, trabecular bone, and periodontal ligament space. Note the presence of caries in the teeth and a small restoration, as well as a partially erupted third molar.

bone apposition, and resorption that are constantly occurring at a slow rate.[4]

ALVEOLI

The alveoli are the tooth sockets. They are lined by the cribiform plate, which has thousands of pores through which the tooth and periodontal ligament are supplied with nerves and blood vessels. Each root of a multirooted tooth has its own alveolus.[6]

The bone lining the alveoli contains Sharpey's fibers. It is referred to as a "bundle bone" because of the presence of many fibrils entering into the bone. This type of bone exists elsewhere in the body in locations where tendons or ligaments attach to bone.[10]

COMPACT BONE

Compact bone makes up the cortical plates on the facial and lingual sides of the jaws. This bone is dependent on the alignment of the teeth because it follows the contour of the root surfaces. The height and thickness of the compact bone are determined by this alignment, the angulation of the roots to the bone, and occlusal forces.[10]

CANCELLOUS BONE

Cancellous bone lies between the cortical plates and the alveolar bone, connecting them. It is also known as spongiosum. In general, there is less spongiosum in the mandible than in the maxilla. The cancellous bone of the alveolar bone blends into the spongiosum of the mandible and maxilla without demarcation.[6]

VARIATIONS IN NORMAL STRUCTURE

There are two variations of the normal bone structure that are nonpathologic and of importance to periodontal health: dehiscences and fenestrations. These areas have no alveolar bone so that the course of periodontal disease differs from other areas. Therapeutic efforts are often modified to protect these areas.

DEHISCENCES

A **dehiscence** is a resorbed area of bone over the facial surface of the root. It can occur in patients with labially inclined roots.[6]

FENESTRATIONS

A **fenestration** is an opening, or window, in the bone covering the facial surface of a root[6] or a boneless window between two adjacent roots that almost touch (Figure 2-8).[9]

ATTACHMENT APPARATUS

The periodontal ligament, cementum, and alveolar bone are commonly referred to collectively as the **attachment apparatus.**

Clinical Condition of the Periodontal Tissues

It is primarily the gingival structures that are assessed to determine clinical signs of health or disease. These are also the areas that must be kept free of bacterial plaque, through personal and professional care, to maintain or restore periodontal health. Descriptions of the gingiva must note the clinical condition and either describe these structures as normal or differentiate particular areas from normal appearance. Descriptions should include the color, size, shape or contour, texture, and consistency of the gingiva.

COLOR

The gingiva is uniformly light pink or coral pink. Variations in color are produced by the vascular supply, the thickness and degree of keratinization, and the presence of pigment.[4] The mucogingival junction should be a clearly demarcated line, and the tissue apical to that line, the alveolar mucosa, should be bright red and shiny. The increased redness is caused by

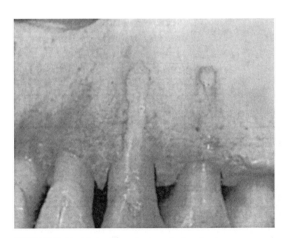

FIGURE 2-8. Variations of normal alveolar bone are seen in this skull. The defect on the left (over the canine) is a dehiscence, and the window through the bone is a fenestration. (Used with permission from Carranza F. Glickman's Clinical Periodontology, 8th ed. Philadelphia: WB Saunders, 1996:747.)

increased vascularization, nonkeratinized epithelium, and a less organized system of collagen fibrils. The alveolar mucosa should blend without demarcation into the vestibule or floor of the mouth. There is no mucogingival junction on the palate because all of the tissue of the palate is keratinized masticatory mucosa.

Melanin pigmentation may be present. Melanin is a non-hemoglobin–derived brown pigment[4] that is more often seen in black and Asian individuals than in white people.[6] The amount of pigmentation may vary greatly. It is uniform in some individuals but appears blotchy or irregular in others. Clinically, these appear as normal variations in the color of the gingiva.

SIZE

The gingiva should not be enlarged; its size should equal the total of its cellular elements and vascular supply.[4] Clinically, size is assessed by the presence or absence of swelling or enlargement.

SHAPE OR CONTOUR

The shape of the gingiva depends on the size and alignment of the teeth.[2, 4] The marginal gingiva should follow a scalloped line around the crowns and lie flat to the tooth. This contour is called knife-edged by some.[3] In general, papillae should fill the interdental spaces. The contour can be influenced by the shape, size, and position of the teeth as well as the relationship of the tooth contact areas.

TEXTURE

The stippled outer texture of the gingiva should provide a matte appearance (not shiny) when dried. The free gingiva should be smooth, and the attached gingiva may appear stippled, resembling an orange peel. Stippling reflects protuberances of connective tissue into the epithelium, called rete pegs, and both stippled and nonstippled gingiva are keratinized.[4, 5] Stippling varies with age. It appears in children at approximately 5 years of age, increases in adulthood, and becomes less pronounced in old age.[4]

CONSISTENCY

The consistency, or tone, of the healthy, attached gingiva is firm because of the tight attachment of the fiber bundles in the underlying connective tissue to the bone and cementum.[2] It should also be resilient[4, 5] when touched by an instrument. The free gingiva should also be firm in texture, not soft or spongy.

SULCUS DEPTH

The normal clinical sulcus depth, when measured by a periodontal probe, is 1 to 3 mm.[2] The sulcular epithelium should be intact, not ulcerated, and should not bleed on gentle probing.[2, 3, 5]

HOST RESPONSE

Each human being reacts to disease processes within a range of responses that are mediated by the individual's ability to react to assault by bacteria, viruses, tumor growth, injury, and a myriad of other influences. The immune system is responsible for the body's reaction, called the host response. Immunology is the study of the immune system and host response.

The development of disease in the healthy periodontium is dependent upon both the microbial assault from dental plaque, which is described in Chapter 4, and the host response. The amount of pathogenic bacteria present in disease does not explain the variation seen in the degree of response. One cannot minimize the contribution of the microbial population to periodontal diseases because infectious agents must be present for the disease to occur.[10] This section provides a brief introduction into the complex discipline of immunology, so that the student can begin to understand how reactions of the human body are related to the etiology and pathogenesis of periodontal diseases. Not only does microbial interaction with the individual patient play an important role in the development of disease, the immune responses alone can manifest as disease processes in gingival and periodontal tissues. The actions of microbes and cells in the host form inflammatory reactions, or inflammation. Inflammation is protective in that it leads to destruction of bacterial assault, but the complex immune system defenses can also lead to tissue alteration and destruction. The consequences of inflammatory response can damage and destroy periodontal tissues, often leading to irreversible changes in the architecture of the periodontal tissues.

The host response acts to wall off infections, localizing them to the specific tissues, in this case the periodontal tissues. These responses are also likely to result in some local tissue destruction which in turn results in what we know as periodontal disease.[11] Bacterial plaque and its products infect the root surface. The inflammatory response attempts to get the infected root away from the body. This extremely complex response is the focus of much investigation. An introductory knowledge is most easily gained by understanding the host response components and their actions. These components consist of the inflammatory cells, antibodies, **complement,** and the **hypersensitivity (allergic) reactions.** Figure 2-9 shows examples of periodontal destruction resulting from various influences.

Inflammatory Cells

Inflammatory cells are attracted to areas of the body by stimuli such as trauma or microbial influences; this signaling process is call **chemotaxis.** Cells such as polymorphonuclear leukocytes (PMNs or neutrophils), macrophages, lymphocytes, and plasma cells are chemotactically attracted to areas of the tissue damage. In periodontal diseases, the cells are attracted to the gingiva, connective tissue, periodontal ligament, and bone. Once concentrated at the area of stimulus, the cells perform several functions: they phagocytize bacteria, they consume bacterial components, and they remove damaged tissues. Inflammatory cells also produce products that affect the permeability of blood vessels, cause cell disintegration (referred to as **lysis**),

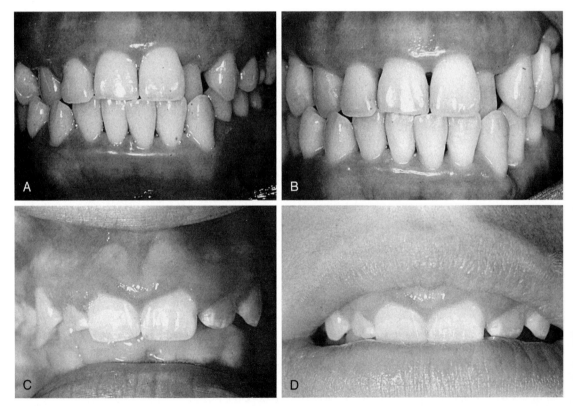

FIGURE 2–9. Inflammatory responses of the gingiva. **A,** Dental plaque-induced gingivitis caused the inflammatory response seen here, including intense redness and edema. The tissue bled very easily when probed, and the patient stated the gingiva bled when he brushed his teeth. **B,** Removal of plaque by instituting good oral hygiene and dental hygiene treatment resolved the inflammation completely. The redness has disappeared so that the gingiva looks pink, and resolution of the edema has left noticeable spaces in some of the interdental papilla areas. **C,** Inflammation occurs for reasons other than the presence of dental plaque (see Chapter 6). This child demonstrated inflammation of the marginal gingiva around the anterior teeth. **D,** Further observation of the child revealed that he did not fully close his lips much of the time. The inflammation resulted from constant drying of the marginal gingiva; a condition referred to as "mouth breathing." This condition did not resolve with plaque removal.

or cause the destruction of alveolar bone by inducing osteoclastic activity. Some of these cells, such as certain lymphocytes, divide to increase their numbers in a process called blastogenesis, thus cascading their effects. The following is a brief description of the cells involved in these inflammatory reactions.[12]

LYMPHOCYTES

Lymphocytes recognize foreign molecules, which are functionally called **antigens.** Cells, usually macrophages, take up antigen and present it to the lymphocytes. The recognition of antigen by lymphocytes is specific; they react to an individual antigen, then retain a memory so that the antigen is recognized again months or years later.

There are three types of lymphocytic cells, T-lymphocytes, B-lymphocytes, and killer or natural killer (NK) cells. T-lymphocytes are derived from the thymus, have several subsets, and are active in cell-mediated (humoral or antibody mediated) immune responses. They occur as helper T-cells, which assist B-cells in the production of **antibody** (protein that binds and disables antigen), or as cytotoxic T-cells, which stimulate cytotoxic activity in other cells such as macrophages. The B-lymphocytes are derived from the liver, spleen, and bone marrow. They serve as receptor sites for antigens and are the precursors of plasma cells. Helper T-cells stimulate B-cells to differentiate into plasma cells, which produce antibodies. In addition, B-cells stimulate other T-cells so that the immune response grows. Antigen processing by macrophages leads to the development of NK cells. The NK cells produce antibodies and a variety of products to stimulate microbicidal effects of the immune response, and they are effective against viruses and tumor cells.[12]

POLYMORPHONUCLEAR LEUKOCYTES

Polymorphonuclear leukocytes (PMNs), also called neutrophils, are attracted to periodontal lesions, particularly acute lesions, by chemotaxis. They make up about 70% of the circulating leukocytes.[12] PMNs **phagocytize** (engulf) and digest microorganisms, and they contain destructive substances that are very important in periodontal infections. PMNs contain granules, which are filled with enzymes such as collagenase or elastase. These enzymes are released and cause tissue destruction when the PMN cells degranulate. Abnormalities in PMNs can lead to more severe periodontal disease if the cells are unable to perform their functions or lack specific granules.

MACROPHAGES

Macrophages are scavenger cells with important phagocytic activity. They can engulf and digest a wide variety of bacteria. Macrophages are thought to differentiate from monocytes in the blood that are carried to the lesion area by the blood stream.[12] The functioning of macrophages is stimulated by the complement reaction (see discussion further on). They are protective in that they phagocytize bacteria, but they produce enzymes and other substances that may play a significant role in collagen destruction, which leads to the loss of periodontal tissues.

AUXILIARY CELLS

Many cells can become involved in the immune response because they react to **cytokines** (a type of effector substance described next), which are released by the lymphoid cells and phagocytes. These cells include mast cells, basophils, eosinophils, and platelets. Mast cells and basophils contain histamine and other substances important in hypersensitivity reactions (discussion follows). When these cells are activated, histamine and other substances are released that mediate hypersensitivity reactions and may enhance collagen destruction and bone resorption. Both eosinophils and platelets also produce a variety of mediating substances.[12]

Effector Molecules

The human body responds to tumor cells, bacteria, or their expressed products by plasma cell production of antibodies (immunoglobulins). First, antigens, foreign molecules of the invading cell or substance, are recognized, then effector molecules are stimulated as part of systems that eliminate foreign substances. Major **effector molecules** are antibodies, complement, and cytokines. There are many effector molecules present in the complex immune system. Three of the most well understood and important aspects, antibodies, complement, and cytokines, are briefly described.

ANTIBODIES

Antibody (**immunoglobulin**) production is a complex process involving macrophages processing antigen and presenting the fragments to T-cells, which interact with B-cells that differentiate into plasma cells, which produce the antibodies. The antibodies are found in blood, tissue fluids such as gingival fluid, and secretions. Antibodies are highly specific and sensitive. Human immunoglobulins are divided into five classes based on structural differences, IgG, IgM, IgE, IgD, and IgA. The structural differences are responsible for variation in effects.

IgG. This antibody has four identified subsets, IgG1, IgG2, IgG3, and IgG4. It is the most abundant of the antibodies and is present in both blood and extravascular fluids. It neutralizes bacterial toxins and enhances their phagocytosis. It is highly concentrated in serum, but much less concentrated in secretions. IgG makes up 80% of the total serum immunoglobulin, passes the placental barrier, and therefore provides immunity that newborns receive from their mothers.

IgM. This antibody develops early in the immune reaction, then is present in very low levels in the later stages of infection. IgM is probably important in the early stages of the immune response and is important in activating complement (discussion follows).

IgE. This antibody is present in very low amounts but is responsible for acute allergic reactions (discussion follows). Antigen reaction with this antibody leads to histamine release, among other substances.

IgD. This antibody is present in very low levels and is thought to be important in triggering the immune response.

IgA. This antibody is the immunoglobulin principally secreted in saliva, tears, and other body fluids. Secretory IgA is thought to activate complement and interfere with bacterial adhesion to tissue surfaces. Gingival tissue and gingival fluid contain IgA, but it is a serum substance and different from the secretory IgA. Secretory IgA may play a role in dental caries, but probably not in periodontal disease because the secretory IgA would not usually penetrate into periodontal pockets.[10]

COMPLEMENT

Complement is made up of proteins and glycoproteins that account for about 10% of the proteins in human serum. It has many functions. The proteins are not antibodies so their concentration is not affected by immunization, as is the case with immunoglobulins. Complement reacts in concert with IgG and IgM, causing lysis and functional alteration of cell walls, which encourage phagocytosis. Bacteria can help protect themselves from this effect by developing a coating. Complement also mediates the degranulation of mast cells, which cause the release of histamine and other substances that increase permeability of small blood vessels. Increased permeability permits migration of PMNs and increased phagocytic activity in the area. The complement reaction occurs in a sequenced and cascading way; once begun the reaction grows until it is complete. This allows for tremendous amplification of the immune response to a relatively small insult by antigen. The reaction also leads to a variety of effects that can result in destruction of periodontal tissues.

CYTOKINES

Cytokines are substances produced by the stimulated immune cells. They provide the communication between cells that mediates the complex interactions among cells and cellular elements. Cytokines assist in development and regulation of immune effector cells (such as increasing the number of T-cells so that their effects increase), cause cell-to-cell communication, and are themselves effector molecules. This is a very complex communication system. Many cytokines have been identified; they have effects on all cells of the immune system, act on many target cells, and play a major role in both the pathogenesis of disease and healing. Cytokines can affect the cells that produce them, neighboring cells, or distant cells. Cytokines are thought to affect pathologic periodontal changes because of the heavy infiltration of plasma cells and lymphocytes found in periodontal diseases.[10]

Cytokines used to be named for their action, such as MAF (macrophage activating factor) or OAF (osteoclast activating factor). Currently, newly identified cytokines are referred to as interleukins, describing their communication function between leukocytes. They are referred to by number, Il-1, Il-2, etc. Other cytokines are still named for their specific function, such as lymphotoxin or interferon. Interferon is of special interest because of its antiviral properties. Cytokines, specifically lymphotoxin, are found in large amounts in response to plaque bacteria antigens in periodontal disease. Lymphotoxin is important because it can stimulate bone and cartilage resorption, leading to the destructive changes seen in periodontal diseases. Cytokines can also have general cytotoxic effects on host cells in the chronic presence of plaque bacteria antigens.

Figure 2-10 presents a diagrammatic scheme of the complex interrelationships between the major components of the host response.

Hypersensitivity (Allergic) Reactions

Allergic reactions are usually protective in nature. They are reactions to foreign bacteria, viruses, or other substances. They may also cause tissue destruction by triggering overreactions called **hypersensitivity reactions**. Tissue damage can occur in a host who has been sensitized by one exposure to a substance, then challenged again by the same substance. There are four types of hypersensitivity reactions, anaphylaxis or type I, cytotoxic or type II, immune complex or type III, and cell-mediated, delayed, or type IV. Types I, II, and III are immediate reactions and occur within minutes or hours; they are the more likely reactions to affect the periodontal tissues. Type IV reactions are delayed and can occur days later or beyond.

Histamine is released in Type I hypersensitivity reactions. This can be a generalized or localized reaction. Generalized reaction can lead to serious life-threatening consequences, as can be

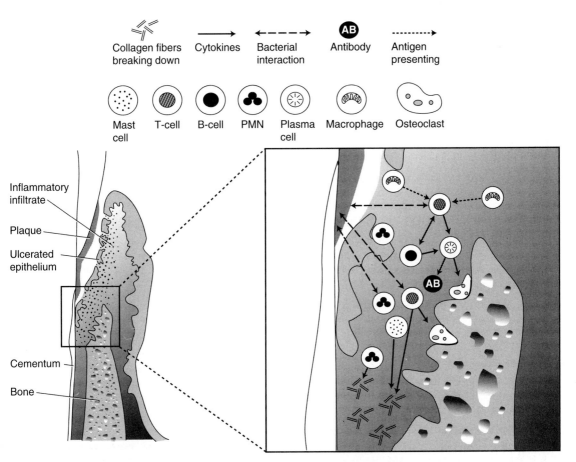

FIGURE 2–10. Interaction and effects of cells in the immune response. PMNs are attracted to the site to phagocytize bacteria and neutralize toxic substances. Mast cells degranulate and produce substances that effect collagen destruction. Macrophages are phagocytic and present antigens to T-cells and B-cells in order to amplify the immune response. T-cells produce cytokines, which regulate the immune response. B-cells proliferate and mature to become plasma cells. Plasma cells produce antibodies that provide both local and systemic immune responses. Antibodies also alter bacteria so they can be phagocytized. Cytokines and bacterial interactions mediate this cascading cellular response. (Courtesy of Randal W. Rowland, MS, DMD, MS.)

seen in individuals with food or drug allergies. A localized reaction can result in increased tissue destruction in an area such as the periodontium. Histamine is found in higher concentrations in chronically inflamed gingiva than in healthy gingiva. The histamine causes many actions, including increased capillary and venule permeability, which attract more immune cells to an area and increase the inflammatory response.

Cytotoxic reactions, Type II hypersensitivity responses, result in the breakdown of tissue or blood cells. They are the products of antibodies that react directly to antigens tightly bound to the surfaces of cells. These reactions are not seen in gingival or periodontal diseases but are manifested in other oral diseases such as pemphigus, where antibodies react directly with epithelial cell membranes.

Immune complex (Arthus) reactions, or Type III hypersensitivity reactions, occur when high levels of antigen persist in an area without being eliminated. The reaction occurs around small blood vessels, activates complement, and can cause extensive localized tissue damage. An example of a Type III or Arthus reaction is the wheal and flare response seen in skin tests for tuberculosis.

Cell-mediated, delayed, or Type IV hypersensitivity reactions are related to the reaction of antigens with the surface of T-lymphocytes. Once sensitized to an antigen, these lymphocytes can undergo blastogenesis, or transformation, resulting in mitotic division and increasing the number of immunocompetent cells sensitized to the specific antigen. These reactions explain why, upon a second exposure to an allergic agent such as a bee sting, the reaction can be greatly increased and possibly life threatening.

The host response aspects of periodontal diseases are expanding areas of inquiry in dentistry. As these complex interactions are better understood, the disease process, particularly why it affects individuals differently, will become clearer. As understanding grows, the therapies to be discussed in later chapters in this book will also be refined and made more patient specific. It is important to appreciate the significance of the host response. In treating periodontal disease, therapeutic scaling and root planing of one quadrant of teeth appears to invoke healing in untreated areas. This phe-

nomenon is seen is clinical trials where "no treatment" areas of the mouth show significant improvement in the course of the study.[13] It is thought that the stimulation of the host response against plaque antigens results in the unforeseen healing in untreated areas.[14]

Other Protective Responses in the Oral Environment

The normal function of oral epithelium is protective in nature, acting as a very effective barrier to mechanical and microbial assault. The host response acts to wall off infections when they do occur. The presence and amount of gingival fluid and the ameliorating effects of saliva affect the interface between the surface of the tissues and the host. These two substances play a protective role in the host[15] and are briefly described here.

GINGIVAL OR SULCULAR FLUID

Gingival or sulcular fluid is considered an inflammatory exudate because it is present in much greater amounts when the gingiva is inflamed than when in the healthy state. It also increases with normal, physiologic functions, such as the mastication of coarse foods, tooth brushing, female sex hormones, smoking, and after periodontal surgery.

The sulcular epithelium permits migration of molecules into the gingival sulcus, although in very small amounts. The resulting fluid contains enzymes, cellular elements, electrolytes, and compounds such as glucose. Leukocytes, primarily PMNs, are excreted, making up about 92% of the cellular content of the fluid. These cells appear extravascularly in the connective tissue, travel across the epithelium, and are expelled into the sulcus. It is presumed that these cells protect against the extension of plaque into the sulcus.[15]

The antibiotic tetracycline is concentrated in the gingival fluid at a higher rate than found circulating in the blood stream. This property has made tetracycline more useful in some cases for treating periodontal diseases than other antibiotics. As discussed in chapter 7, antibiotics are useful as adjunctive therapy in some aggressive forms of periodontal disease but are not used routinely. The drugs most commonly prescribed are tetracycline or its derivatives for this reason. They are not indicated for the treatment of gingivitis.[16]

SALIVA

Saliva exerts several major protective influences in the oral environment. These include lubrication, physical protection, cleansing, buffering, remineralization of teeth, and antibacterial actions.[15] Saliva contains organic elements that can cause structural damage to oral organisms, antibodies to inactivate bacteria so they can be engulfed by leukocytes, and enzymes to inhibit tissue breakdown. Saliva has an important buffering action to maintain the pH level in the mouth and thus reduce the demineralization of teeth. It contains coagulation factors to hasten blood coagulation and protect wounds from bacteria, and minerals to remineralize teeth.[15]

Saliva is an extremely complex substance and its functions are far from fully understood. However, the importance of saliva in periodontal disease and dental caries has been demonstrated in experimental animals. When salivary glands have been removed, the incidence of caries and periodontal disease increases, and wound healing is delayed. Increased incidence of these diseases is also seen in humans who have xerostomia, reduced salivary function, which may occur for many reasons.[15]

Conclusion

The interrelationship of the anatomic characteristics of the periodontium and the host response is dynamic and evolving. New research will continue to uncover more information on this fascinating aspect of human health and disease, and will permit the development of improved therapies.

STUDY QUESTIONS

MULTIPLE CHOICE

1. The attached gingiva is demarcated from the alveolar mucosa by the:

   a. gingival sulcus
   b. marginal groove
   c. mucogingival junction
   d. unattached gingiva

2. The name of the structure that surrounds the tooth and creates a cuff or collar of epithelium extending approximately 1.5 mm coronally is:

   a. free attached gingiva
   b. free marginal gingiva
   c. free gingival groove
   d. stippled gingiva

3. The slight depression in the gingiva appearing between the buccal and lingual interdental papillae is called the:

   a. col
   b. embrasure space
   c. gingival groove
   d. gingival space

4. The histologic sulcus depth is approximately:

   a. 1 mm to 3 mm
   b. 2 mm to 5 mm
   c. 3 mm to 4 mm
   d. 3 mm to 5 mm

5. The principal fiber bundles in the connective tissue that run from the cementum to the alveolar crest and protect the periodontal ligament are called the:

   a. alveologingival group
   b. circular group
   c. dentoperiosteal group
   d. transseptal group

6. The window in the normal bone structure covering the surface of the root is called a dehiscence. The dehiscence is a significant structure in periodontal disease.

   a. Both statements are TRUE.
   b. Both statements are FALSE.
   c. The first statement is TRUE, the second is FALSE.
   d. The first statement is FALSE, the second is TRUE.

7. Cells attracted to areas of the body by stimuli such as microbial influence or trauma are referred to as:

   a. chemotactic cells
   b. cytokines
   c. inflammatory cells
   d. blood cells

8. Inflammatory cells perform all of the following functions EXCEPT one. Which one is the EXCEPTION?

   a. remove damage tissue
   b. reduce osteoclastic activity
   c. phagocytize bacteria
   d. lyse cells

9. B-lymphocytes differentiate into plasma cells. Plasma cells are important in producing the antigen/antibody response.

   a. Both statements are TRUE.
   b. Both statements are FALSE.
   c. The first statement is TRUE, the second is FALSE.
   d. The first statement is FALSE, the second is TRUE.

10. Effector molecules perform all of the following functions EXCEPT one. Which one is the EXCEPTION?

    a. stimulate systems to eliminate foreign substances
    b. cause cell-to-cell communication
    c. decrease the immune response by cascading the reaction
    d. cause the production of antibodies

11. Hypersensitivity reactions:

    a. can be delayed or immediate
    b. cause no tissue damage
    c. are not life-threatening
    d. are only localized in nature

SHORT ANSWER

12. Why is the term "probing depth" more accurate than the term "sulcus depth"?

    _____

    _____

13. List the functions of the periodontal ligament.

    _____

    _____

14. Describe the color, size, shape, texture, and consistency of normal gingiva.

    _____

    _____

15. Describe the protective effects of gingival fluid.

_____

_____

16. Describe the protective effects of saliva.

_____

_____

REFERENCES

1. Dorland's Medical Dictionary, 29th ed. Philadelphia: WB Saunders, 2000.
2. Löe H, Listgarten MA, Terranova VP. The gingiva structure and function. In Genco RJ, Goldman HM, Cohen DW, eds. Contemporary Periodontics St. Louis: CV Mosby, 1990:3-32.
3. Wilkins EM. Clinical Practice of the Dental Hygienist, 8th ed. Philadelphia: Lippincott Williams and Wilkins, 1999;186-199.
4. Itoiz ME, Carranza FA Jr. The gingiva. In FA Carranza and MG Newman eds. Clinical Periodontology, 8th ed. Philadelphia: WB Saunders, 1996;12-29.
5. Fedi PF Jr. The gingiva. In The Periodontal Syllabus, 2nd ed. Philadelphia; Lea & Febiger, 1989:1-13.
6. Hassell TM. Tissues and cells of the periodontium. Periodontology 2000 1993;3:9-38.
7. Armitage GC. Clinical recognition and assessment of chronic inflammatory periodontal disease. In Biologic Basis of Periodontal Maintenance Therapy. Berkeley: Praxis, 1980:1-32.
8. Terranova VP, Goldman HM, Listgarten MA. The periodontal attachment apparatus structure, function, and chemistry. In Genco RJ, Goldman HM, Cohen DW, eds. Contemporary Periodontics. St. Louis: CV Mosby, 1990:33-54.
9. Carranza FA Jr, Ubios AM. The tooth supporting structures. In FA Carranza and MG Newman, eds. Clinical Periodontology, 8th ed. Philadelphia: WB Saunders, 1996:30-51.
10. Offenbacher S. Periodontal diseases: pathogenesis. Ann Periodontol 1996;1:821-878.
11. Genco RJ. Host responses in periodontal diseases: current concepts. J Periodontol 1992;63:338-355.
12. Nisengard RC, Newman MG, Sanz M. Host response: basic concepts. In Carranza FA and Newman MG, eds. Clinical Periodontology, 8th ed. WB Saunders Co., Philadelphia; 1996:111-120.
13. Kaldahl WB, Kalkwarf KL, Patil KD, Dyer JK, Bates RE Jr. Evaluation of four modalities of periodontal therapy. Mean probing depth, probing attachment level and recession changes. J Periodontol 1988;59:783-793.
14. Ebersole JL, Taubman MA, Smith DJ, Haffajee AD. Effect of subgingival scaling on systemic antibody responses to oral microorganisms. Infect Immun 1985;48:534-539.
15. Carranza FA Jr, Bulkacz J. Defense mechanisms of the gingiva. In Carranza FA and Newman MG, eds. Clinical Periodontology, 8th ed. WB Saunders Co., Philadelphia; 1996:103-110.
16. Drisko CH. Non-surgical pocket therapy: Pharmacotherapeutics. Ann Periodontol 1996;1:491-566.

3

Dorothy A. Perry

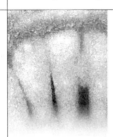

Epidemiology of Periodontal Diseases

Chapter Objectives

1. Define epidemiology and explain the relationship of this discipline of study to the identification and treatment of gingival and periodontal diseases.
2. Compare and contrast the plaque, calculus, bleeding, and periodontal indices that are used to quantify conditions in the oral cavity and explain how these scoring systems are applied to diagnosis and treatment of disease.
3. Briefly describe the national prevalence data and how information of this type is used to understand the status of periodontal health in the United States.
4. List the risk factors and determinants that are related to periodontal diseases.
5. Describe the disease prevalence trends revealed for gingival and periodontal diseases.
6. State the prevalence of juvenile periodontitis and HIV-associated periodontitis and describe their unique characteristics.

Key Terms

Calculus Index
Community Index of Periodontal Treatment Needs
Determinant
Gingival fluid flow
Gingival Index
Incidence
Periodontal Disease Index
Periodontal Screening and Recording

Prevalence
Risk factors
Russell's Periodontal Index
Severity
Simplified Oral Hygiene Index
Sulcus Bleeding Index
Miller Index of Tooth Mobility
Volpe Manhold Index

DEFINITION OF EPIDEMIOLOGY

Epidemiology is the study of health and disease in human populations and associated factors. Epidemiology deals with the **prevalence** of disease, the number of cases of a disease present in a given population at one time; **incidence** of disease, the rate of occurrence of new disease in a population over a given period of time;[1] **severity** of disease, the level of disease; and **risk factors** (also referred to as **determinants**), which are exposures, behaviors, and characteristics associated with disease. Determinants are risk factors that cannot be modified, i.e., gender as opposed to smoking.[1] Epidemiologic research differs from clinical research in that entire groups are the focus of study, not individuals; and that persons without the disease are included in the study in order to quantify risk.[2] Prevalence alone, simply counting the number of individuals with disease, is not sufficient to understand periodontal disease in the population.[3]

Periodontal disease is a complex interaction of bacterial infection, host response, and patient behavior. Epidemiologic research provides information on another dimension of disease. It describes how much of the population is affected by periodontal disease and how severe it is likely to be, and identifies characteristics or behaviors likely to be found in persons with the disease. In order to make these observations about populations of individuals, the researcher must define what constitutes disease. This is done by clinical assessment of individuals in the population using measurement scales or indices. The indices are interpretations of measurements such as probe measurements, plaque assessments, or the presence of bleeding. For example, periodontal disease can be defined as having probe depths of greater than 4 mm in at least one site in the mouth. It can also be defined as having one or more probe depths of 7 mm, or having the gingival tissue bleed when probed in one or more sites.

Once the definition of the disease has been set, the researcher has to have an examiner or team of examiners trained to apply the indices to members of a population. This means the indices have to be calibrated, or standardized, so that what one examiner would interpret as a 4 mm probing depth, all would interpret the same way. It is impossible to have 100% agreement between examiners at all times, but with training they can agree most of the time. This agreement is essential for the information collected to be meaningful, so you will know that these data can be accurately interpreted. Imagine the difficulty if one examiner probed 7 mm and another probed 5 mm in the same pocket and your definition of periodontal disease is 6 mm. That patient might not be accurately classified in your population as either

with or without the disease. The calibration process permits the epidemiologic data collected by all examiners to be evaluated together as a group and to provide meaningful information to the audience.

Another important point about epidemiologic research is related to the population of individuals to be examined. It is not possible to examine every human being in large epidemiologic studies, so representative samples are selected. This can be done through random selection of subjects, or very sophisticated sampling techniques using subsets of the population. In either of these cases, the results found in the sample can be generalized to a much larger group of the population, but rarely to everyone. As an example, epidemiologic studies of heart disease were conducted in the past solely on men, so although the findings could be generalized to men, there was real concern about applying the findings to women. These studies now include women because treatment effects or risk factors need to be assessed based on differences in populations such as gender.

Although it is complex, epidemiologic research gives us important insights into health problems. It is of interest to dental hygienists to understand the number of people in the population with periodontal disease, how severe it is, and what behaviors or characteristics are associated with the disease.

Epidemiologic data do not provide absolute values for a population, and studies differ in their findings on the same matters due to differences in population or examiners or measuring scales. But well designed and run epidemiologic studies provide us with much information that is distinct from information gained from clinical studies. Epidemiology provides a general understanding of the disease occurring in patients. For example, we know that periodontal disease occurs in a relatively small but significant percentage of the U.S. population, so not everyone seeking dental hygiene treatment has periodontal disease. However, it is also important to remember that in clinical practice, when a patient with periodontal disease requires dental hygiene care, the disease affects 100% of that person. Dental hygiene care is dictated by the specific findings for that person, not general population findings.

This chapter reviews important epidemiology indices so the dental hygienist can understand the yardsticks by which periodontal disease is defined. One very large, well run epidemiologic study will be reviewed to describe the overall periodontal health of U.S. populations. Several risk factors associated with more severe disease will be described, and other population studies will be presented.

REVIEW OF IMPORTANT INDICES

Epidemiologic data are collected with well defined measuring systems known as indices. These indices have defined scales, are easily applied to populations of individuals, and measure some specific aspect of the disease or condition of interest—in this case, signs of periodontal disease.

The presence of the signs of periodontal disease, as measured by these indices, does not mean that the individual examined has a specific amount of periodontal disease; this information makes up part of a picture of the prevalence and severity of disease in the evaluated population. The use of multiple indices permits the association of various signs and symptoms in the population. Several indices have been used to evaluate the periodontal status of populations. In each case, the units are defined with upper and lower limits. This section explains what it means to say that the population had a mean (average) plaque index of 2 or that 7 percent of the population had severe periodontal disease characterized by one or more deep pockets.

Many indices are used in research. The following indices are commonly used in longitudinal studies and surveys. This section explains what these scores mean. It is important to consider the scoring system used when interpreting research results, because they are all different. For a detailed discussion of all indices, see Wilkins.[4]

Plaque and Debris Indices

Plaque is an important quantity to define because it is the etiologic agent in periodontal disease. Screening populations for the presence of plaque determines whether all of the people have plaque, how much, and how it relates to other signs of disease. Sometimes plaque is measured by a simple scale, presence (scored as 1) or absence (scored as 0). If all plaque caused periodontal disease, this approach might be sufficient. However, the quantity of plaque provides only a picture of oral hygiene, such as where the accumulation is greatest and how good or poor oral hygiene practices are in a given population. It does not correlate well with periodontal disease.[1]

PLAQUE INDEX OF SILNESS AND LÖE (PL I)[5]

The Plaque Index (Pl I) places the most significance on the amount of plaque at the gingival margin because of the importance of the proximity and relationship of plaque in that location to gingival inflammation. This index, which has been used in many studies, can be used to measure all teeth or selected teeth in a study, or can be applied to selected surfaces of the teeth. The following criteria are used for scoring.

0 = The gingival area of the tooth is free of plaque; the surface is tested by running a probe across the tooth surfaces at the gingival margin; if no soft material adheres, then the area is considered free of plaque.

1 = No plaque is observed in situ by the unaided eye, but plaque is visible on the point of a probe after the probe has been moved over the tooth surface at the entrance of the gingival crevice.

2 = The gingival area is covered by a thin to moderately thick layer of plaque that is visible to the naked eye.

3 = The accumulation of soft matter is heavy, and it fills the crevice produced by the gingival margin and the tooth surface.

The "tooth score" is determined by adding the scores for the measured surfaces on each tooth and dividing this number by the number of surfaces. The "whole mouth score" is determined by adding the tooth scores and dividing this number by the number of teeth. These data can be evaluated by tooth, by groups of teeth, or over individuals in the population. In a population with an average plaque score of 2, a moderate level of plaque is present in most of the individuals. Alternatively, if a tooth has a plaque score of 1, little plaque is present and the plaque cannot be seen by the naked eye.

SIMPLIFIED ORAL HYGIENE INDEX (OHI-S) OF GREENE AND VERMILLION[6]

The **Simplified Oral Hygiene Index** (OHI-S) has both a debris index (DI-S) and a **calculus**

index (CI-S). The scores can be used singly to provide a plaque index or a calculus index, or they may be combined to provide an oral hygiene index.

The DI-S, the plaque portion of the index, is a numeric assessment of plaque and debris on the teeth. As representative of the entire dentition, six selected teeth are scored: the buccal surfaces of the maxillary first molars, the lingual surfaces of the mandibular first molars, and the labial aspects of the maxillary and mandibular left central incisors. Scoring criteria are:

0 = No debris or stain.
1 = Soft debris covering as much as one-third of the tooth surface, or extrinsic stain without debris.
2 = Soft debris covering one-third to two-thirds of the tooth surface.
3 = Soft debris covering more than two-thirds of the surface.

The debris score for the individual is obtained by adding the scores for all surfaces and dividing this number by the number of surfaces scored. An average score across the population can be determined by adding the individual scores and dividing this number by the number of individuals. When this index is interpreted, a DI-S score of 2 has considerably different meaning than a Pl I score of 2. If an individual has an average DI-S score of 2, two-thirds of the teeth are covered with plaque. In contrast, a Pl I score of 2 means that there is a thin to moderately thick layer of visible plaque at the gingival margin.

Calculus Indices

Calculus is a significant factor associated with periodontal disease, although it is not an etiologic agent (see Chapter 5). It has been measured in many epidemiologic studies, and the amount of calculus present is significant to the practice of the dental hygienist. Knowing the extent of calculus formation in the population helps to explain why so much practice time is spent removing it. Longitudinal studies can help to determine what to expect, in general, when patients return after 6 months, or 6 years, for their next dental hygiene appointment.

CALCULUS INDEX OF THE OHI-S[6]

The selection of teeth to be measured is the same as with the DI-S described earlier. Scoring

for the CI-S is similar. A score of 2 on the CI-S indicates a considerable quantity of supragingival calculus, some subgingival calculus, or both. The criteria are as follows:

0 = No calculus.
1 = Supragingival calculus covering up to one-third of the tooth surface.
2 = Supragingival calculus covering one-third to two-thirds of the tooth surface, or flecks of subgingival calculus.
3 = Supragingival calculus covering more than two-thirds of the surface, or a continuous heavy band of subgingival calculus.

To determine the OHI-S score, the combined score of DI-S and CI-S, the mean scores on both indices for all subjects are added, then divided by the total number of subjects. These OHI-S scores are higher, ranging from 0 to 6. A score of 6 is the highest score possible on the DI-S, 3, plus the highest score possible in the CI-S, 3. A combined OHI-S score does not indicate how much debris or how much calculus is present. An OHI-S score of 3 could indicate heavy calculus accumulation, heavy debris accumulation, or a combination. For this reason, it is often helpful to consider both components of the OHI-S score.

VOLPE MANHOLD PROBE METHOD OF CALCULUS ASSESSMENT (VM)[7]

The **Volpe Manhold Index** scoring system measures only supragingival calculus. It was designed to measure the mandibular incisors, but also has been applied to other teeth. It has been used in studies of "tartar" control toothpastes. A periodontal probe with millimeter markings is used to bisect each of the three parts of the lingual surface of the incisor, and a measurement of the height of calculus is made for each. Scores for the direct lingual, mesial lingual, and distal lingual surfaces are averaged to provide a tooth score. Tooth scores are averaged to provide a score for the individual. The score can be interpreted as indicating the approximate height of calculus, in millimeters, on the measured surfaces.

Indices of Gingival Disease or Bleeding

Indices of gingival disease are assessments of bleeding of the gingiva. These indices are commonly used in epidemiologic studies and other clinical research in periodontology. Bleeding is an important sign to monitor because it is associated with inflammation, bleeding on probing is the most common sign used in clinical practice to monitor gingival health, and bleeding precedes periodontal destruction. Bleeding is not the ideal index of periodontal disease because most gingival bleeding does not progress to periodontitis: however, periodontitis is always preceded by gingivitis, which is characterized by bleeding.

GINGIVAL INDEX OF LÖE AND SILNESS (GI)[8]

The **Gingival Index** is an evaluation of each of four sides of the tooth: mesial, distal, lingual, and facial. The index is scored by visual inspection of the gingiva and by gentle probing, stroking, or sweeping motion into the sulcus. A score is assigned to each surface, and an average score is assigned to the tooth. GI scores for areas of the mouth, for selected teeth, or for the full mouth are computed by adding the tooth scores and averaging that number by the number of teeth examined. The following criteria are used for scoring:

0 =   Absence of inflammation.
1 =   Mild inflammation characterized by slight color change, little change in texture, and no bleeding on probing.
2 =   Moderate inflammation characterized by redness and swelling of the gingiva and accompanied by bleeding on probing.
3 =   Severe inflammation characterized by significant redness and hypertrophy, a tendency to bleed spontaneously, and ulceration.

With this index, a score of 2 indicates bleeding on probing. In general, a tooth score, individual score, or population score greater than 1 suggests some level of moderate inflammation characterized by bleeding on probing.

SULCUS BLEEDING INDEX (SBI)[9]

The **Sulcus Bleeding Index** (SBI) is also a measure of bleeding on probing. Like the GI, measurements are taken at four points around each tooth: the mesial, distal, buccal, and lingual surfaces. A probe is gently inserted in the sulcus area and withdrawn. The gingival units

are scored 30 seconds after probing. The scoring units are:

0 =   Healthy appearance with no bleeding on probing.
1 =   Healthy appearance, with no color or contour change, but bleeding on probing.
2 =   Bleeding on probing and color change in tissue, but no swelling.
3 =   Bleeding on probing, color change, and slight swelling of the gingival unit.
4 =   Bleeding on probing and obvious swelling, with or without color change.
5 =   Spontaneous bleeding, bleeding on probing, color change, and significant swelling, with or without ulceration.

A score of 2 on the SBI scale indicates moderate inflammation characterized by bleeding on probing. This scale differentiates between the more severe signs of inflammation, including significant swelling and color change. It has been argued that the important distinction is when the tissue bleeds, so the usefulness of identifying grades of inflammation beyond that point depends on the purpose of the study.

Indices of Periodontal Disease

Indices of periodontal destruction measure factors beyond gingival changes and include bone loss around the teeth. They have been used to estimate periodontal health for individuals, communities, and populations. More recent national data have relied on millimeter measures of periodontal probing depth and attachment loss rather than on an encompassing index of periodontal disease. Millimeter data are more easily translated and understood by clinicians than index scores. However, important data have been collected with index scores. Two important indices are described here.

RUSSELL'S PERIODONTAL INDEX (PI)[10]

Russell designed and used the **Periodontal Index** in the 1950s and 1960s. It is a progressive scale that assigns a numeric score to each tooth. This scale is weighted more toward bone loss than toward gingival inflammation. The score for each tooth is added and averaged by all teeth examined in the individual, providing a score for each person. Population scores are determined by averaging the scores of individuals. The criteria for scoring are:

0 = Negative, with no inflammation or loss of function.
1 = Mild gingivitis, with inflammation in the free gingiva, but not circumscribing the tooth.
2 = Gingivitis, with inflammation circumscribing the tooth, but normal probing depths.
6 = Gingivitis, with pocket formation; the gingival sulcus is deepened, function is normal, and there is no drifting.
8 = Advanced destruction, with loss of masticatory function; the tooth may be loose, may sound dull on percussion, and may be depressible in the socket.

The higher scores indicating bone loss weight this scale so that it does not discriminate as to attachment loss, probe depth measurements, or other gingival indices. However, it was developed early in the 1950s, and it provided important information that was not previously quantified. A PI score of 6.5 or 7 indicates periodontal destruction, but not the extent of probing depths or attachment loss. Suggested interpretations of the PI are: a score of 1.6 to 5.0 indicates reversible disease and higher scores indicate irreversible disease.[2]

PERIODONTAL DISEASE INDEX OF RAMFJORD (PDI)[11]

The PDI evaluates the gingival condition and measures probe depths and attachment loss. It is designed to evaluate six teeth: #3, the maxillary right first molar; #9, the maxillary left central incisor; #12, the maxillary left first bicuspid; #19, the mandibular left first molar; #25, the mandibular right central incisor; and #28, the mandibular right first bicuspid. Measurements from these teeth have been shown to be representative of the entire dentition. Scoring is determined on the following scale:

GINGIVITIS
0 = Negative.
1 = Mild gingivitis involving the free gingiva.
2 = Moderate gingivitis involving the free and attached gingiva.
3 = Severe gingivitis with hypertrophy and hemorrhage.

PERIODONTAL DISEASE (THE GINGIVITIS SCORE IS DISREGARDED)
4 = Pocket depths on two or more of the surfaces measure up to 3 mm apical to the cementoenamel junction.

5 = Pocket depths on two or more of the surfaces measure 3 to 6 mm apical to the cementoenamel junction.
6 = Pocket depths on two or more of the surfaces measure more than 6 mm apical to the cementoenamel junction.

The scores for each of the six teeth are added, then averaged to provide a score for the individual. Individual scores can be averaged to compute a population score. With this system, as with the PI, much information is compressed into a single number that provides an impression of the overall level of disease, but little information about the needs of any individual. For this reason, these scoring systems are reserved for survey and screening purposes and are not employed in dental hygiene practice, where detailed and individualized assessments are needed (see Chapter 9).

Other Indices

A number of other indices have been developed and used. This section describes four of the most important, all of which have different goals.

CIPTN[12]

One of the most significant indices used in epidemiologic research is the **Community Index of Periodontal Treatment Needs** (CIPTN), which was developed by the World Health Organization. This index assesses the periodontal treatment needs in the community, not simply the level of disease. A specially designed periodontal probe is used for this assessment. It is a color-coded probe with a black band extending from 3.5 to 5.5 mm. It has a rounded ball tip, 0.5 mm in diameter, that helps to prevent excessive penetration of the probe tip into the connective tissue. Excessive penetration would lead to overestimation of pocket depths. Ten teeth are examined, two in each posterior sextant and one in each anterior sextant. The teeth examined are #2, #3, #8, #14, #15, #18, #19, #25, #30, and #31. There are routines for scoring in the case of missing teeth. The use of substitute teeth is permitted, and if a sextant has only one tooth, it is considered part of the next sextant. The worst finding for each tooth is coded, and the worst finding for the sextant is the treatment category for that sextant. Individual tooth codes are as follows:

0 = No signs of inflammation or pocketing.
1 = Gingival bleeding after probing.
2 = Supra- or subgingival calculus present.
3 = Pathologic pockets of 4.0 to 5.5 mm.
4 = Pathologic pockets of 6 mm or more.

After the codes are assigned to teeth, the treatment categories are assigned per sextant based on the highest score for each sextant. The treatment categories are as follows:

0 = No treatment (code 0 only).
I = Improvement in oral hygiene (code 1 only).
II = Category I + scaling (codes 2 and 3).
III = Categories I + II + complex periodontal treatment (code 4).

This information can be presented in a variety of ways. Treatment needs can be expressed as the percentage of subjects in each treatment category or as the percentage of sextants needing specific treatment. For example, if 85 percent of the population is scored as category II, the population is in need of scaling and oral hygiene instruction: the services of both the dental hygienist and the general dentist are required. The percentage of the population scored as category III may be in need of the services of the periodontist.

A study by Lang[13] suggested a weakness in the CIPTN system: It may overestimate the need for treatment. This highlights the difference in focus between the epidemiologist and the clinician in private practice. CIPTN treatment categories suggest the need for the population to be brought to a complete state of health. This individualized dental care model is used in the United States and in many other countries. However, when dealing with different populations and limited resources, the epidemiologist may choose to target individuals who are at greatest risk for tooth loss. Lang suggested that the use of radiographs with defined bone loss criteria might be better suited to determining the minimal treatment needs of the population and also could specify treatment for those at greatest risk for losing the teeth. It is unrealistic to expect that certain populations, such as the Sri Lankan tea workers studied by Anerud and co-workers[14] who have no oral hygiene practices and no dentists, would receive treatment at the level of industrialized populations. CIPTN might not provide a useful measure for such a population if the goal of the researcher was to direct resources to preserve teeth.

GINGIVAL FLUID FLOW[15]

Another important index is the measurement of **gingival fluid flow** from the sulcus. This index is primarily used in periodontal research studies to identify early inflammation. An increase in the flow of crevicular fluid is one of the first measurable changes in the inflammatory process of the periodontium. Fluid is measured on filter paper strips placed within the sulcus. The measurement is made on a calibrated machine called a Periotron (IDE Interstate, New York, NY). Comparisons of fluid flow can be made over time in a study population to estimate changes in the amount of inflammation present, or the information can be used in a cross-sectional comparison study of a larger population.

PERIODONTAL SCREENING AND RECORDING (PSR)[4]

The **Periodontal Screening and Recording**, was developed by the American Academy of Periodontology and the American Dental Association. This screening system enables the clinician to identify which patients need a full examination and which patients require only a screening examination in the private practice setting. The utility of the PSR system in practice has not been established.

The World Health Association CIPTN probe, with one black band extending from 3.5 to 5.5 mm, is used to assess PSR scores. The probe is inserted around all areas of all teeth in the sextant, and the periodontium is examined for inflammation, plaque, and calculus. Sextants are graded individually, and only the worst score for the sextant is recorded. The sextant evaluation is coded in the following manner:

0 = The colored section of the probe is completely visible in the deepest probe depth of the sextant; no calculus, defective margins, or bleeding.
1 = The colored section of the probe is completely visible in the deepest probe depth of the sextant; no calculus or defective margins, but bleeding after probing.
2 = The colored section of the probe is completely visible in the deepest probe depth of the sextant; supra- or subgingival calculus or defective margins present.

3 = The color-coded section of the probe is only partly visible in the deepest probe depth in the sextant (indicating at least one 3.5 to 5 mm probe depth); calculus, defective restorations, and bleeding may or may not be present.

4 = The color-coded section of the probe completely disappears into the deepest probe depth in the sextant (indicating at least one pocket of 6 mm or deeper).

* = An asterisk is added to any of the preceding sextant codes if any notable features—such as furcation involvement, pathologic mobility, mucogingival defect, or marked recession—are identified.

The highest score in any sextant for the individual patient determines the case management. If any score of 3 or 4 is identified, a complete, full mouth periodontal examination should be performed. General management guidelines are associated with the sextant codes. Codes 0 and 1 require plaque control and preventive care. Code 2 indicates plaque control, prevention, calculus removal, and correction of defective restorations. Codes 3 and 4 require complete assessment and a periodontal treatment plan. Regardless of code, any sextant that has an abnormality asterisk (code*) requires a specific treatment plan.

It will be interesting to see whether this system is widely adopted in dental practices. It is a screening examination with criteria for identifying patients who need complete evaluations.

MILLER INDEX OF TOOTH MOBILITY[16]

Miller described the system that is most commonly used to quantify tooth mobility **(Miller Index of Tooth Mobility)**. It is used both in epidemiologic studies and in the clinical assessment of individual patients. Two metal instrument handles are placed on either side of the tooth to be tested, and the tooth is moved in a facial-lingual direction. It is not advisable to assess mobility with the fingers because the soft pads may not provide enough resistance to detect slight mobility. The mobility grading scale is 0 to 3 as follows:

0 = No movement when force is applied.
1 = Barely distinguishable tooth movement.
2 = 1 mm movement in any direction.
3 = > 1 mm movement in any direction, or

tooth is depressible or can be rotated in the socket.

This index is often modified with plus or minus signs, or identified with Roman numerals. However, the more used (1+, 2−, 2, etc.), the less reproducible and meaningful the scale becomes. A simple way to apply Miller's index is practiced by Taggart: if you think it is mobile, score it 1; if you are sure it is mobile, score it 2; and if it is depressible in the socket, score it 3.

NATIONAL PREVALENCE DATA

A large scale national study reporting the oral health of United States adults was published in 1987.[17] This complex study evaluated employed adults. The sample was drawn from businesses of various sizes and from healthy seniors older than 65 years who attended senior centers around the country. Minors and household workers were excluded. This study was a stratified, multistage probability sample that included all racial and socioeconomic groups across all regions of the United States. Of employed adults 18 to 65 years old, 15,132 were examined, representing approximately 100,000,000 of the United States population. The senior population examined included 5686 subjects, representing approximately 4,000,000 older adults in the United States. In the employed group, more men than women were examined; the ratio was 1.24. In the senior sample, more women were examined; the ratio was 0.52.

This information provides an overview of the periodontal health of adults in the United States, a snapshot in time rather than a long-term study designed to evaluate changes over time. The findings likely underreport prevalence to some degree because the scoring system did not evaluate all surfaces of all teeth. Examiners scored buccal and mesial buccal surfaces only in two randomly selected quadrants, one maxillary and one mandibular. However, most of the sites that were eligible to be examined were evaluated. This study provides a snapshot of the oral health of more than half of the adults in the United States. The percentage of the population with at least one site of a specific sign is the prevalence, and the average percentage of sites per individual with the sign is the extent of disease measured in the population.

Edentulism

Edentulism is decreasing significantly in the United States. Younger age groups have dramatically more teeth than older groups. By the age of 29, fewer than 1 percent of the United States population was edentulous; by age 34 fewer than 2 percent had lost all of their teeth. Of those 60 to 64 years old, 15 percent had lost all of their teeth.

In contrast, 32 percent of seniors defined as 65 years of age or older were edentulous at age 65, and 45 percent were edentulous at age 80. Almost 50 percent of the adult employed population had 27 or 28 teeth; only 4 percent had no teeth. The average number of teeth for employed adults, excluding those who were edentulous, is 25. Those 50 to 60 years old had 20 teeth remaining. Seniors have lost more teeth: only 2 percent had 28 teeth, 2.5 percent had 27 teeth, and 42 percent were edentulous. The average number of teeth in dentate seniors was 19 (Figure 3–1).

Gingival Bleeding

Gingival bleeding was prevalent in approximately 50 percent of the overall population, 47

Percent of Edentulous Persons
among Adult Population, U.S.

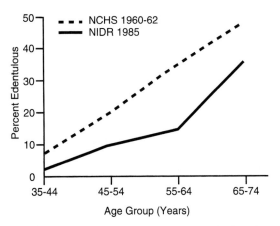

FIGURE 3–1. Edentulousness. Percentage of edentulous persons among the United States adult population. (Used by permission from Oral Health of United States Adults, National Findings, 1987.)

Prevalence of Persons with Gingival Bleeding

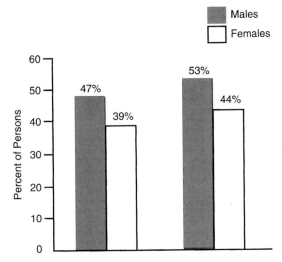

FIGURE 3–2. Gingival bleeding. Prevalence of persons with gingival bleeding. (Used by permission from Oral Health of United States Adults, National Findings, 1987.)

percent of the employed population and 53 percent of seniors. These individuals had one or more bleeding sites, equivalent to a GI score of 2. In terms of extent of disease, adults had an average of 6 percent of sites that bled, whereas 10 percent of sites in each senior bled. Figure 3–2 shows the prevalence of gingival bleeding in the population.

Probing Depths and Periodontal Pockets

Periodontal pockets were defined as probing depths of 4 mm or more. Four percent of 18-year-old subjects, 15 percent of the adult population aged 18 to 65, and 22 percent of seniors had at least one pocket. The extent of pocketing ranged from 5 sites in the average 18-year-old subject to 15 sites in those aged 65. In seniors, 15 percent of sites had pockets of 4 mm or greater.

The average pocket depth in adults was 4.25 mm, and in seniors the average depth was approximately 5 mm. Fewer than 2 percent had one pocket of 6 mm or greater. Fewer than 1 percent of subjects had one pocket that was deeper than 7 mm. Figure 3–3 shows probing depths in the population.

Attachment Loss

Attachment loss was defined as 2 mm or greater. The prevalence of attachment loss (at

Percent of Employed Persons by
Greatest Pocket Depth

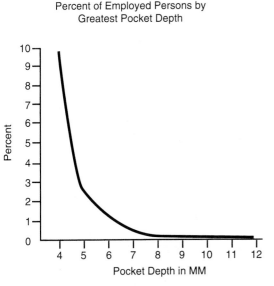

FIGURE 3–3. Pocket depth. Percentage of employed persons by greatest pocket depth. (Used by permission from Oral Health of United States Adults, National Findings, 1987.)

least one site meeting the criterion) was 80 percent in employed men, 73 percent in employed women, 98 percent in senior men, and 94 percent in senior women. The average amount of loss was 2.04 mm in employed subjects, 3.5 mm in senior men, and 2.99 mm in senior women. Forty-four percent of adults had no site with more than 3 mm of attachment loss. Attachment loss of 6 mm was found in 7 percent of adults; 3 percent had one area of 7 mm; and fewer than 1 percent of adults had one site with 8, 9, or 10 mm of attachment loss. Attachment loss increased in severity (the deepest site) with age. Those with one site of more than 6 mm of loss at age 18 made up 0.3 percent of the population, whereas 13.23 percent of the population 60 years or older had at least one site of attachment loss of 6 mm or more.

The extent of attachment loss also increased with age: 10 percent of all surfaces exhibited loss at age 18, and the percentage rose to 50 percent for those 60 to 64 years old and to 60 percent by age 80. Figure 3–4 describes attachment loss in United States adults.

Calculus

Approximately one-third of all adults had some calculus. In the United States study, this number

increased with age, especially with respect to the presence of supragingival calculus. Approximately one-half of all tooth surfaces in seniors had calculus. Figure 3–5 quantifies calculus in the adult population.

Other National Data

Data recently published from the third National Health and Nutrition Examination Survey (NHANES III) reported periodontal conditions on 9689 dentate persons between the ages of 30 and 90 who participated in the study between 1988 and 1994, representing 105.8 million U.S. adults.[18] The authors estimated that 35% of the representative sample had periodontal disease, 12.6% having a moderate or advanced form. Moderate periodontitis was defined as one or more teeth with $\geq$ 5 mm probe depth, two or more teeth with $\geq$ 4 mm probe depth, or one or more posterior teeth with grade II furcation involvement. Mild periodontitis that characterized 21.8% of the population was defined as one or more teeth with $\geq$ 3 mm probe depth, or one or more posterior teeth with grade I furcation involvement. The percentage of the population with at least one probe depth of $\geq$ 5 mm was about 9%. The data were also analyzed for the presence of

Percent of Employed Persons by Most
Severe Site of Attachment Loss

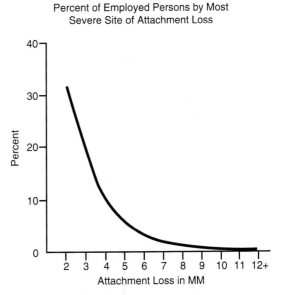

FIGURE 3–4. Attachment loss. Percentage of employed persons by most severe site of attachment loss. (Used by permission from Oral Health of United States Adults, National Findings, 1987.)

Percent of Person with Calculus
U.S. Adult Population, 1985

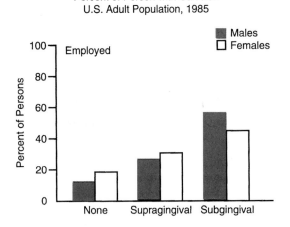

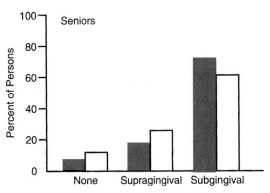

FIGURE 3–5. Calculus. Percentage of persons with calculus in the United States adult population. (Used by permission from Oral Health of United States Adults, National Findings, 1987.)

recession, gingival bleeding, and calculus.[19] The results indicated that 22.5% had at least one area of $\geq$ 3 mm gingival recession, 50.3% exhibited gingival bleeding, 91.8% had calculus that was either supragingival or extended no more than 1 mm subgingivally, and 55.1% had subgingival calculus.

EXTENT OF PERIODONTAL DISEASE

It is impossible to directly compare the results from these large epidemiologic studies, or any others. However, some similarities are evident. It is possible to conclude that 5% to 20% of the population suffers from more severe periodontal disease.[1] Many more people, possibly 35%, have some moderate pocketing, gingival bleeding, and attachment loss.[3] Most people will be keeping their teeth longer and will probably exhibit more pocketing and attachment loss as they age. Most individuals have calculus.[3, 17]

In terms of tooth mortality in Western coun-

tries, a revealing study of Norwegian men who were examined as young adults then again in midlife provided survival rates for their teeth over a period of 45 years. The survival of teeth did vary among teeth in the arch and between individuals. Molars were more likely to be lost than anterior teeth and bicuspids. But the overall mortality (tooth loss) rate was less than one tooth (0.9 teeth) per 1000 teeth per year, and teeth were most likely to be lost during the first decade after eruption.[20]

The dental hygienist continues to play an important role in treating periodontal conditions because most people retain their teeth and have the signs and symptoms of gingivitis, a significant portion of the population exhibits the earlier stages of periodontal disease, and a much smaller proportion has advanced periodontal disease. These people can benefit from dental hygiene care to help control their disease, retain teeth, and prevent new disease from occurring.

RISK FACTORS AND OTHER DETERMINANTS

Several determinants and risk factors are related to periodontal diseases. They are more prevalent in groups or populations with periodontal diseases than those without. These determinants and risk factors are associated with periodontal disease, but they do not necessarily cause disease.

There are differences between groups on determinants such as gender and age. As an example, males are more likely to have periodontal diseases than females. However, as a group, males tend to go to the dentist less often and have poorer oral hygiene, which may explain the differences noted in epidemiologic studies rather than gender. It is also known that disease worsens as populations age, as reported in cross-sectional studies. This may better reflect a lifetime accumulation of disease effects rather than more or more severe disease.[2] Socioeconomic status is also related to periodontal disease; those in lower groups tend to have more disease. They also tend to have less dental insurance coverage, be less educated, and visit the dentist less often. Better-educated people have less periodontal disease.[21] This dichotomous situation may exist because people with more education tend to have better paying jobs, which may lead to better access to dental care.

Significant risk factors for periodontal disease also exist. They include use of tobacco and certain systemic conditions such as HIV infection and diabetes. Tobacco use, primarily smoking, has been associated with increased levels of periodontal disease since the first National Health and Nutrition Evaluation Surveys in 1971–75 (NHANES I). It has been confirmed in subsequent large-scale studies, including the 1987 U.S. adult data previously reviewed. It appears that the vascular reaction to gingivitis is reduced in smokers, masking the inflammatory response.[2, 3] Other studies of smaller scale than the national data emphasize the likelihood that periodontal disease will develop in smokers. Smokers have been reported to have the same levels of plaque as nonsmokers, but they have more calculus and deeper pockets. Severe attachment loss characterized by pockets of 6 mm or greater was present in 19% of smokers, compared to 3% of non-smokers.[22] Another study reported that young adult smokers who regularly attended dentists' offices were 14 times more likely to have periodontal disease than a similar group of non-smokers.[23] The American Academy of Periodontology consensus report affirms that smokers have more sites with deeper pockets and more attachment loss.[24] Certain systemic conditions are also associated with an increased risk of periodontal disease. It has been shown that diabetic individuals, particularly those with insulin-dependent diabetes, are two to three times as likely to have more pocketing, more calculus, and more tooth loss than similar groups of individuals without diabetes.[2, 3] HIV infected individuals have been shown to be more at risk for periodontal diseases but the evidence is not clear cut.[2] Recently, the presence of periodontal disease has been associated with both heart disease[25] and low birth weight babies.[26]

All of these associations are of great interest and significance. Oral infections such as periodontal diseases are not isolated from the rest of the body, and data such as these provide clues to better understanding of the diseases and their effects. For a further discussion of risk factors in periodontal diseases, see Chapter 7.

Other Population Studies

Other population studies provide further insight into periodontal conditions in the United States and other countries. One long-term study by Ismail and co-workers[27] reported the periodontal changes over time in 167 residents in Michigan between 1959 and 1987. At the start of the study, 325 subjects, aged 5 to 60 years, were examined. Of these subjects, 28 (8.6 percent) lost all of their teeth over the ensuing 28 years. In all, 10.9 percent of the teeth present at the baseline evaluation were lost after 28 years. Most individuals had a slow progression of attachment loss over the study period. Approximately 13 percent of those re-examined in 1987 had attachment loss of 2 mm or more, 3 percent had loss of 3 mm or more, and 1.2 percent had loss of 4 mm or more. Attachment loss in 59.3 percent of all sites did not vary more than 1 mm over this period.

Studies such as this confirm that progression of periodontal disease tends to be slow. In addition, several risk factors were associated with subjects who experienced greater attachment loss. They were older, smoked, had high plaque scores, and had tooth mobility at the initial examination.

Studies of populations of seniors in various parts of the United States also provided important information. A study of elderly Iowa residents[28] found that more than 60 percent had teeth. The mean loss of attachment was 2.1 mm. A relatively small percentage of the population, 15 percent, had one or more sites with attachment loss of 7 mm or more. Approximately 32 percent of subjects had one or more pockets on a mesial surface with a probe depth of 4 mm. Only 2 percent had mesial pocketing of 7 mm or more, which was similar to results reported in the NIDR data.[17] In general, moderate periodontal disease was common, but there was much less severe disease.

Seniors attending day centers in Florida also had extensive amounts of moderate periodontal disease, but relatively little severe disease.[29] A sample of 671 adults 65 years and older was evaluated. The average number of teeth remaining per subject was 17, with older subjects having fewer teeth. In the sample, 24 percent of subjects had one or more sites of 7 mm of attachment loss. Most of those subjects had only one or two severely involved sites. Moderate disease characterized by attachment loss of 4 to 6 mm was present in 62 percent of the sample.

A study of 542 New England seniors reported that 66 percent of the population exhibited moderate periodontal disease, with pocketing of 4 to 6 mm, and 39 percent had attachment loss of 4 to 6 mm. Greater pocketing, indicating severe disease, was observed in 21 percent of the subjects, and severe attachment loss was reported in 56 percent of the subjects. However, severe loss was seen in only 2.7 teeth per subject. Gingival bleeding was present in 85 percent of the population. The predictors associated with severe disease in this population were sex (women had less disease than men) and income (higher income was associated with better health).

Studies from Other Countries

A Swiss population of 206 subjects 20 to 69 years old showed similar findings in terms of the prevalence of pocketing and attachment loss.[30] The subjects had an average of 20.7 teeth, a Pl I score of 1.16 (not much visible plaque), and a GI score of 1.34 (some bleeding sites). The Pl I and GI scores increased with age. Seventy-two percent of all pocket depths were 3 mm or less, 26 percent were 4 to 6 mm, and 2 percent were greater than 6 mm. Attachment loss findings were similar: 76 percent of sites showed loss of 3 mm or less, 21 percent had loss of 4 to 6 mm, and 3 percent of sites exhibited loss of 6 mm or more. This was in contrast to the findings in third world countries. In those populations, gingivitis with extensive amounts of plaque and calculus was the norm.[2]

TRENDS IN DISEASE PREVALENCE

It is difficult to compare the results of these studies directly. They have different populations and were scored with different tools, indices, and examiners. However, the trends in the data suggest that a relatively small proportion of the population is in need of extensive periodontal therapy. The United States data found that 3 percent of employed adults and 13 percent of seniors had severe attachment loss.[17] NHANES data suggest the prevalence of deeper pockets to be about 4%.[3] Fifteen percent of the Iowa seniors had severe attachment loss,[28] and 56 percent of the Florida seniors had severe attachment loss, but in just three teeth per person.[29] The Swiss study showed that just 3 percent had severe attachment loss.[30] The majority of probing depths were within the normal range, up to 3 mm, or showed moderate involvement, with pockets of 4 to 6 mm. Much calculus was present in these populations, and gingival bleeding was a consistent finding.

These studies confirm the trends seen in the larger national surveys. They also suggest a significant role for the dental hygienist in meeting treatment needs of the population.

Studies of Ancient Data

The theories regarding the prevalence of periodontal disease in ancient times have recently been reconsidered. It was long thought that periodontal destruction was ubiquitous in ancient populations. Clarke[31] provided evidence that tooth wear, supereruption, and pulpal diseases, rather than periodontal destruction, gave the impression from fossils that periodontitis was rampant in ancient times. His re-evaluation of skull data indicated that only approximately 10 percent of ancients had the bone destruction of periodontal disease. In a study of Scottish skulls from medieval times, Kerr[32] reported that the presence of septal bone changes caused by periodontal disease accounted for fewer than 50 percent of the changes seen in the younger population. However, these changes increased with age. In the older groups, more than 90 percent exhibited bone destruction from periodontal disease, but in relatively few sites. Between 6 and 16 percent of the sites in the older skulls showed bone loss from periodontal disease in 50 percent of septa. The studied population had lived in a time of primitive oral hygiene, if any, and no dental care. However, the prevalence of destructive periodontal disease was similar to that found in Great Britain in the 1960s[32] and strikingly similar to epidemiologic data reviewed in this chapter.

Comparisons Between Modern Studies

Capilouto and Douglass[22] compared the results of the 1987 National Institute of Dental Research (NIDR) study of oral health in the United States and those of the National Center for Health Statistics (NCHS) surveys taken from

1960 to 1962 and from 1971 to 1974. Their analysis suggested that the prevalence of gingivitis has probably decreased, but that the magnitude is difficult to assess because of differing scoring systems. This decrease was probably related to improved oral hygiene, greater education levels, more dental care, less smoking, increased use of fluorides, and increased use of systemic antibiotics. Oliver and colleagues suggested the incidence of gingivitis had not decreased but that the extent of the disease, measured by the mean number of sites per individual, was reduced.[3]

Periodontal disease seemed to affect about the same proportion of younger adults in both surveys. More older adults were affected in the NIDR study, probably because the sample contained more adults older than age 74. No one older than 74 was included in the NCHS survey. The severity of periodontal disease appeared to have decreased. The NCHS study reported that 14.9 percent of men and 10.8 percent of women had Russell's index scores of 3.1 to 8.0, disease with pockets (periodontitis), and the NIDR study reported that 9.46 percent of men and 5.18 percent of women had pocket depths of more than 6 mm. The authors concluded that the prevalence and severity of periodontal disease increased with age and that calculus was an important factor that was present in a high proportion of those with disease. These cross-study comparisons are difficult to make precisely, but the trends also suggest decreasing prevalence of periodontal disease as measured by deeper probing depths, those $\geq$ 4 mm.[3]

EPIDEMIOLOGY OF SPECIFIC PERIODONTAL DISEASES

The periodontal disease associated with young people, in the past known as periodontosis, now called juvenile periodontitis, and referred to as a form of aggressive periodontitis is a distinct entity in periodontal therapy. It has been associated with a specific bacterium, *Actinobacillus actinomycetemcomitans,* and has a prescribed therapy, including the use of antibiotics. This disease led to the understanding that periodontal diseases are different and have different pathogenic flora, but share common signs and symptoms, such as bone loss and pocketing. Periodontal infections associated

with human immunodeficiency virus (HIV) may also differ from other infections because of the reduced ability of the host to fight the infection. These disease entities have been studied to assess their prevalence and other characteristics.

Juvenile Periodontitis

A comprehensive evaluation of the epidemiology of juvenile periodontitis, now considered a form of aggressive periodontitis, was based on the national survey of adolescents and children sponsored by the NIDR in 1986 and 1987.[33] It was learned that 0.53 percent of adolescents exhibited signs of juvenile periodontitis localized to the first molars and incisors (LJP). Generalized juvenile periodontitis (GJP), or bone loss throughout the mouth, was evident in 0.13 percent of adolescents examined. Blacks were at greater risk for juvenile periodontitis, and boys were more likely than girls to experience this attachment loss.

These were significant numbers, representing approximately 70,000 individuals with LJP and 17,000 with GJP. In addition, 1.61 percent of adolescents had incidental attachment loss, representing 212,000 teenagers. However, 97 percent of this group had three or fewer sites of attachment loss, and 76 percent had only one area.

HIV-Associated Periodontal Conditions

The prevalence of HIV-associated gingival and periodontal diseases has been studied in the 1990s. In a group of 181 heterosexual intravenous drug users and heterosexual partners of persons with acquired immune deficiency syndrome (AIDS), periodontal disease was common. It might be more severe in women, but that is not clearly established.[2] It was reported that 91 percent of women and 73 percent of men had periodontal disease. Moderate to advanced disease was present in 75 percent of women and 53 percent of men. Other oral manifestations of HIV infection, hairy leukoplakia, candidiasis, Kaposi's sarcoma, and ulcers were present in 92 percent of the population.[34]

In an AIDS clinic in San Francisco, 136 patients were examined for periodontal disease. Of these patients, 31 percent had gingivitis and 50 percent had bleeding on probing. Periodontal destruction associated with HIV infection was found in 6 percent of patients, whereas destruction not related to HIV was found in 44 percent of subjects.[35] In reviewing the epidemiologic data regarding HIV, Oliver and colleagues reported a likely increased risk for HIV-infected individuals. Although not representative of every sample of HIV-infected patients, the risk of attachment loss of 3 mm or greater was six times higher in immunosuppressed homosexual and bisexual men than non-HIV infected counterparts.[3]

Periodontal disease and gingivitis appear to be common findings in HIV-infected individuals. HIV infection itself also appears to be related to increased risk for periodontal destruction.

TREATMENT NEEDS

These data show that there is a great deal of gingival and periodontal disease in the United States population. Most adults have bleeding sites indicative of gingivitis, and almost all have calculus. In addition, many individuals have 4 to 6 mm probing depths with equal amounts of attachment loss. In terms of treatment needs, Oliver and co-workers[36] suggested in 1989 that almost 90 percent of the treatment needed to address all periodontal needs over a 4-year period would be prophylaxis and that 11 percent of treatment time would be devoted to extensive scaling and surgical intervention. Even with the population living longer and retaining more teeth, these estimates will probably remain stable. Ainamo and co-workers[11] suggested that this situation will be in part the result of good preventive strategies that are dramatically limiting the number of interproximal restorations. The presence of fewer interproximal lesions and fillings simplifies cleaning and prevention so that practitioners can anticipate general improvements in periodontal health.

In 1998, Oliver and colleagues pointed out that there has been a great increase in managed care dental programs resulting in more periodontal procedures, including scaling and root planing, being performed in general dentists' offices. They cited studies and expressed concern that these procedures may not be done as well for patients if the expertise of the periodontist is excluded.[3] This remains a challenge for dental hygienists who must participate in the accurate assessment of all patients, provide expert treatment to the level of their capabilities, and encourage the referral of all appropriate cases to specialists, whether they are employed in private general practices, community clinics, or specialty practices.

The preponderance of these data suggest that much of the periodontal treatment needed by most individuals can be provided by dental hygienists. Special populations with aggressive forms of periodontal disease and HIV-associated forms of disease also fit into this category. Collaboration with dentists and periodontists, proper assessment of individual needs, calculus and plaque removal, prevention education, and appropriate referral are essential to provide comprehensive dental hygiene care. This comprehensive care is the periodontal care that will restore most patients to periodontal health.

As noted by Löe[37] "modern dentistry has changed the face of America." Individuals have more and healthier teeth, less tooth decay, and less periodontal and gingival disease. This change is a significant accomplishment for the dental hygienists, dentists, and periodontists in the United States.

STUDY QUESTIONS

MULTIPLE CHOICE

1. Which plaque scoring system evaluates the amount of plaque at the gingival margin?

   a. Gingival Index of Löe and Silness
   b. O'Leary Index
   c. Plaque Index of Silness and Löe
   d. Simplified Oral Hygiene Index of Greene and Vermillion

2. Which index has both a debris and a calculus index that can be combined for an oral hygiene index?

   a. Gingival Index of Löe and Silness
   b. O'Leary Index
   c. Plaque Index of Silness and Löe
   d. Simplified Oral Hygiene Index of Greene and Vermillion

3. Which index uses a specially designed periodontal probe called the World Health Organization probe?

   a. Community Index of Periodontal Treatment Needs
   b. Periodontal Disease Index of Ramfjord
   c. Russell's Periodontal Index
   d. Sulcus Bleeding Index

4. The 1987 national data on the oral health of United States adults showed that calculus is present in approximately:

   a. one-fourth of all adults
   b. one-half of all adults
   c. one-third of all adults
   d. two-thirds of all adults

5. Tobacco use is associated with increased levels of periodontal disease. It changes the vascular reaction to the inflammatory process.

   a. Both statements are TRUE.
   b. Both statements are FALSE.
   c. The first statement is TRUE and the second is FALSE.
   d. The second statement is FALSE and the first is TRUE.

6. Several epidemiological studies have shown that moderate periodontal disease is present in a large portion of the elderly population. They also show that advanced periodontal disease is present in a much smaller proportion of the elderly population.

   a. Both statements are TRUE.
   b. Both statements are FALSE.
   c. The first statement is TRUE and the second is FALSE.
   d. The second statement is FALSE and the first is TRUE.

7. What percentage of the U.S. adult population suffers from severe periodontal disease?

   a. 35%
   b. 45%
   c. 3% to 20%
   d. 3% to 45%

8. Capilouto and Douglass concluded that the prevalence and severity of gingivitis over the last two decades:

   a. has probably increased over time.
   b. has probably decreased over time.
   c. has probably remained the same

9. What is a significant risk factor for periodontal disease?

   a. gender
   b. race
   c. smoking
   d. economic level

10. Which group is at greatest risk for juvenile (aggressive) periodontitis?

    a. Blacks
    b. Caucasians
    c. Pacific Islanders
    d. Hispanics

SHORT ANSWER

11. Why are indices used in dental hygiene and dentistry? _____

_____

12. Bleeding is not an ideal index of periodontal disease because _____

_____

13. Describe the technique for determining tooth mobility with the Miller Index of Tooth Mobility.

_____

_____

14. List the reasons for a decrease in the prevalence of gingivitis as suggested by Capilouto and Douglass.

_____

_____

15. Project the role of the dental hygienist in the deliv-

ery of periodontal care based on the data provided in this chapter. ———————————————

———————————————

REFERENCES

1. Spolsky VW. Epidemiology of gingival and periodontal diseases. In FA Carranza and MG Newman eds. Clinical Periodontology, 8th ed. WB Saunders, Philadelphia 1996; 61-81.
2. Committee on Research, Science, and Therapy, American Academy of Periodontology. Epidemiology of periodontal diseases. J Periodontol 1996;67:935-945.
3. Oliver RC, Brown LJ, Loe H. Periodontal disease in the United States population. J Periodontol 1998;69:269-278.
4. Wilkins EM. Indices and scoring methods. In Clinical Practice of the Dental Hygienist, 8th ed. Philadelphia. Lippincott Williams and Wilkins; 1999:293-313.
5. Silness J, Löe H. Periodontal disease in pregnancy: II. Correlation between oral hygiene and periodontal condition. Acta Odontol Scand 1964;22:121.
6. Greene JC, Vermillion JR. The simplified oral hygiene index. J Am Dent Assoc 1964;68:7.
7. Manhold JH, Volpe AR, Hazen SP, Parker L, Adams SH. In vivo calculus assessment: II. A comparison of scoring techniques. J Periodontol 1965;36:299.
8. Löe H. The gingival index, the plaque index, and the retention index systems. J Periodontol 1967;38:610.
9. Muhlemann HR, Son S. Gingival sulcus bleeding: a leading symptom in initial gingivitis. Helv Odontol Acta 1971;15:107.
10. Russell AL. A system of classification and scoring for prevalence surveys of periodontal disease. J Dent Res 1956;35:350.
11. Ramjford SP. Indices for prevalence and incidence of periodontal disease. J Periodontol 1959;30:51.
12. Ainamo J, Barmes D, Beagrie G, Cutress T, Martin J, Sardo-Infirri J. Development at the World Health Organization (WHO) Community Index of Periodontal Treatment Needs (CIPTN). Int Dent J 1982;32:281.
13. Lang, NP. Epidemiology of periodontal disease. Arch Oral Biol 1990;35(suppl):9S-14S.
14. Anerud A, Löe H, Boysen H. The natural history and clinical course of calculus formation in man. J Clin Periodontol 1991;18:160-170.
15. Defense mechanisms of the gingiva. In FA Carranza and MG Newman eds. Clinical Periodontology, 8th ed. Philadelphia: WB Saunders, 1996:103-111.
16. Miller SC. Textbook of Periodontia, 3rd ed. Philadelphia: Blakestone, 1950.
17. Miller AJ, Brunelle JA, Carlos JP, Brown LJ, Löe H. The national survey of oral health in U.S. employed adults and seniors: 1985-1986; NIH publication no 87-2868; August 1987.
18. Albandar JM, Brunelle JA, Kingman A. Destructive periodontal disease in adults 30 years of age and older in the United States, 1988-1994. J Periodontol 1999; 70:13-29.
19. Albandar JM, Kingman A. Gingival recession, gingival bleeding and dental calculus in adults 30 years of age and older in the United States, 1988-1994.
20. Hujoel PP, Löe H, Anerud A, Boysen H, Leroux BG. Forty-five-year tooth survival probabilities among men in Oslo, Norway. J Dent Res 1998;77:2020-2027.
21. Löe H, Morrison E. Epidemiology of periodontal disease. In Genco RJ, Goldman HM, Cohen DW, eds. Contemporary Periodontics. St. Louis: CV Mosby, 1990:106-116.
22. Capilouto ML, Douglass CW. Trends in the prevalence and severity of periodontal diseases in the US: a public health problem? J Public Health Dent 1988;48:245-251.
23. Linden GJ, Mullally BH. Cigarette smoking and periodontal destruction in young adults. J Periodontol 1994;65:718-723.
24. American Academy of Periodontology. Tobacco use and the periodontal patient, position paper. J Periodontol 1999;70:1419-1427.
25. Beck J, Garcia R, Heiss G, et al. Periodontal disease and cardiovascular disease. J Periodontol 1996; 67 (Suppl):1123-1137.
26. Offenbacher S, Katx V, Fertik G, et al. Periodontal infection as a risk factor or preterm low birth weight. J Periodontol 1996;67(Suppl):1103-1113.
27. Ismail AI, Morrison IC, Burt BA, Caffesse RG, Kavanagh MT. Natural history of periodontal disease in adults: findings from the Tecumseh periodontal disease study, 1959-87. J Dent Res 1990;69:430-435.
28. Hunt RJ, Levy SM, Beck JD. The prevalence of periodontal attachment loss in an Iowa population aged 70 and older. J Public Health Dent 1990;50:251-256.
29. Gilbert GH, Heft MW. Periodontal status of older Floridians attending senior activity centers. J Clin Periodontol 1992;19:249-255.
30. Schrüch E Jr, Minder CE, Lang NP, Geering AH. Periodontal conditions in a randomly selected population in Switzerland. Community Dentistry and Oral Epidemiology 1988;16:181-186.
31. Clarke NG. Periodontal defects of pulpal origin: evidence in early man. Am J Phys Anthropol 1990;82:371-376.
32. Kerr NW. Prevalence and natural history of periodontal disease in Scotland: the mediaeval period (900-1600 AD). J Periodontal Res 1991;26:346-354.
33. Löe H, Brown LJ. Early onset periodontitis in the United States of America. J Periodontol 1991;62:608-616.
34. Klein RS, Quart AM, Small CB. Periodontal disease in heterosexuals with acquired immune deficiency syndrome. J Periodontol 1991;62:535-540.
35. Masouredis CM, Katz MH, Greenspan D, Herrera C, Hollander H, Greenspan J, Winkler J. Prevalence of HIV-associated periodontitis and gingivitis in HIV-infected patients attending an AIDS clinic. J Acquir Imm Def Synd 1992;5:479-483.
36. Oliver RC, Brown LJ, Löe H. An estimate of periodontal treatment needs in the US based on epidemiologic data. J Periodontol 1989;60:371-380.
37. Löe H. Periodontics of tomorrow. Dent Clin North Am 1988;32:395-405.

Dorothy J. Rowe

4

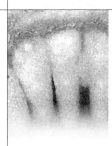

Microbiology of Periodontal Diseases

*C*hapter *O*bjectives

1. Describe and compare the composition and development of supragingival and subgingival plaque.
2. Describe the role of salivary factors in pellicle formation.
3. Describe the influence of bacterial surface components (e.g., capsules, append-ages) on bacterial colonization or coaggregation.
4. Discuss microbial succession in terms of oxygen and nutrient requirements and bacterial adherence.
5. Distinguish the nonspecific and specific plaque hypotheses and the implication of each to plaque control and periodontal therapy.
6. Describe and classify the specific bacteria associated with the various periodon-tal diseases and their characteristics that contribute to their virulence.
7. Describe the significance of dental plaque to the dental hygienist.

*K*ey *T*erms

Actinobacillus actinomycetemcomitans
Adherence
Bacterial coaggregation
Corncob formation
Facultative and obligate anaerobes
Glucan
Gram-positive and Gram-negative cell wall
Lipopolysaccharide or endotoxin

Nonspecific and specific plaque hypotheses
Pellicle
Porphyromonas gingivalis
Salivary glycoproteins
Spirochetes
Subgingival plaque formation
Supragingival plaque formation
Test-tube brush formation

Dental plaque is the major etiologic factor in the initiation and progression of inflammatory periodontal diseases. For decades, dental hygienists have been in-structing patients in proper oral hygiene practices as a preventive measure against dental diseases. Epidemiologic studies showed that poor oral hygiene increases the prevalence and severity of periodontal diseases. However, calculus was thought to be the primary factor causing gingival inflammation, with plaque playing only a contributory role by providing an organic matrix for the attachment of calculus.

In the mid-1960s, researchers began to recognize the significance of plaque in the disease process. Löe and co-workers[3] provided the first direct scientific evidence of the causal relationship between plaque and gingival inflammation. In this study, when subjects with excellent gingival health and little plaque did not perform oral hygiene procedures, plaque accumulation increased and gingivitis developed. Reinstituting oral hygiene practices eliminated dental plaque, resolved gingival inflammation, and restored gingival health. This experimental protocol, known as the experimental gingivitis model, is discussed later in this chapter. Further incriminating evidence was provided by additional studies in which mechanical or chemical plaque control arrested or prevented the progression of periodontal diseases. Because dental plaque is central to the etiology of periodontal diseases, a thorough understanding of its composition and mechanisms of formation is essential.

Dental plaque is often defined as an accumulation of bacteria on the surface of the teeth or other solid oral structures, not readily removed by rinsing. The distinguishing feature between dental plaque and material alba is the strength of the **adherence** of the deposit. Material alba, being a loosely adherent mass of bacteria and cellular debris, can be removed by the mechanical action of a strong water spray.

Biofilm is a term currently being used to describe a microbial ecosystem adherent to a solid surface. In the dental literature, biofilm most often refers to bacterial accumulations on waterlines and dental biomaterials. Dental plaque may also be considered as an example of a biofilm.

Based on its relationship to the gingival margin, plaque can be classified as supragingival or subgingival. Supragingival plaque is deposited on the clinical crowns of the teeth, whereas subgingival plaque is located in the gingival sulcus or periodontal pocket. Small amounts of plaque are difficult to detect clinically without placing a disclosing, or dye, solution on the teeth or scraping the tooth surfaces with an instrument. As plaque accumulation continues, the deposit appears as a white-yellow globular

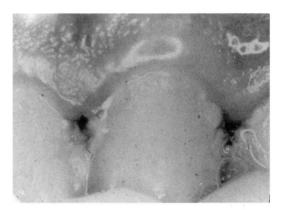

FIGURE 4–1. Supragingival dental plaque on mandibular bicuspids. Note the white mass at the gingival margins and the interproximal surfaces.

mass (Figure 4-1). Subgingival plaque cannot be visually detected; its presence is only revealed by observing its removal from the gingival sulcus or pocket with an instrument. Supragingival plaque forms particularly in sites protected from the normal cleansing action of the tongue, cheek, and lips. Plaque deposits are usually present in pits and fissures of occlusal surfaces and on restorations, artificial crowns, orthodontic bands, removable orthodontic appliances, and dentures.

BACTERIAL CHARACTERISTICS

Dental plaque consists primarily of bacteria. One cubic millimeter of plaque, weighing about 1 mg, may contain more than 10^{10} bacteria, of which there may be several hundred species. Plaque is not a random accumulation of assorted types of bacteria, but a specific and complex arrangement based on bacterial characteristics. To facilitate an understanding of the microbial succession in plaque formation, this section reviews fundamental microbiologic concepts that are used to classify or describe bacteria.

Morphotypes

Several morphologic forms of bacteria are involved in plaque formation. (1) Cocci are spherical. The most common coccoid form in plaque is streptococci (cocci in chains). (2) Rods or bacilli are generally rectangular. Many types are present in plaque: some curved, some with uneven diameters, and some with club-shaped ends. Filaments are thread-like and branching rods. Fusiforms are also thread-like, but are distinguished by their tapered ends. (3) **Spirochetes** are spiral, with one or more axial fibrils incorporated in their cell wall.

Cell Wall Characteristics

The role of specific bacteria in plaque formation and pathogenicity often reflects the **cell wall** structure of the bacteria. A bacteriologic technique, known as Gram staining, divides bacteria into **Gram-positive** and **Gram-negative** types. When organisms are stained and counterstained with specific dyes, the organisms are stained differentially on the basis of the permeability of their cell walls. Gram-positive organisms retain the initial crystal violet (purple) stain, whereas Gram-negative organisms are decolorized by the organic solvent and hence show the safranin (red) counterstain.

As shown in Figure 4–2, the capsule is the outer surface component of Gram-positive bacteria. Also called a slime layer or glycocalyx, it is usually a loose gel-like polysaccharide substance. This polysaccharide is frequently a glucose polymer, called a **glucan**, which participates in bacterial adherence and aggregation. Another characteristic of the Gram-positive cell

wall is the thick peptidoglycan layer, composed of repeating units of two amino sugars. Lysozyme, an enzyme in the saliva, can split the bonds that link these units, causing bacterial cell lysis.

A distinguishing characteristic of the cell wall of Gram-negative bacteria is the outer membrane, which is composed of receptor proteins, involved in adherence (to be discussed later), and complex **lipopolysaccharides.** Lipopolysaccharides are often known as **endotoxins** because of their within-cell location and toxic function. They are released when the integrity of the cell is disrupted. They are potent destructive substances that affect host tissue directly or through activation of host responses. Vesicles (often called microvesicles or blebs) are surface appendages that are eversions or evaginations of the outer membrane and, hence, contain endotoxin. All of the putative Gram-negative periodontal pathogens release vesicles into their surroundings.

Cell surface appendages are also important in adhesion. Fimbriae, or pili, are small proteinaceous projections attached to the external surface of both Gram-negative and Gram-positive bacteria. They appear to mediate the processes of adhesion to hydroxyapatite and coaggregation between different species of bacteria, such as *Actinomyces viscosus* and *Streptococcus san-*

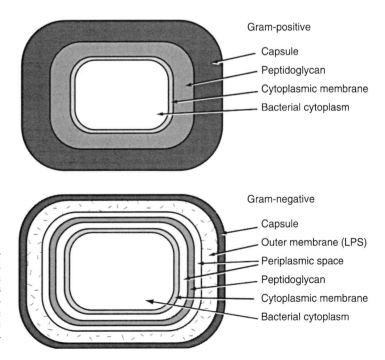

FIGURE 4–2. Structures of Gram-positive and Gram-negative bacterial cell walls. Note the larger peptidoglycan layer in the Gram-positive cell wall as well as the presence of an outer membrane containing lipopolysaccharide (LPS), endotoxin, in the Gram-negative cell wall. (Courtesy of Dr. P. W. Johnson.)

guis. Flagella are long, fine, wavy filamentous structures that are used for motility. They are longer than fimbriae, with a larger diameter. Bacteria may have single or multiple flagella, arranged at either or both poles or distributed around the cell.

Oxygen Environment

Oxygen tension influences the ability of bacteria to grow and multiply. Bacteria that require oxygen for growth are termed **aerobes. Facultative** anaerobic organisms can use oxygen when it is present, but can use anaerobic fermentation when oxygen is absent. They can grow or multiply in both aerobic and anaerobic environments. Aerotolerant anaerobes, which do not use oxygen but can tolerate oxidizing environments, can also grow in both types of environment. Others, **obligate** anaerobes, cannot survive in an aerobic environment. Capnophiles require or prefer carbon dioxide for growth.

Bacterial Metabolism

All bacteria must be supplied with sources of nutrients, but their requirements and end products vary. Many Gram-positive organisms, such as streptococci and actinomyces, are fermentative, or saccharolytic. They obtain their energy from the breakdown of complex organic compounds, such as sugars, to smaller end products, such as lactic acid. Some bacteria that colonize gingival pockets do not ferment sugars and are known as nonfermentative or asaccharolytic. They frequently use amino acids, simple peptides, and proteins for growth.

CLASSIFICATION OF COMMON PERIODONTAL BACTERIA

Gram-negative bacteria
  Rods
    Nonmotile
      Facultative
        Actinobacillus actinomycetemcomitans
        Capnocytophaga ochraceus
        Eikenella corrodens
      Anaerobic
        Porphyromonas gingivalis
        Prevotella intermedia
        Bacteroides forsythus
        Fusobacterium nucleatum
        Leptotrichia buccalis
    Motile
      Facultative
        Campylobacter (Wolinella) recta
      Anerobic
        Selenomonas
  Cocci
    Anaerobic
      Veillonella alcalescens
  Spirochetes
    Anaerobic, motile
      Treponema denticola
Gram-positive bacteria
  Rods
    Irregular morphology
      Facultative
        Actinomyces israelii and *naeslundii*
        Corynebacterium matruchotii
      Anaerobic
        Eubacterium
    Straight rod; facultative
      Lactobacillus
  Cocci
    Facultative
      Streptococcus
    Anaerobic
      Peptostreptococcus micros

CLASSIFICATION OF PERIODONTAL BACTERIA

Previously discussed characteristics form the basis of the classification scheme seen in Classification of Common Periodontal Bacteria. This outline, with examples of specific bacteria, provides a framework for the specific organisms discussed later in this chapter.

The advent of modern molecular genetic methods, such as deoxyribonucleic acid (DNA) homology testing, has contributed to the continual re-evaluation of microbiologic taxonomy and nomenclature. For example, analyses of the

Bacteroides genus of Gram-negative anaerobic rods resulted in the reclassification of several species. Organisms previously in the genus *Bacteroides* are now classified as *Porphyromonas, Prevotella, Capnocytophaga*, or *Eikenella*, based on fermentation, oxygen requirements, and specific DNA similarities. ***Porphyromonas gingivalis***, shown in Figure 4–3, has been studied extensively because it is considered a major periodontal pathogen.

The nomenclature of the *Actinomyces* species has also been revised. Human strains of *Actinomyces viscosus* serotype II are now included with *Actinomyces naeslundii* serotypes II and III in *A. naeslundii* genospecies 2, while

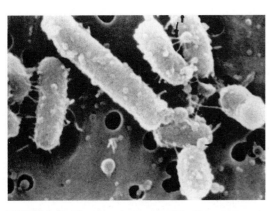

FIGURE 4–3. Electron micrograph of *Porphyromonas gingivalis*. Note the pili or fimbriae extending from the cell surface. (Courtesy of Dr. T. E. Bramanti.)

A. naeslundii serotype I is designated as *A. naeslundii* genospecies 1.

SUPRAGINGIVAL PLAQUE FORMATION

The development of dental plaque is a complex and dynamic process. In-depth, detailed discussions of this subject are reviewed by Liljemark and Bloomquist and by Kolenbrander and London.[1, 2] Understanding **supragingival plaque formation** is facilitated by dividing the process into various stages.

Pellicle Formation

Pellicle, often called acquired or salivary pellicle, is an amorphous, tenacious membranous film that forms on the surfaces of teeth, restorations, calculus, and other solid surfaces. Polishing the teeth with an abrasive agent removes the pellicle, but it reforms on the tooth surface within minutes. Bacteria are not required for its formation, but they adhere to it shortly after it is formed. The pellicle influences the colonization of bacteria on the tooth surface.

The chemical composition of pellicle is similar to that of saliva. This similarity is a reflection of its formation from the glycoproteins of saliva. The adsorption of glycoproteins from saliva is probably an ionic interaction between the calcium and phosphate ions of the hydroxyapatite and the oppositely charged groups of the salivary macromolecules. Many glycoproteins are present in the saliva, of which many are rich in the amino acid proline. Among the proline-rich glycoproteins are acidic glycoproteins that enhance the ability of specific microorganisms, such as *Actinomyces* species, to bind to tooth surfaces. The specificity of the adsorption process is important: pellicle is formed only from glycoproteins that bind selectively to the tooth, and not all of the bacteria available in the saliva can attach to the pellicle. Only those with binding sites for pellicle constituents and occurring in sufficient numbers in saliva are adsorbed.

Initial Colonization of Pellicle by Bacteria

Bacterial cells are continually transported to the pellicle-coated tooth surface through the saliva, in association with dietary materials, or through some other contact with the external environment. However, the only microorganisms that can colonize the pellicle are those that can adhere to the pellicle-coated tooth surface or are in some other way retained. Otherwise, saliva flow, chewing forces, and oral hygiene procedures would eliminate or clear them from the oral cavity. Some bacteria are retained in pits and fissures, tooth surface irregularities, and other areas that are relatively sheltered from oral cleaning mechanisms. Other bacteria that rely on specific mechanisms of adherence interact specifically with the pellicle during initial colonization. Their attachment to pellicle is determined by specific characteristics. Oral bacteria vary significantly in their ability to adhere to different surfaces, and their prevalence at a specific oral site reflects that ability. For example, *Streptococcus mutans* and *S. sanguis* preferentially colonize supragingival plaque, whereas *Streptococcus salivarius* is present in high proportions on the tongue and in the saliva, but only in low proportions on teeth.

RECEPTOR MOLECULES

Salivary components promote adherence by a specific reaction between the bacterial surface and the pellicle-coated tooth surface. The specificity of the reaction is caused by the biochemical differences in cell surface coatings among the bacteria. Molecules, called adhesins, are located on the cell surfaces, usually on the fimbriae or pili. Adhesins that are proteins and that recognize carbohydrate structures are called lectins. These adhesins, or lectins, recognize and then link to specific carbohydrate struc-

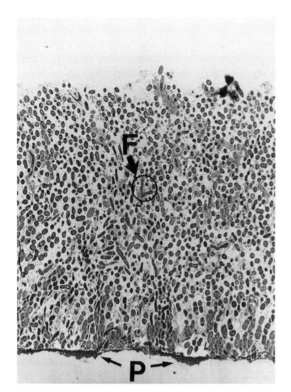

FIGURE 4–4. Electron micrograph of 1-day-old supragingival plaque. Coccal forms predominate, exhibiting differing sizes and morphologic features. Note the pellicle (P) at the plaque–crown interface and a branching filament (F). (Used with permission from Listgarten MA, Mayo HE, Tremblay R. Development of dental plaque on epoxy resin crowns in man. J Periodontol 1975;46:10–26.)

tures in the glycoproteins of the pellicle. These specific lectin-like interactions promote the attachment of specific bacteria. For example, *S. mutans* binds to one type of sugar residue of **salivary glycoproteins**, whereas *S. sanguis* requires another. Lectin-like interactions are also involved in bacterial coaggregations, which will be discussed later.

Adherence can also be inhibited by certain salivary components that bind to bacterial surfaces and coat and, thus, block their surface receptors. Still other salivary polymers agglutinate specific bacteria, thereby blocking their receptors for binding to pellicle. Thus, they facilitate clearance of the bacterial aggregates from the oral cavity. Secretory immunoglobulin A, which is secreted by the salivary glands, is the predominant antibody class in saliva. It also coats the bacterial surfaces, promoting agglutination of bacteria and preventing their attachment to tooth surfaces. Therefore, the composition of saliva plays both a facilitative and an

inhibitory role in the attachment of bacteria to the acquired pellicle.

Initial plaque is characterized by a predominance of coccal bacterial cells, with occasional branching filaments (Figure 4-4). The first organisms form a monolayer of cells, either individually or in small groups. During the first few hours, the attached bacteria proliferate and form small colonies of morphologically similar organisms. Microcolonies of cocci usually form a series of columns that extend out from the pellicle (Figure 4-5). Bacillary and filamentous bacteria are usually aligned with their long axes perpendicular to the tooth surface, and they are often attached to the surface of the predominantly coccal flora (see Figure 4-5). As the colonies expand, they meet and coalesce to form a continuous bacterial mass.

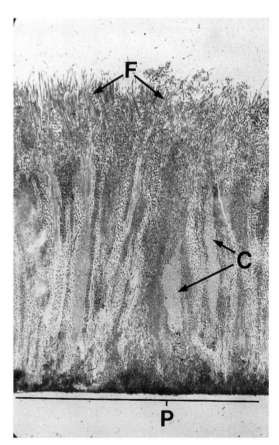

FIGURE 4–5. Electron micrograph of 1-week-old supragingival plaque. Note the microcolonies of cocci (C) extending outward from the pellicle (P) and the numerous filaments (F) attached to the plaque surface. (Used with permission from Listgarten MA, Mayo HE, Tremblay R. Development of dental plaque on epoxy resin crowns in man. J Periodontol 1975;46:10–26.)

Growth and Maturation of Plaque

Although adhesive processes dominate in the initial colonization phase, during maturation, there is an increase in plaque mass and thickness. This increase predominantly results from the proliferation of attached bacteria. Maturation of plaque also requires cohesion of bacterial cells. This cohesion is accomplished by the formation of the intermicrobial matrix. This material among the bacteria is composed of salivary material, gingival exudate, and microbial substances, such as polysaccharides.

EXTRACELLULAR POLYSACCHARIDES

A variety of oral bacteria, such as *S. mutans, S. sanguis, Streptococcus mitis*, and *S. salivarius*, have the capability to form extracellular polysaccharide polymers, or capsules, from sucrose. As shown in Figure 4-6, by the action of the glucosyltransferase enzymes, sucrose is cleaved and the glucose moiety is converted into a highly branched glucose polymer, or glucan, whereas the fructose moiety is available as an energy source. Dextran is a term frequently used in the dental literature to describe a type of glucan with specific linkages. The manner in which the glucoses are linked determines the solubility of the glucan. Linkages between carbon 1 of one glucose and carbon 3 of the next glucose confer greater insolubility. More branching also confers greater insolubility; branch linkages frequently are $\alpha(1-6)$ and $\alpha(1-4)$.

Accumulation of more of this insoluble material results in increased bacterial aggregation of organisms such as *S. mutans*, which can bind glucan molecules. Furthermore, it may also mediate nonspecific entrapment of other microorganisms, promoting the accumulation of cohesive bacterial masses. *Actinomyces* species also can form copious amounts of plaque because of their synthesis of an extracellular heteropolysaccharide. Other polysaccharides are produced by oral streptococci as a source of energy. The levans (polymers of fructose) and soluble glucans, such as dextrans, all of which are synthesized from sucrose, can be used as an energy source in bacterial metabolism.

The matrix protein component is provided by salivary glycoproteins, which promote bacterial adherence when adsorbed to the tooth surface, as previously discussed. The small amount of lipids present in plaque probably represents lipopolysaccharide or endotoxin from Gram-negative cell walls. The concentration of inorganic components, primarily calcium and phosphate, is low in early plaque, but increases significantly as plaque is transformed into calculus.

BACTERIAL COAGGREGATION

Plaque accumulation also results from the aggregation of bacteria to previously attached cells. Certain bacteria adhere to other bacterial species and thus form complex aggregations. This attachment is a direct interaction between

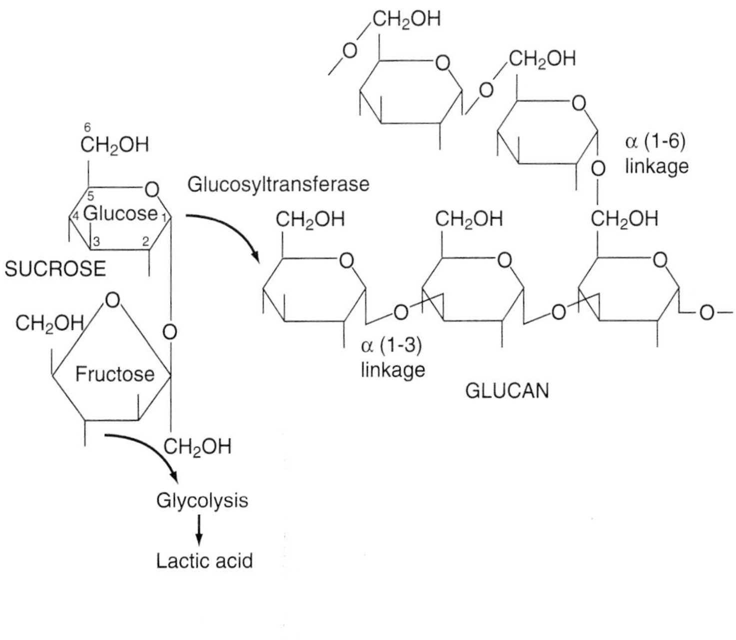

FIGURE 4–6. Chemical reaction of the synthesis of glucan from sucrose catalyzed by the enzyme glucosyltransferase. Glucosyltransferase cleaves sucrose and transfers the glucose moiety to the growing glucan polymer, which has a backbone of $\alpha(1-3)$ linkages and $\alpha(1-6)$ and $\alpha(1-4)$ branch linkages. (Courtesy of D. L. Del Carlo.)

the surface components of the two species. **Bacterial coaggregation** between the filamentous *A. naeslundii* genospecies 2 (previously *A. viscosus*) and coccoid *S. sanguis* appears to be dependent on fimbriae. *A. naeslundii* has two types of fimbriae, based on their function: type 1, associated with attachment, interacts with the proline-rich proteins in salivary pellicle through protein-protein interactions; and type 2, associated with coaggregation with *S. sanguis*, interacts with a specific polysaccharide in the cell wall of *S. sanguis* through a lectin-carbohydrate interaction.

Filaments at the salivary, or external, plaque surface often become coated with cocci, presenting a corncob appearance, so called because of their resemblance to an ear of corn

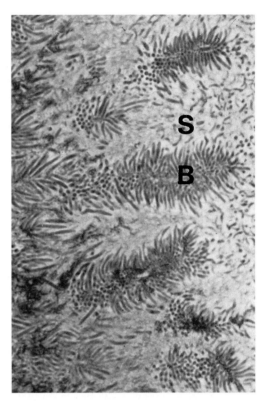

FIGURE 4–8. Electron micrograph of subgingival plaque from an inflamed periodontal pocket. Test-tube brush formations (B), composed of Gram-negative rods attaching to filamentous bacteria, are surrounded by spirochetes (S). (Used with permission from Listgarten MA. Structure of the microbial flora associated with periodontal health and disease in man. J Periodontol 1976;47:1-18.)

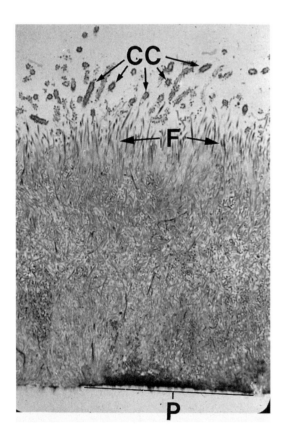

FIGURE 4–7. Electron micrograph of supragingival plaque adhering to a periodontally compromised tooth. A dense, predominantly filamentous mass (F) is adherent to the enamel surface, and corncob formations (CC) extend from the surface (P, pellicle). These complexes consist of filamentous bacteria surrounded by adherent cocci. (Used with permission from Listgarten MA. Structure of the microbial flora associated with periodontal health and disease in man. J Periodontol 1976;47:1-18.)

(Figure 4-7). **Corncob formation** is restricted to species with mutually attractive surface molecules that can mediate binding. The complex is composed of a central filament surrounded by cocci, usually a type of *S. sanguis*. The filaments could be either the facultative Gram-positive *Actinomyces* species and *Corynebacterium matruchotii* or the anaerobic Gram-negative *Fusobacterium nucleatum*. Other bacteria can aggregate to form structures that resemble test-tube or bristle brushes (Figure 4-8). These coaggregates consist of a central axis that is composed of a filamentous bacterium and bristles that are composed of Gram-negative rods. Interbacterial coaggregation may be the only means by which these organisms adhere to plaque. In addition to these examples, there are many other coaggregating pairs of organisms. Generally, early colonizers coaggregate with streptococci and/or *Actinomyces* species, while late colonizers primarily coaggregate with *Fuso-*

bacteria species, which bridges these coaggregations with early colonizers.

In another type of bacterial aggregation, one organism acts as a bridge between two other bacteria that do not interact. For example, some strains of *S. sanguis* aggregate with both *A. naeslundii* genospecies 2 and *Prevotella loescheii*, which do not coaggregate with each other. These multigeneric interactions may be an important mechanism for the attachment of new organisms within plaque and for the ability of organisms to resist the forces that would remove them.

OTHER INTERBACTERIAL INTERACTIONS

In addition to aggregation into complex structures, a number of other interactions occur between microbial species within plaque. Certain bacteria facilitate the colonization of other bacteria by producing substances used by others as nutrients. For example, the lactate produced by streptococci and actinomyces is used by *Veillonella* species as an energy source. In turn, the lactate is converted to hydrogen gas, which is used by a number of other organisms in the gingival pocket, such as *Campylobacter*. Also, *Veillonella* and many Gram-positive organisms can synthesize menadione (vitamin K), which is required by *P. gingivalis* and *Prevotella intermedia*.

MICROBIAL SUCCESSION

As plaque ages, the composition of the flora changes.[3, 4] The initial colonizers proliferate, and this growth alters the environment at the tooth surface, thereby enabling new and different bacterial species to inhabit the developing plaque. After the first day of plaque growth, the proportion of Gram-positive streptococci decreases, and *Actinomyces* and *Veillonella* strains become more prominent. During the next 3 weeks of undisturbed plaque formation, the cocci continue to decrease in relative numbers, particularly because of the increase in filamentous bacteria which, in addition to *Actinomyces* species, include *Rothia*, *Fusobacterium*, and *Corynebacterium* species. These filaments actually invade the plaque and replace many of the streptococci that inhabit the deeper levels. As the plaque increases in thickness, further changes occur in the environment.

When plaque is allowed to grow undisturbed, it becomes more anaerobic. The level of oxygen diminishes as a result of oxygen consumption by facultative organisms. This lower oxygen level allows the growth of obligate anaerobes. Thus, the more mature plaque harbors increasing numbers of obligate anaerobic organisms, such as spirochetes and Gram-negative rods. At this point, no additional bacterial species join the plaque, although the absolute numbers of bacteria may continue to increase. There are many differences between early and mature supragingival plaque, including a greater variety of bacterial shapes and the inclusion of Gram-negative and anaerobic bacteria in mature plaque. However, the most important difference is that mature plaque has the potential to invade the subgingival space and to cause localized gingival disease.

SUBGINGIVAL PLAQUE FORMATION

Subgingival plaque formation is usually initiated by the presence of mature supragingival dental plaque, and the bacterial composition of subgingival plaque is partly influenced by that in the adjacent supragingival portion. However, the microflora environment in subgingival plaque is generally more anaerobic, more Gram-negative, more motile, and more asaccharolytic.

Subgingival Environment

The maturation of supragingival plaque is accompanied by inflammatory changes in the gingiva. Because inflamed gingiva is less tightly attached to the tooth surface, the formation of supragingival plaque proceeds apically into the gingival crevice. In addition, edema causes gingival enlargement, which alters the anatomic relationship between the tooth surface and the gingival margin and changes supragingival into subgingival plaque. This newly created subgingival space, which is protected from normal oral cleansing mechanisms, facilitates further bacterial multiplication.

The subgingival environment is bathed in crevicular or gingival fluid, rather than in saliva. Crevicular fluid originates when inflammatory responses to plaque organisms cause an increase in capillary permeability, which allows plasma to escape. When the fluid leaks into the gingival crevice, it is called gingival crevicular fluid. The volume of this fluid is increased with greater inflammation. Serum-derived crevicular fluid and gingival bleeding provide excellent sources of nutrients for bacteria in general. In addition, these fluids contain specific factors that are essential for the growth of some subgingival organisms.

Microbiologic Composition

Subgingival plaque differs in composition from that of adjacent supragingival plaque because of several factors. The limited access to the oral cavity allows the most fastidious anaerobic bacteria to become established. Also, the addition of further salivary bacteria is restricted. The subgingival area is not subject to the mechanical forces that tend to dislodge bacteria at the clinical crown. Thus, the ability to adhere to the tooth or plaque matrix is not important for survival, and so there are many motile organisms that are completely unattached to the plaque matrix.

Nutrients from the crevicular fluid are readily available, so bacteria that use proteins as energy sources are favored over those that require carbohydrates. Hemin-containing compounds, found in crevicular fluid, enhance the growth of *Porphyromonas* and *Prevotella* species. Also, several complex relationships among the bacteria influence their numbers and types in subgingival plaque. Some of the spirochetes require specific products of proteolytic metabolism, decarboxylated amino acids called ptomaines, produced by *Fusobacterium*. As previously mentioned, Vitamin K (menadione) is produced by *Prevotella oralis* and *Veillonella alcalescens* and is used by *P. intermedia* and *P. gingivalis*. Bacteriocins produced by ***Actinobacillus actinomycetemcomitans*** may inhibit *S. sanguis* in some plaque. Thus, the final proportions of various bacteria found in the subgingival area are the sum of these many processes.

TOOTH-ASSOCIATED SUBGINGIVAL PLAQUE

The subgingival plaque associated with the tooth appears to differ from that associated with tissue. The structure of this portion is similar to that of the supragingival plaque. Bacteria are densely packed and are adjacent to the cuticular material covering the tooth surface. The flora is dominated by Gram-positive filamentous bacteria, but Gram-positive and Gram-negative cocci and rods are also present. In the

apical portion, fewer filamentous organisms are found, and the bacterial deposit is dominated by Gram-negative rods without a particular orientation.

TISSUE-ASSOCIATED SUBGINGIVAL PLAQUE

The layers closest to the soft tissues contain a large number of flagellated motile bacteria and spirochetes. The bacteria are not oriented in any specific manner. Also, there is no defined intercellular matrix similar to that found in supragingival plaque. These motile bacteria are loosely adherent to the surface, and the soft tissue walls are probably responsible for their retention. **Test-tube brush** or bristle brush **formations** and Gram-negative bacteria with multiple flagella are also commonly observed.

PERIODONTAL MICROFLORA

Early theories about the etiologic role of dental plaque in periodontal disease suggested that the severity of inflammation was directly related to the quantity of plaque in the mouth. These theories were based on the belief that plaque is a homogeneous bacterial mass and that all plaques in all mouths have equal potential to cause disease. This theory was called the **nonspecific plaque hypothesis**.[5]

Improvements in anaerobic culture technique permitted better identification of additional bacteria residing in mature plaque and stimulated many microbiologic studies that discriminated between the types of bacteria associated with health and disease. The experimental gingivitis model was used to show that as plaque matures and gingivitis develops, the bacterial composition changes. Further studies showed that microflora in diseased and nondiseased sites differed in bacterial composition. These findings led to the **specific plaque hypothesis**. Originally, this theory supported the idea that only certain plaques cause disease because of the presence of a pathogen or a relative increase in the levels of certain indigenous plaque organisms.[5] Current thinking interprets the term specific as including as many as a dozen microbial species that may be responsible for most cases of periodontitis.

Gingival Health

The gingival crevice harbors a microbial flora both in health and in disease. During health, the flora is relatively simple and sparse. It reflects the bacterial types found in the early stages of plaque formation. Most of the bacteria are Gram-positive organisms and facultative anaerobic species (Figure 4-9).[6] Cocci, the predominant morphotype, compose almost two-thirds of the flora. Streptococci are of particular importance because several species adhere to the pellicle and produce extracellular polysaccharides from sucrose. These polysaccharides enhance further bacterial accumulation on the tooth. The Gram-positive facultative anaerobic rods tend to be filamentous forms, such as *Actinomyces*.

Gingivitis

Accumulation of dental plaque along the gingival margins for 10 to 21 days results in localized inflammation (i.e., red and edematous tissue). The experimental gingivitis model of Löe was used to describe the changes that occur in the composition of the microbial community as plaque develops.[4] The initial flora of Gram-positive cocci and rods and Gram-negative cocci becomes more complex. Initially, there is a substantial increase in filamentous bacteria, such as *Actinomyces*. In later stages, the number of anaerobic and Gram-negative species, especially Gram-negative anaerobic rods, such as *Fusobacterium* and *P. intermedia*, increase, and motile rods and spirochetes appear (see Figure 4-9).[4, 6]

Gingival inflammation can be initiated by many bacterial species if they are present in high numbers as a result of poor oral hygiene. The development of many cases of chronic gingivitis probably constitutes a nonspecific infection. This is in contrast with a specific infection in which a limited number of bacteria are known to create a progressive periodontitis lesion.

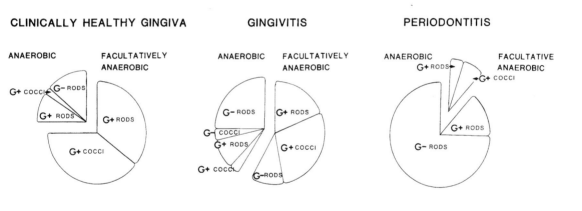

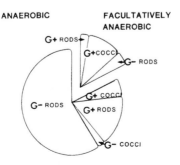

FIGURE 4–9. The relative proportions of various bacterial groups from dental plaque associated with clinically healthy gingiva, gingivitis, adult periodontitis, and juvenile periodontitis. (Used with permission from Carlsson J. Microbiology of plaque-associated periodontal disease. In Lindhe J, ed. Textbook of Clinical Periodontology, 2nd ed. Copenhagen: Munksgaard, 1989.)

Chronic Periodontitis

The continued presence of pathogenic plaque bacteria causes the inflammatory process to extend into the periodontal ligament, cementum, and alveolar bone, leading to the loss of attachment of the gingiva to tooth and to loss of supporting bone. In the early stages of periodontitis, the bacterial flora of the gingival pocket is similar to that of gingivitis, but as the disease becomes more severe, the flora becomes more complex. Clinically, chronic periodontitis has varied manifestations. Accordingly, the composition of the periodontitis flora differs significantly from patient to patient and from pocket to pocket in the same patient. In most cases, there is a greater frequency of a limited number of organisms. However, most patients with periodontitis have high proportions of anaerobes, Gram-negative organisms, and spirochetes, and the predominant organisms are Gram-negative anaerobic rods (see Figure 4-9).[6]

A variety of microbial species, predominantly Gram-negative species, have been implicated in the etiology of periodontitis. *P. gingivalis* seems to be the most important periodontal pathogen based on its numeric presence as well as its possession of specific virulence factors (see Figure 4-3).[7] Other organisms that have been repeatedly found in association with active periodontal lesions include the Gram-negative rods, *P. intermedia, Bacteroides forsythus, F. nucleatum, A. actinomycetemcomitans, Capnocytophaga ochraceus*, and *Eikenella corrodens*; the motile Gram-negative rods, *Campylobacter recta* and *Selenomonas* species; and the spirochetes, *Treponema denticola*.[8, 9]

Many laboratories have studied the subgingival flora of periodontal lesions, particularly comparing active with inactive sites, but no general consensus has been established as to specific pathogens, probably because of the complexity of the periodontal flora and the differing culture and identification techniques among laboratories.[8] The number of longitudinal prospective studies is limited, but results have implicated the presence of some of these same bacteria, *P. gingivalis, P. intermedia, A. actinomycetemcomitans*, and *B. forsythus* with progression of the periodontal lesions.[9]

Refractory Chronic Periodontitis

Refractory chronic periodontitis is defined as the presence of multiple periodontal sites that continue to show attachment loss despite comprehensive periodontal therapy and maintenance care. The subgingival microorganisms recovered from these refractory sites vary according to the study, but they usually include *F. nucleatum, P. intermedia, A. actinomycetemcomitans, Peptostreptococcus micros, P. gingivalis, B. forsythus*, and *C. recta*.[10]

The major reason for unsuccessful therapy appears to be the inability to eradicate the subgingival pathogenic flora. However, recent evidence suggests that host factors, such as smoking contributing to a polymorphonuclear leukocyte (PMN) phagocytic defect, increase the susceptibility of these patients to the pathogenic bacteria.[9]

Localized Juvenile Periodontitis

Classic localized juvenile periodontitis (LJP), now considered a form of aggressive periodontitis, involves alveolar bone destruction around the permanent incisors and first molars in otherwise healthy children with relatively little dental plaque and gingival inflammation. The familial pattern of disease suggests a genetically determined susceptibility. Patients frequently have defective PMN, with impaired ability to migrate to and phagocytose bacteria, thereby increasing the individual's susceptibility to infection.[11]

Gram-negative rods predominate in the microflora of patients with LJP (see Figure 4-9).[6] Most of these rods are *A. actinomycetemcomitans*, which has been strongly implicated as the major pathogen in LJP.[8, 12] Almost all LJP lesions harbor high numbers of *A. actinomycetemcomitans*. This organism is found less frequently and in much lower numbers in periodontally healthy sites of patients with LJP and in adult patients with periodontitis.

Necrotizing Ulcerative Gingivitis

Necrotizing ulcerative gingivitis (NUG) or necrotizing ulcerative periodontitis (NUP) is an infection of the marginal gingiva or periodontium. These conditions are characterized by necrotic, ulcerative lesions of the interdental papillae and severe loss of supporting structures. NUG has a characteristic histopathologic profile: An outer surface similar to the subgingival flora of periodontal lesions, a PMN-rich zone, a necrotic zone with spirochetes and Gram-negative rods, and the underlying connective tissue infiltrated with medium and large spirochetes.

NUG and NUP lesions harbor large numbers of intermediate-sized spirochetes and *P. intermedia*. Although early examinations of NUG lesions identified high levels of fusobacteria, recent culture and immunofluorescence studies have found that most Gram-negative rods are *P. intermedia*.[13]

VIRULENCE OF PERIODONTAL PATHOGENS

The virulence, or pathogenicity, of a microorganism is its ability to cause disease. The factors that contribute to the virulence potential of the major periodontal pathogens are varied and have been extensively discussed in reviews by Slots and Genco[7] and Listgarten.[14] In this chapter, the factors have been divided into three categories:

Proximity to the Tissue

For a microorganism to be virulent, it must be established in close proximity to the periodontal tissue and must be able to withstand the forces of saliva and gingival crevicular fluid that are capable of sweeping it away. Colonization is mediated by cell surface characteristics, for example, fimbriae and extracellular polysaccharides, such as glucan. Bacterial interactions are important for colonization as well as for availability of nutrients.

Evasion of Host Defenses

Normally, the humoral and cellular defense systems are able to rid the microbe from the host. However, periodontal pathogens have developed a variety of strategies to evade or overcome these mechanisms. For example, *P. gingivalis, B. forsythus*, and *T. denticola* have proteases that degrade the immunoglobulin molecule and complement proteins, and thus negate the immunologic protective effects. *A. actinomycetemcomitans* defend themselves from phagocytosis by PMNs by releasing inhibitors of directed migration (chemotaxis), producing antiphagocytosis surface components and inhibiting the PMNs' killing mechanisms. These organisms also produce a leukotoxin that kills or impairs PMNs that enter the periodontal pocket. *P. gingivalis* also releases a factor that interferes with PMN movement to a site of infection.

Tissue Destruction

Bacteria themselves do not need to be present within the tissue to be a major participant in the destructive process. The biologic events that cause periodontal destruction appear to result from the activities of their elaborated molecules. Some bacterial products may directly injure the host cells and tissues. Other components may interact with a variety of cells and activate the humoral and cellular immune reactions that secondarily affect the integrity of the periodontium.

DIRECT EFFECTS

Enzymes. The subgingival microbiota have a vast array of proteolytic enzymes. *P. gingivalis* produces collagenase, the enzyme that degrades native collagen. At least three pathogens—*P. gingivalis, B. forsythus*, and *T. denticola*—produce a trypsin-like protease that is active against various host proteins. The fact that this enzyme also degrades benzoyl-DL-arginine-β-naphthylamide (BANA), a synthetic colorimetric substrate, was used to develop a diagnostic test for periodontal disease.

Toxins. Lipopolysaccharide, or endotoxin, a Gram-negative bacterial cell wall component, induces inflammatory reactions and stimulates osteoclast-mediated bone resorption. Another type of bone-resorbing toxin is released from *A. actinomycetemcomitans*. Toxins that affect fibroblasts and, hence, the synthesis and turnover of collagen are produced by *P. gingivalis, P. intermedia, A. actinomycetemcomitans*, and *Capnocytophaga*. Several pathogens release volatile sulfides that inhibit the synthesis of collagen and noncollagenous substances.

INDIRECT EFFECTS

Some microbial products have the potential to activate nonimmune and immune inflammatory reactions, which in turn cause tissue destruction. For example, endotoxin from *P. gingivalis* and other Gram-negative organisms stimulates the release of prostaglandin E_2 and interleukin-1β from macrophages and fibroblasts, which have the potential to induce inflammation and bone resorption. With regard to the activation of immune reactions, the microbial components act as antigens, initiating the classic humoral and cellular hypersensitivity responses.

SIGNIFICANCE OF DENTAL PLAQUE TO THE DENTAL HYGIENIST

Because of the pathogenic potential of dental plaque, its reduction or control is significant to gingival health. The dental hygienist plays a significant role in this process in terms of both prevention and treatment.

Plaque Control

Historically, a focus of dental hygiene has been oral hygiene instruction (i.e., teaching patients and groups the importance and the techniques of toothbrushing and flossing to achieve plaque control). Extensive plaque control programs, popular in the 1970s, emphasized reducing the quantity of plaque because of the belief in the nonspecific plaque hypothesis and the homogeneity of dental plaque. The development of the specific plaque hypothesis has shifted emphasis to specific microbes. The importance of plaque control has not changed, only its scientific rationale. The current thinking is that thorough plaque removal should be performed daily to keep the plaque perpetually in the initial stages of formation. As discussed, the bacteria that colonize plaque at this stage do not possess the same pathogenic potential as the bacteria that dominate in plaque that has accumulated for more than 24 hours. Instituting thorough plaque control before the mature plaque develops prevents the initiation of the disease process.

Periodontal Therapy

Because subgingival plaque is inaccessible to home care procedures, professional debridement is necessary to remove plaque or at least disrupt its formation. Frequent recall intervals for professional plaque control procedures may be effective because physical disruption of the plaque converts the pathogenic flora back to flora more compatible with health. However, studies have shown that debridement often does not remove *P. gingivalis, P. intermedia, B. forsythus, P. micros*, and *A. actinomycetemcomitans*. These organisms may be colonizing gingival tissues and other areas that are inaccessible to instrumentation and subgingival irrigation with medicaments.

In these cases, mechanical removal may not be the major therapeutic approach for treatment. These cases would require systemic therapy whereby the antimicrobial agent enters the periodontal tissue and pocket through the bloodstream. The choice of antimicrobial therapy would be based on analyses of the subgingival flora because several organisms with different drug susceptibilities may produce periodontal destruction. A new role for the dental hygienist may be to collect the subgingival flora and interpret the results of the microbiologic analyses as a means of monitoring the effects of treatment.

Just as the understanding of how dental plaque is related to periodontal diseases has evolved over time, so may the role of the dental hygienist in the prevention and treatment of the plaque-related periodontal diseases. Plaque assessment and control remains an integral part of the practice of dental hygiene.

STUDY QUESTIONS

MULTIPLE CHOICE

1. What distinguishes supragingival dental plaque from material alba?

   a. the amount of calcium and phosphate ions
   b. the location of the deposit on the tooth
   c. the number of bacteria
   d. the strength of adherence of the deposit to the tooth structure

2. Endotoxin is:

   a. a component of normal saliva
   b. a component of the cell wall of Gram-positive rods
   c. easily degraded by salivary enzymes
   d. probably a cause of incipient root caries
   e. released from Gram-negative cocci at death

3. Fermentative bacteria:

   a. cannot survive in an oxygen environment
   b. obtain energy from carbohydrate metabolism
   c. produce amino acid end products
   d. usually possess fimbriae

4. Which of the following is not a characteristic of salivary glycoproteins?

   a. They enhance binding of bacteria to tooth surfaces
   b. They interact with calcium and phosphate in hydroxyapatite
   c. They promote bacterial aggregation
   d. They result from lysis of the bacterial cell wall

5. Which characteristic ability of bacteria influences their relative numbers in early plaque?

   a. the ability to adhere to pellicle
   b. the ability to form bacterial coaggregations
   c. the ability to multiply in an aerobic environment
   d. the ability to multiply rapidly
   e. the ability to survive in an acid environment

6. Which process facilitates bacterial aggregation?

   a. decreased oxygen tension
   b. formation of levans
   c. interaction of fimbriae with endotoxin
   d. nonselective attachment of Gram-negative bacteria
   e. formation of the product from the glucosyltransferase reaction

7. Which factor facilitates the formation of subgingival plaque?

   a. greater formation of highly branched extracellular polysaccharides
   b. greater production of fermentation end products
   c. predominance of filamentous bacteria
   d. presence of hemin-containing proteins in crevicular fluid

8. Based on the specific plaque hypothesis, gingival health can be monitored by:

   a. determining the total number of bacteria in plaque samples
   b. distinguishing the various types of bacteria in plaque samples
   c. measuring the amount of plaque
   d. recording the number of times the teeth are brushed daily

9. Which characteristic describes the primary periodontal pathogens?

   a. filaments
   b. fimbriae on the cell surface
   c. Gram-negative nonmotile rods
   d. motile organisms

10. What do the following bacteria have in common: *Porphyromonas gingivalis, Bacteroides forsythus,* and *Treponema denticola*?

    a. black pigmentation
    b. capsule
    c. flagella
    d. leukotoxin
    e. trypsin-like protease

SHORT ANSWER

11. Describe changes in the microflora as plaque matures in terms of the following bacterial characteristics:

    a. morphotype
    b. cell wall classification
    c. oxygen requirements
    d. nutrient requirements

    _____

    _____

12. Describe two types of bacterial aggregation.

    _____

    _____

13. Name and describe the probably primary pathogens in the following periodontal diseases:

    a. chronic periodontitis

b. aggressive periodontitis

c. necrotizing ulcerative gingivitis

_____

_____

14. Describe the major virulence factor of Gram-negative bacteria.

_____

_____

15. Describe the chemical reaction in which glucan is synthesized from sucrose.

_____

_____

REFERENCES

1. Liljemark WF, Bloomquist C. Human oral microbial ecology and dental caries and periodontal diseases. Crit Rev Oral Biol Med 1996;7:180-198.
2. Kolenbrander PE, London J. Adhere today, here tomorrow: Oral bacterial adherence. J Bacteriol 1993;175: 3247-3252.
3. Löe HE, Theilade E, Jensen SB. Experimental gingivitis in man. J Periodontol 1965;36:177-187.
4. Theilade E, Wright WH, Jensen SB, Loe HE. Experimental gingivitis in man: II. A longitudinal clinical and bacteriological investigation. J Periodont Res 1966;1:1-13.
5. Loesche WH. Chemotherapy of dental plaque infections. Oral Sci Rev 1976;9:65-107.
6. Slots J. Subgingival microflora and periodontal disease. J Clin Periodontol 1979;6:351-382.
7. Slots J, Genco RJ. Black-pigmented *Bacteroides* species, *Capnocytophaga* species, and *Actinobacillus actinomycetemcomitans* in human periodontal disease: virulence factors in colonization, survival, and tissue destruction. J Dent Res 1984;63:412-421.
8. Moore WEC. Microbiology of periodontal disease. J Periodontol 1987;22:335-341.
9. Wolff L, Dahlen G, Aeppli D. Bacteria as risk markers for periodontitis. J Periodontol 1994;64:498-510.
10. Slots J, Rams TE. New views on periodontal microbiota in special patient categories. J Clin Periodontol 1991;18:411-420.
11. Van Dyke TE, Levine MJ, Genco RJ. Neurophil function and oral disease. J Oral Pathol 1985;14:95-120.
12. Zambon JJ. *Actinobacillus actinomycetemcomitans* in human periodontal disease. J Clin Periodontol 1985;12:1-20.
13. Loesche WJ, Syed SA, Laughon BG, Stoll J. The bacteriology of acute necrotizing ulcerative gingivitis. J Periodontol 1982;53:223-230.
14. Listgarten MA. Nature of periodontal diseases: pathogenic mechanisms. J Periodontal Res 1987;22:172-178.

5

Dorothy A. Perry

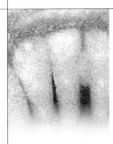

Calculus and Other Disease-Associated Factors

*C*hapter *O*bjectives

1. Describe the role of dental calculus and other disease-associated factors in the initiation and perpetuation of gingival and periodontal diseases.
2. Describe the formation and attachment of supragingival and subgingival calculus in the oral environment.
3. Describe the distribution of calculus deposits and list the characteristics involved in the rate of formation.
4. Explain how anti-calculus agents work in reducing calculus formations in humans.
5. List the factors that are linked to periodontal disease and health and explain the role of the dental hygienist in recognition and treatment.

*K*ey *T*erms

Acquired pellicle
Amalgam overhangs
Calculus
Diphosphonate
First molar loss syndrome
Malocclusion
Mouth breathing
Overcontoured crowns

Pyrophosphate
Salivary calculus
Serumal calculus
Subgingival calculus
Submarginal calculus
Supragingival calculus
Supramarginal calculus
Tartar

A thorough understanding of **calculus**, what it is and why it is important, places calculus removal in perspective in dental hygiene practice. A good deal of time is spent removing calculus and preventing its formation. Calculus removal has an important place in dental hygiene care, but is not the definition of dental hygiene practice.

CALCULUS

The removal of calculus occupies much of the treatment time of the dental hygienist. Perfecting the skills necessary to achieve calculus removal can take years. Calculus removal too often becomes the focus of dental hygiene care for this reason: anything that requires so much time and effort must be more valuable than activities that require less treatment time. Calculus removal is important, but it is only a part of dental hygiene care. Calculus is not a benign substance unrelated to the pathogenesis of gingival and periodontal disease, but it plays a much smaller part in these diseases than bacterial plaque. The dental hygienist may spend 90 percent of treatment time on calculus removal and 5 percent on plaque control, but must not lose sight of the significance of each. Calculus removal is passive treatment for the patient that is provided by a dental hygienist. Daily plaque control, taught by the dental hygienist and performed by the patient, requires active participation by the patient. Daily plaque control allows the individual to limit calculus formation and maintain gingival health for a lifetime.

Tartar

"**Tartar**" is the common name for dental calculus. This term is often used by patients when referring to calculus. The term was introduced by Paracelsus, a Swiss–German physician in the 16th century. He referred to all stony accretions in humans as tartars because he observed that dental calculus, stones in the bladder or gallbladder, and gout-affected joints resembled potassium bitartrate deposits, called tartar, on the bottom of wine casks. He described tartars as the cause of the malady.[1]

The name tartar will no doubt continue to be used for a long time because it is often used in advertising. Products referred to as "tartar control" toothpaste and rinses are popular and reinforce the use of the common name.

Significance

Calculus is formed by the deposition of calcium and phosphate salts in bacterial plaque. It has long been thought to be the cause of periodontal diseases. Its appearance was easily associated with gum infection, and efforts to remove accretions from teeth resulted in better gingival health. As reviewed by Mandel and Gaffar,[2] early epidemiologic studies also associated calculus with periodontal diseases, but could not establish causality, although the data were often interpreted as establishing cause. This interpretation probably occurred because epidemiologic studies tend to compare mean values for calculus and gingival disease, not specific sites. Therefore, calculus may be present in most patients with gingival disease, but not necessarily at all or most of the diseased sites. One study, published in 1960 and reviewed by Mandel and Gaffar,[2] reported that 11 percent of sites with calculus also had gingivitis, whereas 75 percent of tooth surfaces with plaque had gingivitis. This finding was an early suggestion that calculus may be a result of disease, not the cause.

However, calculus contributes to the development of disease, even though bacterial plaque is the etiologic agent. Calculus forms in germ-free laboratory animals, but it is far more abundant in germ-infected animals.[1]

It is also clear that even in young people, the presence of calculus is associated with increased levels of gingival disease. A study of Thai children aged 11 to 13 showed a very significant association between gingivitis, plaque status and calculus accumulation, but no association between calculus status and caries.[3] An evaluation of data from 1,285 young people aged 13 to 20 who participated in the 1986–87 national survey of the oral health of U.S. adolescents indicated that **subgingival calculus** is associated with both incidental attachment loss and those with juvenile periodontitis. Both groups of young people had significantly more gingival bleeding and subgingival calculus than matched control subjects. Importantly, the juvenile periodontitis group had significantly more subgingival calculus than those with incidental attachment loss, suggesting an association between this disease and the presence of subgingival calculus. (See Chapter 7 for a discussion of juvenile periodontitis.)[4]

The role of the bacteria in relation to calculus formation is not completely understood. As the understanding of this relationship increases, dental hygienists are likely to be better able to help patients to control calculus formation.

Definition

Calculus is usually divided into supragingival and subgingival types of accumulations, even

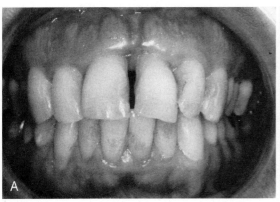 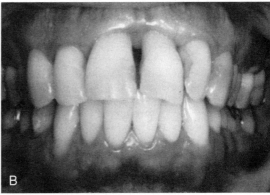

FIGURE 5–1. The effects of plaque-associated calculus on periodontal tissues. Calculus removal results in reduction in the signs of inflammation and easier plaque control. **A.** Before nonsurgical calculus removal and periodontal therapy. **B.** After nonsurgical calculus removal and periodontal therapy.

though both types often occur together. There are significant differences between the two types that have direct bearing on the treatment approaches of the dental hygienist.

Dental hygienists commonly describe patients as light, moderate, or heavy calculus formers, depending on the amount of supragingival calculus that forms between recall visits. This distinction is useful in terms of estimating treatment time, if little else. Patients may have light, moderate, or heavy deposits of subgingival calculus alone, **supragingival calculus** alone, or both. Figure 5-1 highlights the effects of dental hygiene care, including calculus removal.

SUPRAGINGIVAL CALCULUS

Supragingival calculus is found on the clinical crowns of the teeth, above the margin of the gingiva. It is readily visible as a yellowish-white accumulation, although it may darken with age. Figure 5-2 shows an extreme deposition of supragingival calculus.

Formation and Components. Supragingival calculus is tightly adherent to the teeth and may occur on any tooth in the mouth. Supragingival calculus is most abundant near the openings of Wharton's ducts, the lingual surfaces of the lower anterior teeth, and Stenson's ducts, the buccal surfaces of the maxillary molars. Other names for supragingival calculus are **supramarginal calculus**, extragingival, or coronal calculus, indicating location, or **salivary calculus**, reflecting the source of the mineral content.[3]

In supragingival calculus formation, mineral crystals are deposited in an organic matrix of plaque microorganisms, glucans, glycoproteins, and lipids. The calculi (calcified nodules) are stratified, suggesting that supragingival calculus is deposited in layers. Inorganic mineral content makes up 70 to 90 percent of supragingival calculus. The minerals are primarily calcium phosphate (75.9 percent), calcium carbonate (3.1 percent), traces of magnesium,[5] sodium, potassium, and trace elements of fluoride, zinc, and strontium.[1]

The main crystal types in calculus are: 58 percent hydroxyapatite ($Ca_{10}[PO_4]_6 \cdot OH_2$), about 21 percent octacalcium phosphate ($Ca_8[HPO_4]_4$), about 21 percent magnesium whitlockite ($Ca_3[PO_4]_2$), and approximately 9 percent brushite ($Ca[HPO_4] \cdot 2H_2O$).[6] Brushite appears in large proportions, up to 50 percent, in young calculus. After a few weeks or months, the predominant crystal type becomes hydroxyapatite.[1]

The organic component of calculus makes up to 15 to 20 percent of the dry weight of calculus. Half is protein from the bacterial cells, but it also includes carbohydrates and lipids from bacteria and saliva. Small amounts of glycosaminglycans are also found, probably as a result of tissue breakdown.[1] Salivary proteins make up 5.9 percent to 8.2 percent of the organic component of supragingival calculus. Dental calculus, salivary duct calculus, and calcified dental tissues are all similar in organic composition.[6]

Attachment to the Tooth Structure. Attachment to the tooth surface occurs in relationship to bacterial plaque. **Acquired pellicle**

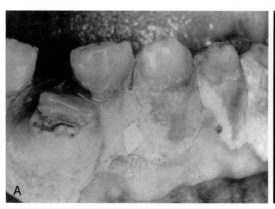
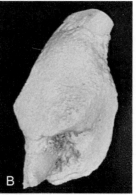

FIGURE 5–2. A. Supragingival calculus can accumulate in huge amounts and may obliterate the structure of the teeth. The white area is food debris. **B.** Only the root tip and incisal edge of this tooth are visible because of the extensive calculus accumulation. The tooth simply fell out.

is strongly bound to the tooth surface, bacterial plaque formation begins with Gram-positive coccoidal organisms, and then calcification occurs. After about 5 days, the plaque becomes filamentous and resembles decalcified mature calculus.[1] Pellicle can grow into microscopic pores and openings and form a dendritic structure below the tooth surface. This structure increases the tenacity of calculus attachment.[1] Mechanical locking of mineral structure into tooth surface irregularities and close adaptation to tooth shape add to its tenacity.[6]

Mineralization in plaque can begin within 24 to 72 hours. Maturation time averages 12 days. It occurs more rapidly in some individuals and more slowly in others.[5] Supragingival calculus can form on occlusal tooth surfaces when the teeth are out of occlusion or in crossbite.[7] It also occurs on fixed and removable prosthetic devices such as fixed bridgework and dentures.[5]

in rings or ledges on root surfaces, but may also appear as veneers. Subgingival calculus is also called **submarginal calculus** because of its location or **serumal calculus** because of the source of the mineral content.[5] Figure 5–3 shows a periodontal patient with subgingival calculus.

Formation and Components. Like supragingival calculus, subgingival calculus forms from mineralized plaque. Pellicle forms, subgingival plaque is seeded by or forms by extension of supragingival plaque, and then mineralization occurs. The mineral content is derived from crevicular fluid rather than from saliva, differentiating it from supragingival calculus.

The organic components of subgingival calculus are similar to supragingival calculus but contain more calcium, magnesium, and fluoride because of the higher concentrations of these

Subgingival Calculus

Subgingival calculus forms on root surfaces below the gingival margin and can extend into the periodontal pockets. Subgingival calculus is likely to be tenacious and black in color. Subgingival calculus is typically dark green or black probably because of the organic matrix products of the subgingival plaque. The subgingival matrix contains blood products associated with subgingival hemorrhage that have dark pigment. These matrix products differ from supragingival calculus, where the organic matrix components come primarily from saliva and do not contain blood.[8] It is commonly deposited

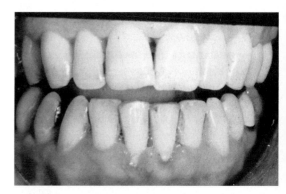

FIGURE 5–3. Subgingival calculus may be difficult to detect from clinical appearance alone. Explorer examination is required for accurate assessment. This case presented with heavy deposits of subgingival calculus that were not readily apparent by visual inspection.

minerals in crevicular fluid.[1] There is no salivary protein present in subgingival calculus, and, interestingly, the sodium content of subgingival calculus increases with the depth of the periodontal pockets.[6]

The pocket contents are composed of subgingival calculus adjacent to the root surface. Then there is a layer of attached plaque, which is covered by loosely adherent bacteria in the pocket. In addition, cells from the pocket wall and inflammatory exudate may be present. Figure 5-4 shows the contents of the periodontal pocket, including calculus.

Attachment to the Tooth Structure. Pellicle attachment to cementum is the mode of subgingival calculus adherence. Deposits also form in and around microorganisms on the more irregular cemental surfaces, possibly caused by the loss of Sharpey's fibers, resorbtion lacunae, or arrested caries.[1] Crystals can grow deeply into cemental irregularities. They appear morphologically similar to cementum, termed calculocementum,[6] and exhibit in-

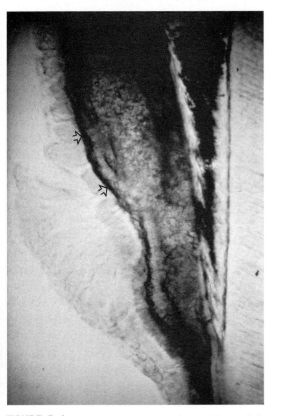

FIGURE 5–4. Histologic section of the contents of the periodontal pocket. Arrows indicate the surface of calculus. Organized bacterial masses are attached to the surface of the calculus (arrows). (Courtesy of Dr. Edward Green.)

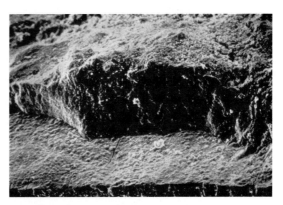

FIGURE 5–5. Scanning electron micrograph of subgingival calculus attached to a cemental surface. (Courtesy of Dr. John Sottusanti.)

tercrystalline bonding.[1] The various methods of attachment make subgingival calculus more tenacious and difficult to remove than supragingival calculus. Figure 5-5 shows a scanning electron micrograph of subgingival calculus adapted to a cemental surface.

Unlike supragingival calculus, the location of subgingival calculus is not site specific.[9] It is found throughout the mouth, and both radiographic examination and explorer detection are required to evaluate the extent and location of deposits. Radiographs alone tend to show mesial and distal deposits and underestimate the amount of calculus present because of technique-related artifacts. Overangulation of film, cervical burnout, and poor processing techniques can limit the reliability of radiographic detection of subgingival calculus. Explorer detection provides the dental hygienist with buccal and lingual estimates of deposits, along with proximal estimates, but it is also subject to the vagaries of technique. It is advisable to use both radiographs and tactile skill to evaluate the amount of calculus present. Figure 5-6 shows calculus embedded in a root surface.

Distribution

The distribution of calculus formation on teeth has been described. Supragingival calculus appears most commonly on the mandibular incisors and maxillary molars, especially the first molar, in relation to the opening of the major salivary ducts. Subgingival calculus is more evenly distributed throughout the mouth.[9, 10] It is a common mistake to assume that no calculus deposits occur around the maxillary anterior teeth. Although less frequent than other loca-

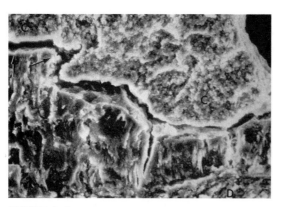

FIGURE 5–6. Scanning electron micrograph of calculus embedded in cemental irregularities. Arrows indicate the surface of the cementum. C is calculus mass, and D is dentin. (Courtesy of Dr. John Sottosanti.)

tions, both subgingival and supragingival calculus can occur there in as many as 10 percent of patients. Figure 5–7 shows calculus distribution.

The course of calculus formation and its distribution in humans has also been described. A landmark study by Anerud and colleagues[11] compared 480 Sri Lankan male tea laborers, 14 to 31 years old, over a 15-year period with

Norwegian men and boys, 16 to 30 years old, over a 20-year period. Anerud and co-workers[11] described the natural history of calculus formation. Findings from Sri Lanka, a society with no dental care and in which tooth brushing was not performed, were compared with the clinical course of calculus formation in Norwegian subjects, who had optimum dental care. Natural history referred to the course of calculus formation over time without any intervention, as in the case of the Sri Lankan subjects. The Norwegian subjects had ample opportunity to receive regular care in school clinics and private dental practices. The Norwegian data represented the course of calculus formation tempered by regular, modern dental treatment. These data, summarized in Table 5–1, clearly show the importance of calculus removal for long-term gingival health and emphasize the importance of thorough calculus removal by the dental hygienist.

For reasons that are not completely understood, there is tremendous individual variation in calculus formation rates. Plaque has shown evidence of mineral precipitation occurring in 1 to 14 days, but it can occur as quickly as within 4 hours. Calcifying plaques may become

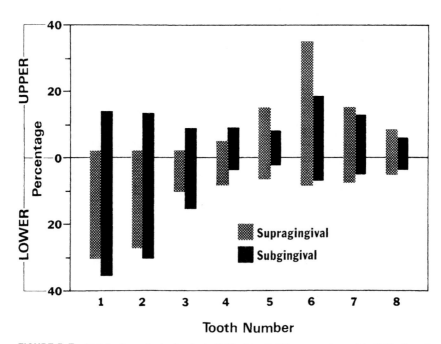

FIGURE 5–7. Distribution of calculus by individual teeth. The percentage of individual teeth with supragingival and subgingival calculus is shown by tooth number and arch. Tooth #1 is the central incisor and tooth #8 is the third molar in each quadrant. (Adapted with permission from Schroeder HE. Formation and Inhibition of Dental Calculus. Vienna: H. Huber Publishers, 1969.)

TABLE 5–1. Calculus Formation in Adult Male Population Based on the Findings of Anerud, Loe, and Boysen[11]

Natural History	Clinical Course
Sri Lankan tea workers with no dental care	Norwegian men with regular dental care
Calculus	
All had some; amount increased over the years	Generally low levels over the years
Supragingival	
Formed early in life on maxillary molars and mandibular anterior teeth	Found in same locations, but at low levels
Continued to grow until age 25 or 30; was present on all teeth	Rarely found in other locations; did not increase in amount with age
Subgingival	
Formed 6–8 years after eruption; continued to increase in extent and severity	Seen at low levels around age 20–29; no predilection for specific teeth
Leveled off at age 30	Increased somewhat with age
Tobacco Effects	
Smokers and betel nut chewers had more calculus than nonsmokers or nonchewers	Not associated with increased amounts of calculus
Loss of Attachment	
Subgingival calculus associated with more attachment loss than teeth with no subgingival calculus	Accumulation of supragingival and subgingival calculus that were removed regularly had no effect on attachment loss

up to 50 percent mineralized in 2 days, and 60 percent to 90 percent mineralized in 12 days.[6] Heavy calculus formers have higher levels of calcium and phosphorus (from the saliva) in the plaque within a few days after a prophylaxis. In addition, differences in diet and in the composition of the microbial flora may contribute to formation rates. Mandel[1] reviewed a number of characteristics that may be related to an increased rate of calculus formation:

1. Elevated salivary pH.
2. Concentration of calcium in saliva.
3. Concentration of salivary bacterial protein and lipid.
4. Low individual inhibitory factors.
5. Higher salivary urea and protein from the submandibular glands.
6. Higher total salivary lipid levels.

Light calculus formers have higher levels of parotid **pyrophosphate**. It has been suggested that dental patients who are taking some medications, such as beta blockers, diuretics, and thyroid supplements, form less supragingival calculus than comparable individuals who are not taking any medications.[12, 13] Research will provide further understanding of this complex interrelationship and will lead to better control of calculus formation.

Pathogenesis

Through the 1960s, calculus was considered a mechanical irritant to the tissues and thus part of the etiology of inflammation. Now that the cause of gingival and periodontal diseases is understood to be pathologic bacterial plaques, calculus is recognized to play a role in plaque formation and retention.

Supragingival calculus is porous and rough and provides an excellent lattice on which plaque can grow. It is not clear whether calculus plus plaque creates greater tissue reaction than plaque alone. However, calculus clearly assists in bringing the bacteria close to the tissue, interfering with oral self-cleansing mechanisms, and making plaque removal more difficult for patients, if not impossible in some areas.[1, 6]

Subgingival calculus is associated with the chronicity and progression of periodontal disease. Periodontal pockets virtually always contain subgingival calculus, even if in microscopic amounts.[6] Subgingival calculus can provide a reservoir for bacteria and endotoxins that are significantly related to the disease process. In addition, it has been shown that subgingival calculus covered by bacterial plaque can cause greater disease progression than plaque alone.[1]

Long-term studies clearly support the removal of all calculus to promote healing and prevent further loss of attachment.[14]

Anticalculus Agents

A number of agents have modest effects on reducing supragingival calculus formation in humans. These agents work through inhibition of hydroxyapatite crystal growth by pyrophosphates or the analogue, **diphosphonate**.[1] Studies in the 1980s showed reduced supragingival calculus in several hundred subjects considered to be heavy calculus formers. Supragingival calculus was reduced by 26 percent after 2 months,[15] and by 37 percent[16] and 21.4 percent[17] after 6 months. All three studies found that pyrophosphate-containing dentrifices were safe and well tolerated by the oral soft tissues of the subjects. Only one comparison study of three types of pyrophosphate toothpastes found greater calculus reduction by one product over another. One case of oral ulcers was reported among 118 subjects who used the products over a 3-month period.[18] Anticalculus toothpastes with fluoride apparently have little negative effect on tooth remineralization and thus do not interfere with caries inhibition by fluorides.

It is important for the dental hygienist to understand and educate patients about the limited effectiveness of these preparations. They appear safe to use and provide for caries prevention (from fluoride in the preparations). However, they only reduce the formation of new supragingival calculus, have no measurable effects on subgingival calculus, and do not reduce the quantity of calculus already present in the mouth. In addition, improved toothbrushing alone can reduce the formation of new supragingival calculus by as much as 50 percent on the lingual surfaces of the lower anterior teeth.[1]

These commercially available "tartar control" anticalculus toothpastes and mouthwashes may be helpful for periodontal patients who accumulate supragingival calculus and for patients using chlorhexidine mouth rinse. Chlorhexidine is associated with increased calculus deposition in addition to staining of the teeth. The dental hygienist should be aware of the usefulness of these products, but should not expect them to provide complete calculus control

or to replace needed instrumentation. As knowledge in this area grows, new and better products will become available to help both the patients and the dental hygienist who is faced with removing copious amounts of calculus.

PLAQUE RETENTIVE FACTORS

Individual factors, such as restoration contour, **poor restorations**, and orthodontic bands and brackets, are clearly linked to periodontal health. This section provides an overview of dental treatment and patient behavior in relation to dental hygiene care.

Dental Restorations

It is clear that plaque retention occurs on the porous surface of calculus. Other factors can also modify the patient's ability to control the accumulation of plaque or the response to plaque. Dental restorations can significantly alter dental plaque growth, retention, and gingival health. Marginal discrepancies between the edges of the restorations and the remaining tooth surface, particularly those margins placed subgingivally, are associated with detrimental periodontal changes. A recent review emphasized that the fit of restorations is generally less than perfect. Studies show that up to 80 percent of restorations examined radiographically exhibit marginal defects, and that those larger than 0.2 mm are always associated with bone loss. In addition, 69 percent of fillings and 82 percent of bridges show evidence of ill-fitting margins.[19] Not only is it important to appreciate how difficult it is to create good fitting margins, patient habits and life styles can also affect susceptibility to periodontal diseases.

CROWN CONTOURS AND MARGINS

Rough-surfaced and **overcontoured crowns**, bridges, and other cast and ceramic restorations have been associated with gingival inflammation and periodontal disease. Plaque accumulation, the etiology of inflammation, is enhanced by subgingival placement of fixed restorations for a variety of reasons: greater surface roughness of the materials, fit of the margin to the remaining tooth structure, and contour of the restoration.[20] One study of 831 private practice dental patients in North Carolina showed that crown margins placed subgingivally were almost always associated with increased gingival inflammation and probing depth compared with uncrowned surfaces. This finding was true even in the case of subjects who had regular maintenance visits.[21]

Sorensen[20] described the problems that result in increased plaque accumulation and retention. Ragged subgingival margins of restorations are difficult for the dentist or dental hygienist to remove, even more so than calculus. These ragged margins provide a sheltered place for plaque growth. Adequate patient plaque control is also more difficult on restorations than on smoother, unrestored surfaces.

All cast margins, even those that fit properly, leave at least a microscopically thin line of cement. This line is next to the gingiva in the case of subgingival margins or open to the oral environment in the case of supragingival margins. The larger the gap, the more it can harbor bacteria like any ragged margin. In addition, the cement is slowly dissolved by saliva, creating a porous space ideal for plaque growth. These observations clearly suggest that the poorer the fit of the subgingival cast restoration margin, the more extreme the gingival reaction is likely to be. The contour of crown restorations is also significant. Bulbous, rounded crowns can impinge on the embrasure space, making plaque control difficult and resulting in increased inflammation of the associated tissues.[20]

Kenney[22] recommended that adaptation of restoration margins be above the gingival margin if possible, that contours of restorations facilitate cleaning, that proximal relationships between the teeth leave space for the gingiva and make cleaning easy, and that restoration surfaces be as smooth as possible so that plaque accumulation is not enhanced.

Specifically, seven items should be kept in mind in relation to dental hygiene care:[22]

1. A healthy gingival sulcus is required before restorative treatment is performed so that the height of the gingiva in relation to the restoration margin can be determined.
2. Margins of restorations should be kept away from the gingiva.
3. Even properly fitting crown margins have a thin line of cement to which plaque can readily adhere.
4. Temporary crowns should have margins that fit as well as possible and should be polished to minimize roughness. Figure 5–8 shows correctly and incorrectly contoured temporary crowns.
5. Restorations should preserve the embrasure space, particularly the interproximal embrasure, so that there is adequate room for the gingiva. Gingiva will fill the space after treatment, and there must be enough room for an adequate collagen attachment.

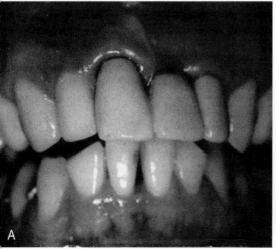
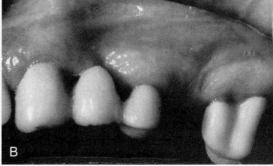

FIGURE 5–8. The plaque-retention effects of temporary crowns on the gingiva. **A.** A poorly contoured temporary crown on tooth #8 resulted in rolled and shiny gingiva. Clinically, the marginal tissue is reddened and swollen. **B.** A well-contoured temporary crown designed for good plaque control. The tissue appears firm and stippled. (Courtesy of Dr. Richard Nagy.)

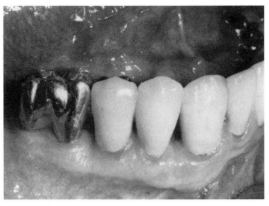

FIGURE 5–9. The hygienically designed gold crown facilitates good plaque control for the periodontal patient. The shape of the crown permits access to an exposed furcation area. (Courtesy of Dr. Richard Nagy.)

6. Crowns must be contoured to facilitate oral hygiene procedures, especially in furcation areas. In some cases, the height of contour of the tooth will be reduced and grooves will be accentuated to allow access to the gingival margin for cleaning. This requirement is especially important in furcation areas. Crowns contoured to allow cleaning of furcation areas are shown in Figure 5-9.

7. Pontics of the old saddle design, overlapping the alveolar ridge on both sides, are hard to keep clean. Newer designs that are bullet-shaped or spheroidal are preferable, and hygienic pontics that leave a 3 mm space between the bottom of the pontic and the gingiva should be used when possible. Figure 5-10 shows a hygienic pontic.

AMALGAM OVERHANGS

Amalgam restorations are one of the most common forms of dental restoration. Unfortunately, they are also the source of **amalgam overhangs**, one of the most common forms of poorly contoured restorations, which cause plaque traps and increased gingival inflammation. Their major contribution to pathology is as a source of plaque retention, and they complicate plaque control for patients. They are associated with increased plaque mass and with plaque colonized by likely periodontal pathogens (Figure 5-11).[23]

The 1990 review by Brunsvold and Lane[23] of the prevalence of amalgam overhangs showed startling statistics. The prevalence of overhanging amalgam margins over a number of studies and several thousand subjects ranged from 25 to 76 percent of all amalgam-restored proximal surfaces. They also reported that at least 33 percent of adult dental patients had one or more overhanging amalgams. In addition, studies showed that bone loss was increased under overhangs by 0.16 to 0.87 mm; probing depth was increased by 0.2 to 0.67 mm; and attachment loss was increased 0.2 to 0.5 mm. Kells and Linden[24] found overhangs in 57 percent of a young dental population, aged 20 to 29 years. However, they did not find increased bone loss in this population.

Recognition of overhanging amalgam restorations is a critical element in dental hygiene care. Pack[25] noted that overhangs exist in an alarming quantity and also that removal of the

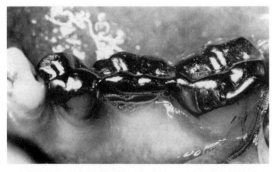

FIGURE 5–10. Hygienically designed pontics, such as the one shown here, facilitate plaque control. This pontic is elevated off the gingiva, leaving space. The space permits the patient to clean under the pontic with floss or an interproximal brush. (Courtesy of Dr. Paulo Camargo.)

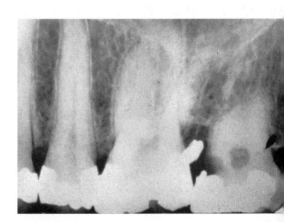

FIGURE 5–11. A large overhanging amalgam restoration can contribute to periodontal destruction because of plaque accumulation. This huge overhang would be very difficult to remove and recontour. The restoration was replaced on the first molar. Note the recurrent caries apical to the restoration on the second molar.

overhangs, scaling of the areas, and oral hygiene instruction resulted in significant improvements in oral health.

Amalgam finishing and overhang removal is a legally permitted duty for many dental hygienists. Certainly, evaluation of amalgam margins for possible overhangs is a responsibility of all dental hygienists because it is an important part of disease prevention and maintenance care. Overhangs are best detected by a combination of radiographic observation and clinical examination with explorers.[23-25] Small overhangs can be removed by hand instruments such as dental knives, ultrasonic instruments, rotary burs, or reciprocating polishers. If removed, large overhangs may leave poorly condensed amalgam with voids that will continue to act as plaque traps. Poor restorations must be replaced.[25] Figure 5-12 shows tools used for overhang removal.

Clearly, the dental hygienist must learn to evaluate amalgam margins, remove and smooth small overhangs, and educate patients about the detrimental effects of poor restorations.

Partial Dentures

Many individuals have lost teeth as the result of periodontal disease, injury, or other conditions. These patients often have the missing teeth restored by removable partial dentures. According to Kenney,[22] the restorations of choice for the periodontally involved dentition are fixed bridges and crowns. However, in some situations, a mouth with many missing teeth may not be restorable with bridgework. Some patients may select removable appliances because of financial or other considerations. Partial dentures make excellent functional and esthetic restorative solutions for many individuals. As mentioned previously, partial dentures, complete dentures, and all other removable devices can collect supragingival calculus. The dental hygienist can remove this calculus during the hygiene appointment by using powered or hand scalers and polishing. Partial denture wearers should also be instructed to clean the appliance daily at home with an accepted denture cleaner, denture brush, and clasp brush.

Natural teeth in function with removable partial dentures tend to have more periodontal pockets, and deeper pockets.[26] Increased susceptibility to caries is also associated with abutment teeth for partial dentures.[22] Clearly, excellent oral hygiene and caries prevention measures must be part of the dental hygiene care provided to these patients. In addition,

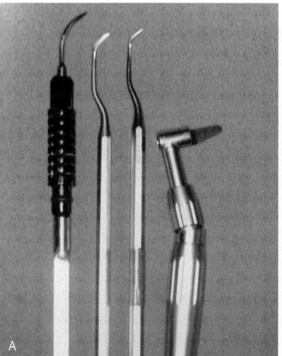
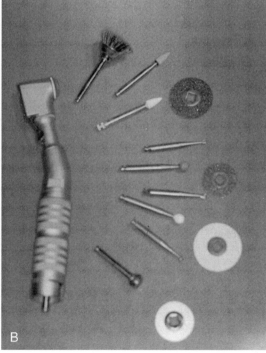

A

B

FIGURE 5–12. **A.** Armamentarium used for removal of amalgam overhang include ultrasonic instruments, hand instruments, and handpiece-mounted files. **B.** Slow-speed handpieces with associated burs and disks can also be used to modify excess amalgam.

regular recall maintenance appointments for thorough examination, calculus removal, oral hygiene reinforcement, and caries prevention should be emphasized.

CONDITIONS THAT AFFECT PERIODONTAL HEALTH

A number of dental conditions affect the periodontal health of patients who are routinely seen by dental hygienists. These include the presence of orthodontic appliances, oral habits such as **mouth breathing**, early loss of the first molars in children, and tobacco use. This section describes these conditions.

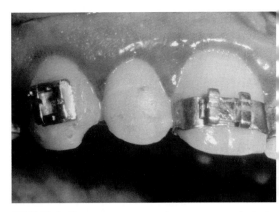

FIGURE 5–13. Orthodontic appliances can result in increased plaque accumulation and periodontal inflammation. The shiny, rolled marginal gingiva appears reddened clinically. The archwire has been temporarily removed to facilitate cleaning.

Orthodontic Appliances

Orthodontic appliances have long been associated with increased plaque accumulation, gingivitis,[27] and caries susceptibility in children and adolescents.[28, 29] Lang and Siegrist[30] reviewed studies evaluating the quantity and quality of plaque in orthodontically treated adolescents. The quantity was less affected than the microbial composition, and there was a shift to a plaque containing more potential periodontal pathogens. In addition, molar bands are more highly associated with gingival inflammation than bonded brackets, suggesting that plaque retention in the sulcus was decreased by bonded attachments that did not enter the sulcus.[31] However, little evidence implicates orthodontic therapy as a condition that causes severe periodontal consequences (Figure 5–13).

Currently, more than 20 percent of orthodontic patients in the United States are adults. That percentage is expected to grow. Boyd and others[32] showed that adult periodontal patients undergoing orthodontic therapy were no more likely to have increased attachment loss than adolescents or adults without periodontal disease if they received normal periodontal maintenance therapy at 3-month intervals.

Evidence suggests that dental hygienists find increased gingivitis and pathogenic plaque in all patients who are undergoing orthodontic treatment. All orthodontic patients, especially adults with periodontal disease, should receive regular dental hygiene care and maintain adequate plaque control.

Malocclusion

Malocclusion is not a cause of periodontal disease. Poorly aligned teeth can leave spaces and complicate daily plaque control and dental hygiene care, but malocclusion is not an initiator of pathology. A 20-year study of 176 adolescents examined for malocclusion in the teen years and subsequently examined in their 30s suggested a risk for periodontal disease, but no greater risk than that seen in men versus women and in lower socioeconomic groups versus higher socioeconomic groups. Specifically, subjects with crossbite, overjet, and crowding had higher gingivitis scores and more pocketing than did the comparison group with no malocclusion.[33] Severe periodontal destruction was rare and most pocketing was in the 3.5 to 5.5 mm range, suggesting that dental hygiene care would be sufficient to control the disease process. The dental hygienist must be aware of malocclusion and recognize the additional responsibility of both the patient and the clinician to create a clean, plaque-free environment. Figure 5–14 shows a patient with malocclusion contributing to the difficulty of plaque removal.

Unreplaced Missing Teeth

Unreplaced missing teeth can cause problems for the patient undergoing periodontal treatment. Missing teeth can allow more occlusal pressure on the remaining teeth and thus contribute to migration. Migration in periodontally

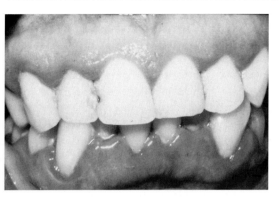

FIGURE 5-14. Malocclusion increases the difficulty of plaque control and can result in periodontal inflammation. The deep overbite and crowded mandibular teeth made plaque control difficult for this patient.

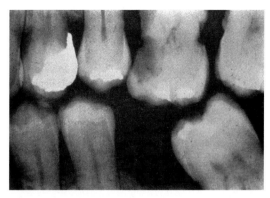

FIGURE 5-16. Radiograph of the consequences of an unreplaced mandibular first molar. Drifting, extrusion, and plaque retention resulted in altered occlusion, caries, and periodontal disease.

involved dentitions usually occurs in a mesial direction, and tilting or extrusion is common in the anterior areas. Premolars can drift distally.[27] Migrating teeth create spaces that complicate plaque control, and many patients find the extrusion and spreading of anterior teeth unsightly (Figure 5-15).

FIRST MOLAR LOSS SYNDROME

Often, permanent first molars are lost in childhood or the teen years. If the molar is not replaced, a classic set of changes occur in the dentition referred to as **first molar loss syndrome**. These changes do not predispose individuals to periodontal disease. Other than an association with gingivitis, first molar loss and other malocclusions have not been proven to initiate periodontal disease, but appear to affect the progress and severity of the disease.[27]

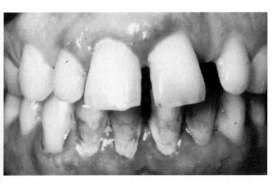

FIGURE 5-15. Pathologic migration of the anterior teeth resulted from the inflammatory process that reduced periodontal support for the teeth. This patient was very concerned about the changes in her appearance and was quite embarrassed by the spaces between the teeth.

The typical course of events after the loss of the permanent first molar is the following:[27]

1. The second and third molars drift mesially and tilt, creating spaces and causing loss of the vertical dimension.
2. The mandibular premolars drift distally and can tilt.
3. The maxillary first molar extrudes into space on the mandibular arch.
4. The anterior overbite is increased, causing the lower anterior teeth to strike the maxillary incisors on or near the gingiva. They can drift lingually, and the increased pressure can cause splaying or spreading of the maxillary anterior teeth.

Although they are not primarily responsible for initiating periodontal disease, these changes create areas of food impaction and spaces that are difficult to clean. In addition to providing periodontal treatment, the dental hygienist must identify these problems, educate the patient about them, and encourage replacement of missing molars. Figure 5-16 shows the classic radiographic appearance of first molar loss syndrome.

Mouth Breathing

Mouth breathing leads to localized gingival inflammation that is usually confined to the labial gingiva of the maxillary anterior teeth. The tissue becomes reddened and swollen, and it bleeds easily. The surface of the gingiva is shiny.[27, 34] Mouth breathing is also associated with higher levels of plaque and gingivitis.[29]

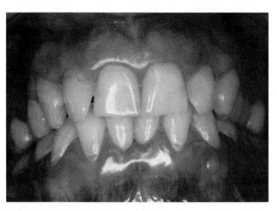

FIGURE 5–17. Mouth breathing results in swollen, shiny gingiva that bleeds easily and appears reddened on clinical examination. The inflamed appearance is unrelated to the amount of plaque present and does not respond to improved plaque control measures.

The gingival inflammation does not respond to periodontal therapy: inflammation persists despite dental hygiene care and plaque control. The inflammation is thought to occur because of the constant drying of the tissues; however, drying of tissue in laboratory animal studies has not reproduced the inflammation.[27] The best care for this condition is palliative, possibly placing petrolatum over the tissue. Figure 5–17 shows the gingival effects of mouth breathing.

Tobacco Use

The use of tobacco products, particularly cigarette smoking, has recently been strongly identified as a risk factor for periodontal disease. Tobacco smoking has long been associated with increased amounts of calculus and dental stains and the development of acute necrotizing ulcerative gingivitis.[35] The 1971–1974 National Health and Nutrition Examination Survey (commonly called NHANES) showed that adults with the highest levels of periodontal disease were also current smokers. Those with the lowest levels of periodontal disease were among the nonsmokers.[10] However, even stronger evidence has been found in the last decade. Bergstrom[36] compared a group of Swedish periodontal patients with a random sample of city dwellers and determined that smokers were 2.5 times more likely to have periodontal destruction. In addition, the prevalence and severity of diseased sites was greater in smokers than in nonsmokers with periodontal disease, even though the subjects had similar amounts of plaque and gingivitis. Bergstrom and Eliasson[37] also reported greater alveolar bone loss in smokers. Haber and others[38] compared smoking as a risk factor for periodontal disease in patients with insulin-dependent diabetes mellitus and in healthy subjects of similar age groups, 19 to 40 years old. The primary finding was that periodontitis was more severe and more prevalent among smokers than among nonsmokers, regardless of diabetic condition, although the prevalence and severity were slightly higher among subjects with diabetes. The findings also indicated that young smokers, aged 19 to 30, were 3.9 times as likely to have periodontal disease characterized by attachment loss of $\geq$ 2 mm and at least one site of probing depth of $\geq$ 5 mm. Smokers aged 31 to 40 were 2.8 times as likely to have periodontal disease. Statistically, smoking accounted for 56 percent of the periodontal disease in the 19- to 30-year-old subjects and 32 percent of the periodontal disease in the 31- to 40-year-old group. Even former smokers had a higher percentage of probing depths > 4 mm than those who had never smoked, but this finding was considerably less than that for current smokers.[38]

Haber and Kent[39] studied the extent of cigarette smoking among patients treated in periodontal offices compared with general dental offices. They reported that smokers were more often found in periodontal practices and that periodontal patients with moderate to advanced periodontal disease were 2.6 times more likely to be smokers. In addition, the frequency of current smoking was associated with increased disease severity.

The toxic effects of tobacco use, whether from forms of smoking or smokeless tobacco are recognized and of importance to dental hygienists and patients. Research has suggested a number of tobacco-induced changes that may be responsible for the increased periodontal disease seen in tobacco users. The epithelial cells of the gingiva show increased keratinization, and the buccal mucosa demonstrates altered oxygen consumption. Nicotine metabolites are found in saliva and gingival crevicular fluid. Polymorphonuclear leukocytes in smokers have a reduced ability to phagocytize substances, and the vascular reaction to inflammation is reduced in smokers. Users of smokeless tobacco, also called spit tobacco, are not safe from these harmful effects. In fact, a specific type of gingivitis, gingivitis toxica, is associated with the destruction of gingiva and bone underlying the location where smokeless tobacco rests in the mouths of users. Our understanding of the effects of tobacco is growing, and it is no longer considered an innocuous social habit, or one that affects only the heart and lungs (Figure 5–18).[27]

An interesting study identified the presence of nicotine or cotinine, the metabolic by-product of nicotine, on the root surfaces of recently extracted teeth from periodontal patients. The nicotine was absent from a sample that had been root planed before extraction.[40] This observation suggests that nicotine can be removed during periodontal therapy, leaving tooth surfaces more compatible with wound healing. However, the nicotine would be quickly replaced by the next cigarette, one likely consumed outside the dental practice door.

It is becoming clear that one responsibility of the dental hygienist is to recognize the serious effects of tobacco use on periodontal patients, educate patients about this relationship, and encourage them to quit using tobacco. The dental hygienist cannot take total responsibility for a tobacco cessation program, but should recognize that nicotine is an addiction and quitting a process. Education and positive reinforcement may help tobacco users to move toward the goal of quitting. It may be especially helpful to recommend that the periodontal patient who uses tobacco abstain during periodontal therapy, to maximize healing after therapy and encourage a move toward quitting.

CONCLUSION

Calculus and its removal are significant elements in guiding patients toward improved oral

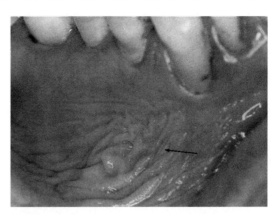

FIGURE 5–18. The effects of chewing tobacco on the oral mucosa. The arrow indicates wrinkled leukoplakia of the buccal mucosa caused by repeated placement of a chewing tobacco plug. Note the recession and staining on adjacent teeth also associated with habitual use of spit tobacco.

health. The dental hygienist must understand the importance of calculus and perfect the technical skills required to remove it in order to provide the best possible care for patients. It is important to note that regardless of the primary or secondary role of calculus in relationship to pocket formation, and although its principal irritating feature is surface plaque, calculus is a significant pathogenic factor in periodontal disease.[6]

Many local factors can also cause plaque retention, inhibit plaque control, and contribute to the development of periodontal inflammation. This chapter described a few major factors that are of particular importance to the dental hygienist. Awareness of these situations can help the dental hygienist to design more specific plaque control activities, encourage patients to seek further treatment, and contribute to the comprehensive care of the periodontal patient.

STUDY QUESTIONS

MULTIPLE CHOICE

1. The common name for calculus, tartar, was introduced in the 16th century by:

   a. Alfred Fones
   b. Irene Newman
   c. Paracelsus
   d. Pierre Fauchard

2. Which type of calculus is tightly adherent to the tooth and found near openings of the salivary ducts?

   a. supragingival
   b. subgingival
   c. serumal
   d. submarginal

3. The mineral content of subgingival calculus is derived from:

   a. crevicular fluid
   b. food particles
   c. saliva
   d. salivary ducts

4. How long does it take for plaque to begin to mineralize?

   a. 4 to 24 hours
   b. 24 to 72 hours
   c. 36 to 48 hours
   d. 72 to 96 hours

5. Each of the following characteristics is related to increased rates of calculus formation EXCEPT one. Which one is the EXCEPTION?

   a. concentration of calcium
   b. concentration of salivary bacterial protein and lipid
   c. elevated pH
   d. higher individual inhibitory factors

6. Subgingival calculus is always covered with dental plaque, and it causes greater progression of periodontal disease than plaque alone.

   a. Both statements are TRUE.
   b. Both statements are FALSE.
   c. The first statement is TRUE, the second is FALSE.
   d. The first statement is FALSE, the second is TRUE.

7. Adequate plaque control is more difficult to achieve with restored teeth because poorly contoured restorations do not retain plaque.

   a. Both statements are TRUE.
   b. Both statements are FALSE.
   c. The first statement is TRUE, the second is FALSE.
   d. The first statement is FALSE, the second is TRUE.

8. Significant tissue improvement occurs with calculus removal, and tissue health is unchanged by poorly contoured restoration.

   a. Both statements are TRUE.
   b. Both statements are FALSE.
   c. The first statement is TRUE, the second is FALSE.
   d. The first statement is FALSE, the second is TRUE.

9. The loss of the first molar is associated with periodontal disease because the condition can effect the extent and severity of disease.

   a. Both the statement and reason are correct and related.
   b. Both the statement and reason are correct but NOT related.
   c. The statement is correct but the reason is NOT.
   d. The statement is NOT correct but the reason is correct.
   e. NEITHER the statement NOR the reason is correct.

10. The toxic effects of tobacco use are caused by:

    a. changes in gingival and mucosal cells.
    b. decrease in the vascular reaction to inflammation.
    c. reduced ability of PMNs to phagocytize substances.
    d. all of the above.

SHORT ANSWER

11. Why was calculus believed to be an etiologic agent of periodontal disease?

    _____

    _____

12. What are the two main minerals found in calculus?

    _____

    _____

13. What do the landmark studies of Sri Lankan and Norwegian subjects and dental care demonstrate?

_____

_____

14. How does an anticalculus toothpaste work?

_____

_____

15. List and describe the plaque retentive factors that are linked to periodontal tissue problems.

_____

_____

REFERENCES

1. Mandel ID. Dental calculus (calcified dental plaque). In Genco RJ, Goldman HM, Cohen DW, eds. Contemporary Periodontics. St. Louis: CV Mosby, 1990:135-146.
2. Mandel ID, Gaffar A. Calculus revisited: a review. J Clin Periodontol 1986;13:249-257.
3. Pattanaporn K, Navia JM. The relationship of dental calculus to caries, gingivitis, and selected salivary factors in 11- to 13-year old Thai children in Chiang Mai, Thailand. J Periodontol 1998;69:955-961.
4. Albandar JM, Brown LJ, Brunelle JA, Löe H. Gingival state and dental calculus in early-onset periodontitis. J Periodontol 1996;67:953-959.
5. Wilkins EM. Dental Calculus. In Clinical Practice of the Dental Hygienist, 8th ed. Philadelphia: Lippincott Williams & Wilkins 1999;277-284.
6. Carranza FA Jr. Dental calculus. In FA Carranza, MG Newman, eds. Clinical Periodontology, 8th ed. Philadelphia: WB Saunders, 1996;150-160.
7. Allen DL, McFall WT Jr, Jenzano J. Microbiology and pathogenesis of inflammatory periodontal disease. In Periodontics for the Dental Hygienist, 4th ed. Philadelphia: Lea & Febiger, 1987;30-55.
8. Haake SK. Periodontal microbiology. In FA Carranza, MG Newman, eds. Clinical Peridontology, 8th ed. Philadelphia: WB Saunders, 1996:84-103.
9. Corbett TL, Dawes C. A comparison of the site-specificity of supragingival and subgingival calculus deposition. J Periodontol 1998;69:1-8.
10. Spolsky V. The epidemiology of gingival and periodontal disease. In FA Carranza, MG Newman, eds. Clinical Periodontology, 8th ed. Philadelphia: WB Saunders, 1996:61-81.
11. Anerud A, Löe H, Boysen H. The natural history and clinical course of calculus formation in man. J Clin Periodontol 1991;18:160-170.
12. Turesky S, Breuer M, Coffman G. The effect of certain systemic medications on oral calculus formation. J Periodontol 1992;63:871-875.
13. Breuer MM, Mboya SA, Moroi H, Turesky SS. Effects of selected beta-blockers on supragingival calculus formation. J Periodontol 1996;67:428-432.
14. Ramfjord SP. Long-term assessment of periodontal surgery versus curettage or scaling and root planing. Int J Technol Assess Health Care 1990;6:392-402.
15. Mallatt ME, Beiswanger BB, Stookey GK, Swancar JR, Hennon DK. Influence of soluble pyrophosphate on calculus formation in adults. J Dent Res 1985;64:1159-1162.
16. Zacherl WA, Pfeiffer HJ, Swancar JR. The effect of soluble pyrophosphates on dental calculus in adults. J Am Dent Assoc 1985;110:737-738.
17. Kazmierczak M, Mather M, Ciancio S, Fischman S. A clinical evaluation of anticalculus dentifrices. Clin Preventive Dent 1990;12:13-17.
18. Kohut BE, Rubin H, Baron HJ. The relative clinical effectiveness of three anticalculus dentifrices. Clin Preventive Dent 1989;11:13-16.
19. Leknes KN. The influence of anatomic and iatrogenic root surface characteristics on bacterial colonization and periodontal destruction: a review. J Periodontol 1997;68:507-516.
20. Sorensen JA. A rationale for comparison of plaque-retaining properties of crown systems. J Prosthet Dentistry 1989;62:264-269.
21. Bader JD, Rozier RG, McFall WT Jr, Ransey DL. Effect of crown margins on periodontal conditions in regularly attending patients. J Prosthet Dentistry 1991;65:75-79.
22. Kenney EB. Restorative-periodontal inter-relationships. In FA Carranza Jr, ed. Philadelphia: WB Saunders, 1990:924-955.
23. Brunsvold MA, Lane JJ. The prevalence of overhanging dental restorations and their relationship to periodontal disease. J Clin Periodontol 1990;17:67-72.
24. Kells BE, Linden GJ. Overhanging amalgam restorations in young adults attending a periodontal department. J Dent 1992;20:85-89.
25. Pack ARC. The amalgam overhang dilemma: a review of causes and effects, prevention, and removal. N Z Dent J 1989;85:55-58.
26. Tuominen R, Ranta K, Paunio I. Wearing of partial dentures in relation to periodontal pockets. J Oral Rehabil 1989;16:119-126.
27. Carranza FA Jr. The role of iatrogenic and other local factors. In FA Carranza, MG Newman, eds. Clinical Periodontology, 8th ed. Philadelphia: WB Saunders, 1996;161-173.
28. Wilkins EM. Care of dental prostheses. In Clinical Practice of the Dental Hygienist. Lippincott Williams & Wilkins 1999;394-410.
29. Wagaiyu EG, Ashley FP. Mouthbreathing, lip seal, and upper lip coverage and their relationship with gingival inflammation in 11-14 year-old school-children. J Clin Periodontol 1991;18:698-702.
30. Lang NP, Siegrist BE. Mechanical plaque retention factors. In Genco RJ, Goldman HM, Cohen DW, eds. Contemporary Periodontics. St. Louis: CV Mosby, 1990:170-183.
31. Alexander SA. Effects of orthodontic attachments on the gingival health of permanent second molars. Am J Orthod Dentofacial Orthop 1991;102:337-340.
32. Boyd RL, Leggott PJ, Quinn RS, Eakle WS, Chambers D. Periodontal implications of orthodontic treatment in adults with reduced or normal periodontal tissues versus those of adolescents. Am J Ortho Dentofacial Orthop 1989;100:191-199.
33. Helm S, Petersen PE. Causal relation between malocclusion and periodontal health. Acta Odontol Scand 1989;47:223-228.
34. Wilkins EM. Disease development and contributing factors. In Clinical Practice of the Dental Hygienist, 8th ed. Lippincott Williams & Wilkins 1996;224-235.
35. Carranza FA Jr. Acute gingival infections. In FA Carranza, MG Newman, eds. Clinical Periodontology, 8th ed. Philadelphia: WB Saunders, 1996;249-259.

36. Bergstrom J. Cigarette smoking as risk factor in chronic periodontal disease. Community Dent Oral Epidemiol 1989;17:245-247.
37. Bergstrom J, Eliasson S. Cigarette smoking and alveolar bone height in subjects with a high standard of oral hygiene. J Clin Periodontol 1987;14:446-469.
38. Haber J, Wattles J, Crowley M, Mandell R, Joshipura K, Kent RL. Evidence for cigarette smoking as a major risk factor for periodontitis. J Periodontol 1993;64:16-23.
39. Haber J, Kent RL. Cigarette smoking in a periodontal practice. J Periodontol 1992;63:100-106.
40. Cuff MJA, McQuade MJ, Scheidt MJ, Sutherland DE, Van Dyke TE. The presence of nicotine on root surfaces of periodontally diseased teeth in smokers. J Periodontol 1989;60:564-569.

6

Edward J. Taggart

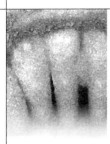

Gingival Diseases

Chapter Objectives

1. Define the types of gingivitis.
2. Relate the events in the pathogenesis of gingivitis to the clinical signs and symptoms.
3. Describe the role of the dental hygienist in the treatment of gingivitis.
4. Identify the medications that can cause gingival hyperplasia in patients.
5. List the similarities and differences in the clinical presentation of chronic gingivitis and other gingival conditions.

Key Terms

Dental plaque-induced gingivitis
   Gingivitis associated with dental
     plaque only
   Gingival diseases modified by systemic
     factors
   Gingival diseases modified by
     medications
   Gingival diseases modified by
     malnutrition

Non-plaque induced gingival lesions
   Gingival diseases of specific bacterial
     origin
   Gingival diseases of viral origin
   Gingival diseases of fungal origin
   Gingival lesions of genetic origin
   Gingival manifestations of systemic
     conditions
   Traumatic lesions
   Foreign body reactions

The dental hygienist plays a crucial role in the treatment of gingivitis and prevention of its recurrence. Diseases of the gingival tissues range from common forms, such as **dental plaque-induced gingivitis**, to rare, but potentially life-threatening forms, such as squamous cell carcinoma or acute leukemia. The dental hygienist may be the first member of the health care team to observe these lesions and bring them to the attention of the patient and other dental health professionals.

A description of the gingival tissues in health is presented in Chapter 2. To review, the gingival epithelium is usually described as pink or coral pink in color, with significant variation based on racial and genetic factors. The attached gingiva is tightly bound to the underlying connective tissue and is not movable. The papillae fill the interdental spaces completely. The surface epithelium of the attached gingiva is often

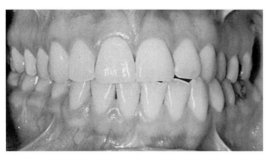

FIGURE 6-1. Normal gingiva. The clinical appearance of healthy gingiva: tissue is pink and uniform in color, stippling can be seen, and the papillae fill the interdental spaces. (See color figure.)

stippled and shows no signs of inflammatory color changes. The marginal gingiva reaches the tooth surface in a knife-edge pattern, and there are measurable sulcus depths of less than 3 mm. The gingival epithelium consists of a keratinized oral epithelium, a nonkeratinized or parakeratinized sulcular epithelium, and a junctional epithelium that forms the attachment to the root surface. Beneath the gingival epithelium, there is dense connective tissue coronal to the alveolar bone. This tissue is laced with bundles of collagen fibers. The normal appearance of healthy gingiva is shown in Figure 6-1 and appears in the color supplement.

GINGIVITIS

Gingivitis is inflammation of the gingival tissues. It occurs on a periodontium with no attachment loss or on a periodontium with attachment loss that is not progressing. Gingivitis manifests as color change (redness), edema (swelling of the tissues), exudate (drainage of gingival fluid from the sulcus), and a tendency to bleed readily (hemorrhage in response to gentle periodontal probing).[1] In addition, there may be changes in gingival contour, loss of tissue adaptation to the teeth, and an increased flow of gingival crevicular fluid.[2] Gingivitis is perhaps the most common human disease and among the easiest to treat and control. However, gingivitis is painless and often unrecognized. Many patients are unaware that they have it, and because it is so common, dentists and dental hygienists frequently do not emphasize its importance. Perhaps the best approach that dental hygienists and dentists can take is to

inform their patients that they have a disease, gingivitis, and that it is easily treated and cured. When the balance between disease and health is understood, patients often cooperate with dental hygiene care and improve their daily oral hygiene practices to cure the disease.

Pathogenesis of Gingival Disease

Pathogenesis is the events in the development and progression of a disease. The pathogenesis of gingivitis is best explained by describing the histology events as they relate to clinical signs. Extensive research on the pathogenesis of gingivitis over the last several decades has explained most of the events in the development of gingival inflammation. This information was obtained by observing humans and animals when bacterial plaque was allowed to accumulate. With these histologic observations, scientists have classified the development of gingival inflammation into three separate stages: an initial stage, an early stage, and an established stage.[3]

STAGE I GINGIVITIS (INITIAL OR SUBCLINICAL STAGE)

The initial stage of gingivitis occurs in the first few days of contact between microbial plaque and the gingival tissues. This stage is an acute inflammatory response that is characterized by dilation of the blood vessels. At this stage, the polymorphonuclear leukocytes (PMNs or neutrophils) attach to the vessel walls and begin to migrate into the surrounding connective tissues. Polymorphonuclear leukocytes (white blood cells with multi-lobulated nuclei) are the principal defense in acute inflammation. They phagocytize (engulf) bacteria, their products, and other products of destroyed tissue. Small amounts of plasma also leak into the surrounding tissues, causing edema in the tissues. PMNs amass in the connective tissue and migrate through the sulcular epithelium into plaque, forming exudate. Exudate from early gingival inflammation is composed mostly of serum and is referred to as "gingival fluid flow." The gingival fluid is clear, not yellow like pus, because few cells are present. A significant number of lymphocytes appear in the gingival connective tissues. These are almost all T-lymphocytes, the type that do not cause tissue damage but maintain a homeostatic response to bacterial infection.[4] In addition, there are epithelial cell changes and collagen degradation caused by activation of the host immune system. These first tissue reactions to plaque infection are not visible in the gingival tissues because they do not cause obvious clinical changes. This initial inflammatory response with no outwardly observable clinical signs is a subclinical infection. This initial lesion of gingivitis is also often referred to as stage I gingivitis.[5]

STAGE II GINGIVITIS (EARLY STAGE)

The next stage is known as early gingivitis. These lesions begin to form 4 to 7 days after plaque has accumulated in the gingival sulcus. The T-lymphocytes increase in number and are localized in the connective tissue under the epithelium of the gingival sulcus. The inflammatory exudate increases and may appear white or yellow. Clinically, the tissues appear slightly red and swollen. The increase in gingival fluid flow (exudate) reaches its peak 6 to 12 days after clinical redness is observed. The perivascular collagen fibers in the connective tissues are destroyed by the inflammation and replaced by blood plasma and inflammatory cell infiltrate. Collagen fibers that attach the underlying connective tissue to the gingival epithelium are also destroyed, and gingival stippling, if present, begins to disappear, causing the gingiva to appear shiny. The junctional epithelium begins to lengthen against the root surface, and it is disrupted by the migrating PMNs and lymphocytes. The gingival tissues tend to bleed when gently probed. Cellular changes occur in the connective tissue fibroblasts, leading to their destruction, probably related to interaction with the lymphoid tissues. The early stage of gingivitis may continue for 21 days or longer. It is the earliest clinical evidence of gingivitis. Early gingivitis has also been called stage II gingivitis.[5]

STAGE III GINGIVITIS (ESTABLISHED STAGE)

After 15 to 21 days, the gingival inflammation reaches the established stage, also called stage III gingivitis.[5] There is a distinct change in the type of white blood cells seen in histologic specimens. Plasma cells, usually associated with an intense antigen–antibody response, are present. T-lymphocytes and B-lymphocytes are found in equal amounts, indicating that tissue destruction by the inflammatory reaction is taking place. B-lymphocytes are related to cell surface immunity and release lymphokines that accelerate the tissue destruction in inflammation. More connective tissue collagen is destroyed, and the junctional epithelium begins to thicken and extend apically on the root surface as well as deep into the underlying connective tissues. This activity represents a conversion of the junctional epithelium into one correctly described as pocket epithelium. The clinical probing depth increases for two reasons. The periodontal probe penetrates more deeply through the junctional epithelium into the connective tissue by about 1 mm because of the loss of collagen, and edema in the tissues moves the gingival margin coronally, increasing the probe readings.

The blood vessels proliferate into capillary loops that reach nearly to the basement membrane of the epithelium, permitting more seepage of serum into the tissues and through the sulcular epithelium. That change, along with the increased presence and activity of inflammatory cells, causes visible pus formation. Capillary proliferation also causes the gingiva to appear red. In extreme cases of congested blood cells in the gingiva, the tissue appears blue because of the presence of many oxygen-depleted red blood cells. In combination, these changes result in red, swollen, and shiny gingiva that exhibit noticeable pus formation and gingival exudate.

The established gingivitis lesion may persist unchanged for months or years. The condition is reversible when plaque is regularly removed permitting the tissues to return to normal without residual tissue destruction.[2] The pathogenesis of gingivitis is summarized in Table 6–1.

Healing of the Gingiva after Treatment

The sequence of healing events is the reverse of those described for the pathogenesis. Healing of gingivitis begins in the connective tissues. The inflammatory cells are replaced by fibroblasts, which lay down a firm extracellular matrix of collagen. With maturity, these fibers become functionally oriented and produce a dense subgingival connective tissue. This connective tissue does not permit penetration of the periodontal probe tip, thus reducing the clinical periodontal probing depth. The gingival

TABLE 6–1. Correlation of Clinical Signs to the Pathogenesis of Gingivitis

Stage	Clinical Signs	Pathologic Events
Initial (Stage I)	None (subclinical infection)	Blood vessels dilate Polymorphonuclear leukocytes migrate into connective tissue Plasma leaks into connective tissue Gingival fluid exits pockets T-lymphocytes predominate
Early (Stage II)	Gingiva may redden Stippling disappears Exudate may appear Bleeding usually occurs on probing	T-lymphocytes increase Cells congregate under sulcular epithelium Gingival fluid increases Collagen is destroyed Lengthened junctional epithelium is disrupted Fibroblasts are destroyed
Established (Stage III)	Gingiva is reddened Gingiva may appear blue-red Probing depths increase Pus forms Tissue swells	Capillaries proliferate T- and B-lymphocytes occur in equal numbers Extensive collagen destruction occurs Junctional epithelium thickens and rete pegs extend into the connective tissue Plasma cells infiltrate Edema increases

color returns to pink as the proliferation of inflammatory cells resolves, and stippling reappears when serum no longer leaks into the tissues to cause edema.

In some cases, stable gingivitis transforms into progressive disease. This change results in advanced lesions with bone destruction, progressing from gingivitis to periodontitis.[4] Periodontitis is discussed in Chapter 7.

Gingivitis has been classified into a number of categories based on clinical manifestations of the disease, etiology, association with systemic diseases, association with medications, or other causes. The classification of gingival diseases and conditions is presented in Table 6–2.

DENTAL PLAQUE-INDUCED GINGIVAL DISEASE

Gingivitis occurs very commonly in all levels of society, rich or poor, industrial or agricultural. The most obvious symptom is bleeding gums. So many people live with this condition that they are often not aware that it is a disease. Many patients will tell the dental hygienist that they believe that everyone's gums bleed, or they always expect their gums to bleed when they brush their teeth. Despite this common assumption, it is true that the gingiva becomes inflamed due to the presence of dental plaque. The following section describes gingivitis and some factors that contribute to the disease.

GINGIVITIS ASSOCIATED WITH DENTAL PLAQUE ONLY

The most common form of gingivitis found in the general population is **gingivitis associated with dental plaque only**, also called **plaque-associated gingivitis**, or gingivitis. This disease is directly related to the presence of bacterial plaque on the tooth surface.[1]

Clinically, gingivitis causes a reddened gingival margin, with pocket formation as a result of gingival swelling and edema, hypertrophy, and deepened penetration of periodontal probes on clinical evaluation. The surface of the gingiva may appear glazed or smooth, and stippling, when present in health, usually disappears. Microscopically, there is an increase in capillaries along the gingival margin, and the epithelium lining the gingival sulcus is ulcerated. This ulceration results in a tendency to bleed when a periodontal probe is placed in the gingival crevice. Bleeding in response to gentle probing is the major clinical indicator of gingivitis. Another common feature of chronic gingivitis is a clear gingival fluid flow, or exudate, which appears to increase with the severity of the gingivitis. Figure 6–2 shows the typical appearance of dental plaque-induced gingivitis. It also appears in the color supplement.

Gingivitis appears to be directly related to the amount of plaque on the tooth surface and the amount of time that the plaque is allowed to remain undisturbed. The plaque is considered

TABLE 6–2. Classification of Gingival Diseases and Conditions[6] (Including illustrated diseases and conditions)

Dental Plaque-Induced Gingival Diseases
Gingivitis associated with dental plaque only
    Describing the gingival condition
    Experimental gingivitis
    Plaque-induced gingivitis modified by local
      contributing factors
Gingival diseases modified by systemic factors
    Endocrine-influenced gingival disease
Gingival diseases modified by medications
Gingival diseases modified by malnutrition

Non-Plaque Induced Gingival Lesions
Gingival diseases of specific bacterial origin
    Acute necrotizing ulcerative gingivitis
Gingival diseases of viral origin
    Primary herpetic gingivostomatitis
Gingival diseases of fungal origin
    Candidiasis of the gingiva
Gingival lesions of genetic origin
    Gingival enlargement
Gingival manifestations of systemic conditions
    Blood dyscrasias-associated gingivitis
      Acute leukemia
    Gingival manifestations of dermatologic disease
      Lichen planus
      Mucous membrane pemphigoid
      Desquamative gingivitis
Traumatic lesions
Foreign body reactions

nonspecific because it is not associated with any specific type of microorganisms. The mature plaque found in long-standing gingivitis has a large percentage of Gram-negative bacteria. This change from Gram-positive plaque associated with health, or healthy plaque, to predominantly Gram-negative plaque, or pathogenic plaque, is characteristic of gingivitis.

Distribution of Gingivitis. Plaque-associated gingivitis may be further classified by its location and the degree of involvement in the dentition. It may be localized to a few teeth or generalized throughout the mouth. It may be limited to the interdental papilla, spread along the entire gingival margin, or involve all of the attached gingival tissues. By definition, gingivitis does not involve the periodontal attachment tissues, and there is no loss of connective tissue attachment to the tooth and no loss of supporting bone.

Describing the Gingival Condition. Gingival tissue descriptions should be recorded in the patient chart. The location and extent of gingivitis should be noted. The terms commonly used to describe the tissues include localized, generalized, marginal, papillary, slight, moderate, and severe inflammation of the gingiva. These descriptors can be combined depending on the extent and severity of the gingivitis. It is also helpful to describe the color, shape, and shininess of the tissues. An example of a good gingival description is "localized inflammation, redness, and swelling on the buccal and lingual posterior sextants" or "generalized severe inflammation, tissues intensely red, with rounded, shiny marginal and papillary gingiva, bleeds easily on probing." These clinical descriptors reflect the histologic changes that have occurred and permit the dental hygienist to evaluate changes in the clinical appearance at subsequent appointments.

Experimental Gingivitis. Gingivitis has been induced and studied experimentally in healthy patients by discontinuing all oral hygiene procedures and permitting bacterial plaque to accumulate.[7] This disease is called experimental gingivitis. Studies have shown that no one is completely resistant to the activity of dental plaque if sufficient time is allowed for symptoms to develop. In general, clinical signs of inflammation occur in everyone within 10 to 21 days after the cessation of plaque control, but subclinical signs of disease occur much earlier.

Gingivitis is reversible. In the experimental setting, the signs and symptoms of gingivitis disappeared in approximately 1 week when

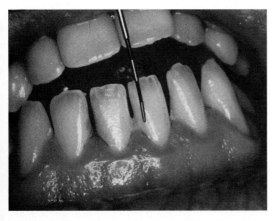

FIGURE 6–2. Plaque-associated gingivitis. The clinical signs of plaque-associated gingivitis are an intense inflammatory response at the gingival margin and bleeding in response to gentle probing. Clinically, the marginal gingiva is very red. (See color figure.)

good plaque control was reinstituted. It is important for the dental hygienist to understand that adequate removal of dental plaque on a daily basis, along with the appropriate periodic recall to remove calculus and other irritants, cures gingivitis and prevents it from recurring.

Evidence of complete resolution of gingival inflammation is presented in Figure 6-3. The importance of regular maintenance appointments, or recalls, is described in Chapter 15.

Many other conditions can lead to gingival inflammation. These are much less common

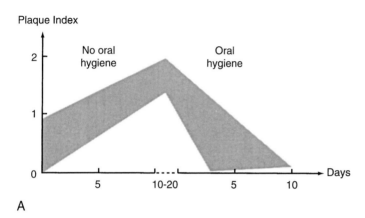

A

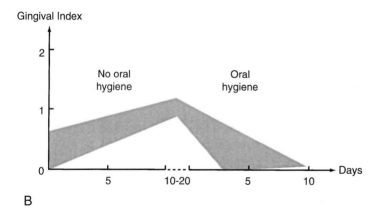

B

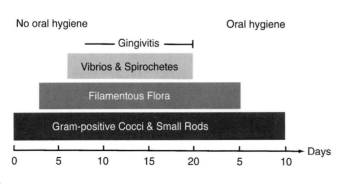

C

FIGURE 6–3. The effects of experimental gingivitis on healthy young adults. **A.** Accumulation of plaque and debris when no oral hygiene procedures were performed. The Plaque Index scores for subjects at the beginning of the experiment ranged from 0 to just under 1. This score indicates that no plaque was visible in any of the subjects. After 10 to 21 days, all subjects had plaque indices above 1 and approaching 2, indicating visible plaque. The shaded area shows the range of plaque scores for subjects. Oral hygiene was reinstituted at day 21, and plaque scores returned to near 0. In some subjects, the score returned to 0 in as little as 3 days, but other subjects took as long as 10 days to achieve a score of 0. **B.** The Gingival Index scores also increased for all individuals during the experiment. The shaded area shows the range of scores among subjects. Scores approached 1, indicating clinical redness (gingivitis), after 10 to 21 days with no oral hygiene. When oral hygiene procedures were reinstituted at day 21, scores returned to baseline levels or below. This finding suggests that all individuals are susceptible to plaque-induced inflammation and that this condition is reversible. **C.** Plaque-induced inflammation is associated with changes in the microflora of the plaque. The graph shows that Gram-positive cocci and small rods persisted in the plaque found at the gingival margin throughout the experiment. However, filamentous forms, vibrios, and spirochetes appeared after the plaque had accumulated for several days. These forms disappeared rapidly when plaque control was reinstituted at day 21. This finding indicates that different floras are associated with gingival health and disease. (Used with permission from Löe H, Theilade E, Jensen SB. Experimental gingivitis in man. J Periodontol 1965;36:177–187.)

than plaque-associated gingivitis, but they are important to recognize. The dental hygienist must distinguish between common gingivitis and conditions with other causes because treatment and healing results differ.

Plaque-Induced Gingivitis Modified by Local Contributing Factors. Although plaque-induced gingivitis may occur with the accumulation of dental plaque alone, there are often tooth-related factors that modify or predispose a localized gingivitis. Such factors include malposed or crowded teeth, dental restorations, or orthodontic appliances. These factors called "plaque traps" usually act to retain plaque and serve to make oral hygiene practices more difficult and less effective. They do not cause the gingivitis, but ordinary daily cleaning practices that may be adequate in other places in the mouth are not sufficient to remove enough plaque in these places, and therefore do not prevent inflammation from occurring. Figure 6-4 shows examples of gingivitis that has occurred in response to plaque accumulation and local contributing factors. These figures also appear in the color supplement.

GINGIVAL DISEASES MODIFIED BY SYSTEMIC FACTORS

Many systemic factors act to modify the manner in which the individual's immune system responds to the assault of accumulated dental plaque. Some conditions that alone do not cause gingivitis may act to intensify it, resulting in **gingival diseases modified by systemic factors.** For example, circulating corticosteroids associated with stress change the environment and may result in a more pathologic

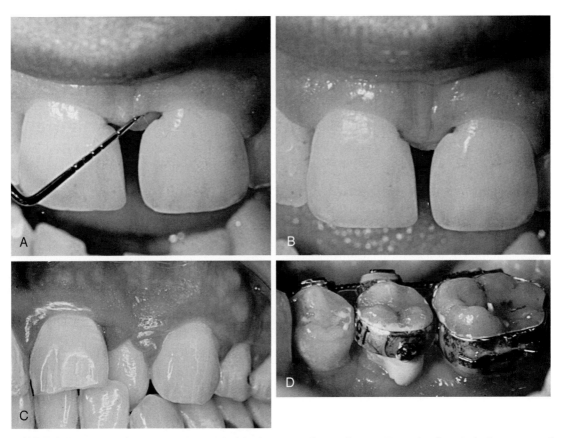

FIGURE 6–4. Plaque-induced gingivitis modified by local contributing factors. (See color figure.) **A.** Overcontoured restorations with probe retracting tissues. In an effort to minimize the large diastema, the dentist constructed acrylic veneers that help fill the space on the mesial surfaces of the central incisors. This created a significant plaque trap. **B.** Overhanging restorations, probe removed. After the probe was withdrawn, the gingival tissues bled, indicating the presence of gingivitis. **C.** Malposed teeth. The lateral incisor is in crossbite and rests palatal to the central incisor and canine. This occlusion resulted in alterations in the size and shape of the embrasure spaces and papilla, making brushing and flossing a challenge. **D.** Orthodontic appliances. Plaque control is poor in this patient and is made more difficult by the presence of orthodontic bands. In addition, excess cement was left protruding over the gingival margin, creating a terrible plaque trap.

plaque.[8] Changes in the endocrine system, such as hormonal changes in puberty, during the menstrual cycle, or pregnancy, are frequently, but not always, associated with inflammatory changes in the gingiva. The following section describes the more commonly seen gingival changes associated with these fluctuations in hormone production.

Endocrine-Influenced Gingival Disease. Gingivitis is often influenced by steroid-type hormones produced by the endocrine glands. These include the hormones associated with puberty, pregnancy, and the use of birth control medications. When female hormone levels are increased, there is an increase in some subgingival bacteria, such as *Bacteroides* species, and gingival inflammation may be greater.[9] There are estrogen receptors in the gingival tissues, and serum concentrations of female sex hormones during pregnancy influence the gingival tissues.[10] Estrogen may also regulate cellular proliferation, keratinization, and vascular proliferation, and vascular fragility in the gingival tissues.[11] The extent of hormone-related changes, like many of the others discussed, is related to the level of plaque control.[12] Poor plaque control aggravates the condition, underscoring the importance of proper home care and regular dental hygiene care.

Several changes in the gingiva have been associated with pregnancy. As hormone levels increase during the second trimester of pregnancy, gingival inflammation may increase significantly. This increase occurs even with good plaque control, but it may be substantial when plaque control is marginal or poor. The gingiva may become dark red and hyperplastic, and may bleed excessively. Figure 6–5 is an example of pregnancy gingivitis. It also appears in the color supplement. Changes may increase as the pregnancy progresses.[13] Most pregnancy-related gingivitis improves or resolves with good home care and removal of local irritants. Sometimes it does not heal completely until after the baby is born and hormone levels return to normal.

Another striking feature in some pregnant women is the presence of a specific type of gingival lesion, a pregnancy tumor. This lesion is not really a tumor, such as a neoplasm, but a localized area of pyogenic granulation tissue. The tissues are highly inflamed, bleed easily, and may cause teeth to be mobile and possibly migrate out of the way. As in other types of

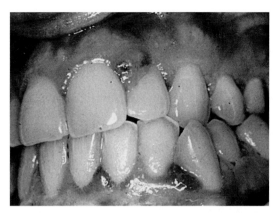

FIGURE 6–5. Pregnancy gingivitis. Hormonally influenced gingivitis was seen in this 27-year-old white female who was 7 months pregnant and had poor plaque control. The gingival margin was intensely red and swollen. This tissue was extremely painful, making oral hygiene practices more difficult and causing the patient to consume a soft diet which resulted in more plaque growth and accumulation. Dental hygiene care improved the condition but it did not completely resolve until after the baby was born. (See color figure.)

gingival enlargement, poor plaque control is related to the severity of the inflammation, and some localized trauma may have occurred. Most lesions resolve after parturition, but in some cases, surgical removal of residual enlargement is required. Figure 6-6 shows an example of pregnancy gingivitis and a so-called "pregnancy tumor." It also appears in the color supplement.

Gingival changes associated with pregnancy have been observed in women who are taking

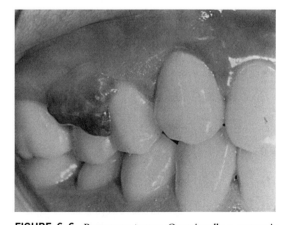

FIGURE 6–6. Pregnancy tumor. Occasionally a pyogenic granuloma, commonly called pregnancy tumor, will appear during pregnancy. Improved oral hygiene and dental hygiene care improved the condition. Many small "tumors" resolve after delivery. In this case, the granuloma was large, and although it shrank after the baby was born, it was surgically removed. (See color figure.)

oral contraceptives or older women who are taking hormone replacement therapy to mitigate symptoms associated with menopause. In general, changes include an increase in gingival inflammation that appears out of proportion to the amount of supragingival plaque present. This condition clearly does not occur in all women. Two mechanisms may cause this significant response: (1) There may be an increase in some potentially pathogenic bacteria, such as *Porphyromonas gingivalis* and *Actinobacillus actinomycetemcomitans*. (2) There may be an increase in prostaglandin E, a mediator of inflammation. Both circumstances would increase the inflammatory response. However, hormone drugs are important to women's health, and their benefits may greatly outweigh any potential side effects to the oral health. For example, evidence suggests that osteoporosis associated with menopause may be a risk factor for periodontal disease.[14] Reducing osteoporosis through the use of hormone supplements may be far more critical than the potential increase of gingival inflammation associated with hormone replacement therapy.

GINGIVAL DISEASES MODIFIED BY MEDICATIONS

A variety of medications can cause changes in the gingival tissues resulting in **gingival diseases modified by medications**. Most commonly, the anti-seizure medication phenytoin has long been associated with gingival overgrowth. This drug is often used to control the seizures that occur with various forms of epilepsy. The gingival tissues may become fibrotic and enlarged. Studies have shown that the enlargement is caused by changes in the epithelial cells and the fibroblasts that create a more dense connective tissue. These changes can be seen even in tissue cultures of cells grown in the laboratory. There is also some evidence that an increase in bacterial plaque causes a concurrent increase in gingival overgrowth in patients taking phenytoin.[15] Therefore, in patients taking this medication, excellent plaque control is necessary to prevent or slow the formation of enlarged gingiva.

Medication-induced gingival enlargement results in gingival contours that enhance plaque accumulation and make plaque removal more difficult. Patients often have heavy calculus formation and increased levels of inflammation because of plaque retention. Treatment of this type of gingival enlargement requires good home care, regular scaling and root planing and, often, surgical reduction of the enlargements with surgical gingivectomy procedures.

Some cardiac medications also cause overgrowth of gingival tissues. These include nifedipine and verapamil, which are commonly used to control blood pressure and reduce recurrence in patients who have had a heart attack. Both of these agents are classified as calcium channel blockers. As these medications become more commonly prescribed, dental hygienists will see more patients with this type of gingival enlargement. As with phenytoin, there is some evidence that excellent plaque control helps to control the symptoms of hyperplasia and gingivitis. Regular dental hygiene care is important to limit the effects of these drugs to the gingiva. Figure 6–7 shows examples of drug-induced gingival enlargement. It also appears in the color supplement.

Another medication that causes gingival overgrowth is cyclosporine, the major drug used for immunosuppression in transplant patients. This medication may also be used to treat multiple sclerosis.[16] Unlike phenytoin- or nifedipine-induced hyperplasia, which is usually limited to the gingiva, cyclosporine can cause excessive accumulation of connective tissue in many other tissues of the body. Most transplant patients take cyclosporine, so this drug is increasingly found in dental patients. In addition, patients with heart, liver, and kidney transplants are taking both cyclosporine and nifedipine. In these cases, gingival enlargement may be extreme. The dental hygienist should remember that many of these patients have complicated medical histories, and the patient should be questioned carefully about the reason for taking these medications. These patients usually require consultation with their physicians before undergoing any dental therapy, including dental hygiene treatment. Figure 6–8 shows gingival enlargement that occurred subsequent to the use of cyclosporin. It also appears in the color supplement.

GINGIVAL DISEASES MODIFIED BY MALNUTRITION

Although relatively rare in developed countries, serious nutritional deficiencies modify the body's response to dental plaque. Deficiencies

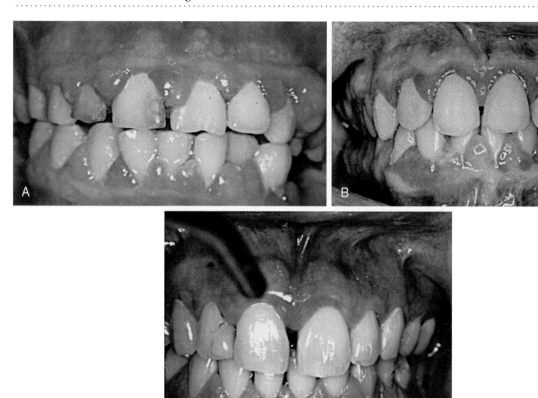

FIGURE 6–7. Drug-induced gingival enlargement. (See color figure.) **A.** Gingival enlargement often results from drug treatment with phenytoin to control seizures. This 23-year-old white male had significant gingival enlargements complicated with intense gingivitis caused by poor plaque control. The patient underwent the surgical procedure gingivectomy (see Chapter 13) one year earlier, and the overgrowth returned. **B.** Another example of phenytoin-induced enlargement, also termed Dilantin hyperplasia, occurred in this young adult male. Gingivectomy was performed and the enlargement recurred in just a few months. (Courtesy of UCSF Division of Periodontology.) **C.** Gingival enlargement has been noted with the use of the drug nifedipine to reduce heart disease and hypertension. This 50-year-old male had been taking nifedipine for two years. Note the swollen interdental papillae particularly on the mandibular anterior teeth. The tissue improved with dental hygiene care but the enlargement remained.

in many vitamins can produce changes in the oral tissues referred to as **gingival diseases modified by malnutrition**. These vitamins include A, B_1, B_2, B_6, and vitamin C. The relationship of ascorbic acid vitamin C, has been the most studied. Vitamin C deficiency causes scurvy, a severe condition resulting in defective collagen formation and maintenance. The gingiva becomes very hemorrhagic and swollen, and the condition rapidly progresses to advanced periodontitis characterized by extensive bone loss and extremely loose teeth.[17, 18] Severe vitamin C deficiency is quite rare today and relatively small amounts of ascorbic acid, largely found in citrus fruits, prevents it. However, sailors on long sea voyages in the 17th and 18th centuries experienced these symptoms quite commonly. As this nutritional deficiency became understood, the British navy stowed limes on its sailing ships to provide the crews with a source of vitamin C. The sailors would suck the limes and became known as "limeys." Figure 6-9 is an example of gingival disease associated with severe malnutrition. It also appears in the color supplement.

NON-PLAQUE INDUCED GINGIVAL LESIONS

Dental plaque is not the only cause of changes in the gingiva. Many systemic infections caused by specific bacteria, such as those found in gonorrhea and syphilis may have gingival signs and symptoms. Fungal infections such as Candida and histoplasmosis may also be manifested in the gingival tissues. Perhaps the most common condition noted in the gingival tissues, usually in young people, is caused by the virus

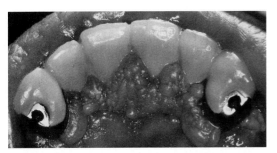

FIGURE 6–8. Drug-induced gingival enlargement. Gingival enlargement occurred in a 54-year-old white male who had undergone a kidney transplant. He was taking cyclosporine to prevent organ rejection and verapamil to control his blood pressure. The lesions developed over a period of 2 years. The bulbous, rounded, bubbly surface of the gingiva is a classic sign of drug-induced gingival enlargement. Verapamil also caused dry mouth in this patient, making him susceptible to tooth decay around the crown margins. Gingivectomy could remove this excess tissue; however, it would expose the crown margins and increase the risk of cervical caries. No gingivectomy was performed. (See color figure.)

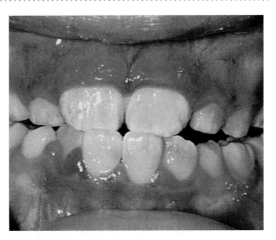

FIGURE 6–10. Streptococcal infection. This 6-year-old presented with a history of high fever and sore throat. Oral examination revealed an acute gingivitis, especially around the erupting incisors. Laboratory culture confirmed streptococcal infection. (See color figure.)

Herpes simplex. These conditions require antimicrobial interventions or, in the case of viruses, usually run their course. Some of the most common **non-plaque induced gingival lesions** are described in the following sections. These are often seen in the dental office because the patients think the infections are of dental origin. In addition, the dental hygienist may be able to help the patient by treating the overlying gingivitis.

GINGIVAL DISEASES OF SPECIFIC BACTERIAL ORIGIN

Many common bacterial infections can occur in the mouth causing **gingival diseases of**

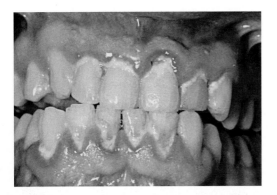

FIGURE 6–9. Malnutrition. This severe gingivitis was seen in an older, homeless female patient who had consumed an extremely restricted diet for many months, noticeably deficient in vitamin C. There was intense redness of the gingiva and thick exudate. The teeth had grade I and grade II mobility. (See color figure.)

specific bacterial origin. An example of concern to parents is streptococcal infection of the throat and oral tissues including the gingiva that may be seen in young children. Figure 6-10 is an example of this condition. It also appears in the color supplement. Sexually transmitted diseases such as meningococcal gonorrhea or syphilis have oral manifestations. These examples are less commonly seen in dental offices. However, the following section describes one disease that was extremely common until about thirty years ago; it is less common now but is still seen and treated by dental hygienists.

Necrotizing Ulcerative Gingivitis. Necrotizing ulcerative gingivitis (NUG) is a disease that occurs occasionally in young adults. This disease was called acute necrotizing ulcerative gingivitis. NUG is a periodontal disease that can occur with no bone loss and a bacterial component. It is common enough that cases are sometimes seen in general dental practices. NUG is related to excessive stress. Outbreaks have been reported after examination periods at colleges and universities. Historically, this relationship to stress is shown by the common name for NUG, "trench mouth." This condition was widespread among soldiers in the trenches during World War I, probably because of stress and poor oral hygiene. NUG is painful. Patients often have sudden onset of burning mouth and inability to eat. The disease most commonly begins in the interdental papillae. After a few days, the tips of the papillae appear punched out and covered by a white necrotic pseudo-membrane. This covering is referred to as a pseudomembrane because the white membrane covering the punched-out papillae is simply a collection of PMNs trapped in the fibrin clot. The attached gingival tissues are usually inflamed. There is often a distinctive breath odor that has been termed "fetor oris" that is unique to this disease. These clinical signs are often all that is needed to make the diagnosis. Figure 6–11 is an example of NUG. It also appears in the color supplement.

A significant feature of NUG infection is the presence of two microorganisms, a fusiform bacillus and a spirochete. These so-called "Vincent's organisms" (the disease was originally identified as Vincent's angina), appear to be present in all cases of NUG. Authorities believe that spirochetes may play an important role in the infection, but a direct causative effect has not been proven.[19] Occasionally, patients have a fever. Antibiotics such as penicillin and metronidazole are useful in the treatment of NUG, but are recommended only if the patient has systemic symptoms of fever and severe malaise.

The treatment for NUG is to completely debride the tissues of plaque and to begin a home regimen of excellent plaque control. Although the gingival tissues are tender, careful scaling with curettes or ultrasonic scalers can be performed, usually over the course of two or more appointments. Patients obtain relief after scaling treatment and postoperatively by rinsing with a dilute solution of hydrogen peroxide and warm water. Repeated bouts of NUG may cause permanent gingival deformation and leave the patient at higher risk for periodontal disease. Untreated, this disease may lead to bone loss and become necrotizing ulcerative periodontitis (NUP).

GINGIVAL DISEASES OF VIRAL ORIGIN

Gingival disease of viral origin may resemble plaque-induced gingivitis. However, these conditions have been studied much less extensively. One viral infection in particular, herpes virus infection, requires deeper understanding because it is highly contagious, very common, and can easily be transmitted to the dental hygienist. The primary form of herpetic infection is described in the following section. There are also secondary forms of the infection that occur around the mouth. These lesions are called "cold sores" or "fever blisters." These are also highly contagious but do not resemble gingivitis. For further information regarding secondary herpetic infections and the various types of herpes viruses, an oral pathology text will provide a full explanation.

Primary Herpetic Gingivostomatitis. Primary herpetic gingivostomatitis, or primary herpes infection, is a common condition, although it is not technically a gingival disease. It must be differentiated from ANUG because the symptoms are similar. This disease is more likely to occur in younger children and adolescents than ANUG, but it is also seen in young adults or middle-aged patients. There are several signs that the dental hygienist may note that differen-

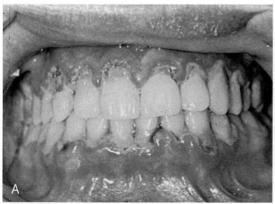
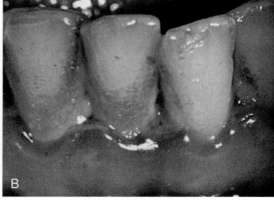

FIGURE 6–11. Acute necrotizing ulcerative gingivitis. **A.** Lesions seen in a 20-year-old male college student characterized by punched-out papillae covered by a pseudomembrane. The patient exhibited fetor oris. **B.** Close-up view of the pseudomembrane and cratering of papillae in the lower anterior area of another male college student. The patient had been under severe stress and smoked two packs of cigarettes per day. (Courtesy of UCSF Division of Periodontology.)

tiate primary herpes from ANUG. Elevated temperature is more common in primary herpes than in ANUG, and the patient usually appears much more ill, exhibiting greater malaise. Perhaps the most important distinguishing feature of primary herpes is vesicle formation. Many vesicles will coalesce into ulcerative lesions located on the gingiva or oral mucosa. This appearance contrasts with the punched-out interdental papillae found in ANUG. Although the patient may have strong breath odor because of poor plaque control, the distinctive fetor oris of ANUG is absent. Figure 6-12 is an example of primary herpetic infection. It also appears in the color supplement.

GINGIVAL DISEASES OF FUNGAL ORIGIN

Fungal organisms have been associated with gingival conditions. Although several fungi species can infect the oral tissues, the most common is *Candida albicans*. It is quite common to observe erythematous and fragile gingival and mucosal tissues under dentures in the mouths of patients who have worn prostheses for long periods of time. These **gingival diseases of fungal origin** are caused by an over-

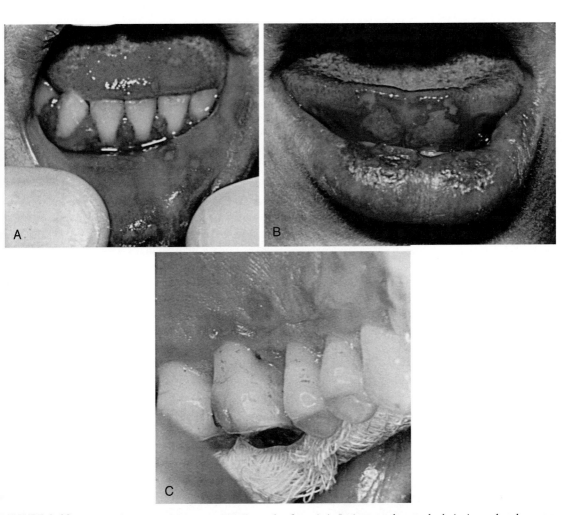

FIGURE 6–12. Primary herpetic gingivostomatitis. (See color figure.) **A.** Lesions on the attached gingiva and oral mucosa characterize this disease. The lip ulcers and inflamed gingiva in this 14-year-old female patient were extremely painful. (Courtesy of Joseph A. Regezi, DDS, MS.) **B.** The vesicles of the herpetic lesions can coalesce to form large ulcers as seen under the tongue of the same patient. (Courtesy of Joseph A. Regezi, DDS, MS.) **C.** Secondary herpetic infections or post-treatment herpetic infection are also seen in the dental office. One week after scaling and root planing, this patient presented with small, painful vesicles on the gingiva adjacent to the area that was treated. The condition resolved without further treatment. Herpes lesions shed virus into the saliva and oral environment. Patients with either primary or secondary herpetic lesions should be reappointed for dental treatment after the lesions have resolved to prevent spread of the lesions and inoculation of the dental hygienist. (Courtesy of the UCSF Division of Periodontology.)

growth of *C. albicans* and must be treated with antifungal or antiseptic therapies, or both.

Candidiasis of the Gingiva. Fungal infections may occur on the gingiva and other oral tissues. The most common are caused by the yeast organism, *Candida albicans*. There have been reports of *Candida* isolated from the gingiva of otherwise healthy patients with periodontitis.[20] In recent years, *Candida* infections have been associated with some of the signs of gingival disease observed in patients with pronounced immunosuppression, such as those with human immunodeficiency virus (HIV). The gingival conditions caused by *Candida* range from initial signs of redness at the gingival margin, called linear gingival erythema, to severe redness with white patches on the gingiva. The white patches are accumulations of organisms and debris that easily rub off the gingiva, exposing ulcerated tissue. Although the exact mechanism for this infection is still under investigation, it has been suggested that HIV infection may alter the lymphocyte response to *Candida albicans*.[21] It is important to remember that individuals who are immunosuppressed for any reason, including organ transplants, are at risk for oral fungal infections. Figure 6–13 is an example of *Candida* infection associated with HIV. It also appears in the color supplement.

GINGIVAL LESIONS OF GENETIC ORIGIN

Some individuals have gingival changes that seem to be genetically predisposed. Research into genetic diseases is a vastly growing disci-

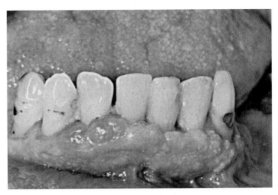

FIGURE 6–14. Idiopathic gingival enlargement (gingival enlargement of unknown origin). These lesions were present in a 61-year-old white male. A pebbled surface and enlarged papillae are seen between the lower right central and lateral incisors, creating a diastema. Periodontal probing depths were within normal limits. (See color figure.)

pline, and much more information will be available as human genome research continues. One disease that may be observed by the dental hygienist is gingival enlargement described in the following section.

Gingival Enlargement. Gingival enlargement, historically termed "hyperplasia" or "hypertrophy," is a pathologic overgrowth of the gingiva. It has a variety of causes, so its actual incidence in the population is not known. Gingival enlargement may be caused by excessive reactions to bacterial plaque, a variety of medications, or infections, or it may occur as a side effect of systemic diseases, as previously described. Gingival hypertrophy related to plaque and other factors is important for the dental hygienist to recognize because there are several important diseases that may be observed in the gingiva. These conditions do not respond to good plaque control with complete healing. However, plaque control through patient education and dental hygiene care is important because poor patient plaque control worsens most of these gingival conditions. A case of gingival enlargement is presented in Figure 6–14. It also appears in the color supplement.

In all cases, when the oral tissues appear dramatically different from what would be expected with chronic plaque-associated gingivitis, the patient should be evaluated for possible systemic disease. If excessive gingivitis is seen, the patient should be treated appropriately and re-evaluated in 2 to 4 weeks to ensure that the clinical situation has resolved. If it has not, the

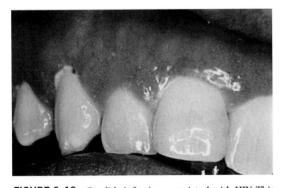

FIGURE 6–13. Candida infection associated with HIV. This 35-year-old white male presented with a severe gingivitis with white, membranous deposits. Note the mass of white material at the gingival margin on the buccal surface of the cuspid. Histologic smear of the white material revealed the characteristic hyphae found in these infections. The patient was treated with antifungal medication and good oral hygiene care. (See color figure.)

dental hygienist and dentist should consider further evaluation and possible referral of the patient to a specialist.

GINGIVAL MANIFESTATIONS OF SYSTEMIC CONDITIONS

Certain systemic conditions can result in changes to the gingival tissues. Although rare compared to plaque-induced gingivitis, they are important and must be considered when evaluating a patient with gingival inflammation that does not appear to be consistent with the amount of plaque observed. The more common of these conditions are related to mucocutaneous disorders or dermatologic diseases. Others include blood dyscrasias. Only the **gingival manifestations of systemic conditions** that are occasionally seen in the dental office will be described in the following sections. For a further discussion of other systemic diseases, please see Chapter 17.

Blood Dyscrasias-Associated Gingivitis.[6] There are many blood dyscrasias. They are of significant health risk to the patient and are not often observed in the dental office. One condition, acute leukemia, is sometimes first seen in the dental office because of the quick onset of gingival changes. These may be the first dramatic symptoms of the disease and will cause the patient to seek dental treatment, not knowing that the problem is medical.

ACUTE LEUKEMIA. Acute leukemia is a life-threatening disease that may be seen initially in the gingival tissues. This condition causes hemorrhagic and swollen gingival tissues, far more pronounced than would be expected from the amount of plaque and calculus present. The patient often reports that the tissues were normal until recently. The gums bleed easily and are swollen and tender. Sometimes the dental hygienist is the first health provider to recognize that this is not dental plaque-induced gingivitis. Figure 6–15 is an example of a gingival condition associated with acute leukemia. It also appears in the color supplement.

Gingival Manifestations of Dermatologic Disease. Many other systemic diseases are manifested in the gingival tissues. The more common diseases are related to dermatologic diseases such as lichen planus and benign mucous membrane pemphigoid. These diseases must be recognized so that patients can receive appropriate therapeutic and palliative care.

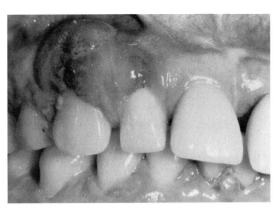

FIGURE 6–15. Acute leukemia. A 35-year-old female presented with severely swollen and painful gingiva that was intensely inflamed with granulation-type tissue. The pain was so severe that the patient could not brush her teeth and was reluctant to eat. In these cases dental hygiene care will not produce normal healing, although it may improve the condition. (See color figure.)

LICHEN PLANUS. Lichen planus is a chronic disease thought to be immune related. It affects the skin and mucous membranes of middle-aged patients. Men and women are equally affected. It occurs in a variety of forms, ranging from the common asymptomatic reticular form with keratotic lines called striae, to the relatively rare erosive and bullous forms in which portions of the lesions become ulcerated and painful.

The reticular form commonly affects the gingival tissues and usually appears as lacy white lines (Wickham's striae) with a bumpy appearance. There may be areas of white lesions alternating with raw, reddened areas in the erosive form of lichen planus. The severity of this disease appears to be related to the stress level of the patient. Most studies suggest that this disease is caused by a cell-mediated immune reaction, although the mechanism is not known. Skin lesions are less common and appear as a rash of small, flat-topped papules that tend to itch. There is concern about the potential of the erosive form of lichen planus to transform into squamous cell carcinoma. For this reason, periodic observation of this chronic condition is warranted. Topical steroids have been used to control this disease during flare-ups, but no known cure has been developed.[22] Figure 6–16 presents an example of gingival changes associated with lichen planus. It also appears in the color supplement.

MUCOUS MEMBRANE PEMPHIGOID. Benign mu-

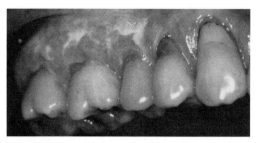

FIGURE 6–16. Lichen planus. Lichen planus on the buccal gingiva in a 71-year-old female appeared as a lacy, white, flat lesion. It was generally asymptomatic, with occasional flare-ups that the patient described as tender. Symptoms were relieved by topical steroid application. Good plaque control should be encouraged in these cases, even if the lesions are sore. (See color figure.) (Courtesy of UCSF Division of Periodontology.)

cous membrane pemphigoid, or more correctly, cicatricial pemphigoid, is a chronic vesiculobullous disease that is seen as blistering and sloughing of the surface of gingival epithelium. Although its etiology is not known, it is considered an autoimmune reaction, similar to lichen planus. It is more common in older individuals and much more common in women than in men. These lesions may also appear on other oral tissues, such as the buccal mucosa and the inner surface of the lips, helping to distinguish them from common plaque-associated gingivitis. Symptoms of the gingival lesions range from mild discomfort to painful raw, bleeding areas because the epithelium actually strips away from the underlying connective tissue. This peeling of the epithelium when rubbed, known as Nikolsky's sign, may prevent the patient from

performing any form of oral hygiene. Eating can be difficult, and the patient may switch to a diet of soft foods to avoid having anything touch the painful gingival surface. Figure 6-17 is an example of mucous membrane pemphigoid. It also appears in the color supplement. Treatment is often palliative at best, but steroid therapy may help to relieve symptoms. Topical corticosteroids may bring gingival lesions under control and allow for better eating habits and plaque control. Chlorhexidine mouth rinses may help to control plaque accumulation and permit the topical steroids to lessen the intensity of these lesions.[22]

DESQUAMATIVE GINGIVITIS. When cicatricial pemphigoid lesions are limited to the gingival tissues, the disease may be termed desquamative gingivitis or gingivosis. This condition is most often described as sloughing of the gingival epithelium, leaving a painfully raw, red surface. Figure 6-18 is an example of desquamative gingivitis or gingivosis. It also appears in the color supplement. The etiology is suspected to be autoimmune, but desquamative gingivitis may also be caused by allergic reactions to drugs, food, or other substances.[23] As with other pemphigoid lesions, meticulous plaque control may help, but it is often difficult for the patient to perform because of the painful erosive lesions. The disease may continue for many years or, particularly in children, may disappear spontaneously. Topical and systemic steroid therapy may help to control the disease process.

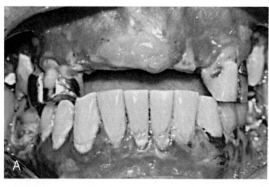
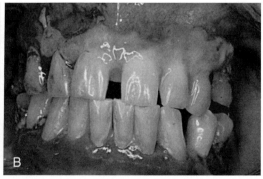

FIGURE 6–17. Benign mucous membrane pemphigoid. (See color figure.) **A.** This case is an 81-year-old woman with highly inflamed gingiva. The epithelium sloughed when rubbed with gauze, leaving a raw, bleeding surface. The maxillary partial denture that replaced the anterior teeth may have irritated the tissue further. The patient experienced significant pain when eating and brushing the teeth, so plaque control was difficult. The condition improved with dental hygiene care. **B.** This 64-year-old female presented with painful and sloughing gingiva. Note the areas she was able to brush have less severe inflammation. (Courtesy of Joseph A. Regezi, DDS, MS.)

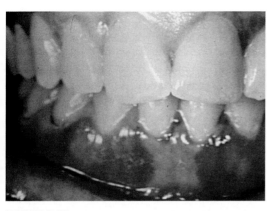

FIGURE 6–18. Desquamative gingivitis. Desquamative gingivitis in this 14-year-old white female exhibited bullous lesions (splits in the tissue). Tissues were intensely inflamed and painful. In these cases, plaque control is important to reduce the inflammation. Oxygenating mouth rinses may also help relieve symptoms. (See color figure.) (Courtesy of UCSF Division of Periodontology.)

TRAUMATIC LESIONS

Often the gingival tissues are damaged by trauma. These **traumatic lesions** can be painful and be a surprise finding made by the patient. Common lesions seen in dental hygiene practice are burns from foods such as hot pizza or burritos, chemical burns from aspirin placed on the gingiva for pain relief, or cuts from chicken bones or hard bread crusts. Some interesting cases of advanced recession caused by trauma are illustrated here in Figure 6–19. The pictures also appear in the color supplement.

FOREIGN BODY REACTIONS

Damage to gingival tissue, similar to traumatic lesions, can be caused by **foreign body reactions** in or near the tissues. A relatively common lesion observed in dental practices is an acute gingival reaction to food impaction

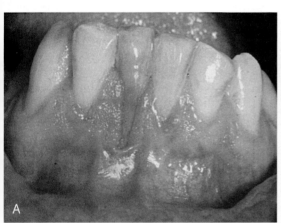

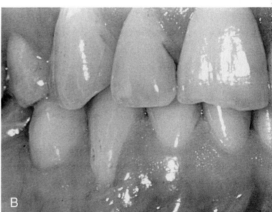

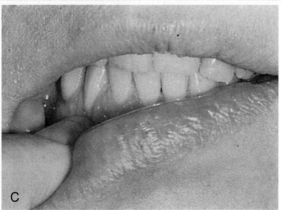

FIGURE 6–19. Traumatic lesions of the gingiva. (See color figure.) **A.** This patient presented with excessive gingival recession on the buccal surface of the mandibular central incisor. His deep overbite caused this recession by actually scraping away the gingival tissue every time the patient closed the teeth together. The condition has stabilized with this amount of recession and has not changed for several years. **B.** The dental hygienist noted an area of unexplained localized gingival recession on the mandibular left cuspid. No etiology could be identified. While questioning this patient, the hygienist noticed her nervous habit of scratching the tooth root with her fingernail. **C.** The cause of the recession was the repeated traumatic injury illustrated in this photograph.

from food particles such as popcorn husks or apple skins. These are localized painful lesions with sudden onset. Often a good dental history will reveal the source, and removal of the foreign substance will bring immediate relief. Figure 6–20 is an example of such an acute gingival reaction. It also appears in the color supplement.

DENTAL HYGIENE CARE

Dental hygiene care is a critical part of the treatment of gingival conditions. In all of the conditions described in this chapter, the dental hygienist can improve the patient's comfort and gingival health, even if the gingival condition cannot be cured.

Plaque-induced gingivitis may be one of the most common human diseases. It is certainly the most common periodontal disease.[24] The relationship between the accumulation of bacterial plaque and gingival inflammation has been well documented. The importance of this relationship cannot be minimized because gingival disease will develop in anyone if plaque is allowed to accumulate. No person is genetically resistant to plaque-induced gingivitis. The bacterial nature of plaque-induced gingivitis appears to be nonspecific. The overall composition of the plaque in gingivitis is different from that in health, but no specific bacteria are usually responsible. Therefore, the control and prevention of gingivitis is a primary responsibility of the patient and the dental hygienist, with therapy and home care aimed at reducing all of the bacterial plaque on the tooth surfaces.

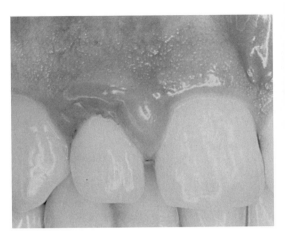

FIGURE 6–20. Foreign body reaction. This patient presented with red, swollen tissue in one interproximal area. The papilla was very painful and bled with slight provocation. The dental history revealed that the swelling and soreness had started suddenly the previous weekend. Exploration of the area using a periodontal probe and curette dislodged a popcorn husk imbedded in the sulcus. When the husk was removed, the patient felt immediate pain relief and the lesion resolved in two days. (See color figure.)

Other gingival diseases or manifestations of systemic diseases can mimic dental plaque-induced gingivitis and may be exacerbated by poor plaque control and the presence of local irritants. For this reason, it is important to recognize unusual conditions and distinguish them from chronic gingivitis. Dental hygiene care will always consist of patient education and the removal of local irritants to promote healing. The level of responsibility, frequency, and results of treatment may vary, but the patient's condition can be improved with dental hygiene care.

STUDY QUESTIONS

MULTIPLE CHOICE

1. Edema is which of the following?

   a. drainage
   b. hemorrhage
   c. redness
   d. swelling

2. Which stage of gingival inflammation begins within 4 to 7 days after plaque has accumulated in the sulcus and may be seen as slightly red and swollen?

   a. initial stage
   b. early stage
   c. established stage

3. At which stage of gingival inflammation can bleeding from the sulcus be detected with a periodontal probe?

   a. initial stage
   b. early stage
   c. established stage

4. Dental plaque-induced gingivitis is reversible when bacterial plaque is removed.

   a. Both statements are TRUE.
   b. Both statements are FALSE.
   c. The first statement is TRUE and the second is FALSE.
   d. The first statement is FALSE and the second is TRUE.

5. Plaque traps cause increased accumulation of dental plaque in specific areas and may contribute to the development of gingivitis.

   a. Both statements are TRUE.
   b. Both statements are FALSE.
   c. The first statement is TRUE and the second is FALSE.
   d. The first statement is FALSE and the second is TRUE.

6. What is the first and major clinical feature of dental plaque-induced gingivitis?

   a. drainage
   b. hemorrhage
   c. redness
   d. swelling

7. Clinical signs of inflammation will appear approximately how many days after all plaque control measures are discontinued?

   a. 5 to 7
   b. 7 to 9
   c. 10 to 21
   d. 21 to 36

8. Which gingival condition is characterized by pain, vesicle formation, burning mouth, and the inability to eat?

   a. acute leukemia
   b. acute necrotizing ulcerative gingivitis
   c. phenytoin hyperplasia
   d. primary herpetic gingivostomatitis

9. Which calcium channel blocker can cause excessive growth of gingival tissues?

   a. cyclosporine
   b. nefidipine
   c. phenytoin
   d. corticosteroid

10. A "pregnancy tumor" is a localized area of pyogenic granulation tissue and is a neoplastic lesion.

    a. Both statements are TRUE.
    b. Both statements are FALSE.
    c. The first statement is TRUE and the second is FALSE.
    d. The first statement is FALSE and the second is TRUE.

SHORT ANSWER

11. List the classifications of gingival diseases.

    _____

    _____

12. Why is the bacterial plaque in chronic gingivitis considered nonspecific?

    _____

    _____

13. Describe the changes in gingival tissues that may occur during pregnancy.

    _____

    _____

14. What is the primary way to treat and prevent chronic gingivitis?

    _____

    _____

REFERENCES

1. American Academy of Periodontology. Proceedings of the World Workshop on Clinical Periodontology. Chicago: American Academy of Periodontology, 1989:I-2.

2. American Academy of Periodontology. The pathogenesis of periodontal diseases. J. Periodontol 1999;70:457–470.

3. Page RC, Schroeder HE. Periodontitis in Man and Other Animals. A Comparative Review. Basel, Karger; 1982:5–45.

4. Page RC, Schroeder HE. Structure and pathogenesis. In Schluger S, Yuodelis R, Page RC, Johnson RH. Periodontal Diseases. Philadelphia: Lea & Febiger, 1990:186,203.

5. Carranza F, Perry DA. Clinical Periodontology for the Dental Hygienists. Philadelphia: WB Saunders, 1986:25.

6. Armitage GC. Development of a classification system for periodontal diseases and conditions. Ann Periodontal 1999;4:1-6.

7. Löe H, Theilade E, Jensen SB. Experimental gingivitis in man. J Periodontol 1965;36:177-187.

8. Atkinson PT. Refractory adult periodontitis: the influence of repressive coping style. Dissertation, Fielding Inst. UMI diss serv #9826502; Ann Arbor MI; 1998.

9. Kornman KS. Age, supragingival plaque, and steroid hormones as eclological determinants of the subgingiva flora. In Genco RJ, Mergenhagen SE, eds. Host-Parasite Interactions in Periodontal Diseases, Washington, DC: American Society for Microbiology, 1982:132-138.

10. Hugoson A. Gingival inflammation and female sex hormones: a clinical investigation of pregnant women and experimental studies in dogs. J Peridontal Res 1970;5:1-18.

11. Vittek J, Hernandez JR, Wenk EJ, Rappaport SC, Southren AL. Specific estrogen receptors in human gingiva. J Clin Endocrinol Metab 1982;54:608-612.

12. Silness J, Löe H. Periodontal disease in pregnancy: Part II. Correlation between oral hygiene and periodontal condition. Acta Odontol Scand 1964;22:121-135.

13. Löe H, Silness J. Periodontal disease in pregnancy: Part I. Prevalence and severity. Acta Odontol Scand 1963;21:533-551.

14. van Wowern N, Kausen B, Kollerup G. Osteoporosis: a risk factor in periodontal disease. J Periodontol 1994;65:1134-1138.

15. O'Neil T, Figures K. The effects of chlorhexidine and mechanical methods of plaque control on the recurrence of gingival hyperplasia in young patients taking phenytoin. Br Dent J 1982;152:130-133.

16. Hefti AF, Eshenaur AE, Hassell TM, Stone C. Gingival overgrowth in cyclosporine: A treated multiple sclerosis patient. J Periodontol 1994;65:744-749.

17. Woolfe SN, Hume WR, Kenney EB. Ascorbic acid and periodontal disease: a review of the literature. J Western Soc Periodontol 1980;28:44-52.

18. Charbeneau TD, Hurt WC. Gingival findings in spontaneous scurvy. A case report. J Periodontol 1983;54:694-697.

19. Listgarten MA. Electron microscopic observations of the bacterial flora of acute necrotizing ulcerative gingivitis. J Periodontol 1965;36:328-339.

20. Rams TE, Slots J. Candida biotypes in human adult periodontitis. Oral Microbiol Immunol 1991;6:191-192.

21. Lamster IB, Grbic JT, Mitchell-Lewis DA, Begg MD, Mitchell A. New concepts regarding the pathogenesis of periodontal disease in HIV infection. Ann Periodontol; 1998;3:62-67.

22. Regezi JA, Sciubba J. Oral Pathology: Clinical-pathologic Correlations, 2nd ed. Philadelphia: WB Saunders, 1993;21-25, 114-120.

23. Nisengard RJ, Neiders M. Desquamative lesions of the gingiva. J Periodontol 1981;52:500-510.

24. Page RC. Oral health status in the United States: prevalence of inflammatory periodontal diseases. J Dent Educ 1985;49:354-364.

7

Edward J. Taggart

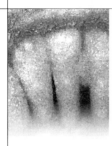

Periodontal Diseases

*C*hapter *O*bjectives

1. Describe the pathogenesis of periodontitis, and list the factors that affect disease progression.
2. List and describe the American Academy of Periodontology categories of periodontal diagnosis and the five case types of periodontal disease.
3. Compare and contrast the following forms of periodontitis as to demographics and clinical characteristics:
   a. aggressive periodontitis
   b. chronic periodontitis
   c. early-onset periodontitis
   d. juvenile periodontitis
   e. necrotizing ulcerative periodontitis
   f. periodontitis as a manifestation of systemic disease
   g. prepubertal periodontitis
   h. refractory periodontitis
4. State the role of systemic antibiotic treatment, locally delivered controlled-release antibiotic treatment, and enzyme suppression treatment in periodontitis.

*K*ey *T*erms

Abscess
Acquired deformities
Aggressive periodontitis
Antibiotic therapy
Bone loss
Chronic periodontitis
Clinical attachment loss
Developmental deformities

Enzyme suppression therapy
Necrotizing ulcerative periodontitis
Pathogenesis
Pathogenicity
Periodontal disease
Periodontitis
Risk factor

Periodontal disease is an inclusive term describing any disease of the tissues surrounding the teeth, including gingival diseases and diseases of the supporting structures. This chapter describes forms of **periodontitis**, the periodontal diseases of the supporting tissues.

Periodontitis is a set of periodontal diseases. It is characterized by inflammation of the supporting tissues of the teeth, specifically the periodontal ligament, cementum, and alveolar bone.[1] Unlike gingivitis, which is limited to the epithelium and gingival connective tissues, periodontitis results in loss of connective tissue attachment to the cementum of the tooth root. Loss of attachment results in deepening of the gingival sulcus to form a periodontal pocket by migration of the junctional epithelium along the root surface. The result is recession, **bone loss**, or both. Left unchecked, periodontitis causes a weakened periodontium characterized by mobile teeth that are susceptible to abscess formation. The disease can be uncomfortable and unsightly. Teeth are lost; they simply fall out, or they are extracted if they become acutely infected or are not treatable by periodontal or restorative dental methods.

Periodontitis is characterized by tissue inflammation, loss of connective tissue, and destruction of collagen fibers. The condition is seen clinically as pocket formation. Loss of alveolar bone also results from the spread of inflammation triggering bone resorption.

Periodontitis occurs in a variety of forms. Most forms of periodontal disease are clearly related to bacterial plaque accumulation and retention. Because of the strong association between plaque and periodontal disease, the most significant determinants of successful treatment are the consistent removal of plaque on a daily basis by the patient (home care, or personal plaque control) and the removal of plaque, the products of plaque, calculus, and plaque retention factors (such as overhanging restorations, open margins, and defects on the tooth surface) at appropriate intervals by the dental hygienist or dentist.

CLASSIFICATION OF PERIODONTITIS

The American Academy of Periodontology has recommended classifying periodontitis into a number of general categories based on its etiology, clinical presentation, **pathogenesis**, progression, and response to therapy.[2] Seven categories of periodontitis are recognized, but they probably represent many different bacterial infections with similar symptoms. An additional category describes **developmental or acquired deformities** that are related to periodontitis. See Classification of Periodontal Diseases and Conditions.[2]

CHRONIC PERIODONTITIS

Chronic periodontitis is the most common form of **periodontal disease**. When most clinicians refer to periodontitis or periodontal disease, they are referring to the diagnosis of chronic periodontitis. In this chapter, the terms are used interchangeably except when the term chronic periodontitis is used to differentiate one disease entity from another.

Chronic periodontitis may have its preclinical onset in adolescence, and, unless halted by therapy, it appears to progress continually for the life of the individual. This disease is characterized by bone resorption that progresses slowly and predominantly in a horizontal direction. It is not usually significant clinically until about the age of 35 years, although recent evidence suggests it may occur at any age. Epidemiologic evidence suggests periodontitis may occur more commonly among United States males than females, but this is not a consistent

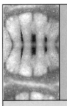

CLASSIFICATION OF PERIODONTAL DISEASES AND CONDITIONS[2]

  I. Gingival Diseases (refer to Chapter 6)
 II. Chronic Periodontitis
     A. Localized ($\leq$30% of involved sites)
     B. Generalized (>30% of involved sites)
III. Aggressive Periodontitis
     A. Localized
     B. Generalized
 IV. Periodontitis as a Manifestation of Systemic Disease
  V. Necrotizing Periodontal Disease
     A. Necrotizing ulcerative gingivitis (NUG) (refer to Chapter 6)
     B. Necrotizing ulcerative periodontitis
 VI. Abscess of the Periodontium
VII. Periodontitis Associated with Endodontic Lesions
VIII. Developmental or Acquired Deformities and Conditions

finding throughout the world. It may be explained by the fact that females visit the dentist more regularly in this country and therefore may benefit from more prevention and earlier treatment (see Chapter 2).

The severity of the disease is directly related to the accumulation of plaque and calculus on the surfaces of the teeth. The rate of periodontal destruction may vary depending on the disease activity and the patient's resistance. Chronic periodontitis is not associated with systemic disease or abnormalities in host defense.

Chronic periodontitis is a prevalent disease that may be either localized or generalized and progresses slowly until the teeth are lost by either exfoliation or extraction. The progression of periodontitis appears to occur in episodic bursts of activity that cause attachment loss.[3] The disease progresses in the presence of pathologic dental plaque, and attachment loss occurs when collagen fibers in the local area are destroyed. Disease activity halts when the host resistance controls the disease process through therapy or natural defenses.

It is difficult to determine when chronic periodontitis is actively causing destruction rather than being in a quiescent state of equilibrium between the disease processes and the host defenses. The most reliable method is to document the loss of periodontal attachment (**clinical attachment loss** or CAL) over time. This measurement documents increases in the distance from the cementoenamel junction to the apical depth of the periodontal pocket. The method requires successive measurements over time, weeks, months, or years. It does not tell you if the disease is actively progressing at the moment you examine the patient.

A subclassification system dividing chronic periodontitis into case types related to the severity of disease has been suggested by the American Academy of Periodontology. This system is convenient for approximate categorization of disease severity. Classifying the disease as slight, moderate, or advanced periodontitis aids in determining appropriate treatment plans and reimbursement levels.[4] Some patients have combinations of disease severity. It is common to find slight or moderate periodontal disease with one area or more of severe periodontitis characterized by much greater attachment loss.

There are also defined case types for gingivitis and refractory periodontitis (a form of aggressive periodontitis). The case types are shown in Classification of Periodontal Disease. This classification is useful for communication and treatment planning purposes, but it is intentionally vague and does not define specific periodontal infections.

Other classifications have been proposed for dental hygienists and dentists to use in assessing

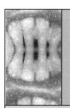

AMERICAN ACADEMY OF PERIODONTOLOGY DISEASE CLASSIFICATION

Case Type I: Gingivitis
Inflammation of the gingiva characterized clinically by changes in color, gingival form, position, surface appearance, and the presence of bleeding, or exudate.

Case Type II: Slight Chronic Periodontitis
Progression of the gingival inflammation into the deeper periodontal structures and alveolar bone crest, with slight bone loss. There is usually a slight loss of connective tissue attachment and alveolar bone.

Case Type III: Moderate Chronic or Aggressive Periodontitis
A more advanced stage of periodontitis, with increased destruction of the periodontal structures and noticeable loss of bone support, possibly accompanied by increased tooth mobility. There may be furcation involvement in multirooted teeth.

Case Type IV: Advanced Chronic or Aggressive Periodontitis
Further progression of periodontitis, with major loss of alveolar bone support, usually accompanied by increased tooth mobility. Furcation involvement in multirooted teeth is likely.

Case Type V: Refractory Chronic or Aggressive Periodontitis
Multiple disease sites that continue to show attachment loss after apparently appropriate therapy. These sites presumably continue to be infected by periodontal pathogens, no matter how thoroughly or frequently therapy is provided. This category includes patients with recurrent disease at a few or many sites.

patients with chronic periodontitis. A sub-classification based on the degree of attachment loss may be more useful for determining the destructiveness of periodontitis in specific cases. This classification system is shown in Table 7-1.[5]

The defining element for classifying periodontal disease is not probing depth, but the level of attachment loss from the cementoenamel junction, indicating bone loss. This concept is important for the dental hygienist to remember. Probing pocket depth (also called probe depth, probing depth, or pocket depth) is significant because the patient's ability to adequately clean deepened pockets is greatly reduced. In addition, deepened periodontal pockets usually require instrumentation of complex root anatomy, including flutes, grooves, and furcation areas. For this reason, instrumentation of the root surface is more difficult and the prognosis for the tooth may be negative. However, the degree of periodontal disease severity is directly related to the amount of periodontal ligament destroyed and the amount of bone lost. The bone does not begin exactly at the cementoenamel junction, but is 1 to 2 mm apical to it in the healthy state. Therefore, viewing radiographs is an indispensable aid in assessing the severity of bone loss in periodontal disease (Figure 7-1, also in color supplement).

Patients with a diagnosis of slight to moderate chronic periodontitis may often be treated in a general dental practice, with the dental hygienist taking a major role in therapy. However, patients with a diagnosis of advanced periodontitis are best treated in a specialty periodontics practice. Although an important part of the treatment may be performed by the dental hygienist in the periodontist's office, the patient should be referred to a specialist for evaluation before any periodontal treatment is begun. With this approach, all signs of the disease will still be evident to assist the periodontist in diagnosis and treatment planning.

Chronic periodontitis is considered a multibacterial disease. Plaque from diseased sites contains high levels of anaerobic and gram-negative organisms. It also contains elevated levels of spirochetes. Of the primary pathogens associated with periodontal diseases, *Porphyromonas gingivalis* is perhaps the most common species identified.[6] Other species commonly found in high levels in chronic periodontitis include *Bacteroides forsythus*, *Prevotella intermedia*, *Camphylobacter rectus*, *Eikenella corrodens*, *Fusobacterium nucleatum*, *Actinomyces actinomycetemcomitans*, and *Treponema* and *Eubacterium* species. In addition, periodontal disease progression is associated with *P. gingivalis*, *P. intermedia*, *B. forsythus*, *C. rectus*, and *A. actinomycetemcomitans*.[7] This extremely complex microbiology is being studied extensively, which will lead to developments in both diagnosis and treatment for periodontal diseases. For further understanding of plaque bacteria, see Chapter 4.

Bacterial diagnosis of periodontal diseases is an exciting area of research in periodontology. But until this complex plaque is better understood, clinical rather than bacteriologic diagnosis remains the best method of classifying periodontal disease. A significant number of cases of chronic periodontitis have been reported without detection of *P. gingivalis* or other suspected forms of periodontal pathogens in the pockets.[8]

The complex plaque in periodontitis constitutes a mixed infection. Antibiotics are not usually indicated in its treatment because the goal of treatment is not the eradication of all bacteria; rather, it is to replace the infection with younger, less established plaque that is associated with health. Healthy plaque can usually be created by mechanical debridement through scaling and plaque removal procedures.

Most patients with periodontal disease have this chronic form of periodontal disease. It affects around 5 percent to 20 percent of the adult population in the U.S. Although this is a very complex disease, the Consensus Report of the World Workshop (AAP) identified the following characteristics of chronic periodontitis:

- Most prevalent in adults, but may appear in children and adolescents
- Periodontal destruction is consistent with the amount of local factors
- Subgingival calculus is frequently found

TABLE 7-1. Severity of Periodontal Diseases[2] Evaluated by Clinical Attachment Loss (CAL)

Severity	CAL Measurements
Slight	1–2 mm
Moderate	3–4 mm
Severe	≥5 mm

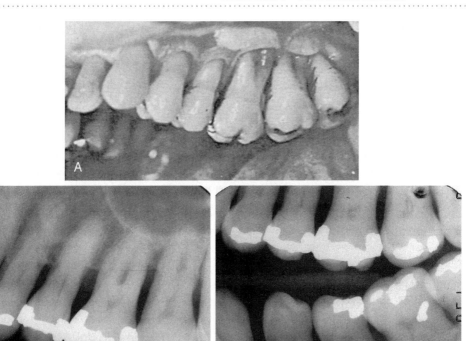

FIGURE 7–1. Clinical attachment loss, not probing depth, is the primary indicator of periodontal bone loss. **A.** This case is a 65-year-old male with advanced bone loss and attachment loss, but minimal probing pocket depths of 2 to 3 mm in the maxillary right posterior sextant. This patient was treated 20 years ago with nonsurgical periodontal therapy. His condition has been stable for 20 years because of good oral hygiene and regular periodontal maintenance at 3- to 4-month intervals. The stain seen on the proximal root surfaces is due to daily use of 0.12% chlorhexidine mouthrinse. (See color figure.) **B.** Periapical radiograph of the maxillary right posterior area. Advanced bone loss and furcation involvement are seen in the first molar. **C.** Bitewing radiograph of the right side. It is not possible to see the level of bone loss in the bitewing; therefore, periapical radiographs or vertical bitewings are required to adequately determine the degree of bone loss. (Courtesy of Calvin S. Lau, DDS.)

- Variable microbial pattern
- Slow to moderate progression, with periods of rapid progression
- Classified on the basis of extent and severity
- Associated with local predisposing factors
- May be modified by systemic diseases
- May be modified by factors such as stress and tobacco use.

Treatment. Treatment of all types of chronic periodontitis requires removal of the local etiologic factors. Steps include education in personal plaque control for the patient's home care, complete removal of all plaque and calculus from the root surfaces by the dental hygienist, and control of associated factors such as overhanging margins and habits such as smoking. As the attachment loss increases from moderate to advanced periodontitis, complete removal of calculus is difficult, and additional procedures, such as periodontal surgery, may be indicated (Figures 7-2, 7-3, and 7-4) (See color figures.)[9] A complete description of the dental hygiene treatment protocol for adult periodontitis is found in Chapter 10.

PERIODONTITIS AS A RISK FACTOR FOR SYSTEM DISEASES

It has long been known that some systemic diseases alter the presentation and progression of periodontal diseases (see Chapter 17). More recent evidence suggests that periodontal diseases may play a role as a **risk factor** in the development and management of serious systemic disease. In particular, periodontal infections have been implicated in cardiovascular diseases,[10] pre-term, low-birth weight infants,[11] and bacterial pneumonia.[12] In addition, it ap-

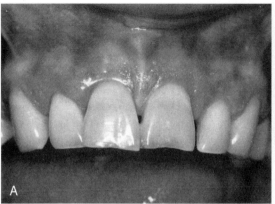
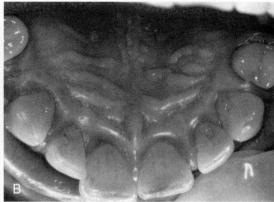

FIGURE 7–2. Slight periodontitis. **A.** The clinical appearance of the maxillary anterior shows normal-appearing gingiva, with little obvious attachment loss. **B.** The clinical appearance of the lingual view suggests inflamed gingiva, but attachment loss must be assessed by careful probing around the teeth. (See color figure.)

pears to be more difficult to control non-insulin dependent diabetes in patients with severe periodontitis.[13] Although the exact mechanisms for these interrelationships have not been determined, several explanations for these increases in risk have been proposed.

Periodontitis and Cardiovascular Disease

Cardiovascular disease, including heart attack and stroke, annually account for almost half of the deaths in the United States and most developed countries. Periodontal disease, along with other factors such as high cholesterol, smoking, diabetes, overweight, and sedentary lifestyle, appears to be associated with increased risk of heart attack and death.[14] Using data from the third National Health and Nutrition Examination Survey (NHANES III) conducted by the National Institutes of Health, scientists evaluated the relationship of periodontal conditions and history of heart attack in people 40 years of age and older. When other factors were controlled, the statistical evaluation of the data indicated a 14 percent increase in the odds of heart attack for every patient with a 10 percent increase in sites with 3 mm or more attachment loss.[15] In addition, tooth loss from all causes appeared to be related to cardiovascular disease. These studies suggest that adverse health effects are related to chronic infections, which are mediated by inflammatory agents that trigger the development of atherosclerosis (plaque development) in the coronary arteries.[16] A possible mechanism of action for this is

that endotoxins from bacteria in dental plaque trigger an increased release of inflammatory mediators from T-cells of susceptible patients. The increase in the amount of inflammation in periodontal tissues is both destructive and reparative, but in the arteries, there is strong evidence that the same inflammatory mediators increase platelet aggregation and adhesion to arterial endothelial walls.[10]

Periodontitis and Pre-term Birth

Pre-term birth (defined as gestation of less than 36 of 40 weeks) and low birth weight (defined as less than 2500 grams) is a major public health problem. It is directly related to infant mortality and other significant problems, and now is implicated in relationship to periodontal disease. An extension of the periodontal inflammatory response, similar to that proposed for cardiovascular disease, has been proposed to explain this relationship. It is thought that some of the inflammatory mediators stimulated in the periodontium produce endocrine-like cytokines (another mediator) that may affect the fetus. In addition, lipopolysaccharides (LPS), also referred to as endotoxins, from dental plaque bacteria may act directly on the placental membrane via the bloodstream. One study suggests that active periodontal disease may account for over 18 percent of all pre-term, low-birth weight babies, which makes it more significant than either cigarette smoking or alcohol use.[11] It is clear that appropriate periodontal care and oral hygiene during pregnancy are extremely important.

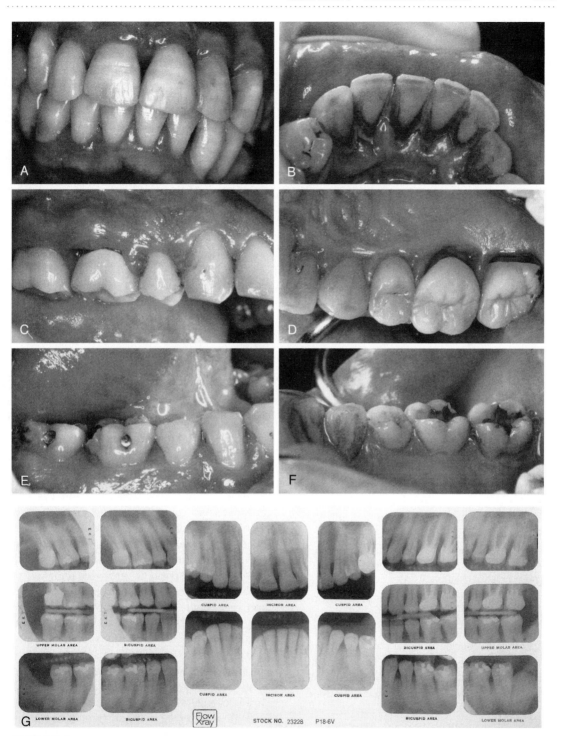

FIGURE 7–3. Moderate periodontitis. **A.** The facial view shows swollen, shiny marginal gingiva, with missing interdental papillae. Recession is visible on the upper right cuspid and lateral incisor. However, the extent of the attachment loss cannot be assessed without radiographs and periodontal probing. **B.** The mandibular lingual view shows heavy deposits of plaque and calculus, with intense inflammation and edema of the marginal gingiva. **C.** The maxillary right buccal view shows recession on the distal surface of the first molar, with gingival hyperplasia on the mesial papilla. The tissue has receded enough to expose the margin of the crowns. **D.** The maxillary right lingual view shows marked swelling of the marginal gingiva. Recession is indicated by the exposed crown margin on the first molar. **E.** The mandibular right buccal view shows boggy interdental tissue. **F.** The mandibular right lingual view shows less obvious interdental swelling, but heavy plaque, calculus, and stain accumulation. **G.** The full mouth radiographs indicate 3 to 5 mm of bone loss generalized throughout the mouth. The maxillary and mandibular right first molars show localized advanced bone loss with furcation involvement. (See color figure.)

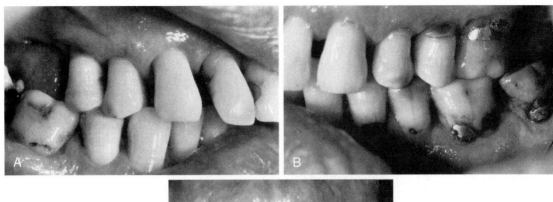

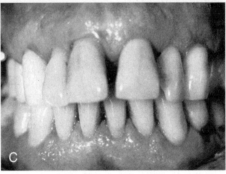

FIGURE 7–4. Advanced periodontitis. Advanced periodontitis presents the clinical characteristics of recession, plaque, calculus, inflammation, and drifting and missing teeth. It is not possible to assess the extent of the disease without radiographs and full mouth probing. However, the clinical signs in this case suggest more severe bone loss because of the visible recession and furcations. The gingiva appears firm and stippled, masking the underlying inflammation. This masking is common in chronic periodontal disease. **A.** The right side. **B.** The left side. **C.** The anterior view. (See color figure.)

Periodontitis and Bacterial Pneumonia

Bacterial pneumonia, bacterial infections of the lung tissues, can be a life-threatening infection, particularly in elderly or immunocompromised patients. This is an important problem in nursing home populations because more antibiotic-resistant infections are emerging, and oral hygiene is often poor among these individuals. Pneumonia occurs in the lower respiratory tract, which is usually sterile, but aspiration or spread of infectious agents can contaminate it. A number of the periodontal pathogenic bacteria found in dental plaque have been associated with pneumonia, and an additional number of other potential respiratory pathogens reside in dental plaque. Since oral hygiene in nursing home patients appears to decrease with the age of the residents, improving oral hygiene in these patients may also decrease the incidence of bacterial pneumonia in this population.[12]

Periodontitis and Control of Non-insulin Dependent Diabetes

Diabetes has long been considered a risk factor for periodontal disease because it appears to increase patient susceptibility to many types of infections. The exact mechanism for this is unclear.[17, 18] A mechanism of action has been proposed for the increases in clinical attachment loss seen in type I diabetes, insulin-dependent diabetes mellitus (IDDM). In patients with IDDM, the periodontal ligament cells may be less able to respond to growth factors in the inflammatory response required to maintain and regenerate the periodontium during healing.[19] These patients tend to be younger and have more aggressive disease, so there are many systemic effects beyond those seen in the periodontium. Increased clinical attachment loss is also associated with the later onset of IDDM, and with cigarette smoking.

Type II diabetes mellitus, non-insulin dependent diabetes mellitus (NIDDM) is usually found in patients over 50 years of age and rarely seen in anyone younger than 40. Evidence suggests that poor glycemic control among patients with NIDDM may be related to periodontal disease and increased clinical attachment loss. Although the mechanism for this has not been established, it is known that cytokines produced by the inflammatory response to periodontal infection can interfere with the action of insulin. It is important to know that the management of NIDDM may be improved through the treatment of periodontal infections and their prevention.[13]

AGGRESSIVE PERIODONTITIS

The diagnosis **aggressive periodontitis** is the appropriate term for those periodontal diseases that progress exceedingly rapidly with massive bone loss.[2] This is in contrast to chronic periodontitis, which has been described as attachment loss progression up to 1 mm per year when untreated.[20] Progression of attachment loss greater than this rate may be considered to be an aggressive type of periodontitis, although there is little clinical evidence to support this as a completely separate diagnosis. Attachment loss progression appears to vary widely by individual, although there clearly is an increase in progression with age.[21]

The microflora associated with both aggressive periodontitis and chronic periodontitis appear to be quite similar, so it is difficult to describe a separate diagnosis based on bacterial identification alone.[22] In fact, it is likely that the interaction of different bacteria in subgingival plaque may be a more important factor in determining the progression of periodontal destruction rather than individual components, reflecting increased understanding of dental plaque as a biofilm (see Chapter 4).[23] In spite of this difficulty, it is possible to distinguish between aggressive periodontitis and chronic periodontitis based on the progression of bone loss; and between different forms of aggressive periodontitis based on other factors, such as age of the patient at clinical detection, relative levels of certain bacterial species, or presence or absence of possible defects in the immune response. Like chronic periodontitis, aggressive forms of the disease can be localized or generalized, which may further help characterize the disease. For convenience, a subclassification of aggressive periodontal diseases based on historical observation is useful. Aggressive periodontal diseases may be classified as 1) early-onset diseases, including juvenile and prepubertal periodontitis, and rapidly progressive periodontitis; and 2) refractory periodontitis. See the Types of Aggressive Periodontitis.

Early-onset Periodontitis

Early-onset periodontitis is a group of periodontal diseases that affect patients younger than 30 years. It includes a number of periodontal disease patterns: prepubertal periodontitis, juvenile periodontitis (both localized and generalized forms), and rapidly progressive periodontitis.[24] These diseases have different clinical and microbiologic characteristics that distinguish them from the more common chronic periodontitis. These identifying features are: (1) associated microbiota, (2) early age of onset, (3) rapid rate of tissue destruction, and (4) the possibility of defects in the immune system.

PREPUBERTAL PERIODONTITIS

Prepubertal periodontitis is a very rare condition that may be localized or generalized, and may affect both the primary and the secondary dentition. Usually, there is severe gingival inflammation, rapid bone loss, and early tooth loss. Deciduous teeth are often lost because of periodontal infection, and permanent teeth become infected as they erupt. Many patients lose all of their teeth at an early age. Many of these young patients have white blood cell defects that also leave them susceptible to other infections.[25] Prepubertal periodontitis responds poorly to conventional treatment techniques, such as scaling and root planing. **Antibiotic therapy** may help. However, treatment usually slows rather than stops the disease progress. Individuals with prepubertal periodontitis frequently become edentulous at an early age (Figure 7–5, also in color supplement).

JUVENILE PERIODONTITIS

Juvenile periodontitis is a form of early-onset periodontitis that is recognized in the periodontal literature because of its specific plaque infec-

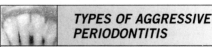

TYPES OF AGGRESSIVE PERIODONTITIS

Early-Onset Periodontitis
  Prepubertal Periodontitis
  Juvenile Periodontitis
    Localized Juvenile Periodontitis
    Generalized Juvenile Periodontitis
    Post-Juvenile Periodontitis
  Rapidly Progressive Periodontitis
Refractory Periodontitis

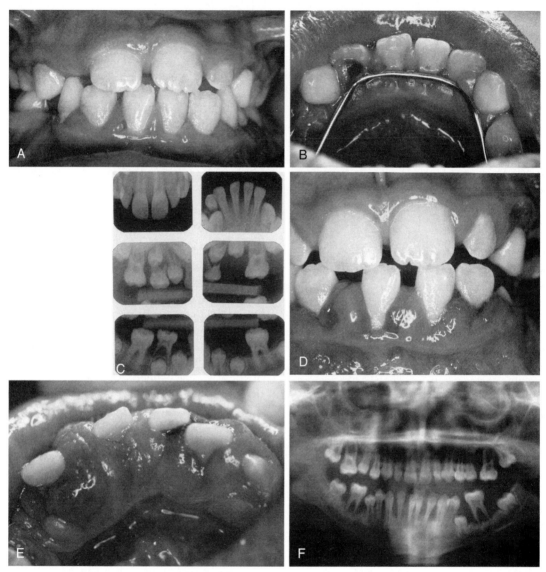

FIGURE 7–5. Prepubertal periodontitis. Prepubertal periodontitis is a rare disease characterized by advanced bone loss and premature tooth loss. This male with prepubertal periodontitis had multiple periodontal procedures performed, including periodontal surgery and several courses of antibiotic therapy. The bone loss continued to progress, and many of these teeth were lost. **A.** At age 8 years, the clinical presentation of the anterior teeth showed erupting teeth and signs of gingival inflammation. Tissue swelling and redness were extensive, and there were heavy deposits of plaque. **B.** The mandibular lingual view showed granulation tissue growing over and around the mandibular space maintainer. **C.** Periapical radiographs at age 8 years showed erupting teeth and significant bone loss around both the permanent and the deciduous molars. **D.** By age 10 years, the clinical presentation of the anterior teeth showed extreme hyperplastic tissue and tooth migration. **E.** The hyperplastic tissue condition was remarkable in the lower anterior area at age 10. **F.** A panographic X-ray taken at age 10 years. Bone loss has proceeded to the apices of the permanent first molars. Treatment included multiple sessions of scaling and root planing, periodontal surgery, and antibiotic therapy. The prognosis for the teeth is poor, and this child will probably be edentulous as a teenager. (See color figure.)

tion.[26] It has been subclassified into localized and generalized forms.

LOCALIZED JUVENILE PERIODONTITIS

The localized form is characterized by extreme bone loss that is usually seen around the permanent first molars and incisors in patients younger than 20 years, but it may also involve other teeth. Often, this disease is not diagnosed until the patient is older. Interestingly, many of these patients do not have high levels of plaque accumulation or inflammation around the affected teeth, and the disease may not be recognized until routine dental X-rays show the advanced bone loss. Many of these patients have loose teeth or teeth that appear to be drifting (Figure 7-6, also in color supplement).

The dental hygienist is in an excellent position to recognize juvenile periodontitis during assessment procedures. Plaque and calculus are often minimal around teeth with deep pockets, and oral hygiene often appears good. The bacteria most often reported in localized juvenile periodontitis is *Actinobacillus actinomycetemcomitans*, which is found in high numbers in the subgingival plaque,[27] in fact up to 90 percent of the plaque mass.[7] This organism does not produce a large amount of extracellular matrix and therefore may be present in large numbers in the periodontal pocket without large amounts of attached plaque. Another interesting feature of localized juvenile periodontitis is the large percentage of neutrophils in the bloodstream that have abnormally slow chemotactic response.[28] A laboratory that uses deoxyribonucleic acid (DNA) probe technology has been developed to confirm the diagnosis of localized juvenile periodontitis. In this test, samples of the gingival fluid or plaque from the sulcus of infected teeth are matched with known DNA from *A. actinomycetemcomitans* bacteria to identify the specific bacterial infection and confirm the diagnosis.

Localized juvenile periodontitis appears to be more common in girls and young women than in boys and young men, and it can run in families. The disease is more commonly reported in blacks than in whites. Interestingly, both amounts of visible plaque and caries rates in affected individuals are often low.

Treatment. Several authors have suggested that controlling localized juvenile periodontitis requires treating the patient until all *A. actino-* *mycetemcomitans* bacteria are gone. Usually, therapy requires mechanical debridement with scaling and root planing while the patient takes systemic antibiotics, usually some form of tetracycline. Periodontal surgery is often required to eliminate the infection and the bony defects in the periodontium.

GENERALIZED JUVENILE PERIODONTITIS

Generalized juvenile periodontitis occurs more rarely than the localized form. It affects most or all of the teeth of young adolescents. The first molars and incisors are often the most severely involved teeth. Generalized juvenile periodontitis is also associated with a neutrophil chemotactic disorder. It differs from localized juvenile periodontitis in that significant clinical inflammation is often present, with heavy plaque and calculus formation. The bacterial flora is also different. It includes larger numbers of *P. gingivalis* and *Eikenella corrodens* along with large numbers of *A. actinomycetemcomitans*.[29]

Treatment. Treatment of generalized juvenile periodontitis consists of improved home plaque control, scaling and root planing, and antibiotic therapy. Periodontal surgery is often required to correct defects in bone architecture and reduce pocket depth (Figure 7-7, also in color supplement).

POST-JUVENILE PERIODONTITIS

A special classification of juvenile periodontitis termed postjuvenile periodontitis has been suggested. This disease has the clinical appearance of either localized or generalized juvenile periodontitis, but it has stopped or significantly slowed. It is seen in adults rather than adolescents. The diagnosis appears to be based on the appearance of severe bone loss around the incisors or first molars more than on any other criterion. This condition is probably a late diagnosis of juvenile periodontitis rather than a different disease, because juvenile periodontitis may spontaneously slow or stop. Also, the lesions of post-juvenile periodontitis often appear much like adult periodontitis, with significant inflammation, plaque, and calculus.

Treatment. This disease is treated by conventional techniques, including scaling and root planing, home care instruction, and periodontal surgery to correct deep pockets and bony defects. Some dentists also prescribe a course of

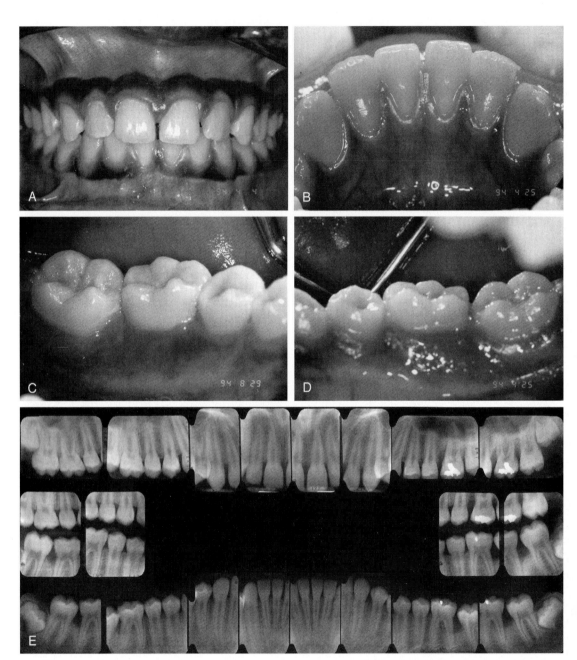

FIGURE 7–6. Localized juvenile periodontitis. Localized juvenile periodontitis is more common than prepubertal periodontitis, but is still a rare disease. This 15-year-old male has deceptively normal-appearing gingiva. Plaque, calculus, and signs of inflammation were minimal. The patient has had nonsurgical and surgical periodontal treatment and a course of tetracycline therapy. The condition has stabilized. **A.** Anterior view of the maxillary and mandibular teeth and gingiva. **B.** Lingual view of the mandibular anterior teeth. **C.** Lingual view of the right mandibular posterior teeth. **D.** Lingual view of the left mandibular posterior teeth. **E.** A full mouth radiographic series showed moderate localized bone loss around both mandibular first molars and the maxillary left first molar. The bone level appeared normal on the other teeth. There was furcation involvement on both maxillary and mandibular first molars. The formation of the third molars appeared normal. (See color figure.) (Courtesy of Lisa T. Grosso, RN, DDS.)

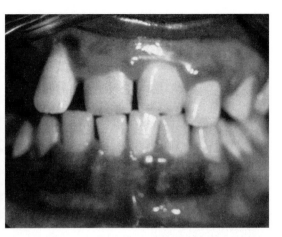

FIGURE 7–7. Generalized juvenile periodontitis. Advanced generalized juvenile periodontitis can be characterized by mobile and drifting teeth, as seen in this 17-year-old black female. (See color figure.)

antibiotic therapy to kill pathogenic bacteria in the plaque.

RAPIDLY PROGRESSIVE PERIODONTITIS

Rapidly progressive periodontitis occurs in young adults, usually between 20 and 30 years old. The disease usually involves most of the teeth, but localized forms of rapidly progressive periodontitis have been reported. Whereas juvenile periodontitis usually shows little clinical inflammation, rapidly progressive periodontitis causes severe gingival inflammation and varying amounts of plaque and calculus. Loss of bone and connective tissue usually occurs rapidly over a period of weeks or months. The loss can be so rapid that it is startling to the treating dental hygienist and dentist (Figure 7-8, also in color supplement).

This disease may have a genetic component because a large percentage of affected patients have altered neutrophil chemotaxis. It has been suggested that a diagnosis of rapidly progressive periodontal disease requires that individuals be younger than 30 years old, with multiple areas of at least 5 mm of attachment loss and pocket depths of 6 mm or greater.[30] For reasons that are not understood, this progression of attachment loss may suddenly cease. Unfortunately, in most cases, the disease progresses to tooth loss if untreated and can only be slowed with treatment.

A number of bacteria have been suggested as related to this disease, including *P. gingivalis,* *Prevotella intermedia, E. corrodens*, and *Campylobacter recta.*

Treatment. Treatment is directed at eliminating the local factors through good plaque control, subgingival scaling and root planing, and possibly periodontal surgery. In addition, antibiotics help when added to the therapeutic regimen. Usually, forms of tetracycline are prescribed. However, metronidazole, amoxicillin/clavulanic acid, ciprofloxacin, and several drug combinations have been used.[31]

Refractory Periodontitis

Refractory periodontitis is periodontal disease that is unresponsive to appropriate treatment. In other words, appropriate and thorough treatment followed by continuing supportive periodontal therapy does not arrest the progress of the disease.[2] The disease may occur at single or multiple sites around the teeth. Presumably, these sites continue to be infected with periodontal pathogens, regardless of what treatments have been tried. These individuals have been classified as "extreme downhill patients." Data suggest that they may represent 8 to 14 percent of patients originally diagnosed as having advanced chronic periodontitis (Figure 7-9, also in color supplement).[32]

Refractory periodontitis has a wide variety of presenting symptoms. In fact, it may represent a number of separate diseases. No single bacterial agent has been identified in refractory periodontitis, and it has been suggested that the disease may be the result of several species working in combination.[33] Most diagnosed patients have undergone repeated attempts to control their disease process, including multiple episodes of periodontal surgery, frequent scaling and root planing, and antibiotic administration. These patients may harbor organisms that are tenacious and resistant to normal therapies. These patients are easily mistaken for those with recurrent periodontal disease. Refractory periodontitis is a continuing disease that is unresponsive to therapy.

PERIODONTITIS AS A MANIFESTATION OF SYSTEMIC DISEASE

Periodontitis may present as a manifestation of systemic disease. A number of systemic diseases

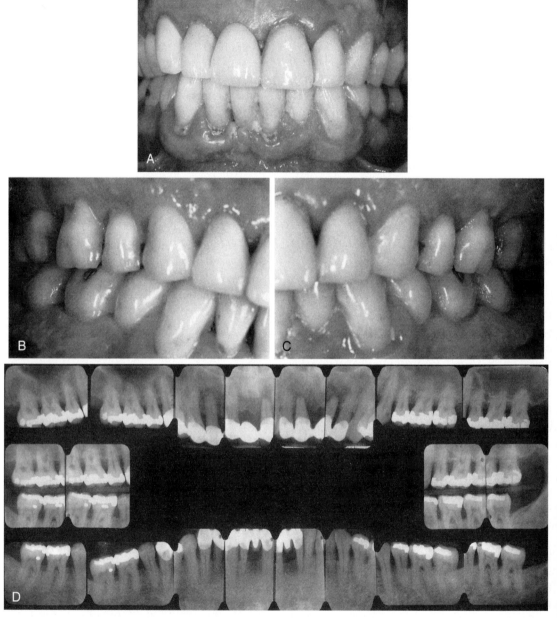

FIGURE 7–8. Rapidly progressive periodontitis. This periodontal disease is characterized by rapid loss of bone in young adults. In this 32-year-old male, clinical assessment showed plaque, calculus, signs of inflammation, and recession. The radiographs showed generalized advanced bone loss. **A.** Clinical presentation of the anterior teeth. There are heavy deposits of plaque and calculus. **B.** Clinical presentation of the right side. **C.** Clinical presentation of the left side. **D.** Full mouth radiographs of rapidly progressing periodontitis. Furcation involvement is seen in all molar regions, and external resorption is seen at the apex of the maxillary left central incisor, probably as a result of past trauma. (See color figure.) (Courtesy of Craig Y. Yonemura, DDS, MS.)

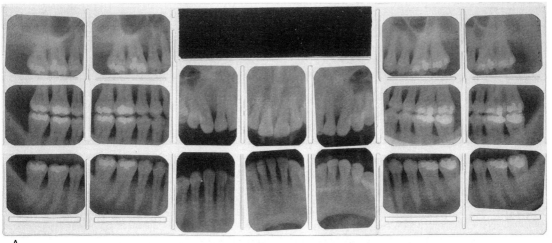

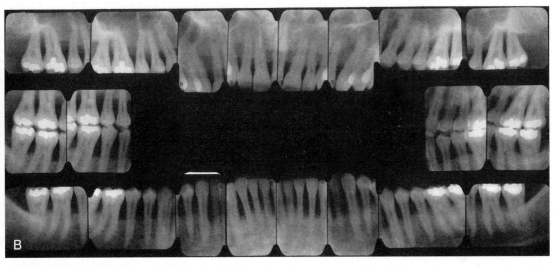

FIGURE 7–9. Refractory periodontitis. This condition is unresponsive to periodontal therapy. Bone and attachment loss continue despite good plaque control and all appropriate treatment. **A.** Radiographs of a 35-year-old male with moderate to advanced bone loss on all teeth. **B.** Two years later, the bone loss continued to progress despite excellent plaque control, nonsurgical and surgical periodontal therapy, systemic antibiotics, and 2- to 3-month periodontal maintenance visits. Bone loss has proceeded almost to the apices of the maxillary molars. (See color figure.)

appear to increase the severity and character of periodontal disease, although most patients with advanced disease can be classified into one of the other categories, most often chronic periodontitis or rapidly progressive periodontitis. Systemic diseases, such as Down's syndrome, insulin-dependent diabetes mellitus, acquired immune deficiency syndrome (AIDS), and Papillon-Lefevre syndrome, can increase the severity of periodontal disease. The use of this diagnosis may be beneficial to the dental hygienist and dentist by emphasizing the presence of an underlying systemic problem and therefore affecting management. For example, diabetes increases both the severity of bone loss and

the rate of progression of periodontal disease. As mentioned earlier, chronic periodontal disease is now considered a major complication of diabetes.[17]

For all patients, significant periodontal disease beyond what would be expected for the level of plaque and calculus should suggest a more thorough medical evaluation. Life-threatening diseases, such as uncontrolled diabetes and leukemia, may first be seen as changes in the gingival and periodontal structures. Other systemic diseases, such as hypophosphatasia, alter tooth development and therefore alter periodontal attachment. These signs and symptoms mimic early-onset periodontal diseases. It is important that the physician be included as a member of the oral health care team to collaborate in the evaluation of patients with unusual forms of periodontitis.

In most cases, systemic factors worsen the symptoms of chronic periodontitis by reducing an individual's resistance to all disease processes. Consideration should be given to protecting patients with systemic diseases by providing antibiotics during periodontal therapy. Any patient with a systemic disease that makes the periodontal disease worse should be informed of the nature of the periodontal situation. Increased levels of personal plaque control and more frequent periodontal recall visits are often required. Treatment considerations for periodontal disease associated with systemic illnesses are described in Chapter 17.

NECROTIZING PERIODONTAL DISEASES

This classification of diseases includes necrotizing ulcerative gingivitis (NUG), described in Chapter 6, and **necrotizing ulcerative periodontitis**. These appear to be different stages of the same disease, and both seem to be related to diminished systemic resistance to bacterial infection in the periodontal tissues. As described in Chapter 6, necrotic gingival tissues, gingival pain, gingival bleeding, and fetid breath odor characterize NUG. At this stage, the infection is thought to be limited to the gingiva. When it extends to involve the attachment apparatus, it is considered to be a periodontal disease rather than a gingival disease.

Necrotizing Ulcerative Periodontitis (NUP)

Acute necrotizing ulcerative periodontitis (NUP) is the most appropriate term for the massive tissue-destroying process that is an extension of acute necrotizing ulcerative gingivitis. By definition, when bone loss and loss of connective tissue attachment to the root surface are present, the disease is periodontitis, not gingivitis. Therefore, most cases of necrotizing ulcerative disease should be considered NUP.

This disease causes severe progressive destruction of the gingiva and alveolar mucosa that spreads rapidly to the deeper tissues. The

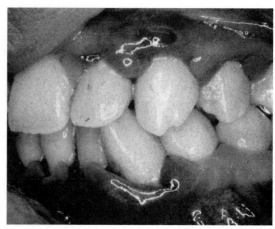

FIGURE 7–10. Necrotizing ulcerative periodontitis. The clinical presentation of a patient with necrotizing ulcerative periodontitis. Characteristics of the disease include intense inflammation, punched-out interdental papillae, and attachment loss. In this patient, the attachment loss was most obvious on the mesial aspect of the mandibular cuspid. The condition was painful, and the patient had severe breath odor. (See color figure.) (Courtesy of UCSF Division of Periodontology.)

gingiva is intensely red, and there is extensive necrosis of the soft tissues, which form a white pseudomembranous surface. There may be severe loss of connective tissue attachment, but periodontal pockets are usually not present.[2] NUP is characterized by pain, a distinctive fetid mouth odor (fetor oris), punched-out tips of the interdental papilla, and spontaneous bleeding. This clinical presentation is often diagnostic. NUP is associated with systemic immune deficiency diseases, such as human immunodeficiency virus (HIV) infection. In these patients, NUP may indicate deterioration of the immune system and be a predictor for the diagnosis of AIDS.[34] NUP may also occur in patients with nutritional deficiencies and has been related to extreme stress (Figure 7–10).

Some periodontists have suggested an additional classification of chronic necrotizing periodontitis to describe periodontitis in adults that exhibits regions of punched-out and retracted interdental papillae with extreme root sensitivity. Other signs of NUP are often absent. This condition is not yet well defined, and most dental scientists believe that the correct diagnosis of this set of symptoms is still most often chronic periodontitis.

ABSCESS OF THE PERIDONTIUM

Periodontal abscess is an acute, localized purulent infection of the periodontium. Although discussed in greater detail in Chapter 16, Periodontal Emergencies, abscesses are presented here because the American Academy of Periodontology recognizes them as a separate diagnosis of periodontal diseases and conditions in the most recent classification of disease.[2]

Periodontal abscesses most often occur in patients with chronic periodontitis, usually cases that have been untreated (Figure 7-11, also in color supplement). They may be acute or chronic in nature. The abscess is thought to occur because the periodontal pocket containing pathologic bacterial plaque becomes occluded, allowing the infection to become localized into an acute infection in the adjacent tissues. Acute periodontal abscesses are associated with rapid bone loss, and should be treated immediately (Figure 7-12, also in color supplement). Acute periodontal abscesses are commonly thought to occur more frequently following periodontal scaling or prophylaxis,[35] however other studies dispute this finding.[36]

If the acute abscess is left untreated, the infection will seek a route to drain. It then becomes a chronic abscess, constantly inflamed, and will result in continued bone loss. Chronic periodontal abscesses are frequently asymptomatic and the patient is unaware of any draining pus. Upon questioning, patients often recall vague symptoms such as episodes of localized swelling in the area, or "funny" feelings in the gingiva around the chronic abscess. These symptoms may be related to episodes of acute infection, when the chronic abscess has lost its ability to drain.

Usually periodontal abscesses occur in deep-

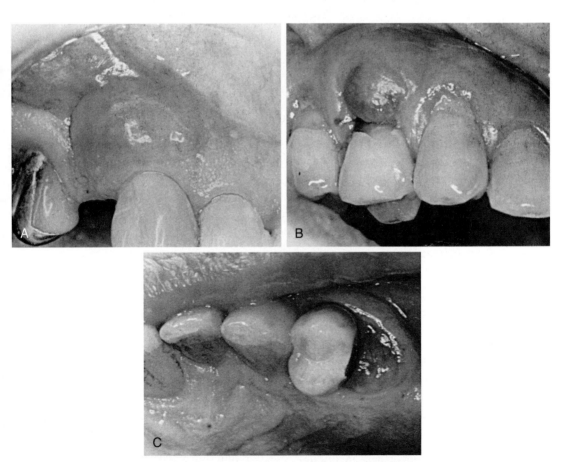

FIGURE 7–11. Acute periodontal abscess. **A.** This large painful abscess arose in the proximity of a 9mm pocket on the distal surface of the cuspid. Note the significant color change and fluctuant appearance of the overlying gingiva. **B.** The acute abscess can also arise very close to the marginal gingiva. This abscess is smaller, possibly because it is partially draining through the orifice of the pocket, and associated with a deep pocket on the facial surface of the maxillary first premolar. **C.** Acute abscesses can occur around any surface of the teeth. This abscess arose on the distal of a first premolar. It was very painful to the patient and the pocketing around the tooth was severe. The tooth was lost after repeated episodes of acute abscess. (See color figure.)

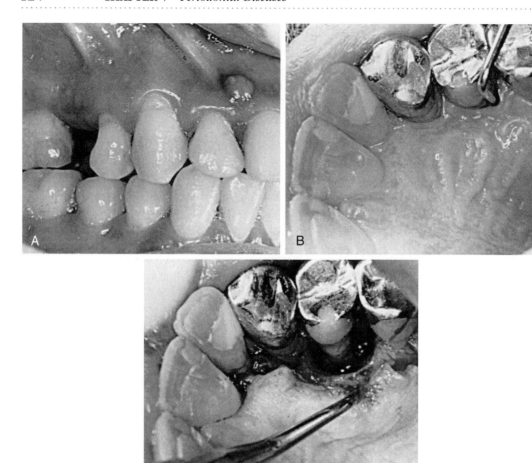

FIGURE 7–12. Acute periodontal abscess. **A.** This acute periodontal abscess drained through a sinus in the mucosa. The swelling associated with this lateral incisor is positioned away from the gingiva in the mucosa, mimicking a lesion of endodontic origin. **B.** Acute periodontal abscesses that drain through the periodontal pocket may exhibit much less swelling but are still very painful. This abscess was associated with a deep pocket on the lingual of the tooth, and drained through the pocket. **C.** Upon retraction of the flap to expose the root surface and treat the abscess, the extent of bone loss can be seen. (See color figure.)

ened pockets, but they may appear only in the gingival tissues, when they are called gingival abscesses (see Chapter 6). Gingival abscess is most often caused by a foreign body being forced into the sulcus. The condition resolves when the material is removed and the area cleaned.

A unique form of periodontal abscess occurs around partially erupted teeth, usually third molars. This abscess occurs around a flap of tissue partially covering the tooth called an operculum. This is called a pericoronal abscess, often referred to as pericoronitis (see Chapter 16, Periodontal Emergencies). The pericoronal abscess may be extremely painful and can spread to the submandibular tissues.

Treatment. The treatment of periodontal abscesses, whether acute, chronic, pericoronal, or localized in the gingiva, involves careful debridement of the pocket. It often includes surgical removal of the lining of the periodontal pocket through open or closed curettage. Systemic antibiotics must be administered if there is evidence of fascial cellulitis, or if the patient has a fever. Definitive treatment for a pericoronal abscess is removal of the operculum or extraction of the partially erupted molar.

Periodontitis Associated with Endodontic Lesions

Periodontal abscesses must be differentiated from abscesses of endodontic origin that may also have signs and symptoms in the periodontium. An abscess may be entirely periodontal, or entirely endodontic in origin, or it may be a combined lesion. In the case of periodontitis associated with an endodontic lesion, a chronic periodontal pocket may have progressed to join an endodontic lesion, it may have infected the pulp of the tooth through the apex or lateral canals in the tooth root, or the endodontic lesion could drain out through the periodontal ligament infecting the surrounding tissue. An overview of endodontic lesions and combined lesions is presented in Chapter 16.

Treatment. The treatment of periodontitis associated with endodontic lesions generally requires endodontic therapy. Root canal treatment alone is sufficient if the lesion is only of endodontic origin. Occasionally the lesions require both endodontic and periodontal therapy because of the combined nature of the disease. It is important to know that scaling and root planing should not be performed on a combined abscess until after the endodontic lesion has healed. This is because scaling and root planing disrupts the attachment of the collagen fibers to the root surfaces. There is a higher likelihood of periodontal reattachment if the draining sinus tract through the periodontal ligament is not disturbed. Leaving the infection undisturbed permits all the cellular elements to remain in place, so the healing potential in the area is preserved.

DEVELOPMENTAL OR ACQUIRED DEFORMITIES AND CONDITIONS

There are a number of acquired or developmental conditions that are seen in the periodontium that may or may not require periodontal treatment. These include pseudopockets, where the gingival margin is coronal to the cementoenamel junction. This developmental condition is often seen on the distal of second or third molars. Pseudopockets make plaque control difficult and can result in gingivitis or chronic periodontitis. Gingival recession may be a developmental condition if it is the result of underlying osseous defect, or may represent an acquired defect resulting from trauma from toothbrush abrasion. Whether developmental or acquired, gingival recession may lead to root sensitivity, root caries, gingivitis, and possibly

be an esthetic problem. Examples of developmental conditions, altered tooth development resulting in a cemental spur and another of a lateral developmental groove, are illustrated in Figure 7-13, and appear in the color supplement.

METHODS OF DETECTING PERIODONTAL DISEASE

The most common and accepted method of detecting periodontal disease is careful assessment of the attachment level around all surfaces of all teeth with a graduated periodontal probe. Probing depths are recorded at six points around the tooth. Pocket depths of greater than 3 mm may indicate attachment loss and periodontal disease. The location of the gingival margin on a tooth as well as the degree of bone loss determines the classification of the disease. Probing pocket depth itself is secondary in diagnostic significance to clinical attachment level.

The presence of bleeding in response to probing and visible color change in the gingival tissue are also important factors in the diagnosis of periodontal disease. The relationship between bleeding and progression of disease is not strong, but there is evidence that this information, in conjunction with the probing attachment level and radiographic signs of bone loss, assists in the diagnosis and classification of the disease. Areas that do not bleed are not likely to show progressive bone loss and attachment loss. Other diagnostic data and tests include mobility and comparison of probing data over time.[37]

ETIOLOGY OF PERIODONTITIS

As in gingivitis, dental plaque is the principal cause of all forms of periodontitis. Treatment that is directed at elimination or reduction of the amount and quality of dental plaque is the most effective. However, the pathogenicity of plaque bacteria varies widely, as does the susceptibility of each patient. This variability makes the causes of periodontitis less clear-cut than the direct relationship between dental plaque and gingivitis. Many other factors are involved. Studies on animals, when dental plaque formation had been arrested or con-

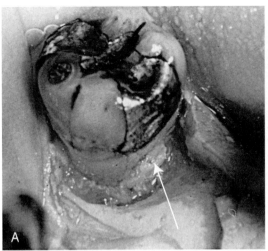
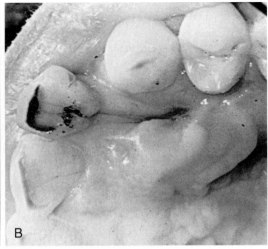

FIGURE 7–13. Developmental conditions associated with periodontitis. **A.** Cementicle. In this case, a cementicle or cementum spur on the mesial of the mandibular molar was located just apical to the CEJ. This caused plaque retention and resulted in an infrabony defect. Treatment with scaling and root planing was impossible, and the spur required surgical removal. Healing was uneventful and the periodontal problem was resolved. **B.** Lingual Developmental Groove. Maxillary lateral incisors often have lateral grooves extending apically from the cingulum. In this case, the groove extended to near the apex of the tooth, retaining plaque and permitting calculus to form in the groove. After repeated instances of periodontal abscess, the tooth required extraction. There was no other periodontal disease present in this patient's mouth. Most developmental grooves are not this extensive and can be treated successfully with surgical removal of bone to the apical extent of the groove, and placement of a tissue-compatible restoration in the groove. (See color figure.)

trolled, have indicated that nutritional deficiencies, hormonal alterations, and trauma from occlusion cannot in themselves cause periodontal pocket formation. However, in the presence of dental plaque, these situations may worsen the progression of periodontitis (see Chapter 4).

Dental calculus is calcified dental plaque. It does not by itself cause periodontal disease; however, it is covered with millions of organized bacteria. Because of its large surface area and rough surface, its associated plaque is difficult to remove and regrows at a rapid rate. The presence of calculus on a root surface indicates that there is always plaque present. For this reason, scaling and root planing, or periodontal debridement to remove the calculus and associated plaque, is the cornerstone of periodontal treatment (see Chapter 5).

Conditions that retain plaque or make dental plaque difficult to remove by either the patient or the dental hygienist play significant roles in the etiology of periodontitis. Overhanging or poorly contoured dental restorations, food retention or impaction areas (plaque impaction), furcations, spaces between teeth, missing and drifted teeth, and alterations in tooth morphol-

ogy (such as fluting and grooves), increase the likelihood of periodontitis. Furthermore, deepened periodontal pockets harbor large amounts of subgingival plaque that is difficult to control with home care. Deep pockets must be carefully debrided, often by the dental hygienist, to control periodontitis.

Hormonal changes associated with pregnancy, menopause, and oral contraceptive use have been studied extensively. These hormones may change the environment of the gingival sulcus and alter the types of bacteria that grow in the plaque, therefore increasing the likelihood of pathogenic plaque.[38] Hormones definitely increase the flow of gingival fluid by causing proliferation and increased permeability of the microcirculation. However, good plaque removal appears to control the level of gingival inflammation.

TOBACCO USE

Tobacco use is a known risk factor for periodontal disease.[39] It has been clearly associated with increased attachment loss. Young smokers have been demonstrated to have more progression of disease than nonsmokers, even when controlled for the level of plaque present.[40] Smokers have also been shown to be at higher risk for tooth loss than nonsmokers.[41] Smoking also has an effect on healing after periodontal therapy. Studies have shown that smokers have less probing depth reduction and less attachment gain than nonsmokers following scaling and root planing.[42]

There are several possible explanations for this increased risk, including both direct and indirect effects of tobacco smoke. Tobacco smoke contains a large number of cytotoxic and vasoactive components, including nicotine. Nicotine ingestion causes vasoconstriction, possibly explaining why smokers have less gingival bleeding than nonsmokers. Smokers also have diminished neutrophil function, possibly explaining why smokers rather than nonsmokers are more likely to have refractory periodontitis.[43] Smoking is also thought to impair fibroblast function and reduce the capacity of the periodontal tissues to heal. Reduced healing characterized by slower turnover in gingival tissues may upset the balance between the disease process and the healing process, resulting in progression of periodontal diseases.

The role of other forms of tobacco, cigar smoking, and spit tobacco use, is less clear. The particular effects of cigars have been much less studied than cigarettes, although the effects are likely to be quite similar. Localized gingival recession is commonly seen in the oral areas where spit tobacco is held, often between the gingiva and the vestibular mucosa.[44]

Treatment. It is important for patients to refrain from smoking during periodontal therapy in order to maximize the healing potential. All patients who smoke or use any form of tobacco should be informed of the effects of tobacco on the disease process. Presented with this information, some will be encouraged to reduce their tobacco use or to stop entirely.[45]

PATHOGENESIS OF PERIODONTITIS

It is not known exactly when periodontitis begins. Many scientists believe that periodontitis

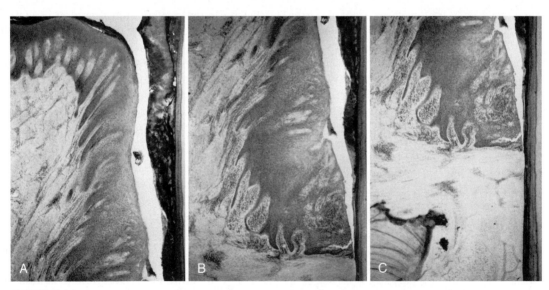

FIGURE 7-14. The histology of a periodontal pocket. **A.** The coronal portion of the periodontal pocket is adjacent to a plaque- and calculus-covered root surface. The sulcular epithelium is thickened, with exaggerated rete pegs. There is a dense inflammatory cell infiltrate under the sulcular epithelium and surrounding the blood vessels. **B.** The base of the same periodontal pocket shows the apical termination of the thickened junctional epithelium, which has separated from the root surface during specimen preparation. The epithelium precisely follows the contours of the root surface and calculus. A large amount of inflammatory cell infiltrate is seen within the thickened junctional epithelium. Microulcerations appear on the epithelium lining the pocket, and the dense infiltrate has replaced the collagen fibers in the connective tissue. **C.** A lower-power view of the same specimen shows the crest of the alveolar bone and the periodontal ligament space. The inflammatory cells have migrated along the vascular channels into the periodontal ligament, spreading the infection. The structure on the lower left side is the crest of the alveolar bone. There is a single osteoclast seen in its resorbtion bay at the crest of the bone; the cell appears pale. (Courtesy of Gary C. Armitage, DDS, MS.)

begins as gingivitis that progresses to attachment loss. However, careful clinical studies have not shown if and when this transition occurs. In periodontitis, the **pathogenicity** is that the inflammation extends into the attachment apparatus and results in periodontal pocket formation. Two mechanisms have been proposed for the initiation of the spread of infection: (1) the bacteria and their products may break down the interface between the sulcular epithelium and cause detachment of the junctional epithelium, and (2) the bacterial products may interfere with the normal growth and maintenance of the junctional and sulcular epithelium, permitting it to break down. In either case, as inflammation progresses, the sulcular epithelium increases in thickness and begins to infiltrate into the underlying connective tissue.

Pockets deepen because of the breakdown of the collagen fibers in the gingival connective tissue by enzymes such as collagenase, which is released by some of the plaque bacteria and the host's inflammatory cells. Periodontal pockets form and deepen as the junctional epithelium elongates, then separates from the root surface at the coronal end. The plaque bacteria release a number of chemotactic substances that increase the flow of neutrophils into the gingival sulcus. The neutrophils react with bacteria, producing the suppuration, or exudate, often seen in progressing periodontal disease (see Figure 7-14).

Periodontitis begins when there is apical migration of the junctional epithelium and loss of crestal alveolar bone. Because bone is an active tissue, with continuous resorption and formation, it is not possible to determine histologically exactly when bone loss has occurred as a result of periodontitis. When bone resorption exceeds apposition, a net decrease in the amount of bone occurs. Loss of crestal alveolar bone is called periodontal bone loss. There is limited evidence that systemic bone thinning, such as seen in osteoporosis, is related to increased alveolar bone loss and tooth loss. Clearly, most of the bone loss seen in periodontal disease is caused by local inflammation rather than by systemic changes.

When periodontal disease is established, both plasma cells and lymphocytes are present in the periodontal tissues. Plasma cells are important in antigen–antibody reactions, a major

activity of the immune system. Antigen–antibody reactions activate a cascade of events that attract additional inflammatory cells to the periodontal tissues. These cells also produce active molecules that cause additional destruction of the collagen fibers in the periodontal connective tissue. Lymphocytes, when stimulated by bacterial plaque, release lymphokines, another class of active proteins. Lymphokines have many effects on the inflammatory system, including the production of chemical factors that activate osteoclasts and thus increase osseous resorption.[46] For a more complete description of the host response, see Chapter 2.

Other products of the interaction of bacterial plaque with inflammatory cells include prostaglandins, which stimulate bone resorption. In combination, these and other factors, such as activated complement, appear to cause bone loss in progressing periodontitis. Interestingly, understanding the mechanisms of bone resorption may provide a clue to new methods of periodontal disease treatment. For instance, nonsteroidal anti-inflammatory drugs inhibit prostaglandins, and current research suggests that these drugs may inhibit some of the bone loss seen in periodontitis.[47] However, in combination, these processes result in varying degrees of deepened pockets, tissue inflammation, bone loss, exposed furcations, and mobile teeth seen in periodontitis.[48]

Genetic Factors Promoting Periodontitis

There is increasing evidence that susceptibility to periodontal disease, including chronic periodontitis and aggressive periodontitis, may be genetically determined. Studies on European individuals suggest that increases in production of interleukin 1 (IL-1) are associated with increased periodontal destruction.[49] This finding has led to the potential for genetic testing to determine if an individual is susceptible to chronic periodontitis.

ANTIBIOTICS IN THE TREATMENT OF PERIODONTAL DISEASES

The treatment of periodontal infections involves altering the subgingival bacterial flora to remove the cause of infection and allow tissues to heal and inflammation to resolve. Because of the nonspecific nature of the infection, this goal is most often accomplished through mechanical procedures, such as scaling and root planing, and possibly periodontal surgery.

Some forms of periodontal disease, however, continue to progress, and therapy may be augmented by antibiotic treatment. Antibiotic treatment may be either systemic (given to the patient orally or by injection) or applied locally to the specific site of infection.

Systemic Antibiotics

Systemic antibiotics are indicated in the treatment of periodontal diseases when mechanical therapy has not been successful or when specific microorganisms have been identified. In general, treatment for chronic periodontitis, with its mixed infection of multiple bacteria and its relatively straightforward response to mechanical therapy, does not benefit from antibiotic treatment. However, the treatment of aggressive forms of periodontitis may benefit from systemic antibiotic administration in addition to mechanical periodontal therapy. Antibiotics used for systemic administration in the treatment of periodontal diseases include the tetracyclines, metronidazole, penicillins, clindamycin, and the cephalosporins. In addition, several of these antibiotics have been used in combination, with varying results. A summary of the uses for these antibiotics follows.

TETRACYCLINE

Tetracyclines are a particularly useful group of antibiotics for treating periodontal diseases because they are concentrated in the gingival sulcus fluid. In other words, when administered orally, a higher concentration of the antibiotic is available in the gingival fluid than in the circulating plasma. *A. actinomycetemcomitans* is usually susceptible to tetracycline. Therefore, this antibiotic is particularly helpful in the treatment of localized juvenile periodontitis. The drug is usually prescribed in the form of minocycline, which has a long serum half-life, or doxycycline, which tends to have a lower incidence of gastrointestinal side effects than generic forms of tetracycline. In addition to their antimicrobial effect, tetracyclines may be helpful in periodontal therapy because they inhibit collagenase activity and thus help to control the spread of disease.[50]

METRONIDAZOLE

Metronidazole has been used to treat periodontal diseases because of its ability to inhibit several periodontal pathogens, including spirochetes, *Porphyromonas* species, and *Prevotella* species. Because metronidazole kills anaerobic bacteria, its use in treating rapidly progressing periodontitis seems logical. It is not effective against *A. actinomycetemcomitans*, so it is not prescribed to treat juvenile periodontitis.[50]

PENICILLIN

Penicillin is less effective against periodontal disease infections than other drugs because many periodontal pathogens are resistant to it. Resistance occurs when bacteria produce enzymes that break down the antibiotic. These enzymes are produced by other bacteria in the periodontal pocket. This resistance may be overcome by the addition of other chemicals to the antibiotic. One penicillin-type drug, a combination of amoxicillin and potassium clavulanate, has been useful in the treatment of refractory periodontitis.[51]

OTHER DRUGS

Other agents, such as clindamycin and ciprofloxacin, have been recommended for use in controlling refractory periodontitis and rapidly progressive periodontitis based on limited studies. However, their effectiveness and place in periodontal therapy is still being investigated. A promising supplemental treatment has been to use several of these agents in combination. Although metronidazole and amoxicillin are not effective alone in eliminating *A. actinomycetemcomitans* in localized juvenile periodontitis and rapidly progressive periodontitis, studies have shown that they may work well when used together.[52]

Treatment Considerations

Systemic antibiotic treatment is not without risk. There is the possibility of allergic reactions and the development of resistant strains of pathogenic bacteria. In addition, all antibiotics have side effects that may cause unpleasant reactions or toxicity.[53] Side effects include stomach upset, diarrhea, abdominal pain, dizziness, and muscle weakness. An important side effect of tetracycline is that it interferes with the effectiveness of birth control pills.

It is always wise to determine which organisms are associated with the disease and whether they are susceptible to the specific antibiotic being considered before prescribing antibiotics. This permits use of a drug to target the correct pathogens. Laboratory tests can provide information about microbiologic culture and antibiotic sensitivity. However, these tests are expensive and time consuming. Laboratories have developed methods of DNA analysis to determine which species of predominant bacteria are found in periodontal pockets, and a number of diagnostic kits for in-office identification have been developed.[54] The major drawback of these assays is that they are only available for a few pathogens, and these few may not be present at high levels in all periodontal infections.[55]

Rapid chairside identification of the predominant microbial forms in periodontal infections will facilitate the appropriate use of antibiotics in the treatment of periodontal diseases. Until the microbiology of periodontitis is better understood, and rapid testing is available for all pathogens, antibiotics are prescribed at the discretion of the dentist and periodontist. They are most often used to augment the treatment of juvenile periodontitis and in cases that respond poorly to mechanical therapy.

Locally Delivered Controlled-Release Antibiotics

Locally delivered controlled-release antibiotics are now available to assist in treating periodontal diseases. A controlled-release tetracycline fiber can be packed into isolated periodontal pockets that do not respond to other methods of treatment. The fibers effectively control the number of periodontal pathogens in periodontal pockets and reduce the clinical signs of refractory diseases. Tetracycline fibers deliver a continuous high level of antibiotic directly to the site of infection, an advantage over systemic delivery.[56] They have been shown to reduce bleeding and periodontal pocket measurements by about 2 mm in pockets over 7 mm deep. The results were favorable but less dramatic in shallower pockets (Figure 7–15).

Other approaches to local delivery utilize other drugs. Doxycycline hyclate, an analogue of tetracycline, is available for use in the form of a biodegradable polymer gel. The gel preparation is liquid when mixed, applied to infected pockets using a syringe, and becomes a semisolid gel as it heats to body temperature. Clinical trials indicate this preparation has similar treatment results to those obtained using tetracycline fibers. It is also similar to the results of meticulous scaling and root planing.[57] Metronidazole, an antibiotic effective against gram negative organisms and protozoans, and minocycline, a broad spectrum antibiotic, are also being tested for local use. These forms of local treatment are not yet available.

The antimicrobial disinfectant chlorhexidine can be employed for local therapy in the form of a biodegradable chip containing 2.5 mg of chlorhexidine. The chip is relatively large, it measures 5 mm high by 4 mm wide, so it can really only be used in deep pockets. This delivery system has the obvious advantage of ease in placement. It is also biodegradable and contains no antibiotic. Using a disinfectant rather than an antibiotic removes the risk of potential side effects or the development of resistance to drugs that might one day be needed for lifesaving procedures. One study has compared the effectiveness of the chips to scaling and root planing alone in patients with 5 mm to 8 mm pockets. When the chip was applied after scaling and root planing, the results showed about 1 mm improvement in probing depth and 0.75 mm improvement in attachment loss measurements compared to 0.65 mm probe depth reduction and 0.58 mm improvement in attachment loss for scaling followed by placebo treatment.[58]

There are major advantages of locally delivered antimicrobial agents over systemically delivered ones. First, local delivery results in much lower amounts of the drug present in the serum. The drug is still absorbed through the periodontium into the serum, but at a very low rate. The total dose required is also much lower than doses required for systemic administration, and this greatly reduces any risk of systemic side effects. Second, the active agent is present in high concentration at the site of infection, rather than having to be diffused through the entire circulatory system.[59]

The agents used for local delivery produce small clinical changes, but they can be significant, especially in deep pockets and hard-to-instrument areas such as furcations. More effective agents will be identified and delivery

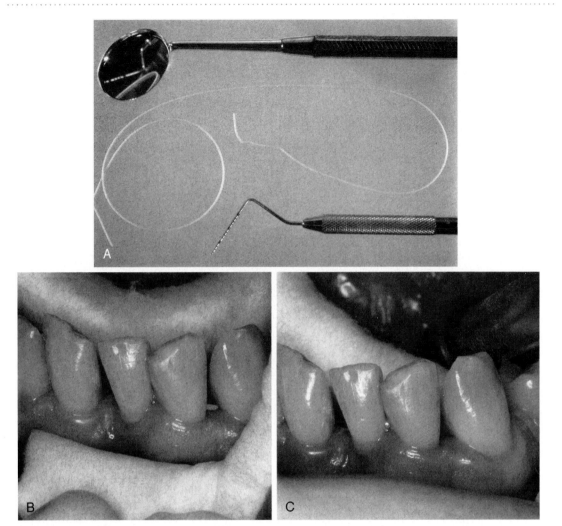

FIGURE 7–15. Local delivery of antibiotics. Tetracycline fibers are available to treat periodontal diseases. When packed into the periodontal pockets, they provide a dose of antibiotic directly to the site of infection. Tetracycline fibers are used to treat isolated pockets and areas that are unresponsive to conventional treatment techniques. **A.** Fiber placement requires a probe or other instrument to pack the fibers into a dense mass in the periodontal pocket. **B.** Tetracycline fibers placed on the distal aspect of the mandibular left lateral incisor. The tip of the fiber protrudes from the pocket. The fiber is pushed completely into the pocket and held in place with a tissue adhesive for 10 days. **C.** Two weeks after fiber removal, the tissue appears firm and healthy. The pocket depth has been reduced from 7 to 5 mm as a result of tissue shrinkage and connective tissue healing.

systems will no doubt improve over time, so this form of treatment will continue to be useful in periodontal therapy. At this time, these agents hold particular promise for treatment of isolated recurrent periodontitis in patients who are on periodontal maintenance therapy,[60] or the treatment of medically compromised patients who cannot tolerate the spectrum of conventional periodontal therapies.[61]

Enzyme Suppression Therapy

A significant portion of the tissue destruction observed in the pathogenesis of periodontal disease results from the enzymes released by the inflammatory response to bacterial plaque.[62] These enzymes are cytokines that mediate the destruction of collagen and therefore damage gingival and periodontal fibers. They also have effects on the alveolar bone and trigger resorption by stimulating osteoclastic activity (refer to Chapter 2, Host Response section). Studies have been directed toward identifying the cytokines present in gingival fluid (an early inflammatory reaction to periodontal infection) and finding ways to reduce or eliminate them in the inflammatory process.[63]

This knowledge has led to exploring **enzyme suppression therapy**. Some types of tetracycline antibiotics, such as doxycycline, have both antibiotic and enzyme inhibition effects.[64] Sub-antimicrobial doses of doxycycline have been shown to produce enzyme inhibition that is not related to antibiotic activity. A 12-month protocol of this medication, doxycycline hyclate taken orally twice per day in 20 mg doses, enhanced the results of scaling and root planing in patients with moderate periodontal disease. The drug protocol contributed to greater reductions in probing depths in deep pockets, and more attachment level gains. These changes equaled about 0.5 mm improvement in the drug treatment group over scaling and placebo control. The effects were more dramatic, up to 2 mm improvement, in deeper pockets. Bacterial resistance did not develop in the subjects because of the low dose regimen.[65] Although these changes were small, there were substantial and clinically significant improvements in deeper pockets. This is a promising new treatment for periodontitis and will lead to many developments in the future.

CONCLUSION

Periodontitis is a collection of diseases that are characterized by destruction of the attachment apparatus of the teeth. They have been classified according to age of onset, clinical manifestations, and rate of progression. These diseases are caused by an overgrowth of bacteria that inhabit the oral cavity and subgingival environment. Specific types of bacteria may be increased in different forms of periodontal disease.

The dental hygienist often provides the first line of recognition and treatment for chronic periodontitis, which is among the most common human diseases. It is important for the dental hygienist to be familiar with all of the forms of periodontal diseases, recognize diseases that are unusual or may represent systemic involvement, and suggest referral to specialists when symptoms suggest advanced or unusual periodontal diseases or conditions.

STUDY QUESTIONS

MULTIPLE CHOICE

1. What is the principal etiologic agent of periodontitis?

   a. a neutrophil deficiency
   b. dental plaque
   c. subgingival calculus
   d. antigen-antibody reactions

2. Gingivitis and periodontitis share all the following characteristics EXCEPT one. Which one is the EXCEPTION?

   a. tissue inflammation
   b. pocket formation
   c. alveolar bone loss
   d. collagen fiber destruction

3. All of the following conditions contribute to the retention of dental plaque EXCEPT one. Which one is the EXCEPTION?

   a. subgingival calculus
   b. cigarette smoking
   c. deep pockets
   d. overhanging restoration margins

4. Chronic periodontitis is:

   a. a rare disease
   b. usually significant before age 35
   c. either localized or generalized
   d. not treatable with antibiotics

5. Localized juvenile periodontitis is associated with all the following characteristics EXCEPT one. Which one is the EXCEPTION?

   a. bone loss around the molars and incisors
   b. patients younger than 20 years old
   c. a neutrophil defect
   d. *Porphyromonas gingivalis*

6. Periodontal disease can be assumed to be progressing when:

   a. there is bleeding on gentle probing
   b. pockets are present
   c. attachment loss increases over time
   d. bone loss is evident in radiographs

7. Cigarette smoking is a risk factor for periodontal disease because:

   a. smokers have poor plaque control
   b. gingival bleeding is increased
   c. fibroblast function increases
   d. gingival healing is retarded

8. All of the following diseases are forms of aggressive periodontitis EXCEPT one. Which one is the EXCEPTION?

   a. chronic periodontitis
   b. refractory periodontitis
   c. rapidly progressive periodontitis
   d. localized juvenile periodontitis

9. Systemic antibiotic therapy may be useful in the treatment of some forms of periodontitis because the microbial flora in chronic periodontitis is composed of known amounts of specific pathogens.

   a. Both the statement and the reason are correct and related.
   b. Both the statement and the reason are correct but NOT related.
   c. The statement is correct, but the reason is NOT.
   d. The statement is NOT correct, but the reason is correct.
   e. NEITHER the statement NOR the reason is correct.

10. The most useful antibiotic for augmenting the treatment of juvenile periodontitis is penicillin because the microbial flora of this form of the disease is composed of up to 90% *A. actinomycetemcomitans*.

    a. Both the statement and the reason are correct and related.
    b. Both the statement and the reason are correct but NOT related.
    c. The statement is correct, but the reason is NOT.
    d. The statement is NOT correct, but the reason is correct.
    e. NEITHER the statement NOR the reason is correct.

SHORT ANSWER

11. Describe the differences between refractory periodontitis and recurrent adult periodontitis.

    _____

    _____

12. List the four identifying characteristics of early-onset periodontitis.

    _____

    _____

13. Which type of bacteria is associated with localized juvenile periodontitis?

    _____

    _____

14. Why are tetracyclines so useful in the treatment of some periodontal infections?

_____

_____

15. What are the three main roles of the dental hygienist in the treatment of periodontal diseases?

_____

_____

REFERENCES

1. American Academy of Periodontology. Glossary of Periodontal Terms. Chicago: American Academy of Periodontology, 1992:37-38.
2. Armitage GA. Development of a classification system for periodontal diseases and conditions. Ann Periodontal 1999;4:1-6.
3. Goodson JM, Tanner ACR, Haffajee AD, Sornberger GC, Socransky SS. Patterns of progression and regression of advanced periodontal disease. J Clin Periodontol 1982;9:472-481.
4. American Academy of Periodontology. Current Procedural Terminology for Periodontics and Insurance Reporting Manual. Chicago: American Academy of Periodontology, 1991:19.
5. Workshop on Quality Assurance in Dentistry. J Dent Educ 1994;58:659-662.
6. Christersson LA, Zambon JJ, Denford RG, Grossi SG, Genco RJ. Specific subgingival bacteria and diagnosis of gingivitis and periodontitis. J Dent Res 1989;68:1633-1639.
7. Haake SK. Periodontal microbiology. In FA Carranza and MG Newman, eds. Clinical Peridontology, 8th ed. WB Saunders Co. Philadelphia; 1996:84-103.
8. Slots J, Listgarten MA. *Bacteroides gingivalis, Bacteroides intermedius,* and *Actinobacillus actinomycetemcomitans* in human periodontal diseases. J Clin Periodontol 1988;15:85-93.
9. Rabbani GM, Ash MM, Caffesse RG. The effectiveness of subgingival scaling and root planing in calculus removal. J Periodontol 1981;52:119-123.
10. Beck J, Garcia R, Heiss G, Vokonas PS, Offenbacher S. Periodontal disease and cardiovascular disease. J Periodontol 1996;67:1123-1237.
11. Offenbacher S, Katz V, Fertik G, Collins J, Boyd D, Maynor G, McKaig R, Beck J. Periodontal infection as a possible risk factor for preterm low birth weight. J Periodontol 1996;67:1103-1113.
12. Scannapieco FA, Mylotte JM. Relationships between periodontal disease and bacterial pneumonia. J Periodontol 1996;67:1114-1122.
13. Taylor GW, Burt BA, Becker MP, Genco RJ, Shlossman M, Knowler WC, Pettitt DJ. Severe periodontitis and risk for poor glycemic control in patients with non-insulin-dependent diabetes mellitus. J Periodontol 1996;67:1085-1093.
14. SUNY Buffalo School of Dental Medicine. Gum disease and heart attacks: a connection. Oral Health Newsletter 1998;1:1-3.
15. Arbes SJ, Slade GD, Beck JD. Association between extent of periodontal attachment loss and self-reported history of heart attack: an analysis of NHANES III data. J Dent Res 1999;78:1777-1782.
16. Joshipura KJ, Douglass CW, Willett WC. Possible explanation for the tooth loss and cardiovascular disease relationship. Ann Periodontol 1998;3:174-183.
17. Löe H. Periodontal disease the 6th complication of diabetes mellitus. Diabetes Care 1993;16:329-334.
18. Moore PA, Weyant RJ, Mongelluzzo MB, Myers DE, Rossie K, Guggenheimer J, Block HM, Huber H, Orchard T. Type I diabetes mellitus and oral health: assessment of periodontal disease. J Periodontol 1999; 70:409-417.
19. Hobbs HC, Rowe DJ, Johnson PW. Periodontal ligament cells from insulin-dependent diabetes exhibit altered alkaline phosphatase activity in response to growth factors. J Periodontol 1999;70:736-742.
20. Löe H, Anerud A, Boysen H, Smith M. The natural history of periodontal disease in man. The rate of periodontal destruction before 40 years of age. J Periodontol 1978;49:607-620.
21. Albandar JM. A 6-year study on the pattern of periodontal disease progression. J Clin Periodontol 1990;17:467-471.
22. Haffajee AD, Socransky SS. Microbial etiological agents of destructive periodontal diseases. Periodontal 2000 1997;14:12-32.
23. Socransky SS, Haffajee AD, Cugini MA, Smith C, Kent RI. Microbial complexes in subgingival plaque. J Clin Periodontol 1998;25:134-144.
24. Nevins M, Becker W, Kornman K, eds. World Workshop in Clinical Periodontics. Chicago. American Academy of Periodontology, 1989:123-131.
25. Page RC, Bowen T, Altman L, Page RC, Bowen T, Altman L, Vandesteen E, Ochs M, Mackenzie P, Osterberg L, Engel D, Williams BL. Prepubertal periodontitis: I. Definition of a clinical disease entity. J Periodontology 1983;54:257-271.
26. Ranney RR. Diagnosis of periodontal disease. Adv Dent Res 1991;5:21-36.
27. Löe H, Brown LJ. Early onset periodontitis in the United States of America. J Periodontol 1991;36:177-187.
28. Suzuki JB, Collison BC, Falkler WA, Nauman RR. Immunologic profile of juvenile periodontitis: II. Neutrophil chemotaxis, phagocytosis and spore germination. J Periodontol 1984;55:461-467.
29. American Academy of Periodontology. Periodontal diseases of children and adolescents. Chicago: American Academy of Periodontology, 1992:1.
30. Ranney RR. Immunological studies of young adults with severe periodontitis: I. Medical evaluation and humoral factors. J Periodontal Res 1981;16:390-402.
31. Genco RJ. Systemic antimicrobials in the management of periodontal diseases. In Periodontal Disease Management. Chicago: American Academy of Peridontology, 1994:237-252.
32. Hirschfeld L, Wasserman B. A long-term survey of tooth loss in 600 treated periodontal patients. J Periodontol 1978;49:225-227.
33. Haffajee AD, Socransky SS, Goodson JM. Clinical parameters as predictors for destructive periodontal disease activity. J Clin Periodontol 1983;10:257-265.
34. Glick M, Muzyka BC, Salkin LM, Lurie D. Necrotizing ulcerative periodontitis: a marker for immune deterioration and a predictor for the diagnosis of AIDS. J Periodontol 1994;65:393-397.
35. Dello Russo MM. The post-prophylaxis periodontal abscess. Etiology and treatment. Int J Perio Restor Dent 1985;5:29-34.
36. Perry DA, Taggart EJ. Occurrence of periodontal abscess in incompletely treated periodontal disease. J Dent Res 1996;76:[Abstract 568].
37. Lang NP, Joss A, Orsanic T, Gusberti FA, Siegrist BE.

Bleeding on probing: a predictor for the progression of periodontal diseases? J Clin Periodontol 1986;13:590-596.

38. Kornman K, Loesche W. The subgingival microflora during pregnancy. J Periodontol Res 1980;15:111-122.

39. Haber J, Wattles J, Crowley M, Mandell R, Joshipura K, Kent RL. Evidence for cigarette smoking as a major risk factor for periodontitis. J Periodontol 1993;64:16-23.

40. Linder GJ, Mullally BH. Cigarette smoking and periodontal destruction in young adults. J Periodontol 1994;65:718-723.

41. Holm G. Smoking as an additional risk for tooth loss. J Periodontol 1994;65:996-1001.

42. Renvert S, Dahlen G, Wikstrom, M. The clinical and microbiological effects of non-surgical periodontal therapy in smokers and non-smokers. J Clin Periodontol 1998;25:153-157.

43. Kenny EB, Kraal JH, Saxe SR, Hones J. The effects of cigarette smoke on human oral polymorphonuclear leukocytes. J Perio Res 1997;12:227-234.

44. Robertson PB, Walsh M, Greene J, Ernster V, Grady D, Hauck W. Periodontal effects associated with the use of smokeless tobacco. J Periodontol 1990;61:438-443.

45. American Academy of Periodontology. Tobacco use and the periodontal patient. J Periodontol 1999;70:1419-1427.

46. Horton JE, Raisz LG, Simmons HA, Oppenheim JJ, Mergenhagen SE. Bone resorbing activity in supernatant fluid from cultured human peripheral blood lymphocytes. Science 1972;177:793-795.

47. Williams RC, Jeffcoat MK, Howell TH, Bolla A, Stubbs D, Teoh KW, Reddy MS, Godhaber P. Altering the progression of human alveolar bone loss with nonsteroidal anti-inflammatory drugs. J Periodontol 1989;60:485-490.

48. Listgarten MA. Pathogenesis of periodontitis. J Clin Periodontol 1986;13:418-425.

49. Korman KS, Crane A, Wang H-Y. The interleukin-1 genotype as a severity factor in adult periodontal disease. J Clin Perio 1997;24:72-77.

50. Gordon JM, Walker CB. Current status of systemic antibiotic usage in destructive periodontal disease. J Periodontol 1993;64:760-771.

51. Manusson I, Clark WB, Low SB, Maruniak J, Marks RG, Walker CB. Effect of non-surgical periodontal therapy, combined with adjunctive antibiotics in subjects with "refractory" periodontal disease: I. Clinical results. J Clin Periodontol 1989;16:647-653.

52. Pavicic MJ, van Winkelhoff AJ, Douque NH, Steures RWR, DeGraaf J. Microbiological and clinical effects of metronidazole and amoxicillin in *Actinobacillus actinomycetemcomitans* associated periodontitis. J Clin Periodontol 1994;21:107-112.

53. Genco RJ. Antibiotics in the treatment of periodontal diseases. J Periodontol 1981;52:545-558.

54. Greenstein G. Diagnosis of periodontal diseases. Compend Contin Educ 1994;15:750-770.

55. Newman MG, Sanz M. Advanced diagnostic techniques. In FA Carranza and MG Newman eds. Clinical Periodontology, 8th ed. WB Saunders. Philadelphia; 1996:375-390.

56. Tonetti M, Cugini MA, Goodson JM. Zero-order delivery with periodontal placement of tetracycline-loaded ethylene vinyl acetate fibers. J Periodontol Res 1990; 25:243-249.

57. Garrett S, Johnson L, Drisko CH. Two multi-center studies evaluation of locally delivered doxycycline hyclate, placebo control, oral hygiene, and scaling and root planing in the treatment of periodontitis. J Periodontol 1999;70:490-503.

58. Jeffcoat MK, Bray KS, Ciancio SG. Adjunctive use of a subgingival controlled-release chlorhexidine chip reduces probing depth and improves attachment levels compared with scaling and root planing alone. J Periodontol 1998;69:989-997.

59. Rapley JW, Cobb CM, Killoy WJ, Williams DR. Serum levels of tetracycline during treatment with tetracycline-containing fibers. J Periodontol 1992;63:817-820.

60. Newman MG, Kornman KS, Doherty FM. A 6-month multicenter evaluation of adjunctive tetracycline fiber therapy used in conjunction with scaling and root planing in maintenance patients: clinical results. J Periodontol 1994;65:685-691.

61. Jolkovsky DL, Ciancio SC. Antimicrobial and other chemotherapeutic agents in periodontal therapy. In FA Carranza and MG Newman eds. Clinical Periodontology, 8th ed. WB Saunders. Philadelphia 1996;511-512.

62. American Academy of Periodontology. The pathogenesis of periodontal disease. J Periodontol 1999;70:457-470.

63. Ingman T, Tervahartiala T, Ding Y, Tschesche H, Haerian A, Kinane DF, Konttinen YT, Sorsa T. Matrix metalloproteinases and their inhibitors in gingival crevicular fluid and saliva of periodontitis patients. J Clin Periodontol 1996;23:1127-1132.

64. Golub LM, Lee HM, Greenwald RA, Ryan ME, Sorsa T, Salo T, Giannobile WV. A matrix metalloproteinase inhibitor reduces bone-type collagen degradation fragments and specific collagenases in gingival crevicular fluid during adult periodontitis. Inflamm Res 1997; 46:310-319.

65. Caton J, Blieden T, Adams D, Crout R, Hefti A, Killoy W, Nagy R, O'Neal R, Quinones C, Taggart E, Wolff M, Ciancio S. Submicrobial doxycycline therapy for periodontitis. J Dent Res 1997;76:[Abstract 1307].

8

Phyllis L. Beemsterboer

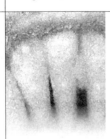

Occlusion and Temporomandibular Disorders

Chapter Objectives

1. Define the role of the dental hygienist in the detection of occlusal abnormalities and jaw dysfunction.
2. Describe the biologic basis of occlusal function and the adaptive capability of the oral system.
3. Compare and contrast the classification of primary and secondary traumatic occlusion in periodontal diagnosis and treatment.
4. Describe the cause and list the common signs and symptoms of temporomandibular disorders.
5. Describe the procedures for clinically assessing jaw function and occlusion in a screening examination.
6. Identify the various modalities used to treat temporomandibular disorders.

Key Terms

Bruxism
Dysfunction
Myalgia
Occlusal function

Orthofunction
Trauma from occlusion
Trismus

The dental hygienist has an important role in the detection of occlusal abnormalities and jaw dysfunction. The application of true prevention principles includes attention to the form and function of all aspects of the head and neck. Form is the morphology of the teeth, bones, and temporomandibular joint (TMJ), whereas function includes the jaw muscles and neuromuscular system. Good oral health requires the functional harmony of the teeth, muscles, and TMJ.

Bacterial plaque is the causative factor in periodontal diseases. However, numerous local and systemic factors can affect the response of the body to inflammatory periodontal diseases. This chapter describes the relationship of normal and abnormal form and function to provide a better understanding of **occlusal function** and dysfunction in periodontal treatment. In addition, it describes a method of screening for temporomandibular disorders (TMDs). The classification and treatment of these disorders are also discussed. The role of the dental hygienist is to *recognize* the signs and symptoms of pain and dysfunction, *record* the parameters of these signs and symptoms, and *refer* the patient for diagnosis and treatment.

BIOLOGIC BASIS OF OCCLUSAL FUNCTION

The oral cavity in function—during talking, chewing, and swallowing—is in a dynamic rather than a static state. **Orthofunction** is a state of morphofunctional harmony in which the forces developed during function are within an adaptive physiologic range. In orthofunction, which means health and comfort for the patient, there are no pathologic changes in the oral tissues. Another term used to describe a range of morphologic variability is physiologic occlusion. This term indicates psychologic and physical comfort for the patient, a normal adaptive situation. An occlusal relationship that functions for the patient is considered optimum and does not follow a particular occlusal configuration.[1, 2] For example, a malocclusion, although not ideal, can still be in orthofunction.

Dysfunction is a state of morphofunctional disharmony in which the forces developed during function cause pathologic changes in the tissues. These changes result in abnormal function or pain. The degree of dysfunction can be slight, with no great disturbance to the patient, or significant, making daily activity difficult or impossible.

The range of morphofunctional harmony to disharmony is dependent on the adaptive capability of the oral system.[1, 3-7] At one end of the spectrum is the normal range, orthofunction. When the forces directed through the teeth and periodontol attachment in function and parafunction exceed what an individual system can handle, dysfunction may result. This trauma occurs where the greatest force is exerted against a weakened periodontal apparatus. Axial forces directed along the tooth and periodontium usually meet the demands necessary for normal function. Parafunctional activity, such as grinding or clenching, can stress this system. Antiaxial forces directed along the tooth and periodontium can cause resorption or a hypertrophic response. For this reason, some areas in the oral cavity will break down as a result of these forces, whereas other areas will not show any injury.

Certain factors affect the response of the teeth and periodontal structures to normal and abnormal functions. These factors include the size and shape of the roots, the quantity and quality of the alveolar bone, and the presence of microbial plaque.[8, 9] Oral habits and other occlusal situations, such as missing or shifting teeth, can increase the frequency and force on the teeth. When periodontal disease has weakened the periodontium, these forces may exceed the individual's adaptive capability, causing injury. At this point, a treatment intervention can correct an existing problem and prevent further damage. An occlusal contact relationship that is harmonious does not produce a painful response in the masticatory system.

When the condyles of the TMJ rest in the normal closed superoanterior position and the mandible has a well-distributed, even contact with the maxilla, the maxillary system is in a stable relationship. This situation allows the TMJ system to tolerate such activities as hyperfunction and possibly some trauma. The structures of the masticatory system can tolerate a certain amount of functional change. When functional changes exceed a certain level, alteration to the tissues begin. This structural breakdown will vary depending on the individual and on systemic and local factors.[5]

Trauma from Occlusion

A traumatic occlusion is an occlusion that has caused injury to the teeth, muscles, or TMJ.[10] A classification of primary traumatic occlusion is made when heavy occlusal forces exceed the adaptive range in a normal periodontium, causing injury to tissues and bone. A classification of secondary traumatic occlusion is made when normal occlusal forces exceed the capability of a periodontium that is already affected by periodontal disease. **Trauma from occlusion** does not initiate gingivitis and periodontal disease. When inflammation is present, occlusal trauma can increase tissue attachment loss and supporting bone destruction. Therefore, occlusal trauma is of interest in the diagnosis and treatment of periodontal disease.[11]

Traumatic occlusion does not refer to a malocclusion as described by Angle's three classifications. Angle's Class I, II, or III occlusion classifies and describes the skeletal relationship of the maxillary to the mandibular teeth. Because malocclusion of the teeth may interfere with the removal of bacterial plaque, it is a factor in the attainment of good oral hygiene. Common terms used to describe mandibular function and dysfunction are listed in Terms Used to Describe Mandibular Function and Dysfunction.

The occlusal relationship of the teeth is not a predictor of pain or problems in the TMJ. Common occlusal features, such as intercuspal position or midline discrepancies, do not provide the dominant factors in defining TMD populations.[12]

Controversy regarding the clinical significance of trauma from occlusion has existed for some time. It is now widely accepted that in the absence of marginal gingival irritation, trauma from occlusion does not produce gingival inflammation. Trauma associated with orthodontic movement of teeth is self-limiting. Self-limited mobility is greater than normal, but based on the adaptive capacity of the periodontium. Thus, the increased mobility of the teeth is handled through periodontal adaptation to the excessive forces without causing trauma from occlusion.[1] Dentists use this rationale when selectively grinding on the occlusal surface of the teeth after periodontal therapy to create a dentition that does not produce injury. The goal is to establish an occlusal relationship that will foster a favorable periodontal response. True trauma from occlusion (trauma that exceeds the adaptive capacity of the periodontium) increases bone loss and pocket depth formation. This situation may occur with bruxism in a periodontal patient.

Certain tooth relationships can also be detrimental to the attainment of good periodontal

TERMS USED TO DESCRIBE MANDIBULAR FUNCTION AND DYSFUNCTION

Arthralgia   Pain in a joint structure.
Arthrocentesis   Puncture of a joint space with a needle and removal of fluid.
Bruxism   Grinding or gnashing of the teeth, usually during sleep; an oral habit that can cause periodontal injury and pain and discomfort in the jaw.
Clenching   Clamping and forcing the teeth together without grinding.
Clicking   Cracking or snapping noise in the temporomandibular joint because of disk and condyle incoordination; can occur in one or both joints.
Crepitation   Grating noise in the temporomandibular joint because of damage to the disk and articulating joint surfaces.
Dyskinesia   Abnormal movement; can describe masticatory muscle incoordination or spasm.
Excursive movement   Mandible in movement from side to side and forward; movement away from the intercuspal position.
Fremitus   Vibration or movement of a tooth when in function; can be observed or felt by placing a finger over the tooth.
Hypertrophic   Enlargement.
Intercuspal position   The maximum intercuspation of the mandibular and maxillary teeth; also called "centric occlusion" and "habitual occlusion."
Laterotrusion   Mandibular movement away from the midline; the laterotrusive side moves away from the midline in function, and the mediotrusive side moves toward the midline.
Morphofunctional   Relationship of form and function.
Myalgia   Pain in a muscle.
Myositis   Inflammation in a muscle.
Occlusal therapy   Treatment that alters the occlusal contacts or mandibular position of the jaw.
Occlusal trauma   Pathologic changes in the oral cavity as a result of occlusal forces, an occlusion-producing injury.
Orthofunction   A state of mophofunctional harmony in which the forces developed during function are within an adaptive physiologic range.
Parafunctional   Movement of the mandible outside the range of function.
Physiologic occlusion   An occlusion that is free of disease and dysfunction and has adapted to some physiologic changes.
Retruded contact position   The mandible in the end point of the terminal hinge closure, also called "centric relation position."
Spasm   Involuntary contraction of a muscle or muscles, usually painful and interfering with function.
Trismus   Spasm in the masticatory muscles associated with a disturbance in the trigeminal nerve.

health. Open contacts or faulty contacts between teeth can cause areas of food impaction. Food impaction is the forceful wedging of food into the periodontium by occlusal forces. The self-cleansing aspects of the dentition do not exist in these situations, and food impaction can be a contributing factor in periodontal disease.

The dental hygienist must carefully complete the clinical assessment of the patient, noting all of the gingival conditions and determining the reason for the condition if possible. In the past, certain gingival conditions, such as recession, clefting, or thickening of the gingival margin, were thought to be caused by trauma from the occlusion. These causative relationships have not been supported by research.

Understanding the multifactorial origin of jaw dysfunction and how it relates to the treatment of the periodontal patient is important. When an individual can attain and maintain good oral hygiene, malocclusion of the teeth is of no periodontal significance.[1] However, most patients have difficulty with plaque removal, making malocclusion a factor to be considered in the progression of periodontal disease.

TEMPOROMANDIBULAR DISORDERS

TMDs are a grouping of musculoskeletal conditions that produce pain or dysfunction in the masticatory system. When the disorder involves the muscles and not the joint, it is referred to as extracapsular. A problem occurring in the TMJ is known as intracapsular. The percentage of people who have signs or symptoms of a functional disorder can be as low as 5 percent or as high as 60 percent, making the prevalence of TMDs significant.[5, 13, 14] Historically, TMDs have been described with a number of labels, such as TMJ syndrome and myofacial pain dysfunction syndrome. Most orofacial clinicians and researchers agree that TMD is a term that accurately reflects the scope and complexity of the conditions.[3] As part of the diagnosis made by the dentist, a subcondition such as myofacial pain or arthritis further describes the problem. It is important for the dental hygienist to remember that there are many orofacial pain problems besides TMD.

Cause

The etiology of TMDs is multifactorial. Because of the many causes, TMDs are frequently diffi-cult to diagnose and treat. Stress is often a factor in TMDs, and patients with TMDs may have a history of other diseases, such as arthritis and psychological problems. In determining the causes of TMDs, a history of macrotrauma or microtrauma may be discovered by the clinician. A macrotrauma is usually a single event that may have caused damage to the masticatory system. Such an event could be a sports-related injury, a whiplash accident, or a fall. The patient may not even relate such an event to later occlusal or TMJ pain and discomfort. Microtrauma is a number of minor habits or events that cause damage to the masticatory structures. Examples of microtrauma include bruxism, postural, and oral habits.

Categories of Temporomandibular Disorders

There are four main diagnostic categories for TMD. See Diagnostec Categories for Temporomadibular Disorders. They are based on criteria derived from the signs and symptoms gathered in the comprehensive TMD evaluation.[13, 15] The first category is muscle and fascial disorders of the masticatory system. This group includes **myalgia, trismus,** spasm, dyskinesia, **bruxism,** and other muscle disorders. Disorders of the TMJ, the second category, include internal derangements that impair mechanical function of the TMJ such as arthritis conditions. The third category includes disorders of mandibular mobility, such as ankylosis, muscular fibrosis, internal derangement, and adhesions in the joint. The fourth category, disorders of maxillomandibular growth, is less common. These disorders include neoplastic and nonneoplastic conditions.

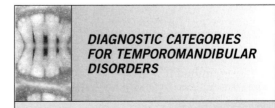

DIAGNOSTIC CATEGORIES FOR TEMPOROMANDIBULAR DISORDERS

Muscle and fascial disorders of the masticatory
  system
Disorders of the temporomandibular joint
Disorders of mandibular mobility
Disorders of maxillomandibular growth

ORAL HABITS

Oral habits can contribute to periodontal and dental damage in the oral cavity. Oral habits are repetitive masticatory activities outside the normal range of function. These parafunctional activities can involve tooth-to-tooth contact or contact with foreign objects. The amount of damage is related to the intensity and duration of the habit. Oral habits can lead to tooth damage, muscular hypertrophy, muscular pain and tenderness, and periodontal tissue injury. Bruxism is the most frequently described oral habit.

BRUXISM

Bruxism is clenching or grinding of the teeth when the individual is not chewing or swallowing. Bruxism can occur as rhythmic side-to-side movements or through a sustained clench. Clenching is continuous or intermittent closure of the jaws under vertical pressure.[6] Grinding and clenching are parafunctional habits that are involuntary and may be destructive. Bruxism is further categorized into nocturnal (nighttime) and diurnal (daytime) types. Bruxism can be identified by the presence of wear facets that are not caused by masticatory function. The results of bruxism may be tooth wear, tooth fracture, restoration fracture, myalgia, hypertrophy of the masticatory muscles, and headache. Bruxism or periodontal disease can cause mobility in the teeth. Researchers have found that bruxism does not cause damage to the periodontium and that periodontal disease and bruxism seldom occur in the same individual.[16]

The prevalence of bruxism is difficult to estimate because most patients are unaware that they grind their teeth. Stress may contribute etiologically to bruxism. Other causes may be neurologic or occupational. Bruxism is common in children between the ages of 3 and 12 years.

There is no absolute cure for bruxism. A variety of treatment approaches have been reported, with varying levels of success. Often, awareness of the problem and its consequences helps the patient to control the habit. Other treatments include occlusal splints, pharmacologic therapy, physical therapy, and behavioral modification therapy.[17-19] Bruxism can be a significant problem with patients who have advanced loss of support in the periodontal mechanism (Figures 8-1 and 8-2).

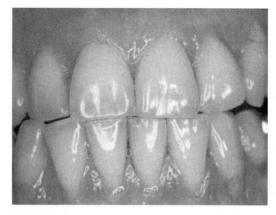

FIGURE 8–1. Bruxism caused mild tooth wear in a 56-year-old female.

Signs and Symptoms of Temporomandibular Disorders

Four primary symptoms are commonly reported in patients with TMDs. These symptoms are pain and tenderness in the muscles of mastication, pain and tenderness in the TMJ, painful clicking of the joint during function, and limitation of mandibular motion. In addition to these primary symptoms, a number of other symptoms are found in patients with TMDs. An uncomfortable bite, incoordination of the jaw (dyskinesia), ringing in the ears, and muscle swelling are described by these patients. In the dentition, signs include tooth wear, tooth mobility, and pulpitis. The presence of one or more of these symptoms does not indicate a positive diagnosis of TMD. A diagnosis can be made only after the patient undergoes a complete clinical examination for the signs of TMD

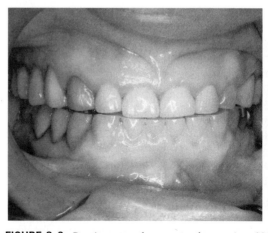

FIGURE 8–2. Bruxism caused severe tooth wear in a 32-year-old male.

and a careful differential diagnosis is completed.[10, 13, 20]

Pain in the masticatory muscles (myalgia) is the most common symptom reported by patients with a muscle disorder. This pain is usually dull, aching, and continuous or recurrent. Muscle pain may be a normal protective response or may be the result of changes in the muscle tissue caused by hyperactivity or trauma. Stress can cause an increase in the tonicity of the head and neck muscles. Associated with muscle pain is a reduction in mandibular function, usually the inability to open the mouth widely. Muscle soreness over a long period may be myofascial pain, an acute pain disorder that can occur in any muscle in the body.

Tenderness or pain in the TMJ (arthralgia) is another common finding in TMDs. The pain in this region arises from the soft tissues surrounding the joint. The articular surfaces of the joint are not innervated. This pain is sharp, sudden, and associated with the jaw in function.

The dysfunction that is common within the TMJ is usually observed in the form of a joint sound. The sound is caused by a disruption of the normal movement of the condyle and articular disk in the joint. A single sound is known as a click or a pop; a grating sound is known as crepitus. Within the joint, problems can be caused by incoordination of the disk condyle, restricted translation of the condyle, or dislocation of the condyle.[5, 13] Another set of problems result from inflammatory joint disorders, such as osteoarthritis and polyarthritis. For these patients, pain in the TMJ is dull, aching, and constant, and is increased in function.

The signs and symptoms of TMDs are observed frequently in the dentition. Mobility or movement of the teeth can result from periodontal disease or excessive occlusal forces. Tooth wear or breakdown of the enamel or dentin is a common sign. The functional or parafunctional origin of the wear is determined by locating the position of the worn surfaces on the teeth.

SCREENING FOR TEMPOROMANDIBULAR DISORDERS

Screening for TMD is an important part of the dental hygiene examination. This screening should be completed for each patient. It is simple to accomplish and does not involve a great deal of additional chair time. Once the clinician is comfortable with performing the screening, it should take approximately 3 or 4 minutes. The screening examination will lead to one of three conclusions:

1. The jaw system is in orthofunction; there are no contraindications to proceeding with dental hygiene treatment.
2. Problems exist in the jaw system; dental hygiene and dental treatment should proceed with caution, and the patient should be informed.
3. The patient should be referred for a comprehensive evaluation before any dental hygiene or dental treatment is administered.

Patients who have signs or symptoms of pain or jaw dysfunction should be referred to the dentist for a comprehensive examination. The dental hygienist is in an excellent position to identify patients with the signs and symptoms of jaw dysfunction and to refer them for treatment. Initial scaling therapy and subsequent maintenance (supportive periodontal therapy) appointments allow the dental hygienist to screen for TMD and to gather subjective information that can aid the dentist in diagnosis and treatment.

The screening examination has subjective and objective portions. The subjective portion is a series of questions that the patient is asked while the medical history is taken or during examination of the oral cavity. The objective portion is performed by the clinician and is divided into the assessment of clinical jaw function and the assessment of occlusion.

Subjective Questionnaire

The questions posed in the subjective questionnaire are designed to screen for patient-reported signs and symptoms of TMDs.[13, 15] A positive response to several of these questions does not necessarily indicate a dysfunctional situation. A comprehensive history and a complete clinical examination are needed to identify dysfunction. The patient should be asked the following questions:

1. Do you have difficulty opening your mouth?

2. Do you hear noises from the jaw joints?
3. Does your jaw "stick," "lock," or "go out"?
4. Do you have pain in or around the ears, temples, or cheeks?
5. Do you have pain when you chew or yawn?
6. Does your bite feel uncomfortable or unusual?
7. Do you have frequent headaches?
8. Have you had a recent injury to your head or neck?
9. Do you have arthritis?
10. Do you have problems chewing, talking, or using your jaws?
11. Do you clench or grind your teeth? Do others hear you grind?
12. Have you previously been treated for a jaw joint (TMJ) problem?

Assessment of Clinical Jaw Function

The techniques in the clinical objective examination are designed to identify certain signs and symptoms of TMDs. These techniques can be added to dental hygiene assessment and documentation procedures. Several positive findings do not necessarily indicate a dysfunctional situation. Dysfunction can be assessed only by a comprehensive history and a complete clinical examination.

MUSCLE PALPATION

Normal muscles are equal in length, and they contract and relax without discomfort or pain. Muscles that have been overworked or injured, are painful, and do not contract properly.[21] The

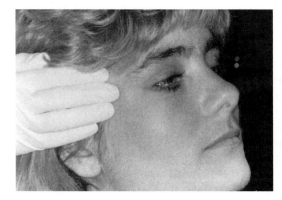

FIGURE 8–4. Palpating the temporalis muscle.

temporalis and masseter muscles are examined bilaterally by palpating the origin, body, and insertion of the muscle. Gentle finger pressure lasting 2 seconds along the muscle may elicit a response from the patient. The patient should be instructed to differentiate pressure from pain. Painful reactions should be recorded (Figures 8-3 and 8-4).

MANDIBULAR MOVEMENT

The normal opening and closing of the jaw should be smooth and symmetrical, and the patient should be able to achieve a minimum of 40 mm opening distance. The interincisal opening (incisal edge to incisal edge) is measured after the patient is asked to open the mouth as wide as possible. Any report of pain should be recorded. If the clinician can passively increase the interincisal distance for a patient (use the thumb and finger to open wider), there may be a muscular problem. The

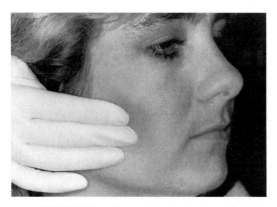

FIGURE 8–3. Palpating the masseter muscle.

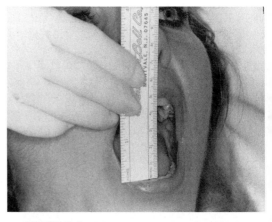

FIGURE 8–5. Measuring the interincisal distance.

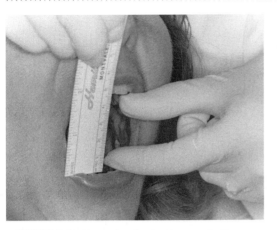

FIGURE 8–6. Measuring the passive stretch distance.

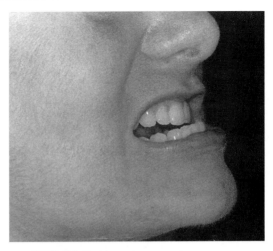

FIGURE 8–8. Measuring protrusive movement.

passive stretch distance should also be recorded (Figures 8-5 and 8-6).

The normal mandibular movement with the teeth not in contact from side to side and forward should be approximately 8 mm. This distance is recorded by measuring the patient's ability to move the mandible laterally and protrusively from the midline. The left lateral movement, right lateral movement, and protrusive movement are measured and recorded (Figures 8-7 and 8-8).

JOINT FUNCTION

Both temporomandibular joints together in function have the ability to rotate, translate, and move excursively forward and side to side. The normal maximum opening of the jaw should be smooth and straight. The pathway during opening and closing is observed for any alteration from the midline. A deviation is a shift in the midline during opening that disappears at some point later in the opening movement. A deflection is a shift in the midline that becomes greater as the opening movement continues. A deviation may be caused by interference in the disk of the joint, whereas a deflection is caused by a restriction in one joint. Any type of alteration is recorded (Figures 8-9 and 8-10).

JOINT SOUNDS

On opening, the condyle and disk of the TMJ move forward (anteriorly) to the articular eminence. The normal joint functions smoothly, without noise, irregularities, or pain. Pain or restrictions in the joint can be detected by palpation. The fingers are placed over the condyles, and slight pressure is applied. Then the patient is asked to open and close the mouth slowly. A sound elicited by the joint in function

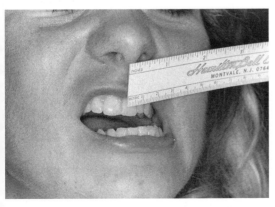

FIGURE 8–7. Measuring left lateral movement.

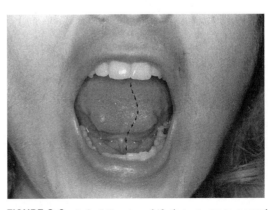

FIGURE 8–9. A deviation is a shift that returns to normal midline at opening.

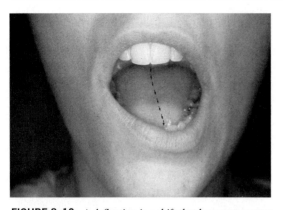

FIGURE 8–10. A deflection is a shift that becomes greater on opening.

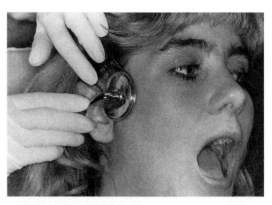

FIGURE 8–12. Listening for joint sounds. A stethoscope is also helpful, but not necessary to determine clicking or crepitus.

is either a click or crepitus. The click is a short sound, whereas crepitus is a grating sound. A sound that occurs on opening and closing is called a reciprocal click. Any irregularity, pain, or sound is noted in the chart (Figures 8-11 and 8-12).

Assessment of Occlusion

INTERCUSPAL POSITION

The normal position of the teeth in maximum intercuspation is called centric occlusion. It should be stable, with a firm, well-distributed pattern of occlusal contact. The patient should be able to open and close several times without searching for a comfortable bite. The dental hygienist should ask the patient to open and close normally, while observing the closure pattern. Any difficulty finding a comfortable bite should be noted in the chart.

The posterior teeth should have firm, even contact when the teeth are together in maximum intercuspation. The anterior teeth may have only light or no contact. To evaluate this contact, polyester film (mylar)—occlusal indicator (shim stock) paper—is placed between the teeth at small intervals. The mylar is held with a hemostat forceps. The patient is asked to close and hold on the mylar while the dental hygienist tugs slightly outward. If the mylar strip holds, there is contact. If the mylar strip slips through the teeth, there is no contact. The presence or absence of intercuspation contact should be noted for the incisors, canines, premolars, and molars on the right and left sides of the mouth (see Figures 8-13, and 8-14).

PROTRUSIVE, LATERAL, AND MEDIAL EXCURSIVE MOVEMENTS

Normal movement of the jaw with the teeth in contact should be smooth, symmetrical, and able to achieve about 8 mm of magnitude. Start-

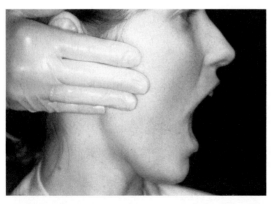

FIGURE 8–11. Palpating the temporomandibular joint. Light palpation is an excellent way to detect substantial clicks and crepitus.

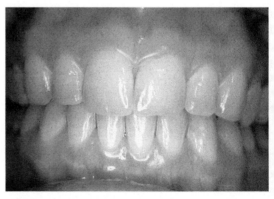

FIGURE 8–13. Teeth in normal maximum intercuspation.

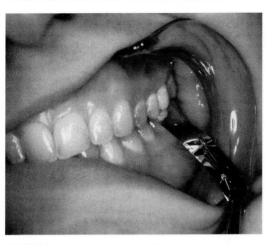

FIGURE 8–14. Determining occlusal contact in the left molar area.

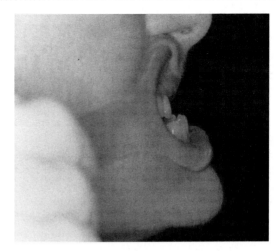

FIGURE 8–15. Determining protrusive movement.

ing in intercuspation, the patient is asked to protrude the jaw as far as possible. Movement that is limited or deviates on protrusion is recorded.

A supracontact (high spot) is an area on a tooth that may prevent well-distributed stable contact between the maxillary and mandibular teeth. Occlusal interferences are supracontacts that are capable of injuring the periodontal tissues or complicating mandibular movement.[10]

Lateral movement is examined starting from the intercuspal position. The patient is asked to move the jaw toward the right shoulder. The movement toward the right lateral side is observed, and any limitations are recorded. The test is repeated on the left side.

Medial movement is also examined starting from the intercuspal position. However, mylar film is used to determine the presence of mediotrusive or laterotrusive contacts. The mylar is placed between the molars on the right side. The patient is asked to move the jaw 2 mm toward the opposite side. If the mylar does not hold, no contact exists. If it holds, a mediotrusive contact exists. This contact may prevent proper movement of the jaw in function. The test is repeated on the left side. Supracontacts or interferences are noted in the chart (Figures 8-15 and 8-16).

TOOTH MOBILITY AND WEAR

The assessment of occlusion also includes an evaluation of tooth mobility and tooth wear as well as full mouth radiographs. These aspects of assessment and documentation are routine

elements of dental hygiene care. The results of the related dental hygiene assessment should be included in the TMD screening.

Slight mobility of the teeth, especially the lower incisors, is normal. This movement is usually charted to monitor any increases over time. Greater mobility can occur when occlusal forces exceed the adaptive capability of the periodontium. Mobility is evaluated along with the presence of disease in the periodontium. A classification of primary traumatic occlusion is made when heavy occlusal forces exceed the adaptive range in a normal periodontium. A classification of secondary traumatic occlusion is made when normal occlusal forces exceed the capability of a periodontium that is affected by periodontal disease.

The visible and palpable movement of a tooth during function or parafunction is called fremitus. The term is used to describe mobility

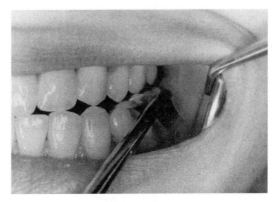

FIGURE 8–16. Determining lateral movement using a mylar strip.

and can be observed or felt. To feel the movement, the dental hygienist places a finger over the tooth root on the attached gingiva (Figure 8-17).

Wear caused by tooth-to-tooth contact is called attrition. A certain amount of wear is normal, but accelerated wear is the result of parafunctional activity, such as bruxism. Excessive wear may result in a flat tooth surface, a cupped-out occlusal surface, or obliteration of the cusps. A facet is a tooth surface worn by attrition from functional or parafunctional causes. A facet is smooth and shiny because it is the result of the enamel rods becoming fractured and polished. A facet that is shiny is known as an active facet, whereas a nonshiny or velvet-like facet is termed passive. When the facet is angular, the occlusal forces are directed laterally and increase the risk of periodontal injury.[10] To determine whether the wear is from functional or parafunctional use, the dental hygienist asks the patient to close the mouth. The dental hygienist observes the position of the mandible. If a pattern for the wear cannot be established, other factors must be considered. Oral habits, such as nail biting or foreign substance abrasion, can also cause tooth wear (Figure 8-18).

RADIOGRAPHIC EVALUATION

Excessive occlusal forces can cause changes in the teeth and periodontium. These changes can be observed in periapical radiographs. The radiographs should be examined for widening of the periodontal ligament, increased density of the surrounding bone (osteosclerosis), or increased cementum at the apical areas of the root (hypercementosis). The widening of the

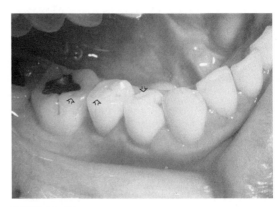

FIGURE 8–18. Wear facets (arrows) on premolars and molars.

periodontal ligament is caused by resorption of bony support from the excessive occlusal forces. Osteosclerosis and hypercementosis are hypertrophic responses to the occlusal forces (Figures 8-19 and 8-20).

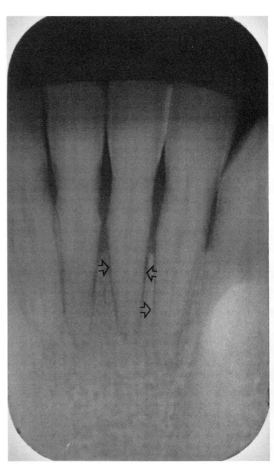

FIGURE 8–19. Widened periodontal ligament (arrows). (Courtesy of Dr. Richard Nagy.)

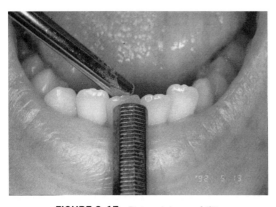

FIGURE 8–17. Determining mobility.

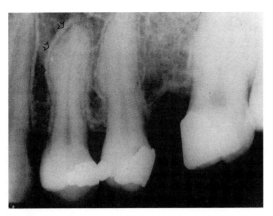

FIGURE 8–20. Hypercementosis. Arrows indicate widened cementum. (Courtesy of Dr. Stewart White.)

A temporomandibular screening form for use by the dental hygienist is provided as Figure 8-21. This form can be modified to suit the needs of a particular clinician or dental health care setting.

The Comprehensive Examination

A comprehensive examination for TMD completed by the dentist or TMD specialist involves an extensive history and physical examination. The physical examination for this expanded evaluation includes examining mandibular motion in all planes, palpating the TMJ, palpating the masticatory muscles, examining and listening to joint sounds, palpating the cervical musculature, and determining the stability of the dentition and skeleton.[13] Additional diagnostic tests and radiographs are used when necessary to aid in the diagnosis and prognosis of TMD.

TREATMENT OF TEMPOROMANDIBULAR DISORDERS

A number of modalities are used to treat TMD. The goal of treatment is to reduce pain and improve the ability of the jaw system to function. The method of treatment of TMD should be based on a clear understanding of the problem and should address the cause as well as the symptoms. Clark[22] established three criteria to be used as guidelines for selecting TMD treatments: The treatments should be based on a correct differential diagnosis, should be selected with reason and purpose, and should be directed toward eliminating or neutralizing the cause of the symptoms.[22] The patient often asks the dental hygienist for advice about treatment choices and referrals. Common treatment methods are as follows.

The approach to TMD treatment that is suggested by most orofacial clinicians and researchers is conservative and reversible.[7, 15, 23-26, 28] This conservative approach uses simple, noninvasive methods rather than irreversible methods, such as open joint surgery. A highly recommended approach uses a physical medicine model with a strong behavioral–educational component.[20, 27] Usually, this approach requires a combination of dental office therapy and home treatments. The first step in the treatment of a patient with TMD is to recommend initial therapy. In this model, initial therapy consists of suggesting a soft diet, limited movement of the jaw, application of moist heat to the affected area, and a nonnarcotic analgesic. The patient also receives a careful explanation of the disorder and the usual outcome of treatment. Patients frequently improve after 2 to 3 weeks of initial therapy. Often, simply understanding the possible reason for the symptoms leads to improvement.

Initial therapy is a set of simple, noninvasive steps that can provide immediate comfort and relief of symptoms. The first step is to instruct the patient to eat only soft foods. Avoiding food such as apples and hard rolls allows the overworked jaw muscles to rest. Moist heat provides relief from muscle pain by increasing circulation. A hand towel folded in thirds and moistened with warm water can be placed under the chin and around the neck. Icing of the muscles can also reduce pain. Ice is rubbed against the area until it is numb, approximately 5 minutes. The skin is allowed to warm between applications.

The use of nonnarcotic analgesics is often valuable in relieving jaw pain. Common over-the-counter drugs, such as aspirin and ibuprofen, can effectively reduce musculoskeletal discomfort. The dentist may prescribe stronger drugs when the symptoms do not respond to the nonnarcotic analgesics. Medications for TMD should be prescribed for a limited time.[1, 5]

Treatment Methods

HOME THERAPY

Home therapy includes initial therapy (soft diet, heat or ice packs, nonnarcotic analgesics), rest, and some jaw movement exercises. The jaw

Temporomandibular Disorders Screening Form

Assessment of Clinical Jaw Function

A.   Muscle Palpation

	Pressure (slight discomfort)	Pain (hurts)
Masseter		
Temporalis		

B.   Mandibular Movement

	Measurement in millimeters (mm)	
Interincisal opening		
Passive stretch		
Lateral movement (left and right)		
Protrusive movement		

C.   Joint Function

Opening Pathway	Normal	Deviation (returns to midline)	Deflection (becomes greater)

Palpation of the joint	No discomfort	Pain
Lateral aspect		
Posterior aspect		

D.   Joint Sounds

Sounds of the joint	No sounds	Click	Crepitus
Left joint			
Right joint			

Assessment of Occlusion

E.   Intercuspal Position

	Easy and repeatable	Difficult and searching
ICP closure pattern		

ICP contact	Right (y/n)	Left (y/n)
Incisors		
Canines		
Premolars		
Molars		

F.   Excursive Movements

Protrusive	Forward (mm)	Deviates on movement (y/n)

	Right (mm)	Left (mm)	Supracontact (y/n)
Lateral movement			
Medial movement			

G.   Tooth Evaluation

	Anterior teeth (y/n)	Posterior teeth (y/n)
Tooth mobility		
Tooth wear		
Radiographic signs		

Clinical action from screening exam and assessment:

No contraindication to dental hygiene treatment   _____

Treat with caution and informed consent for dental hygiene treatment   _____

Refer for consult and dental treatment   _____

FIGURE 8–21. Temporomandibular Disorders Screening Form.

movement exercises are demonstrated to the patient, and a daily program is recommended. The exercises both relax and stretch the sore muscles so that they can regain their original function.

PHYSICAL THERAPY

Physical therapy treatments include ultrasound, massage, electrical stimulation of the muscles, soft tissue manipulation, and exercise programs. The goal of home treatment and office treatment programs is the same: To help the patient to gain pain relief and develop new behaviors that will change any habits that contribute to the problem.

OCCLUSAL APPLIANCES

Occlusal appliances are made of hard acrylic resin. The appliance fits over the occlusal and incisal surfaces of the maxillary or mandibular teeth. The appliance is usually called a splint, nightguard, or biteguard. A splint is used to protect the teeth and to provide a stable position for them. The goal of a therapeutic splint is to reduce symptoms and encourage normal muscle function. The success or failure of a splint depends on its selection, fabrication, and adjustment.[5] The occlusal splint is not a mouthguard. A mouthguard is used by athletes to protect their teeth, head, and neck during contact sports.

In the past, occlusal adjustment was a common form of treatment for TMD. Research has shown that this modality is not as effective as more conservative methods, however. Limited occlusal adjustment may be appropriate in some situations, but it is rarely considered as primary TMD treatment.[3]

BEHAVIORAL THERAPY

Behavioral methods include stress or anxiety counseling, depression counseling, and psychiatric therapy. Pain management clinics and programs, usually offered by universities or hospitals, can provide traditional and nontraditional therapies for patients from a group of multidisciplinary practitioners.

PHARMACOLOGIC THERAPY

The groups of medications that are prescribed for patients include analgesics, antianxiety drugs, anti-inflammatory agents, muscle relaxants, and local anesthetics. These agents are administered orally or by injection.

A trigger point is a painful, hypersensitive band of muscle tissue. A trigger point can refer pain to another area, triggering pain. The use of local anesthetics, such as carbocaine, can aid in the diagnosis and treatment of this myofascial pain.

SURGICAL THERAPY

Arthroscopic and arthrocentesis surgeries can help patients with acute TMJ derangement–induced hypermobility to gain a full range of jaw motion. A condylectomy (removal of the condyle), which is more extensive than a condylotomy (partial removal), may be indicated for severe TMJ growth disturbances or tumors. Any surgical procedure should be completed only after a careful diagnosis and the consideration of a second opinion.

IRREVERSIBLE TREATMENTS

Irreversible treatments for TMD, such as surgery to the joint or disc, are permanent alterations. Surgical treatments are indicated only in a small percentage of patients.[28]

THE DENTAL HYGIENE APPOINTMENT

Dental hygienists will treat patients who have symptoms of or are in treatment for jaw pain and dysfunction. They must adapt the dental hygiene treatment plan to accommodate these patients. See Considerations for Treating the Patient with a Temporomandibular Disorder. The patient with TMD requires a series of short appointments, rather than one long appointment, to minimize trauma to the masticatory

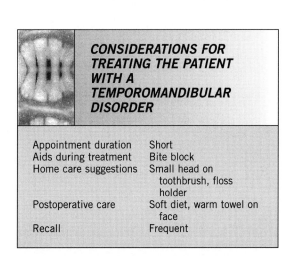

CONSIDERATIONS FOR TREATING THE PATIENT WITH A TEMPOROMANDIBULAR DISORDER

Appointment duration	Short
Aids during treatment	Bite block
Home care suggestions	Small head on toothbrush, floss holder
Postoperative care	Soft diet, warm towel on face
Recall	Frequent

muscles and joint. The use of a bite-block to maintain the oral opening is one alternative for a patient with a history of jaw pain and fatigue. The use of a toothbrush with a small head or the use of other interdental cleaning devices can simplify daily oral hygiene care for patients with limited opening or malpositioned teeth. Occasionally, dental hygiene treatment must be postponed until initial TMD therapy is completed and the patient can tolerate a lengthier appointment. Initial therapy, such as a soft diet and moist heat, may be helpful to a dental hygiene patient after a long scaling appointment.

CONCLUSION

The dental hygienist plays an important role in the detection and recording of occlusal abnormalities and jaw dysfunction. This role is to recognize the signs and symptoms of pain and dysfunction, record the parameters of these signs and symptoms, and refer the patient for diagnosis and treatment. Understanding the many local and systemic factors that can influence the response of the body to inflammatory periodontal diseases helps the dental hygienist to provide the patient with the best possible dental hygiene care.

STUDY QUESTIONS

MULTIPLE CHOICE

1. Which of the following best characterizes ortho-function?

    a. proper arch form in a Class I occlusal relationship
    b. ordinary masticatory forces
    c. few or no occlusal interferences
    d. adaptive capacity of the oro-facial complex

2. The term for heavy occlusal forces that have caused injury to tissues and bone in a normal periodontium is:

    a. physiologic occlusion
    b. dysfunctional occlusion
    c. primary traumatic occlusion
    d. secondary traumatic occlusion

3. The etiology of temporomandibular disorders is described as:

    a. behavioral
    b. neurologic
    c. psychologic
    d. multifactorial

4. An oral habit such as bruxism can result in all of the following EXCEPT one. Which one is the exception?

    a. muscular hypertrophy
    b. muscular pain and tenderness
    c. change in microflora
    d. periodontal tissue injury

5. What are the four primary symptoms of temporomandibular disorders?

    a. muscle pain, muscle swelling, jaw pain, and dyskinesia
    b. muscle pain, clicking, headache, and uncomfortable bite
    c. muscle pain, jaw pain, clicking, and limitation of motion
    d. muscle pain, jaw pain, dyskinesia, and limitation of motion

6. Myalgia is best described as:

    a. pain in the muscles
    b. incoordination of the jaw
    c. clicking in the joint
    d. crepitus in the joint

7. The normal jaw should achieve an opening distance of at least:

    a. 32 mm
    b. 38 mm
    c. 40 mm
    d. 46 mm

8. The term for an opening pathway of the jaw that shifts in the midline and disappears later in the opening movement is:

    a. deviation
    b. deflection

9. A deviation of the mandible to the right on opening suggests:

    a. crepitus
    b. clicking
    c. restriction of the left condyle
    d. restriction of the right condyle

10. The most frequently recommended approach for the treatment of temporomandibular disorders is:

    a. occlusal splint therapy
    b. pharmacologic therapy
    c. physical medicine therapy
    d. occlusal reduction therapy

SHORT ANSWER

11. What is the role of the dental hygienist in the detection of occlusal abnormalities and jaw dysfunction?

    _____

    _____

12. An occlusal relationship that functions for the patient is considered optimum. What is this relationship called?

    _____

    _____

13. What is the range of morphofunctional harmony to disharmony dependent on?

    _____

    _____

14. List several factors that can affect the response of the teeth and periodontium to function.

    _____

    _____

15. What is the term for an occlusion that has caused an injury to the teeth, muscles, or joint?

_____

_____

16. Is the occlusal relationship of the teeth a predictor of pain or problems in the temporomandibular joint?

_____

_____

17. What percentage of people have signs or symptoms of temporomandibular disorders?

_____

_____

18. List the signs and symptoms of bruxism.

_____

_____

19. Describe the eight aspects of the assessment of clinical jaw function and occlusion.

_____

_____

20. Three of the main categories of temporomandibular disorders are disorders of the joint, disorders of mandibular mobility, and disorders of maxillomandibular growth. What is the fourth category?

_____

_____

REFERENCES

1. Ramfjord SP, Ash MM. Occlusion, 3rd ed. Philadelphia: WB Saunders, 1983.
2. Solberg WK. Masticatory function. In Carranza FA Jr. Clinical Periodontics, 7th ed. Philadelphia: WB Saunders, 1990:73-89.
3. Laskin D. The president's conference of the examination, diagnosis and management of temporomandibular disorders. J Am Dent Assoc 1983;106:75.
4. Mohl ND, Zarb GA, Carlsson GE, Rugh JD. A Textbook of Occlusion. Chicago: Quintessence, 1988.
5. Okeson J. Fundamentals of Occlusion and Temporomandibular Disorders, 3rd ed. St. Louis: CV Mosby, 1992.
6. Solberg WK. The role of morphofunctional occlusal factors in periodontal disease. In Carranza FA Jr. Clinical Periodontics, 7th ed. Philadelphia: WB Saunders, 1990:422-431.
7. Solberg WK, Clark GT. Abnormal Jaw Mechanics. Chicago: Quintessence, 1981.
8. Polson AM. The relative importance of plaque and occlusion in periodontal disease. J Clin Periodontol 1986;13:923-929.
9. Schluger S, Yuodelis R, Page R, Johnson RH. Periodontal Disease, 2nd ed. Philadelphia: Lea & Febiger, 1990.
10. Solberg WK. Trauma from occlusion. In Carranza FA Jr. Clinical Periodontics, 7th ed. Philadelphia: WB Saunders, 1990:264-285.
11. Ericsson I. The combined effects of plaque and physical stress on periodontal tissues. J Clin Periodontol 1986;13:918-922.
12. Pullinger AG, Seligman DA, Gornbein JA. A multiple logistic regression analysis of the risk and relative odds of temporomandibular disorders as a function of common occlusal features. J Dent Res 1993;72: 968-979.
13. Clark GT, Seligman DA, Solberg WK, Pullinger AG. Guidelines for the examination and diagnosis of temporomandibular disorders. J Craniomandibular Disord Facial Oral Pain 1989;3:7-14.
14. Dawson PE. Evaluation, Diagnosis and Treatment of Occlusal Problems. St. Louis: CV Mosby, 1989.
15. McNeill C. Temporomandibular Disorders. Chicago: Quintessence, 1991.
16. Hanamura H, Houston F, Rylander H, Carlsson GE, Haraldson T, Nyman S. Periodontal status and bruxism. J Periodontol 1987;58:173-176.
17. Clark GT, Adachi NY, Dornan MR. A review of physical medicine procedures for temporomandibular disorders. J Am Dent Assoc 1990;121:151-162.
18. Clark GT, Beemsterboer PL, Solberg WK, Rugh JD. Nocturnal electromyographic evaluation of myofascial pain dysfunction patients undergoing occlusal splint therapy. J Am Dent Assoc 1979;99:607-611.
19. Clark GT, Beemsterboer PL, Rugh JD. Nocturnal masseter muscle activity and the symptoms of masticatory dysfunction. J Oral Rehabil 1981;8:279-286.
20. Clark GT, Seligman DA, Solberg WK, Pullinger AG. Guidelines for the treatment of temporomandibular disorders. J Craniomandibular Disord Facial Oral Pain 1990;4:80-88.
21. Miller AJ. Craniomandibular Muscles. Boca Raton: CRC Press, 1991.
22. Clark GT. Sequencing of treatment for JAW dysfunction. In Ludeen HC, Gibbs CH. Advances in Occlusion. Acton, MA: Publishing Sci Group, 1980.
23. Clark GT, Lanham F, Flack VF. Treatment outcome for consecutive TMJ clinic patients. J Craniomandibular Disord 1988;2:87-95.
24. Green CS, Laskin DM. Long term evaluation of treatment for myofacial pain-dysfunction syndrome: a comparative analysis. J Am Dent Assoc 1983;107:235-238.
25. Solberg WK, Clark GT. Temporomandibular Joint Problems. Chicago: Quintessence, 1980.
26. Ramfjord SP, Ash MM. Periodontology and Periodontics: Modern Theory and Practice. St. Louis: Ishiyaku EuroAmerica, 1989.
27. Rugh JD. Behavioral therapy. In Mohl ND, Zarb GA, Carlsson GE, Rugh JD. A Textbook in Occlusion. Chicago: Quintessence, 1988.
28. Management of Temporomandibular Disorders. NIH Technol Assess Statement 1996 Apr 29-May 1:1-31.

9

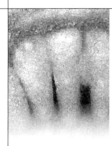

Cheryl A. Cameron / Gina D. Evans / Dorothy A. Perry

Clinical Assessment

Chapter Objectives

1. Define the aspects of clinical assessment in the dental hygiene process of patient care.
2. Describe the components of each assessment in the clinical examination.
3. List and describe the indices used to report plaque accumulation, periodontal status, furcation involvement, tooth mobility, dental caries, root caries, and tooth wear.
4. Describe the normal and abnormal clinical presentation of the periodontum and dentition.
5. Identify the radiographic changes seen in periodontal diseases.

Key Terms

Assessment
Clinical examination
Data collection

Documentation
Evaluation
Radiographic examination

Assessment is the first stage in the dental hygiene process of patient care.[1] It provides the foundation for the subsequent diagnosis, planning, implementation, and **evaluation** of dental and dental hygiene care. Therefore, assessment is a critical part of the overall quality of care delivered to every patient.

Assessment must be accompanied by the **documentation** of information gathered during the assessment process. It is inadequate to assess the patient's status without documenting the information in the patient record. The documentation is a reference tool, an historical record, and a patient educational resource essential to the patient care delivery process. It may also serve an important medicolegal function.

The information and procedures essential to the assessment of a patient's periodontal status include the chief complaint, medical and dental histories, **clinical examination,** and **radiographic examination**.[2] The value of the assessment process is enhanced when **data collection** follows a comprehensive and systematic protocol. This chapter describes the elements of an assessment protocol for dental hygiene

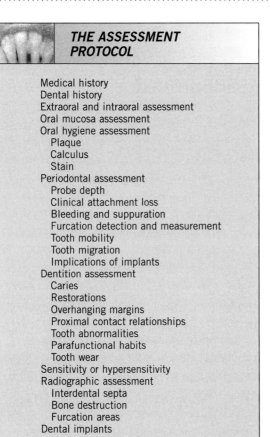

THE ASSESSMENT PROTOCOL

Medical history
Dental history
Extraoral and intraoral assessment
Oral mucosa assessment
Oral hygiene assessment
   Plaque
   Calculus
   Stain
Periodontal assessment
   Probe depth
   Clinical attachment loss
   Bleeding and suppuration
   Furcation detection and measurement
   Tooth mobility
   Tooth migration
   Implications of implants
Dentition assessment
   Caries
   Restorations
   Overhanging margins
   Proximal contact relationships
   Tooth abnormalities
   Parafunctional habits
   Tooth wear
Sensitivity or hypersensitivity
Radiographic assessment
   Interdental septa
   Bone destruction
   Furcation areas
Dental implants

practice. An overview of the assessment process is presented in The Assessment Protocol.

PATIENT HISTORY

Medical History

The medical history is obtained at the initial appointment and is reviewed or updated at each subsequent visit. The importance of the medical history should be explained to all patients because they may omit information that they do not consider relevant to their dental problems. The medical history helps to ensure patient safety, health, and well-being by aiding the clinician in (1) the evaluation of oral manifestations of systemic disease, (2) the detection of systemic conditions that may affect the periodontal tissue response, and (3) the detection of systemic conditions that require special pre-

cautions and modifications in treatment procedures.

Various medical history questionnaires are used by dental professionals. They vary in length, content, and format.[3, 4, 5] Regardless of which questionnaire is used, it is critical to supplement the information through a patient interview. Computer-based medical histories are being developed that automatically request supplemental information when patients provide a positive response to a question. Until this format is routinely available, the dental hygienist will be responsible for the necessary inquiry into areas of risk initially identified by the patient. All patient responses should be documented in the patient record and there should be no unanswered questions on the medical history form.

It is now expected that patient vital signs be taken to augment the medical history document. This includes blood pressure, pulse, and respiration. Some clinics and offices also routinely screen for body temperature using oral thermometer measurements; others take temperatures only if the patient has signs and/or symptoms of infection of an oral nature or anywhere in the body. The taking of vital signs is a simple and important screening process. They should be noted clearly on the medical history form at the initial interview and all subsequent updates.

The medical history must be signed and dated by both the patient and the dental hygienist to validate the patient responses. When a patient has a medical history that significantly affects the delivery of oral health care, the issues of concern should be highlighted in the patient record.

Dental History

Patients should be asked to identify their chief complaints or reasons for seeking oral health care. Chief complaints and problems described by patients include bleeding gums, loose teeth, spreading of the teeth with the appearance of spaces where none existed before, bad taste in the mouth, food catching between teeth, rough spot on tooth, and itchy feeling in the gums relieved by digging with a toothpick. Patients also describe pain of varied types and duration, for example, hurts to bite hard things, hurts to eat sugar or sweet things, hurts to brush teeth at the gumline, constant dull gnawing pain, dull pain after eating, acute throbbing pain, sensitivity to heat and cold, burning sensation in the gums, and sensitivity to inhaled air. Identifying the chief complaint is a critical part of establishing rapport with the patient and developing a treatment plan that meets the patient's personal goals of care.

Patient reports of dental problems often lack descriptive detail. It is essential that the dental hygienist assist the patient in providing the necessary details required for the dental diagnosis. The pertinent information may include, but is not limited to, the specific location, the type of stimulus, the duration on stimulation, the frequency of occurrence, the date of the initial problem, and any changes in the problem since the initial identification. Information about reported dental problems allows the oral health professional to assess the patient's immediate needs and to evaluate the need for radiographs and diagnostic testing.

A dental history should also include information about the patient's previous dental experiences, current oral hygiene practices, and attitudes toward dentistry. It is also helpful to gather information about the patient's family, social history, and habits, such as caffeine consumption, tobacco use, alcohol use, and drug abuse. These factors may affect the plan and delivery of oral health care.

CLINICAL EXAMINATION

The accurate diagnosis of periodontal disease requires a comprehensive clinical examination. This examination should include extraoral, intraoral, oral mucosa, oral hygiene, periodontal, and dentition assessments.

Extraoral and Intraoral Assessment

The head, neck and oral cavity should be visually examined for the presence of pathology. In addition, lymph chains and salivary glands should be palpated to identify swelling or masses. Findings from such an examination may support the development of an oral health treatment plan or the detection of systemic conditions requiring medical attention.

Oral Mucosa Assessment

The oral mucosa assessment requires an understanding of the normal clinical features of the intraoral soft tissues. Three types of oral mucosa line the oral cavity: masticatory mucosa, specialized mucosa, and lining mucosa. The masticatory mucosa covers the gingiva and hard palate. It is attached to the underlying tissues except in the areas of the marginal or unattached gingiva, is unmovable, and has a keratinized epithelial covering. The specialized mucosa covers the upper surface, or dorsum, of the tongue and contains taste buds and many papillae. The lining mucosa covers the inner parts of the oral cavity, such as the floor of the mouth, ventral surface of the tongue, inner lips, cheeks, and alveolar mucosa, including the vestibule and soft palate. It is not attached to the underlying tissues, is movable, and has a non-keratinized epithelial covering.

The gingiva makes up part of the masticatory mucosa that covers the alveolar bone and surrounds and attaches to the necks of the teeth. Anatomically, the gingiva consists of the free gingiva or marginal gingiva, attached gingiva, and interdental papillae.

The free, or unattached, marginal gingiva consists of the gingival margin, gingival sulcus, and free gingival groove. It is the border gingiva that closely surrounds each tooth. The free gingiva connects with the attached gingiva at the free gingival groove and attaches to the tooth at the most coronal aspect of the epithelial junction. The gingival margin is the most occlusal or incisal aspect of the gingiva and represents the entrance into the gingival sulcus. The gingival sulcus, also known as the gingival pocket, is the space between the internal aspect of the free gingiva (the sulcular epithelium) and the tooth. The free gingival groove is a visible, shallow linear depression that demarks the joining of the free gingiva and the attached gingiva. When the gingiva is in the state of health, the free gingival groove approximates the bottom of the gingival sulcus. Figure 9-1 shows the anatomy of normal gingival tissues.

The attached gingiva is firm, resilient tissue, that extends from the free gingival groove to the movable alveolar mucosa. The joining of the attached gingiva and the alveolar mucosa is called the mucogingival junction. The pattern

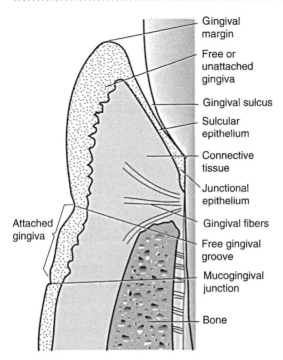

FIGURE 9–1. Diagram of the anatomy of normal gingival tissues.

Gingival margin
Free or unattached gingiva
Gingival sulcus
Sulcular epithelium
Connective tissue
Junctional epithelium
Gingival fibers
Free gingival groove
Mucogingival junction
Bone
Attached gingiva

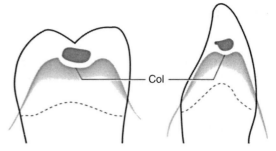

FIGURE 9–3. Location of the col, the nonkeratinized epithelial depression connecting the buccal and lingual papillae of teeth, apical to the contact area.

Col

of the mucogingival junction is usually a slightly scalloped line, as seen in Figure 9-2. The attached gingiva on the buccal aspect of the mandible and maxilla extends from the free gingival groove to the mucogingival junction and is continuous with the vestibule. The width of the attached gingiva is determined by subtracting the sulcus or pocket depth from the total width of the keratinized gingiva (from the gingival margin to the mucogingival junction). This measurement is performed by stretching the lip or cheek to demarcate the mucogingival line while the pocket is probed. The amount of attached gingiva is considered insufficient when stretching the lip or cheek induces movement of the free gingival margin. The attached gingiva on the lingual aspect of the mandible also extends from the free gingival groove to the mucogingival junction, but it is continuous with the lining of the floor of the mouth. On the palatal aspect of the maxilla, the attached gingiva is continuous with the masticatory palatal mucosa.

The interdental papilla is the tissue between two adjacent teeth. It consists of a facial or buccal papilla, a lingual papilla, and a col. The col is the valley, or depression, connecting the facial or buccal papilla and the lingual papilla. The col is shown in Figure 9-3. It is usually

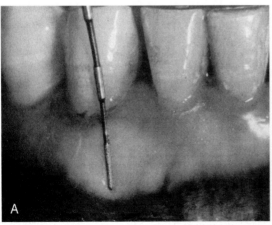

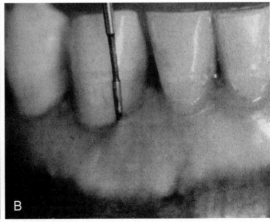

A   B

FIGURE 9–2. The width of the attached gingiva is important to assess. **A.** Probe measuring the clinically apparent width of the attached gingiva. **B.** Probe inserted into the pocket penetrates beyond the apparent width of the attached gingiva, indicating epithelial attachment apical to the mucogingival line.

nonkeratinized, and it conforms to the interproximal contact area. The col is often absent in areas in which teeth are not in contact.

The health status of the gingiva can be determined by considering four universally accepted descriptive categories: color, contour, consistency, and texture. The color of normal marginal and attached gingiva is a pale coral pink, but it can vary as a result of individual skin pigmentation, degree of vascularity, and epithelial keratinization. Bright red gingival tissues indicate acute inflammation. Dark red to cyanotic gingival tissues indicate chronic inflammation. The contour (also referred to as shape or form) of healthy marginal gingiva is uniformly scalloped. Inflamed gingival margins appear swollen, rounded, or shiny, and the scalloped appearance may be lost. Festoons are inner tube–like swellings at the gingival margin. They are thought to be the result of an increase in the number of cells; inflammation may increase the inner tube–like appearance. Clefts, such as a Stillman's cleft, appear as slit-like depressions on the facial or lingual gingival margins. Healthy interdental papillae appear as pointed, knife-like tissues that fill embrasure spaces between teeth. When the papillae are inflamed, their appearance may be flattened, blunted, bulbous, cratered, or hyperplastic. The consistency of marginal and interdental gingiva should be firm when palpated with the side of a blunt instrument, such as a periodontal probe. In the presence of inflammation, the gingiva may be soft and spongy, swollen, shiny, and easily deflected away from the tooth with an instrument or a blast of air. In healthy mouths, attached gingiva has a stippled, orange peel-like texture. When inflamed, the gingiva loses its stippled texture and appears smooth. In the case of very fibrotic tissue, the stippling may still be apparent, even in the presence of inflammation.

The lining mucosa that is of particular concern during a clinical assessment includes the alveolar mucosa and frenum attachments. Alveolar mucosa is loosely attached, movable tissue that is not keratinized. It is darker than the attached gingiva because the mucosa is thinner and the underlying blood vessels are visible. The alveolar mucosa begins at the mucogingival junction and is continuous with the lining mucosa of the oral cavity. Frenum attachments are folds of mucosal tissues, often including muscle fibers, that join the movable mucosa to attached or specialized mucosa. Maxillary and mandibular anterior frenum attachments are located at the midlines of the maxillary and mandibular central incisors, as shown in Figure 9-4. The lingual frenum attachment is located on the underside of the tongue. Maxillary and mandibular buccal frenum attachments are located at the cuspids and premolars.

An assessment of the periodontal health of any dental hygiene patient includes the description and documentation of the oral mucosal features. This documentation provides a baseline for planning dental and dental hygiene treatment interventions and assessing the outcome of treatment. For consistency in evaluation between oral health care providers, it is helpful to provide descriptions of oral mucosal features that are universally recognized. For isolated oral mucosal abnormalities, it is essential to clearly describe their clinical features, location, and severity. When more generalized oral mucosal characteristics are seen, the descriptions can briefly describe the area, which may include much or all of the mucosa. Gingival observations may support the identification of underlying systemic and/or environmental contributing factors that may warrant further investigation (i.e., diabetes, HIV/AIDS, and smoking).[6] Sample gingival descriptions are shown in Figures 9-5 and 9-6 (see color supplement).

Oral Hygiene Assessment

The oral hygiene assessment includes a clinical evaluation of the presence of plaque, calculus,

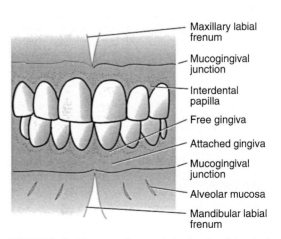

Maxillary labial frenum

Mucogingival junction

Interdental papilla

Free gingiva

Attached gingiva

Mucogingival junction

Alveolar mucosa

Mandibular labial frenum

FIGURE 9–4. The normal anatomic landmarks of the gingival tissue.

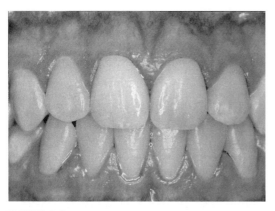

FIGURE 9–5. Gingival description: The gingiva is slightly edematous, showing loss of stippling. Papillae are rounded and fill the interdental spaces. There is a localized rolled margin in the lower anterior area. The marginal gingival tissues appear reddened on clinical examination. (See color figure.)

and stain. The data collected during this assessment helps the dental hygienist to develop a dental hygiene treatment plan, design patient education strategies, and evaluate the outcome of oral hygiene instruction.

PLAQUE

Patient education can be enhanced if the plaque assessment protocol includes a visual representation of the location and presence of plaque. The O'Leary Plaque Control Record provides a simple, commonly used method for recording the presence of plaque on the buccal, lingual, mesial, and distal surfaces of each tooth.[7] When time is limited, dental hygienists may modify this system by limiting the assess-

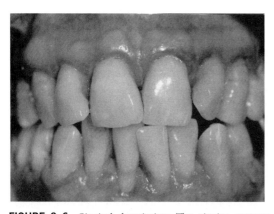

FIGURE 9–6. Gingival description: The gingiva appears inflamed, with generalized rolled borders. Papillae do not fill the interdental spaces, and there is some loss of stippling. The marginal gingival tissues appear reddened. (See color figure.)

ment to specifically identified teeth that are representative of the entire dentition.

Plaque at the gingival third of each tooth surface is noted on a plaque control record that identifies each tooth evaluated. Disclosing solution may be used to stain plaque accumulations. When a tooth is missing or is not included in the assessment protocol, the record should be marked accordingly. When plaque is present at the gingival third of an assessed tooth surface, the corresponding area of the plaque control record should be filled in or marked with a dash or dot. The plaque control record is used to record the presence of plaque regardless of amount. The amount of plaque can be indicated in a narrative description that supplements the plaque control record.

The plaque control record is scored by adding the number of surfaces with recorded plaque. This total is divided by the number of surfaces included in the assessment. The score is reported as a percentage of the number of tooth surfaces with plaque. For example, 20 (number of surfaces with recorded plaque) ÷ 40 (number of surfaces included in the assessment) = .50 or 50% (percentage of total surfaces with plaque). This score should be used to reinforce improved oral hygiene or to emphasize the need for improvement in problem areas. Figure 9–7 shows a plaque control record form.

The inclusion of several plaque control records on a single form permits easy evaluation of trends in plaque control. These records can be valuable motivational tools because they enable patients to see change over time. The plaque control record must provide space for patient identification, the plaque score, and the date of each assessment.

CALCULUS

The assessment of calculus aids the dental hygienist in oral hygiene instruction and treatment planning. The presence of supragingival calculus can be directly observed. Light supragingival calculus deposits are more easily observed when dried with air. Subgingival calculus is detected with careful exploration of each tooth surface to the level of the gingival attachment with an explorer. Figure 9–8 shows the topography evaluated by explorer detection. Gentle blasts of air may be used to deflect the gingiva and permit some visualization of the

PLAQUE CONTROL RECORD

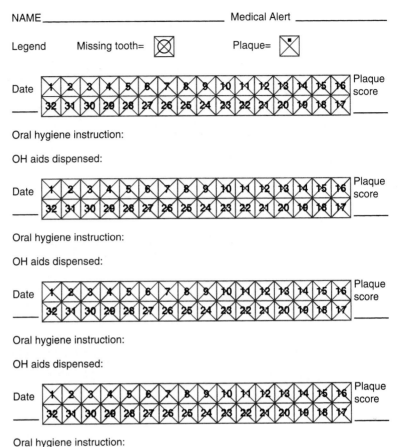

FIGURE 9–7. Example of a plaque control record. Four plaque scores can be recorded to provide the patient with a comparison over time, monitor improvement, and reinforce better plaque control. There is also space to record the oral hygiene instructions given at each session and to list the aids dispensed.

calculus. Radiographs may show heavy interproximal calculus deposits, as seen in Figure 9-9. They cannot be relied on for the thorough detection of calculus because calculus is usually present in greater amounts on the teeth than can be seen on radiographs. The documentation of calculus should include a description of its type (i.e., supragingival or subgingival), location (i.e., tooth, surface, generalized, localized, or interproximal), quantity (i.e., heavy, moderate, or light), and nature (i.e., tenacious, white and chalky, spicules, or dark stained rings).

DENTAL STAIN

Pigmented deposits on the tooth surface are called extrinsic stains. They are primarily esthetic problems that result from the pigmentation of ordinarily colorless acquired pellicle and dental plaque by chromogenic bacteria, foods, and chemicals. These removable stains vary in color, composition, and firmness of adherence to the tooth surface. In contrast, intrinsic stains occur within the tooth structure and cannot be mechanically removed by polishing.

Brown Stain. Brown stain is a thin, translucent, acquired, usually bacteria-free pigmented pellicle. It is frequently associated with insufficient oral hygiene and a failure to use a dentifrice. Brown stain is the most commonly occurring stain and can be very diffuse and at varying intensities throughout the dentition. The occurrence of these discolorations is heightened on surfaces that tend to form concentrated pellicle (i.e., gingival margins and interproximal areas) and in areas of tooth irregularities (i.e., abrasions and attritions).[8] The brown staining is often caused by tannin, which

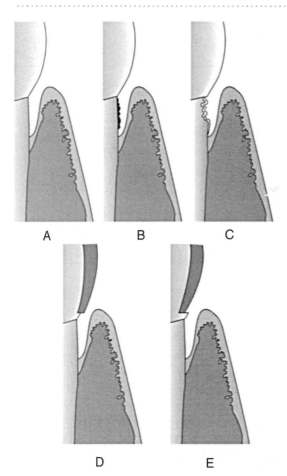

A   B   C

D   E

FIGURE 9–8. The topography of tooth surfaces identified by explorer detection. **A.** Pathologically deepened sulcus with normal topography. **B.** Calculus on the root surface. **C.** Caries on the root surface. **D.** Overhanging restoration margin. **E.** Undercontoured restoration margin.

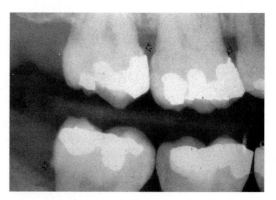

FIGURE 9–9. Bitewing radiograph showing interproximal subgingival calculus. Radiographic appearance of spicules (spurs) of calculus is evident between the teeth.

has a denaturing effect on pellicle proteins, and is found in coffee, tea, fruits, or wines.[8]

Tobacco produces tenacious dark brown or black surface deposits and brown discoloration of tooth structure. Staining is not necessarily proportional to the amount of tobacco used, but depends to a considerable degree on preexisting acquired coatings that attach the tobacco products to the tooth surface.

Chlorhexidine was introduced to United States dental practice in the 1980s as a general antiseptic with broad antibacterial action against Gram-positive and Gram-negative bacteria and yeasts.[9, 10, 11] An undesirable side effect of continued use of chlorhexidine solution is the discoloration of the oral mucosa and staining of the teeth.[9, 10, 12, 13] It imparts a yellow-brown to brown color to the tissues of the oral

cavity.[9] The staining appears in the cervical and interproximal regions of the teeth, on restorations, in plaque, and on the surface of the tongue.[9, 10, 12] Aldehydes and ketones, which are normally intermediates of both mammalian and microbial metabolism, may contribute to the formation of discoloration by chlorhexidine.[8, 12, 13] Chlorhexidine also has a denaturing effect on proteins that may result in increased staining of the acquired pellicle by metal ions.[8, 11, 13] It has also been suggested that there may be increased binding of dietary chromogens after treatment with chlorhexidine.[8, 13, 14] Similar staining occurs with the use of alexidine. Chlorhexidine staining is shown in Figure 9–10.

The anti-caries benefits of stannous fluoride have long been recognized. However, more recently, stannous fluoride is being used for the control of plaque formation,[15] gingivitis,[16] and dentinal hypersensitivity.[17] Stannous fluoride imparts a yellow-brown or golden discoloration

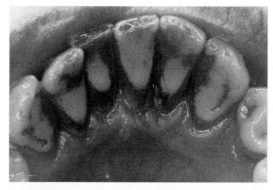

FIGURE 9–10. Chlorhexidine stain on the lower anterior teeth. Note the formation of supragingival calculus, which is also stained.

of the tongue and teeth. It has been suggested that this stain is primarily stannous sulfide.[18]

Black Stain. Black stain usually occurs as thin black lines on the facial and lingual surfaces of the teeth near the gingival margin and also as diffuse patches on proximal surfaces. It is firmly attached, tends to recur after removal, is more common in women, and may occur in mouths with excellent hygiene. The black stain that occurs in children is typically associated with a low incidence of caries[19, 20] The microflora of black stain is dominated by chromogenic bacteria, which may be the cause of the black pigmentation.[19] Another theory is that the black pigmentation is an insoluble ferric sulfide produced as a result of an interaction of hydrogen sulfide producing bacteria and iron from the saliva and gingival fluid.[21]

Green Stain. Green stain is a green-yellow stain, sometimes of considerable thickness. It is most often associated with children. The stain is considered to be stained remnants of the enamel cuticle, but this theory has not been substantiated.[22] The discoloration has been attributed to fluorescent bacteria and fungi, such as *Penicillium* and *Aspergillus*.[23] Green stain usually occurs on the gingival half of the facial surfaces of anterior teeth.[20, 24] It is associated with poor oral hygiene.[20]

Orange Stain. Orange stain is less common than green or brown stain. It may occur on both the facial and lingual surfaces of anterior teeth. Orange stain is often associated with poor oral hygiene and is observed to form on loosely attached debris.[20] *Serratia marcescens* and *Flavobacterium lutescens* have been suggested as the responsible chromogenic organisms.[25]

Extrinsic Stains. Extrinsic stains should be evaluated and documented according to their color (i.e., brown, black, green, yellow, or orange), location (i.e., tooth or surface), extent (i.e., amount of surface or tooth covered by stain), and intensity (i.e., light, moderate, or heavy). Routine documentation of extrinsic stains at dental hygiene appointments can help the dental hygienist develop an oral hygiene instruction plan that responds to patient concerns about the esthetic effects of these stains.

ORAL HYGIENE INSTRUCTION

The oral hygiene assessment including the documentation of the presence of plaque, calculus, and stain, supports the development of oral hygiene instruction programs for patients. To ensure consistency among oral health care providers, the oral hygiene aids that have been prescribed, dispensed, and introduced to the patient, as well as the long-term instructional plan, should be documented in the patient record. To facilitate access, oral hygiene related information (i.e., oral hygiene assessments and oral hygiene instructional plans) should be collectively located in the patient record. Because of its integral role in patient education, the plaque control record should be stored near the oral hygiene instruction plan.

Periodontal Assessment

Periodontal assessment includes a clinical evaluation of the periodontium, looking for signs of inflammation and damage to periodontal tissues. The clinical detection of inflammatory lesions and damage to periodontal tissues is essential for diagnosis, treatment planning, and monitoring therapeutic effectiveness.[26, 27] The clinical procedures most commonly used for periodontal assessment include measuring periodontal probe depths and clinical attachment levels, assessing gingival bleeding and suppuration, identifying and measuring furcations, testing mobility, and recognizing pathologic migration.[28] This assessment should follow an established sequence to ensure that it is comprehensive and complete.

PROBING MEASUREMENTS

Periodontal probing is performed to numerically assess the apical extent of the epithelial attachment in relation to the gingival margin and the cementoenamel junction. These measurements are used to assess periodontal disease status, support treatment planning decisions, design individualized prevention plans, and evaluate the success of treatment. Recorded probings in conjunction with current radiographs provide the dental hygienist with detailed information on pocket depths, clinical attachment loss, furcation involvement, and bone loss. In addition to supporting the periodontal diagnosis, this information is helpful in planning oral hygiene instruction as well as during debridement, scaling, and root planing appointments.

A periodontal probe is used to obtain two

types of epithelial attachment measurements. The most commonly reported measurement is the distance between the gingival margin and the base of the gingival sulcus. This distance is known as the periodontal pocket depth, probing depth or, in the case of periodontal health, gingival sulcus depth. Probing measurements should be taken at six sites on each tooth: distobuccal, buccal, mesiobuccal, distolingual, lingual, and mesiolingual. Probing the periodontal pocket depth is shown in Figure 9–11.

The second epithelial attachment measurement is clinical attachment loss. Clinical attachment loss is the distance between the cementoenamel junction and the most apical extent of the epithelial attachment, as shown in Figure 9–12. When the cementoenamel junction is visible, this measurement is determined by adding the periodontal pocket depth to the gingival recession measurement. Gingival recession is the distance between the cementoena-

mel junction and the gingival margin. When the gingival margin is coronal to the cementoenamel junction, the distance between the gingival margin and the cementoenamel junction is subtracted from the periodontal pocket depth to calculate the clinical attachment loss.

Clinical attachment loss provides a more accurate picture of periodontal status because attachment loss can occur with any gingival probe depth. In many circumstances, other factors such as previous periodontal therapy and surgery, occlusal trauma, occlusal attrition leading to extrusion, and traumatic toothbrushing, can contribute to attachment loss. One of the most accurate and reliable means of assessing the progression and remission of periodontal disease is clinical attachment loss.[29, 30] In addition, the observation of clinical attachment loss may support the identification of underlying systemic and/or environmental contributing factors that may warrant further investigation (i.e., osteoporosis or smoking).[31, 32, 33] Figures 9–13 and 9–14 show the significance of clinical attachment loss versus periodontal probing depth.

Periodontal probe measurements cannot detect disease activity or predict destruction. Unfortunately, clinical attachment loss is only an indication that destructive disease processes have taken place.[34] It is crucial to maintain accurate epithelial attachment measurement records, current and past radiographs, and a history of periodontal disease to allow the detection of changes that may indicate disease processes.[34]

Probing depths may be affected by the clinician's insertion force, the probe's tip shape and size or measurement scale, the insertion point and angulation, and the patient's gingival inflammation status. Inflamed tissues should be carefully probed. The probe tip easily penetrates inflamed epithelial attachment and may result in inaccurate periodontal probing measurements.[35] Pockets with inflamed tissues are generally 1 mm deeper than the histologic depth as determined by the location of the most coronal cells of the epithelial attachment.[36] Therefore it is important to include both pocket depth and a narrative description of the gingival tissues in the patient record.

In the past, bleeding was considered an indicator of active disease; however, studies show that bleeding is not an absolute predictor of

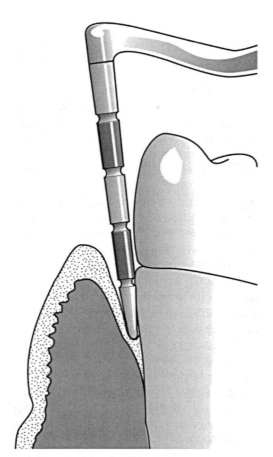

FIGURE 9–11. Diagram of probing the periodontal pocket depth. The millimeter measurement indicates the distance from the margin of the gingiva to the base of the pocket.

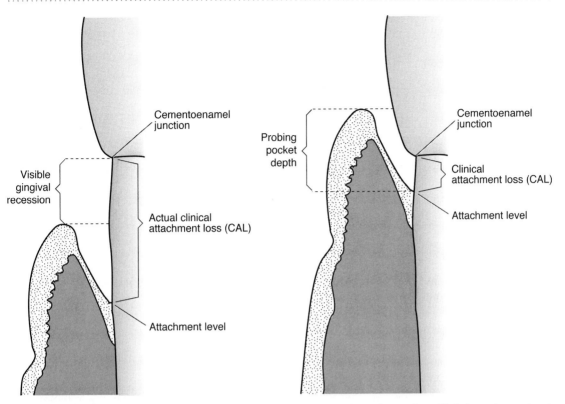

FIGURE 9–12. The difference between probing pocket depth and clinical attachment loss. Clinical attachment loss is often the more critical assessment for the long-term health of the tooth and success of treatment. It is important to understand the distinction between clinical attachment loss, gingival recession, and pocket depth. The 3 mm probing depths represented here depict distinctly different levels of clinical attachment loss.

active disease.[37-39] Therefore, clinical examination alone does not permit the dental hygienist to accurately determine whether periodontal disease is active or imminent.[37] The presence of bleeding, in periodontal maintenance patients, has been shown to be an indicator of disease progression at those sites that continue to bleed.[40] Bleeding and deeper probe depths may indicate active disease in as many as 30 percent of patients.[41] Therefore, the presence of bleeding does not necessarily indicate a site is at increased risk of attachment loss. The ab-

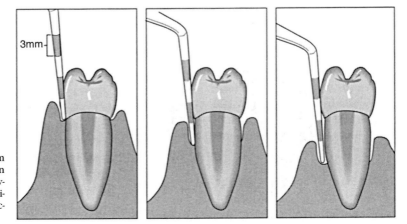

FIGURE 9–13. Diagram of 3 mm probing pocket depths in relation to different clinical attachment levels. Greater attachment loss indicates more periodontal destruction.

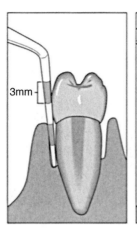
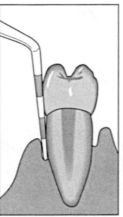
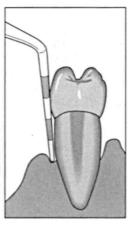

FIGURE 9–14. Diagram of different probing pocket depths related to the same level of clinical attachment loss. Deeper probing pocket depths do not necessarily indicate more periodontal destruction.

sence of bleeding on probing, on the other hand, generally indicates current stability of the periodontium.[37, 39, 40, 42, 43] However, reduced bleeding and suppressed clinical signs of gingival inflammation may be observed in smokers with periodontal disease due to the effects of nicotine on the peripheral circulation.[44]

The documentation of bleeding points during probing is important and should be included in the patient's periodontal record. Gingival bleeding can be assessed during the probing process. This assessment can be as simple as noting and recording the presence or absence of bleeding or can be more detailed and consider the nature of the response (i.e., amount and quickness of bleeding).[43] When the assessment of bleeding is limited to the dichotomous determination of presence or absence, bleeding can be documented by circling or placing a dot above the probing depths, or recording the probing depth in red.

The presence of suppuration or purulent exudate, in combination with periodontal pockets and bleeding on probing, can indicate that the site is subject to periodontal disease progression.[40, 41] Clinical assessment of suppuration, the formation of pus, within a periodontal pocket is performed by gently placing a finger against the marginal gingiva and pressing toward the crown of the tooth as shown in Figure 9–15. Suppuration is formed on the inner pocket wall, but the external appearance of the pocket is unchanged. Therefore, visual examination with digital pressure is required. Suppuration does not occur in all periodontal pockets. However, suppuration may be present, although not visibly detectable, and therefore its clinical absence

is not an indicator of periodontal stability.[37] The clinically detectable presence of suppuration should be documented in the patient's periodontal record.

FURCATION IDENTIFICATION AND MEASUREMENT

A furcation is the location on a multirooted tooth where the root base divides into separate roots. A two-rooted tooth has a bifurcation; a three-rooted tooth has a trifurcation. Normally, a furcation is not clinically visible or detectable. In the presence of attachment loss in the furca-

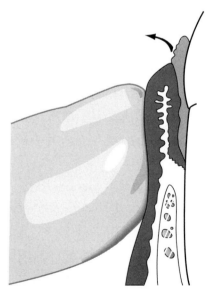

FIGURE 9–15. Suppuration can be expressed from infected periodontal pockets by gentle finger pressure. (Modified with permission from Carranza F, Newman M. Glickman's Clinical Periodontology, 8th ed. Philadelphia: WB Saunders, 1996.)

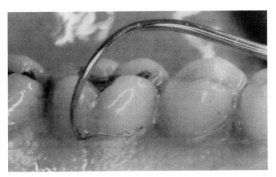

FIGURE 9–16. Naber's probe placed to assess lingual furcation on a lower molar.

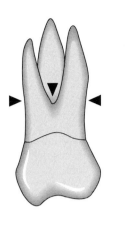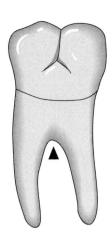

FIGURE 9–17. The locations of furcation areas (arrows) on maxillary three-rooted and mandibular two-rooted teeth.

tion area, a tooth is considered to have furcation involvement. During the periodontal assessment, it is important to evaluate the presence, type, location, and extent of involvement within a furcation area. A furcation probe, such as the Nabers series seen penetrating a furcation area in Figure 9-16, and radiographs (discussed in the section on radiographic assessment) are the primary furcation diagnostic tools.

Furcations may be visually observed, but are most commonly manually detected as an indentation during probing or exploration. Once a furcation is identified, its type must be determined. The type of furcation present in a two-rooted tooth is a bifurcation involvement. The type of furcation present in a three-rooted tooth may be either a bifurcation or a trifurcation involvement. In two-rooted mandibular molars, the locations of potential bifurcation involvement are the buccal and lingual aspects. The locations of potential bifurcation involvement

in two-rooted maxillary premolars are the mesial and distal aspects. The locations of potential bifurcation involvement in three-rooted maxillary molars are the buccal, mesiolingual, and distolingual aspects. The locations of potential trifurcation involvement in three-rooted maxillary molars are the buccomesiolingual and buccodistolingual aspects. Molar furcation areas are shown in Figure 9-17.

Estimations of horizontal and vertical bone loss within a bifurcation or trifurcation are used to determine the degree of involvement. The horizontal component is the measurement of bone loss horizontally under the crown of the tooth. Table 9-1 shows the Glickman Index of horizontal furcation classifications.[45, 46]

The vertical component is the measurement of bone loss within the bifurcation or trifurcation vertically from the roof or dome of the

TABLE 9–1. Glickman Index of Horizontal Furcation Classifications

Grade	Description
Grade I	Pocket formation into the flute of the furca, but the interradicular bone is intact.
Grade II	Loss of interradicular bone, with pocket formation of varying depths into the furca, but not completely through to the opposite side of the tooth.
Grade III	Complete loss of interradicular bone, with pocket formation that is completely probeable to the opposite side of the tooth.
Grade IV	Loss of attachment and gingival recession making the furca clearly visible upon clinical examination.

Used with permission from Kalkwarf KL, Reinhardt RA. The function problem: current controversies and future directions. Dent Clin North Am 1988; 32:243; from Carranza FA Jr., Takei HH. Treatment of furcation involvement and combined periodontal-endodontic therapy. In Glickman I. Clinical Periodontology, 8th ed. Philadelphia: WB Saunders, 1996:640.

TABLE 9–2. Tarnow and Fletcher Vertical Furcation Classification Index

Subclass	Description
Subclass A	0 to 3 mm probeable depth from the roof or crotch of the furca.
Subclass B	4 to 6 mm probeable depth from the roof or crotch of the furca.
Subclass C	7 mm or greater probeable depth from the roof or crotch of the furca.

Adapted with permission from Tarnow D, Fletcher P. Classification of the vertical component of furcation involvement. J. Periodontol 1984;55:284.

furcation (crotch of the tooth) to the current bone level. The vertical component may be difficult to assess if the furcation entrance is covered by soft tissue that obstructs access and vision. The Tarnow and Fletcher vertical furcation classification index is described in Table 9-2 and illustrated in Figure 9-18.[47]

Probing a furcation area with a traditional periodontal probe can provide an accurate measurement as long as the furcation entrance is visible. A curved, calibrated furcation probe is designed to universally adapt to furcations (Figure 9-19). A furcation should be probed with care. The probe tip can easily penetrate through inflamed epithelial attachment and result in inaccurate measurements.[35] The furcation probe should be guided into the furcation entrance by sliding the probe along the hard surfaces of the tooth to ensure that the probe does not penetrate the attached soft tissues within the furcation.[48]

Once a bifurcation or trifurcation is found during clinical assessment, further investigation should be performed to determine its cause. Radiographs can be instrumental in this assessment. They help to visualize anatomic abnormalities, defective restorations, or destruction of the periodontium caused by periodontal or endodontic lesions. Teeth with furcation involvement have been shown to be at greater risk for continued bone loss and tooth loss.[40]

TOOTH MOBILITY

The periodontal assessment should include an evaluation of tooth mobility. Tooth mobility should be distinguished between physiologic mobility and pathologic mobility.

Physiologic tooth mobility is the normal or expected mobility of a tooth. All teeth have a slight degree of physiologic mobility because they are supported by the periodontal ligament. Physiologic mobility varies in different teeth (highest in the central and lateral incisors) and at different times of the day.[49] Mobility is greatest on arising in the morning and progressively decreases during the day. The increased mobility in the morning is attributed to slight extrusion of the teeth because of limited occlusal contact during sleep. During the waking hours, mobility is reduced by chewing and swallowing forces, which intrude the teeth in the sockets. Tooth mobility that occurs beyond the physiologic range is termed pathologic or abnormal mobility. Pathologic mobility is horizontal or vertical movement of a tooth beyond its physiologic limits.

Pathologic tooth mobility is caused by factors affecting the periodontal ligament space and loss of alveolar bone. Loss of tooth support can be the result of horizontal or vertical bone

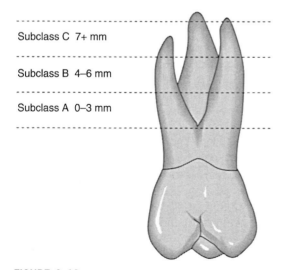

FIGURE 9–18. Tarnow and Fletcher subclassification of furcations indicating the relative bone loss from the dome of the furcation to the bone height for each subclassification. (Adapted with permission from Tarnow D and Fletcher P. Classification of the vertical component of furcation involvement. J Periodontol 1984;55:284.)

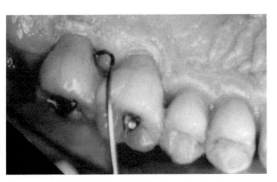

FIGURE 9–19. The curved, calibrated Naber's probe is designed to assess furcations on any tooth surface, including the difficult to assess mesial surface shown.

loss from periodontal disease or periodontal surgical therapy. The amount of mobility depends on the severity and distribution of the bone loss around each tooth, the length and shape of the roots, and the ratio of the crown to root length.[49] Primary occlusal trauma occurs when teeth in a normal periodontium are subjected to excessive occlusal forces that cause pathologic mobility. Abnormal occlusal habits, such as grinding (bruxing) and clenching, are a common cause of tooth mobility. Secondary occlusal trauma occurs when teeth in a compromised periodontium (for example, teeth exhibiting bone loss from previous episodes of periodontal disease) become mobile because they cannot withstand normal occlusal forces. Occlusal forces are described in Chapter 8.

Gingival inflammation extending into the periodontal ligament results in degenerative changes that can increase tooth mobility, even in the absence of bone loss. Therefore, increased tooth mobility can be seen in patients with severe gingivitis or early periodontal disease.[49] The spread of inflammation from an acute periapical abscess produces a temporary increase in tooth mobility in the absence of periodontal disease. Traumatic injury can also result in tooth mobility. Increased mobility is often seen after a blow to the mouth and is sometimes seen after surgical periodontal therapy, restoration placement, or endodontic therapy.[49] Tooth mobility is also associated with pregnancy particularly in the last weeks before delivery, and is probably due to increased hydration of connective tissues.[50, 51] It occurs in women with or without periodontal disease.

Mobility is measured by using the metal handles of two dental instruments placed on the buccal and lingual aspects of the tooth and gently rocked back and forth. The use of two fingertips or one fingertip and one instrument is not recommended because the soft pads of the finger can cushion and disguise movement. Abnormal mobility most often occurs in the faciolingual direction. Mobility is graded according to the ease and extent of tooth movement, using the criteria shown in Table 9-3.[52-54]

PATHOLOGIC MIGRATION OF TEETH

Pathologic migration is tooth displacement that occurs when periodontal disease disturbs the balance among the factors that maintain physiologic tooth position. The teeth may move in any direction, and the migration is usually accompanied by mobility and rotation. Pathologic migration in the occlusal or incisal direction is termed extrusion or elongation.

Pathologic migration may be caused by occlusal forces against weakened periodontal support that renders the teeth unable to maintain normal positions in the arch. The problem arises from the weakened periodontium, not necessarily from abnormal occlusal forces.

Unreplaced missing teeth may cause a change in the occlusal forces by allowing the

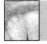

TABLE 9–3. Tooth Mobility Classification	
Grade	**Description**
Grade 0	Physiologic mobility only.
Grade 1/2	Clinical mobility that is slightly greater than physiologic mobility, but <1 mm buccolingually (also designated as a +).
Grade 1	Slight pathologic mobility, approximately 1 mm buccolingually.
Grade 2	Moderate pathologic mobility, approximately 2 mm buccolingually, but no vertical displacement.
Grade 3	Severe pathologic mobility, >2 mm buccolingually or mesiodistally, combined with vertical displacement.

drifting of teeth into the spaces created by their absence. Drifting does not result from destruction of the periodontal tissues, but creates conditions that lead to periodontal disease. Although drifting is common when missing teeth are not replaced, it does not always occur.

Spaces between the teeth, termed diastemas or diastemata, are often created by the separation of the teeth. The disturbed proximal contact relationships lead to food impaction, gingival inflammation, and pocket formation, followed by bone loss and tooth mobility. Occlusal disharmonies created by the altered tooth positions traumatize the supporting tissues of the periodontium and aggravate the destruction caused by the inflammation. Reduction in periodontal support leads to further migration of the teeth and mutilation of the occlusion. See Figure 9-20 for an example of severe pathologic tooth migration.

Pressure from the tongue may cause drifting of the anterior teeth in the absence of periodontal disease or may contribute to pathologic migration of teeth with reduced periodontal support. This correctable problem may be caused by improper swallowing habits. These patients often thrust the tongue against the anterior teeth when swallowing. This habit can be corrected through myofunctional therapy.

PERIODONTAL SCREENING AND RECORDING SYSTEM[55]

In 1993, a simplified system of periodontal assessment known as Periodontal Screening and Recording (PSR) was introduced. PSR is a periodontal disease detection system endorsed by the American Dental Association and the Ameri-

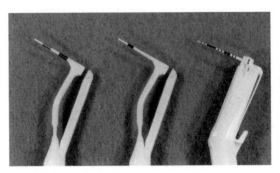

FIGURE 9-21. Disposable probes that can be used for the Periodontal Screening and Recording System. The black bands closest to the probe tips cover a penetration of 3.5 to 5.5 mm. There are 0.5 mm diameter balls on the probe tips.

can Academy of Periodontology.[55] The system was designed to promote efficiency in the periodontal assessment and documentation process without compromising the quality of patient care. However, its value remains to be assessed.

A specially designed periodontal probe with a ball tip and colored calibrations at 3.5 and 5.5 mm is used to probe the standard six sites on each tooth. The probe is shown in Figure 9-21. Bleeding, the presence of overhangs or defective margins, and supragingival and subgingival calculus are assessed while pocket depth is measured. The teeth are divided into sextants. A PSR code is assigned to each sextant and recorded in the patient record. The code that most accurately describes the most periodontally involved tooth in a sextant is assigned to that sextant. The system also provides for the documentation of other periodontal abnormalities, such as furcation involvement, mobility, mucogingival problems, and recession. When two or more sextants are scored Code 3, one sextant is scored Code 3 and Code*, or one sextant is scored Code 4, a comprehensive full mouth periodontal examination and charting should be performed. The PSR system is described in Table 9-4.

PERIODONTAL IMPLICATIONS OF IMPLANTS

Dental implants are an important dental procedure for the replacement of missing teeth. The dental hygienist can play an integral role in the clinical evaluation of implants. Many of the clinical parameters used to assess the periodontium are also used to evaluate dental implants; however, the results may have different significance.

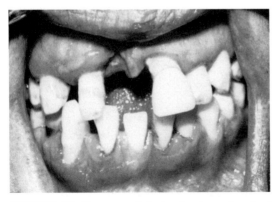

FIGURE 9-20. Extreme pathologic migration and occlusal mutilation seen in advanced periodontal disease.

TABLE 9–4. Periodontal Screening and Recording™ System[55]

Code	Description
Code 0	Colored area of the probe remains completely visible in the deepest crevice in the sextant.
	● No calculus or defective margins are detected.
	● Gingival tissues are healthy, with no bleeding on probing.
Code 1	Colored area of the probe remains completely visible in the deepest probing depth in the sextant.
	● No calculus or defective margins are detected.
	● There is bleeding on probing.
Code 2	Colored area of the probe remains completely visible in the deepest probing depth of the sextant.
	● Supra or subgingival calculus is detected or defective margins are detected.
Code 3	Colored area of the probe remains partly visible in the deepest probing depth in the sextant.
Code 4	Colored area of the probe completely disappears, indicating probing depth greater than 5.5 mm.
Code*	The symbol* is added to the sextant score whenever findings indicate clinical abnormalities, such as:
	● furcation invasion
	● mobility
	● mucogingival problems
	● recession extending to the colored area of the probe (3.5 mm or greater).

Adapted with permission from the American Academy of Periodontology, Chicago, IL, and the American Dental Association, Chicago, IL. Periodontal Screening and Recording and PSR are service marks and trademarks of the American Dental Association.

The first step in the implant assessment process should be to clearly indicate on the periodontal charting records the presence and location of a dental implant. As with the natural dentition, plaque is the primary causative agent in peri-implant gingival inflammation and is associated with implant failure. Therefore, the presence and location of plaque and calculus should be regularly documented. In addition to the oral hygiene assessment of dental implants, it is important to evaluate gingival color, contour, consistency, and texture. The gingival tissue surrounding the implant may be keratinized or non-keratinized. Increased redness and a smoother texture may be associated with healthy non-keratinized gingival tissues. Patients should be interviewed regarding tissue pain or tenderness around the implants. The surrounding gingival tissue should also be assessed for movement in response to retraction of adjacent tissues.[56] Such movement is undesirable because it may adversely affect the implant–soft tissue attachment.

There is some controversy regarding the information that is gained by probing implants as part of implant assessment. Regardless of philosophy, probing should be avoided for the first three months after abutment connection. Special considerations are required when probing an implant. Probing should be performed using a plastic periodontal implant probe to prevent scratching of, or electrochemical interactions with, the implant metal. The probe should be dipped in chlorhexidine between measurements to minimize microbial contamination among sites.[57] Deeper probing depths have been associated with implants surrounded by non-keratinized, alveolar mucosa as opposed to keratinized gingiva.[56] Successful implants generally have probing depths of approximately three millimeters.[58, 59] The assessment of attachment levels requires that probing measurements be taken in relation to a fixed reference point. In the natural dentition, the fixed reference point is the cementoenamel junction. In the dental implant, the fixed reference point should be on the implant or prosthesis. Documentation of the fixed reference point permits repeated assessments of attachment level essential for determining progressive attachment loss.

The anatomic shape of the neck of some implants or the associated restoration complicates the insertion and angling of the periodontal probe. Therefore, when probing of the implant is advocated, removal of the fixed restorations should be considered. The use of the presence or absence of bleeding on probing in assessing the success of an implant has not been validated; however, it is reasonable to record the presence of bleeding when implants are probed.[59] The presence of clinically visible suppuration is likely indicative of an active tissue-destroying process.[59]

Clinical mobility of the implant is an important parameter in evaluating implant health and should be assessed at every visit.[56] Implants with clinically detectable mobility are considered to be failing.[56, 58] Implant mobility is measured with the same technique as prescribed for mobility testing of the natural dentition.[60] However, multiple-unit fixed prostheses may not permit mobility assessment and may require removal for an accurate assessment. Annual removal of fixed prostheses is recommended. Radiographic evaluation of implants is also recommended to monitor bone height.[56]

DOCUMENTATION OF PERIODONTAL ASSESSMENT

The patient record provides a continuous historical accounting of the patient's oral health status and the delivery of oral health care services. The format of the patient record will vary with each clinical setting; however, there are universal methods for documenting oral health status. The content of the patient record will be similar, regardless of whether the record is in a paper or an electronic format.

The patient record must be comprehensive and systematic to provide the information necessary for the diagnosis, planning, implementation, and evaluation of dental and dental hygiene care. A useful periodontal charting record, including a plaque control record is shown in Figure 9-22.

When a patient first seeks oral health care services in a dental practice, an initial assessment of the patient's oral health care status is essential. This documentation includes the chief complaint, medical and dental histories, and clinical and radiographic findings. The patient record may be supplemented by previous dental records. Continuous assessment of the patient's oral health status over the course of the oral health care professional–patient relationship provides a current and historical accounting. The patient's oral health care needs will affect the frequency and detail of these continuing assessments; however, the dental hygienist must be alert to evidence of disease activity or progression.

Dentition Assessment

The dentition assessment includes a clinical evaluation of the teeth for caries, restoration status, proximal contact relationships, anomalies of form, evidence of parafunctional habits, tooth wear conditions, and hypersensitivity. This assessment should follow an established sequence to ensure that the evaluation is comprehensive.

CARIES

Clinical evaluation of the dentition for caries may include visual, tactile, and radiographic assessments. Evidence of defects and anomalies in the tooth structure are of significance for the restoration of the dentition as well as the prevention and treatment of periodontal disease and should therefore be documented. Locations of carious lesions may include pits and fissures, smooth surfaces, interproximal smooth surfaces, and root surfaces. Visual changes in the dentition may include a change of color (i.e., white spot lesion), a change in the density of the tooth structure observed through transillumination, and a break in the surface layer of the tooth structure. Tactile changes in the dentition range from actual cavitation of pits and fissures or smooth surfaces to the tacky, sticky, or leathery sensations of the more intact surface layer. Radiographic changes of caries may appear as radiolucent areas in the tooth structure.

Because of their periodontal structural implications, root surface caries are of particular concern in periodontal assessment. These lesions provide a reservoir for bacteria that can contribute to periodontal inflammation. Root surface caries are usually located below the cementoenamel junction and therefore do not involve the enamel structure. Color changes in the root surface range from yellow to dark brown or black. Incipient lesions may be yellow or light tan, round or oval, and slightly soft, without cavitation or pain. Root surface lesions may rapidly progress and completely encircle the tooth, making restoration difficult. Lesions in remission appear black or dark brown in color and are more leathery in texture than the surrounding normal cementum.[61]

Table 9-5 shows the G.V. Black cavity classification.[62, 63] Table 9-6 shows the classification for assessing and documenting the severity of root surface caries described by Newbrun.[64]

RESTORATION STATUS

Assessment of the restoration status should include documentation of existing restorations,

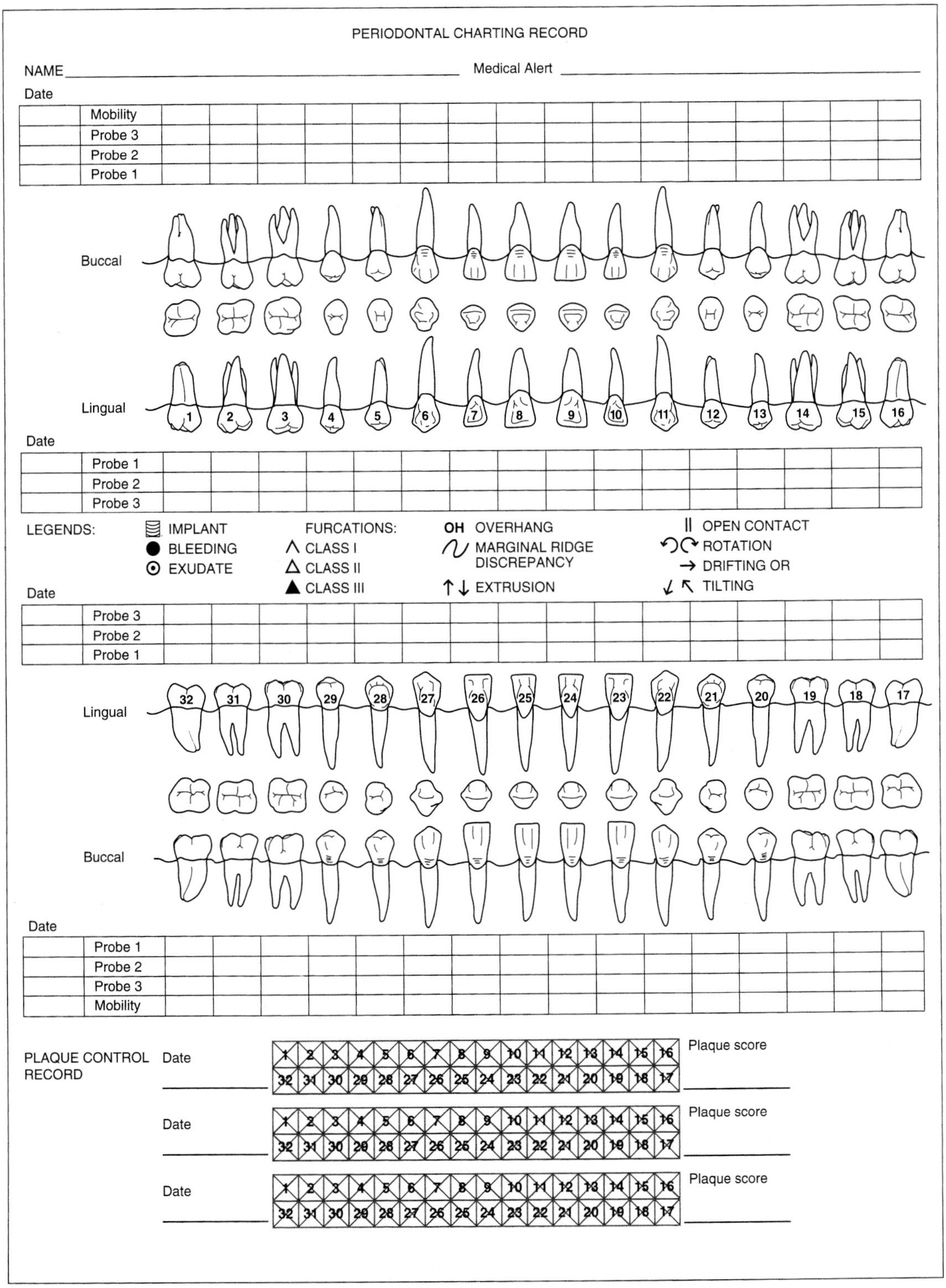

FIGURE 9–22. Periodontal charting record that provides space for multiple probing examinations and plaque assessment. This type of record permits easy comparison of probe depths, recession in order to compute clinical attachment loss, and plaque scores over a series of appointments.

TABLE 9–5. G.V. Black Cavity Classification

Class	Description
Class 1	Pit and Fissure Cavities • occlusal surfaces of premolars and molars • occlusal two-thirds of facials and linguals on molars • lingual surface of maxillary incisors
Class 2	Proximal Cavities in Premolars and Molars
Class 3	Proximal Cavities in Incisors and Canines (does not involve incisal angle)
Class 4	Proximal Cavities in Incisors and Canines (involves incisal angle)
Class 5	Gingival Third Cavities (does not include pit and fissure cavities)
Class 6	Incisal Edge and Cusp Tip Cavities

Used with permission from Black GV. Operative Dentistry, 8th ed. 2 vols. Medico-Dental Publishing Co: Woodstock, IL 1947–48.

poorly contoured restorations, removable prosthetic appliances, and implants. This documentation is essential in the collection of baseline data for comprehensive treatment planning and medicolegal liability protection. The restoration status should be updated periodically to support ongoing treatment planning and to evaluate treatment outcomes.

Overhanging restorations, undercontoured restorations, and poorly fitting crown margins are of particular concern in periodontal assessment because of their direct effect on periodontal health and therapy. Several studies have confirmed that overhanging dental restorations contribute to increased gingival inflammation, attachment loss, and bone loss.[65, 66, 67] Despite major advances in restorative material technology, overhangs continue to be created, are not always clinically detected, and are not always removed when obviously evident in radiographs.[65-67] Patients are often unaware of poor margins and their detrimental effects. The dental hygienist should document these findings and, with the dentist, encourage the patient to undergo treatment for these problems.

PROXIMAL CONTACT RELATIONSHIPS

The dental assessment should include an evaluation of proximal contact relationships. Open contacts permit food impaction that may affect periodontal health. Tight contacts may discourage patient compliance with interproximal plaque removal. Therefore, the tightness of contacts should be assessed to aid in the development of a plan of care and patient education. Proximal contacts are most effectively evaluated with dental floss; however, visual or radiographic observation may provide the necessary

TABLE 9–6. Severity of Root Caries Index by Newbrun

Grade	Description
Grade I (Incipient)	Surface texture is soft and can be penetrated with a dental explorer No surface defect or cavitation Pigmentation from light tan to brown
Grade II (Shallow)	Surface texture is soft, irregular, and rough, and can be penetrated by a dental explorer Surface defect less than 0.5 mm deep Pigmentation ranges from tan to dark brown
Grade III (Cavitation)	Surface texture is soft and can be penetrated with a dental explorer Penetrating lesion with cavitation that is greater than 0.5 mm deep; no pulpal involvement Pigmentation from brown to dark brown
Grade IV (Pulpal)	Deeply penetrating lesion with pulpal involvement Pigmentation from brown to dark brown

Adapted with permission from Newbrun E. Problems in caries diagnosis. Int Dent J 1993;43:136.

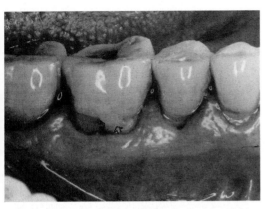

FIGURE 9–23. An enamel projection on the buccal surface of a lower first molar predisposes the patient to periodontal disease because there is no epithelial attachment on enamel.

information. Another condition to be assessed for that causes food impaction is the plunger cusp. This anatomic situation can force food into an embrasure space every time the patient chews food.

ANOMALIES OF TOOTH FORM

Some developmental anomalies directly affect periodontal health and therapy, for example, the enamel projection shown in Figure 9-23. These anomalies include enamel and dentinal defects and anatomic formations that promote plaque retention, inhibit plaque removal, and influence the selection of therapy.

PARAFUNCTIONAL HABITS

Parafunctional habits involve the use of the dentition outside the normal scope of functional occlusion. They may include tooth-to-tooth contact, contact between teeth and soft tissue, and contact between teeth and foreign objects. These interactions may result in damage to the periodontal and tooth structures and soft tissues of the oral cavity. Parafunctional habits include clenching; grinding; biting or chewing of the cheeks, lips, tongue, or fingernails; and using the teeth to open or hold foreign objects, such as office supplies, personal care products, occupational tools, and food or food containers.

TOOTH WEAR

Tooth wear is the loss of tooth structure caused by chronic destructive processes other than dental caries. These destructive processes include abrasion, attrition, and erosion. Determin-

ing the etiology of tooth wear lesions is critical for the prevention of their progression. However identifying the etiology can be complicated because tooth wear conditions may be caused by a combination of destructive processes. In addition to clinical examination, patient interviews may help to identify circumstances that contribute to tooth destruction. Documentation of the presence of tooth wear lesions, the extent of destruction, and the contributing factors is essential to the development of an appropriate plan of care.

Abrasion is the wearing away of tooth structures, usually on the buccal, incisal, and occlusal surfaces as a result of excessive abrasive forces by a foreign object. Buccal lesions are most typically attributed to oral hygiene habits and are "V" or wedge shaped defects and notches at or apical to the cementoenamel junction. Factors that may influence "toothbrush abrasion" include brushing technique, frequency of brushing, amount of time spent brushing, forces applied during brushing, type of toothbrush, and abrasiveness, acidity, and amount of dentifrice used.[68] Figure 9-24 shows abrasion. Personal habits, such as fingernail or thread biting, and holding foreign objects with the teeth (i.e., pipe smoking and seed shelling), may cause incisal and occlusal surface abrasions.

Abfraction is a term used to describe cervical "V" or wedge-shaped lesions that are located apical to the cementoenamel junction. These lesions are located on a single tooth or on non-

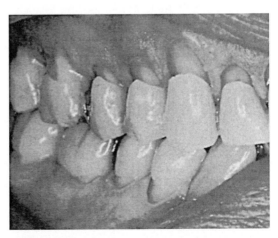

FIGURE 9–24. Severe abrasion and notching of buccal root surfaces. (Used with permission from Carranza F, Newman M. Glickman's Clinical Periodontology. 8th ed. Philadelphia: WB Saunders, 1996.)

adjacent teeth and are hypothesized to be the result of microfractures in enamel and dentin caused by eccentrically applied occlusal forces.[68] For example, during bruxism the changing back-and-forth direction of the occlusal forces bends the tooth, causing side-to-side fatigue and microfracturing at the most flexed area in the cervical region of the tooth.[69]

Attrition primarily occurs on the occlusal and incisal surfaces of the teeth as wear from tooth-to-tooth functional contact. However, attrition can occur on any surface exposed to tooth-to-tooth contact (i.e., buccal and lingual surfaces of anterior teeth in a deep overbite relationship). Parafunctional attrition is often related to excessive grinding motions.[70] Reduced salivary flow may contribute to tooth wear as a result of increased tooth-to-tooth friction.[71]

Erosion is the loss of enamel and dentin primarily by the chemical action of acids other than those produced by oral bacteria.[70] Dietary acids and gastric acids are the most common causes of dental erosion. Dietary erosion is most commonly observed as moderate, generalized erosion of the cervical and buccal surfaces of the maxillary teeth and the occlusal and buccal surfaces of the mandibular teeth, as shown in Figure 9–25.[72] Gastric erosion is more severe than dietary erosion. It is commonly observed on the lingual aspects of the anterior and posterior maxillary teeth, buccal aspects of the mandibular posterior teeth, and occlusal aspects of the mandibular and maxillary posterior teeth.[72] Dietary analysis of the consumption frequency of and duration of exposure to acidic food may help to identify the cause of erosion.[73] Acidic food sources include citrus fruits, other fruits, foods containing vinegar, and carbonated drinks containing citric acid, phosphoric acid, or carbonic acid, acidic sports drinks, salad dressing, herbal tea, and alcohol.[71, 73, 74] Patients who are maintaining a "healthy lifestyle" by exercising and eating a healthy diet with more fruits and vegetables may be inadvertently increasing their risk of dental erosion. Gastric erosion results from vomiting and regurgitation caused by medical conditions such as anorexia nervosa, bulimia, hiatal hernia, ulcers, pregnancy, obesity, and chronic alcoholism.[75]

Medications should not be overlooked as a potential cause of dental erosion. Medications could have the effect of reducing the pH of the oral environment, inducing vomiting, or decreasing salivary flow and its buffering capacity (Table 9-7).

Conventional tooth wear conditions are described as ditching, notching, or flattening of the tooth structure. Less common tooth wear conditions include cupping of the incisal or occlusal surfaces, projection of restorations above the tooth surface, and reduction of tooth length that results in a disproportional width–length ratio. Tooth wear indices have been developed to document tooth wear conditions. The Tooth Wear Index[76] was designed for initial assessment and progressive monitoring of tooth wear conditions, including erosion, abrasion, and attrition. Smith and Knight[76] recommended that each tooth, except heavily restored teeth, be assessed for the presence of tooth wear. The tooth surfaces included in the assessment are the cervical surface, the remainder of the buccal surface, the lingual surface, and the occlusal or incisal surface. The interproximal surfaces are not recorded. An assessment can be performed clinically or from intraoral photographs. The tooth wear scores for each surface of each tooth should be recorded on a chart in the patient record. The tooth wear index is described in Table 9-8.

SENSITIVITY OR HYPERSENSITIVITY

Many patients have areas of thermal (cold or hot) or pressure sensitivity. If the buccal marginal surfaces of the teeth are sensitive to cold, the cause is generally hypersensitive root surfaces as a result of gingival recession. Sensitivity to cold can keep patients from brushing in the area, therefore contributing to the development of gingival inflammation. Thermal sensitivity on

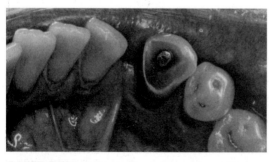

FIGURE 9–25. Severe tooth erosion on the occlusal surface of a mandibular first premolar. The tooth structure has eroded away, leaving the amalgam filling higher than the remaining occlusal surface.

TABLE 9–7. Summary of Tooth Wear Conditions

Tooth Wear, Condition	Location	Description	Etiology
Abrasion	Buccal surface typically at CEJ.	"V" or wedge-shaped defects or notches.	Mechanical process of foreign object—toothbrush.
	Incisal and occlusal surfaces.	Ditches, notches, or indentations.	Mechanical process of foreign object—personal habits.
Abfraction	Cervical surfaces.	"V" or wedge shaped lesion with sharp edges.	Mechanical process involving tooth flexure by eccentric occlusal forces.
Attrition	Incisal or occlusal surfaces.	Flattening or well defined facets.	Mechanical process involving tooth-to-tooth contact.
	Buccal and lingual surfaces.	Facets and ledges.	Tooth-to-tooth contact resulting from deep overbite, crossbite or other functional contact.
Erosion	Cervical and buccal surfaces of maxillary teeth and occlusal and buccal surfaces of mandibular teeth (dietary erosion).	Initial lesions—wide, shallow concavities involving enamel.	Chemical actions of acids other than produced by oral bacteria—predominantly dietary and gastric acids.
	Lingual surfaces of anterior and posterior maxillary teeth, buccal surfaces of mandibular posterior teeth, and occlusal surfaces of mandibular and maxillary posterior teeth (gastric erosion).	Advancing lesions—dentin involvement, restorations rising above adjacent tooth structure, cupping of cusp tips.	

TABLE 9–8. The Tooth Wear Index by Smith and Knight

Score*	Surface	Criterion
0	B/L/O/I	No loss of enamel surface characteristics
	C	No change of contour
1	B/L/O/I	Loss of enamel surface characteristics
	C	Minimal loss of contour
2	B/L/O	Loss of enamel, exposing dentin for less than one-third of the surface
	I	Loss of enamel just exposing dentin
	C	Defect less than 1 mm deep
3	B/L/O	Loss of enamel exposing dentin for more than one-third of the surface
	I	Loss of enamel and substantial loss of dentin, but not exposing pulp or secondary dentin
	C	Defect 1 to 2 mm deep
4	B/L/O	Complete loss of enamel, pulp exposure, or exposure of secondary dentin
	I	Pulp exposure or exposure of secondary dentin
	C	Defect more than 2 mm deep, pulp exposure, or exposure of secondary dentin

*In case of doubt, a lower score is given.
B = buccal; L = lingual; O = occlusal; I = incisal; C = cervical.
Used with permission from Smith BGN and Knight JK. An index for measuring the wear of teeth. Br Dent J 1984;156:436.

the occlusal surfaces may indicate faulty restorations or excessive occlusal wear that affects the nerve of the tooth. Pressure sensitivity or thermal sensitivity can indicate a high or fractured restoration or a fractured tooth. All patients should be asked whether any of their teeth are sensitive. Positive responses should be followed with a thorough examination of the teeth from all angles to detect vertical and horizontal crazing or enamel fractures. The dental mirror can be used for reflection of light. Sensitive areas should be noted in the patient record.

RADIOGRAPHIC EXAMINATION

The radiographic examination serves as an essential adjunct to the clinical examination. Radiographic images of the periodontium play an integral role in assessing the destruction associated with periodontal disease. Due to the episodic nature of periodontal disease, radiographs may permit comparison of changes over time in periodontal status, but they do not indicate the presence of active disease.

Radiographic Assessment

RADIOGRAPHIC SURVEYS OF THE PERIODONTIUM

Radiographs commonly used for periodontal assessment include horizontal and vertical bitewing radiographs, periapical radiographs, and panoramic radiographs. The bitewing radiograph is particularly valuable because of its ability to accurately represent the bone height along the root surface. With proper technique, the x-ray beam is perpendicular to the bone, long axis of the tooth, and film plane, thus minimizing distortion. When a non-perpendicular beam is used, the result may be elongation or foreshortening of the image, causing an inaccurate appearance of an increase or decrease in the bone level. The cusp tips of posterior teeth can assist the dental hygienist in assessing the accuracy of bone height images. When the buccal and lingual cusp tips are level, the x-ray beam was probably correctly angled.[77] Horizontal bitewings are adequate for the assessment of bone height in non-periodontally involved patients; however, vertical bitewings are necessary to capture an image of the existing bone in patients with moderate to advanced periodontal disease. In comparison to periapical radiographs, bitewing radiographs limit the patient's radiation exposure because a reduced number of films is required to capture images of the posterior dentition.

All radiographic surveys should be logged in the patient record. The assessment value of radiographic images is enhanced when the exposure, projection technique, and processing of radiographs are standardized.[78-80] Documentation of the x-ray beam angulation, exposure level and time, type of film, and processing technique enhance radiographic reproducibility, which is important in research. All radiographs should be accompanied by a documented interpretation of the patient's radiographically evident periodontal status.

RADIOGRAPHIC APPEARANCE OF THE PERIODONTIUM

The radiographic evaluation of bone changes associated with periodontal disease is primarily based on the appearance of the interdental septa. In conventional radiographs, the buccal and lingual alveolar crests are obscured by the relatively dense root structure, limiting their use in assessing the patient's periodontal status on the buccal and lingual surfaces. The interdental septum normally has a thin radiopaque border, adjacent to the periodontal ligament space, referred to as the lamina dura. This radiopaque image appears continuous with the alveolar crest, which is the shadow of cortical plate at the crest of the septum. This border appears radiographically as a continuous white line; however, anatomically, it is perforated by numerous small foramina that contain blood vessels, lymphatics, and nerves that pass between the periodontal ligament and the bone. It represents the bone lining the tooth socket. The periodontal ligament space appears as a thin radiolucent line between the lamina dura and tooth root. See Figure 9-26 for an illustration of the radiographic features of the periodontium.

The width and shape of the interdental septum and the angle of the alveolar crest normally vary according to the convexity of the proximal tooth surfaces and the level of the cementoenamel junctions of the approximating teeth.[81] The interdental septa between teeth with prominently convex proximal surfaces (i.e., posterior teeth) are wider anteroposteriorly than are those between teeth with relatively flat proxi-

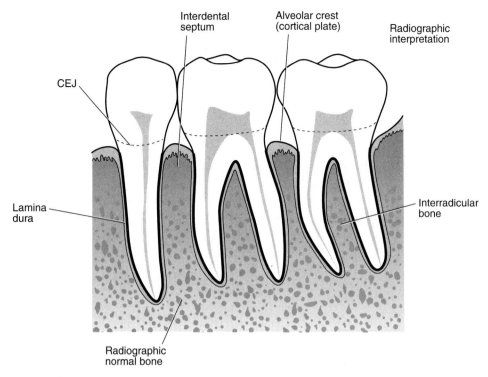

Interdental septum

Alveolar crest (cortical plate)

Radiographic interpretation

CEJ

Lamina dura

Interradicular bone

Radiographic normal bone

FIGURE 9–26. The normal radiographic features of the periodontium in diagrammatic presentation.

mal surfaces (i.e., anterior teeth). The buccolingual diameter of the bone is related to the proximal root width. The alveolar crest generally runs parallel to a line between the cementoenamel junctions of the approximating teeth. When there is a difference in the levels of the cementoenamel junctions (i.e., variation in the degree or inclination of eruption of adjacent teeth), the alveolar crest is angulated rather than horizontal (Figure 9–27).

RADIOGRAPHIC CHANGES WITH PERIODONTAL DISEASE

In periodontal disease, the interdental septa undergo changes that affect the radiodensity of the crestal cortical plate, the size and shape of the medullary spaces, and the height and contour of the bone. When the inflammation process is permitted to progress, fuzziness, loss of radiopacity, and breaks in the continuity of the crestal plate and the lamina dura at the mesial and distal aspect of the alveolar crest may occur (Figure 9–28). These are early radiographic signs of periodontal disease progression. Subsequent formation of wedge-shaped radiolucent areas at the mesial and distal aspect of the crest of the interdental septum are observed (Figure

9–29). The apices of these triangulated areas point apically in the direction of the affected roots. These areas are produced by resorption of the bone of the lateral aspect of the interdental septum and an associated widening of the

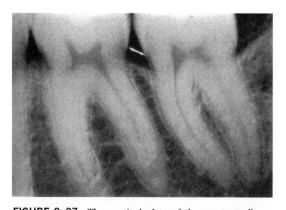

FIGURE 9–27. The cortical plate of the crest usually appears radiographically as a horizontal line running between and slightly apical to the cementoenamel junctions of adjacent teeth. It may appear angled between teeth (arrow) if the cementoenamel junctions of adjacent teeth are not level. This appearance is a variation of normal. The radiograph has been cropped to emphasize the periodontal condition of the teeth. (Used with permission from Carranza F, Newman M. Glickman's Clinical Periodontology, 8th ed. Philadelphia: WB Saunders, 1996.)

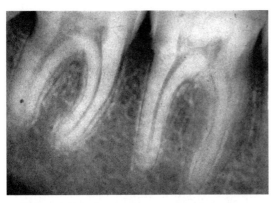

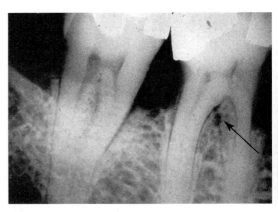

FIGURE 9–28. Radiographic changes in early periodontal disease. There is fuzziness in the lamina dura and an indistinct crest of the interdental septa. The radiograph has been cropped to emphasize the periodontal condition of the teeth.

FIGURE 9–29. Radiographic appearance of horizontal bone loss between two molars. The crestal cortical plate is absent and some wedge-shaped bone loss is apparent next to the tooth roots. The arrow points to an area of furcation involvement. The radiograph has been cropped to emphasize the periodontal condition of the teeth.

periodontal ligament space. As periodontal disease progresses, the height of the interdental septum is reduced by the extension of inflammation and the resorption of bone.

The measurement between the cementoenamel junction and crestal cortical plate is critical for assessing the extent of bone loss. The measurement of normal crestal bone height ranges from 1 to 3 mm from the cementoenamel junction.[82, 83] When the alveolar crest appears to be approximately parallel to the line drawn between the cementoenamel junctions of adjacent teeth, reduction in height of the interdental septum is known as horizontal bone loss. Examples are shown in Figures 9-29 and 9-30

However, horizontal alveolar bone loss has been shown to be a normal physiologic response to aging. Therefore, even in periodontally healthy patients small amounts of bone loss may be observed.[84] When the crest no longer appears parallel to the line formed by the adjacent cementoenamel junctions, the reduction in bone height is known as vertical or angular bone loss. The bone loss is observed to progress vertically along the root to form an angular defect. Vertical bone loss is more common in the posterior that the anterior periodontium.[85] This type of defect is shown in Figure 9-31.

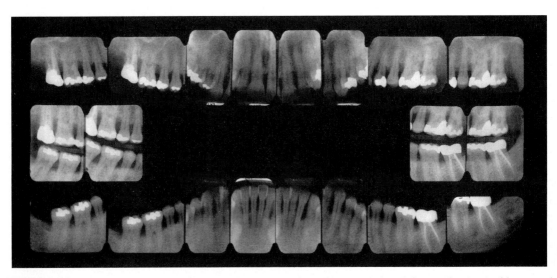

FIGURE 9–30. A full-mouth radiographic survey of a patient with moderate periodontal disease characterized by generalized horizontal bone loss.

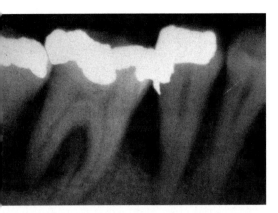

FIGURE 9–31. Radiographic appearance of vertical bone loss. A pronounced vertical defect appears between the mandibular second premolar and the first molar. The radiograph has been cropped to emphasize the periodontal condition of the teeth.

Furcation involvement may be detected by radiographic assessment of the interradicular bone (see Figure 9-29). However, the lack of radiographically detectable furcation involvement is not confirmation of the absence of this type of periodontal destruction (Figure 9-32). The anatomic location of the furcation involvement and variations in radiographic technique may obscure the radiographic image of a furcation. It is not uncommon for one film to show significant involvement, whereas another film of the same tooth shows no involvement because of differences in projection and exposure. To assist in the detection of furcation involvement, the following criteria are suggested:

1. The slightest radiographic change of the periodontal ligament space in the furcation area should be investigated clinically.
2. Diminished radiodensity in the furcation area, as shown by visible outlines of bony trabeculae, suggests furcation involvement.
3. Whenever there is marked bone loss in relation to one root of a molar, it may be assumed that the furcation is also involved.

The radiographic observations associated with the classification of periodontal disease are described in Periodontal Disease Case Types and Associated Radiographic Evidence.

LIMITATIONS OF RADIOGRAPHIC ASSESSMENT OF PERIODONTAL DISEASE

Because conventional radiographs do not show minor changes in bone mass,[86, 87] even slight radiographic changes mean that the periodontal disease has progressed beyond the earliest stages. Since radiographs are two-dimensional images of a three-dimensional structure, they may not reflect the complete extent of bone loss.[89]

Traditional radiographs do not show the internal morphology or depth of the crater-like interdental defects that appear as angular or vertical defects, nor do they show the extent of involvement on the buccal and lingual surfaces. Buccal and lingual crestal bone loss may be obscured by dense root structure. Intact cortical plates on the buccal and lingual surfaces of the interdental septa also obscure detection of destruction in the intermediary cancellous bone. Therefore, it is possible to have a deep crater in the bone between the buccal and lingual plates without radiographic indications of its presence. For destruction of the interproximal cancellous bone to be recorded radiographically, the cortical bone must be involved.

RADIOGRAPHIC ASSESSMENT OF DENTAL IMPLANTS

The radiographic assessment of dental implants includes an examination of the presence of peri-implant radiolucencies and the height of the marginal bone. The accuracy of this assessment is dependent upon the diagnostic quality of the radiographs. Diagnostic quality is enhanced with the use of the paralleling technique where the x-ray beam is perpendicular to the film plane and implant. As with the natural dentition, only proximal bone levels can be

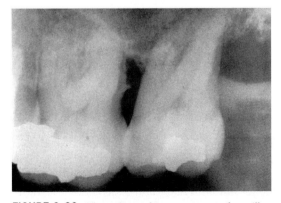

FIGURE 9–32. The radiographic appearance of maxillary molar furcations. The absence of bone on the distal surfaces requires a careful assessment of involvement. Buccal furcations are not obvious. The radiograph has been cropped to emphasize the periodontal condition of the teeth.

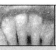

PERIODONTAL DISEASE CASE TYPES AND ASSOCIATED RADIOGRAPHIC EVIDENCE

Type I—Gingivitis	No radiographic defects—soft tissue involvement only. Figure 9–27
Type II—Slight Chronic Periodontitis	Bone destruction isolated to crestal bone. Bone will appear more radiolucent or "fuzzy." Triangulation can be noted in posterior areas. Destruction is usually in isolated areas of the mouth. Figure 9–28
Type III—Moderate Chronic or Aggressive Periodontitis	30–50% of supporting bone has been lost resulting in moderate horizontal and/or vertical bone loss. Bone loss in furcation areas can be seen in posterior areas. Figure 9–30
Type IV—Advanced Chronic or Aggressive Periodontitis	Radiographically characterized with 50% or more bone destruction. Advanced horizontal and/or vertical bone loss. Furcation involvement seen as radiolucencies of interradicular bone. Figures 9–31 and 9–32
Type V—Refractory Chronic or Aggressive Periodontitis	Gradual increases in radiographic bone loss due to unfavorable patient response to conventional periodontal treatment regimens.

distinguished because of the superimposition of the buccal and lingual cortical plates and the implant.

Marginal bone height is the measurement between the marginal bone and an established reference point on the implant (i.e., the implant abutment junction or the top of the abutment). Bone loss of .5 to 1 mm may be observed in the first year following the connection of the abutment to the implant. An annual loss of .05 to .1 mm may be observed in subsequent years.[90] The intervals for radiographic assessment of implants have been suggested to be at six months after loading of the implant, annually for the next three years, and every two years thereafter unless otherwise indicated.

ADVANCEMENTS IN RADIOGRAPHIC ASSESSMENT OF PERIODONTAL DISEASE

Advances in radiographic technique are being pursued to respond to the recognized deficiencies of conventional radiographs. Of particular note for the diagnosis of periodontal disease is digital subtraction radiography (DSR).[91] DSR can reduce the delay between the destruction of bone and its radiographic detection by more efficiently using information captured on the radiograph. It may also be used to assess regen-

eration of bone in response to periodontal therapies. DSR measures changes in bone density over time and therefore requires two standardized radiographs with similar projection geometry, exposure parameters, and processing quality. Structures that have not changed in the time between the two radiographs are subtracted from the image. The remaining visible structure will be bone loss or gain on a neutral background. This is referred to as removing the structural noise.[92] The subtraction image may be further enhanced by superimposing the image on the original radiograph or by using color contrast to illustrate bone gain and loss.[93]

Although DSR permits earlier observation of small levels of bone changes, it is not routinely available in dental practice. The need for radiographs exposed with standardized projection geometry presents a challenge to the practitioner. While methods have been developed for standardizing radiographic images, there are practical limitations to their use in day-to-day practice. Presently, dental practices do not commonly have the image processing equipment required for the conversion of these standardized radiographs to digital images.[94]

Another advance in dental radiography is filmless or digital radiographic systems. The advantages of these systems include instantaneous formation of images, reduction of radiation exposure, elimination of chemical processing, accessibility of backup copies, and availability of size and contrast enhancements. The current disadvantages of these systems include the cost of the equipment; the small size of the active imaging area, resulting in the need for a greater number of radiographs; and the lower resolution, reducing diagnostic quality. However, advances in these digital systems are very promising, and they will no doubt be used more commonly in the near future.

TECHNOLOGIC ADVANCES IN ASSESSMENTS

Scientists and clinicians are working toward the development of cost-effective, efficient technologic advancements to aid in the assessment and diagnosis of periodontal disease. Of particular concern are methods that will enhance the accuracy of the diagnosis of active periodontal disease.

The periodontal literature reports the use of new technologies for the assessment of periodontal disease. These technologies are intended to minimize variation and standardize data collection during clinical examinations. While routinely used in periodontal research, they are not yet practical for use in day-to-day dental practice. Such technologies include controlled-force probes for measuring clinical attachment loss and automated tooth mobility equipment for measuring mobility of teeth and implants.

CONCLUSION

The integration of each component of clinical assessment is critical to the comprehensive diagnosis and treatment of the periodontal patient. This comprehensive approach to oral health care delivery enhances the potential for achieving desirable treatment outcomes and minimizing the effects of periodontal disease.

STUDY QUESTIONS

MULTIPLE CHOICE

1. The first step in the dental hygiene process of patient care is:

   a. assessment
   b. diagnosis
   c. planning
   d. implementation

2. The term for a swelling at the gingival margin that has an inner tube–like appearance is:

   a. cleft
   b. festoon
   c. frenum
   d. tumor

3. The name of a simple, commonly used method for recording the presence of plaque on tooth surfaces is called:

   a. Gingival Index of Löe and Silness
   b. O'Leary Index
   c. Plaque Index of Silness and Löe
   d. Simplified Oral Hygiene Index

4. A type of stain that occurs as a thin black line on the facial and lingual surfaces of the teeth of individuals who have excellent oral hygiene is called:

   a. tobacco stain
   b. chlorhexidine stain
   c. orange stain
   d. black stain

5. The periodontal probe can be used to quantify all of the following EXCEPT one. Which one is the exception?

   a. sulcus and pocket depth
   b. gingival recession
   c. furcation involvement
   d. stain and plaque
   e. clinical attachment loss

6. Bleeding on probing is considered a clinical indication of periodontal disease BECAUSE lack of bleeding on probing means there is stability in the periodontium.

   a. Both the statement and the reason are correct and related.
   b. Both the statement and the reason are correct but NOT related.
   c. The statement is correct, but the reason is NOT.
   d. The statement is NOT correct, but the reason is correct.
   e. NEITHER the statement NOR the reason is correct.

7. The index that can be used to assess the vertical component of bone loss in a bifurcation or trifurcation of a multirooted tooth is the:

   a. Glickman Index
   b. O'Leary Index
   c. Tarnow and Fletcher Index
   d. Simplified Oral Hygiene Index

8. What is the most important parameter for assessment of the failure of an implant?

   a. attachment loss
   b. clinical mobility
   c. probing
   d. radiographs

9. The Newbrun Root Caries Severity Index classification for a lesion with cavitation greater than 0.5 mm is:

   a. Grade I: incipent
   b. Grade II: shallow
   c. Grade III: cavitation
   d. Grade IV: pupal

10. The term for tooth wear on the incisal or occlusal surfaces caused by such habits as fingernail biting, excessive toothbrushing, or pipe smoking is:

    a. attrition
    b. abrasion
    c. erosion
    d. abfraction

11. According to G.V. Black's Cavity Classification, a Class 4 includes:

    a. proximal cavities in premolars and molars
    b. gingival third cavities
    c. proximal cavities in incisors and canines involving the incisal edge
    d. incisal edge and cusp tip cavities

SHORT ANSWER

12. How does assessment of the medical history help the clinician to ensure the safety and health of the patient?

    _____

    _____

13. Describe the steps for completing the O'Leary Index.

    _____

    _____

14. What can cause pathologic tooth mobility?

_____

_____

15. List the aspects included in an assessment of the periodontium and dentition.

_____

_____

16. Describe an early radiographic change present in a patient with periodontal disease.

_____

_____

17. Describe the limitations of conventional radiographs in the detection of bone loss.

_____

_____

18. Describe the radiographic changes seen in AAP Type III-Moderate Periodontitis.

_____

_____

REFERENCES

1. American Dental Hygienists' Association. Standards of Applied Dental Hygiene Practice. Chicago: ADHA, 1985:1.
2. American Academy of Periodontology. Guidelines for Periodontal Therapy. Chicago: AAP, 1992.
3. Minden NJ, Fast TB. The patient's health history form: how healthy is it? J Am Dent Assoc 1993;124:95.
4. Thibodeau EA, Rossomando KJ. Survey of the medical history questionnaire. Oral Surg Oral Med Oral Pathol 1992;74:400.
5. Minden NJ, Fast TB. Evaluation of health history forms used in U.S. dental schools. Oral Med Oral Pathol 1994;77:105.
6. Page RC, Beck JD. Risk assessment for periodontal diseases. Intl. Dent J 1997;47:61.
7. O'Leary TJ, Drake RB, Naylor JE. The plaque control record. J Periodontol 1972;43:38.
8. Eriksen HM, Nordbo H. Extrinsic discoloration of teeth. J clin Periodontol 1978;5:229.
9. Gjermo P. Chlorhexidine in dental practice. J Clin Periodontol 1974;1:143.
10. Löe H, Schiott C. The effect of mouth rinses and topical application of chlorhexidine on the development of dental plaque and gingivitis in man. J Periodontol Res 1970;5:79.
11. Gjermo P. Chlorhexidine and related compounds. J Dent Res 1989;68:1602.
12. Nordbo H. Discoloration of human teeth by a combination of chlorhexidine and aldehydes or ketones in vitro. Scand J Dent Res 1971;79:356.
13. Eriksen HM, Nordbo H, Kantanen H, Ellingsen JE. Chemical plaque control and extrinsic tooth discoloration: a review of possible mechanisms. J clin Periodontol 1985;12:345.
14. Addy M, Moran J. Extrinsic tooth discoloration by metals and chlorhexidine II. Clinical staining produced by chlorhexidine, iron and tea. Br Den J 1985;159:331.
15. Svantun B, Gjermo P, Eriksen HM, Rolla G. A comparison of the plaque-inhibiting effect of stannous fluoride and chlorhexidine. Acta Odont Scand 1977;35:247.
16. Berswanger BB, Doyle PM, Jackson RD, et al. The clinical effect of dentifrices containing stabilized stannous fluoride on plaque formation and gingivitis: a six month study with ad libitum brushing. J Clin Perio 1995;6:46.
17. Thrash WS, Dodds MWJ, Jones DL. The effect of stannous fluoride on dentinal hypersensitivity. Int Dent J 1994;44:107.
18. Rolla G, Ellingsen JE. Clinical effects and possible mechanisms of action of stannous fluoride. Int Dent J 1994;44:99.
19. Slots J. The microflora of black stain on human primary teeth. Scand J Dent Res 1974;82:484.
20. Sutcliff P. Extrinsic tooth stains in children. Dent Pract 1967;17:175.
21. Reid JS, Beeley JA, MacDonald DG. Investigations into black extrinsic tooth stain. J Dent Res 1977;56:895.
22. Ayers P. Green stains. J Am Dent Assoc 1939;26:3.
23. Badanes BB. The role of fungi in deposits upon the teeth. Dent Cosmos 1933;75:1154.
24. Leung SW. Naturally occurring stains on the teeth of children. J Am Dent Assoc 1950;41:191.
25. Bartel HA. A note on chromogenic microorganisms from an organic colored deposit of the teeth. Int J Orthod 1939;25:795.
26. Van der Weijden GA, Timmerman MF, Nijboer A, Reijerse E, Van der Velden U. Comparison of different approaches to assess bleeding on probing as indicators of gingivitis. J Clin Periodontol 1994;21:589.
27. Armitage GC. Clinical evaluation of periodontal diseases. Periodontol 2000 1995;7:39.
28. Consensus Reports From the 1996 World Workshop in Periodontics. Periodontal diseases: Epidemiology and diagnosis. J Am Dent Assoc 1998;129:9-S.
29. Clark WB, Yang MCK, Magnusson I. Measuring clinical attachment: reproducibility of relative measurements with an electronic probe. J Periodontol 1992;63:831.
30. Karim M, Birek P, McCulloch CA. Controlled force measurements of gingival attachment level made with the Toronto automated probe using electronic guidance. J Clin Periodontol 1990;17:594.
31. Mohammad AR, Brunsvold M. The strength of association between systemic postmenopausal osteoporosis and periodontal disease. Int J Prosthodont 1996;9:479.
32. von Wowern N, Klausen B, Kollerup G. Osteoporosis: A risk factor in periodontal disease. J Periodontol 1994;65:1134.
33. Hildebolt CF, Pilgram TK, Dotson M, et al. Attachment loss with postmenopausal age and smoking. J Periodont Res 1997;32:619.
34. Johnson BD, Mulligan K, Kiyak HA, Marder M. Aging or disease? Periodontol changes and treatment considerations in the older dental patient. Gerodontology 1989;8:109.
35. Listgarten MA. Periodontol probing: what does it mean? J Clin Periodontol 1980;7:165.
36. Armitage GC, Svanberg GK, Löe H. Microscopic evalua-

tion of clinical measurements of connective tissue attachment levels. J Clin Periodontol 1977;4:173.

37. Goodson JM. Diagnosis of periodontitis by physical measurement: interpretation from episodic disease hypothesis. J Periodontol 1992;63:373.

38. Haffajee AD, Socransky SS, Lindhe J, Kent RL, Okamoto H, Yoneyama T. Clinical risk indicators for periodontal attachment loss. J Clin Periodontol 1991;18:117.

39. Lang NP, Joss A, Orsanic T, Gusberti FA, Siegrist BE. Bleeding on probing: a predictor for the progression of periodontal disease? J Clin Periodontol. 1986;13:590.

40. Lang NP, Tonetti MS. Periodontal diagnosis in treated periodontitis: Why, when and how to use clinical parameters. J Clin Periodontol 1996;23:240.

41. Baderstein A, Nilveus R, Egelberg J. Scores of plaque, bleeding, suppuration and probing depth to predict probing attachment loss. 5 years of observation following nonsurgical periodontal therapy. J Clin Periodontol 1990;17:102.

42. Lang NP, Adler R, Joss A, Nyman S. Absence of bleeding on probing. J Clin Periodontol. 1990;17:714.

43. Newbrun E. Indices to measure gingival bleeding. J Periodontol 1996;67:555.

44. Preber H and Bergström J. Occurrence of gingival bleeding in smoker and non-smoker patients. Acta Odontol Scand 1985;43:315.

45. Carranza FA Jr, Takei HH. Treatment of furcation involvement and combined periodontal-endodontic therapy. In Carranza FA, Newman MG eds. Clinical periodontology, 8th ed. Philadelphia: WB Saunders, 1996: 640-651.

46. Kalkwarf KL, Reinhardt RA. The furcation problem: current controversies and future directions. Dent Clin North Am 1988;32:243.

47. Tarnow D, Fletcher P. Classification of the vertical component of furcation involvement. J Periodontol 1984;55:283.

48. Zappa U, Grosso L, Simona C, Graf H, and Case D. Clinical furcation diagnosis and interradicular bone defects. J Periodontol 1993;64:219.

49. O'Leary TJ. Tooth mobility. Dent Clin North Am 1969;13:567.

50. Rateitschak KH. Tooth mobility changes in pregnancy. J Periodont 1967;2:199.

51. Folkers SA, Weine FS, Weissman DP. Periodontal disease in the life stages of women. Compend Contin Educ Dent 1992;13:852.

52. Carranza FA, Perry DA. Clinical periodontology for the dental hygienist. Philadelphia: WB Saunders, 1986:132.

53. Miller SC. Textbook of periodontia, 3rd ed. Philadelphia: Blakiston, 1950:125.

54. Schluger S, Yuodelis R, Page RC, Johnson RH. Periodontal diseases: basic phenomena, clinical management, and occlusal and restorative interrelationships, 2nd ed. Philadelphia: Lea & Febiger, 1990:322.

55. American Dental Association and American Academy of Periodontology: Periodontal Screening and Recording™. Chicago: ADA, AAP, 1992.

56. Bauman GR, Mill M, Rapley JW, Hallmon WH. Clinical parameters of evaluation during implant maintenance. Int J Oral Maxillofac Implants 1992;7:220.

57. Koumjian JH, Kerner J, Smith RA. Implants: Hygiene maintenance of dental implants. Illinois Dent J 1991: Jan-Feb: 54.

58. Mombelli A, Lang NP. Clinical parameters for the evaluation of dental implants. Periodontology 2000 1994; 4:81.

59. Lang NP, Mombelli A, Bragger U, et al. Monitoring disease around dental implants during supportive periodontal treatment. Periodontology 2000 1996;12:60.

60. Chavez H, Ortman LF, DeFranco RL, Medige J. Assessment of oral implant mobility. J Prosthetic Dent 1993;70:421.

61. Titus HW. Root caries: some facts and treatment methods. Am J Dent 1991;4:61.

62. Black GV. Operative Dentistry, 8th ed. 2 vols. Medico-Dental Publishing Co.: Woodstock, IL: 1947-48

63. Sturdevant CM, ed. (1995). The Art and Science of Operative Dentistry, 3rd Ed. Mosby: St. Louis.

64. Newbrun E. Problems in caries diagnosis. Int Dent J 1993;43:133.

65. Brunsvold MS, Lane JJ. The prevalence of overhanging dental restorations and their relationship to periodontal disease. J Clin Periodontol 1999;17:67.

66. Machtei EE, Christersson LA, Grossi SG, Dunford R, Zambon JJ, Genco RJ. Clinical criteria for the definition of "established periodontitis." J Periodontol 1992; 63:206.

67. Pack ARC, Coxhead LJ, McDonald BW. The prevalence of overhanging margins in posterior amalgam restorations and periodontal consequences. J Clin Periodontol 1990;17:145.

68. Imfeld T. Dental erosion. definition, classification and links. Eur J Oral Sci 1996;104:151.

69. Grippo JO, Simring M. Dental erosion revisited. J Am Dent Assoc. 1995;126:619.

70. Carranza FA. Aging and the periodontium. In Glickman I. Clinical periodontology, 8th ed. Philadelphia: WB Saunders, 1990:91.

71. Smith BGN. Some facets of tooth wear. Ann R Aust Coll Dent Surg. 1991;11:37.

72. Smith BGN, Knight JK. A comparision of patterns of tooth wear with aetiological factors. Br Dent J 1984;157;16.

73. Lussi A. Dental Erosion. Clinical diagnosis and case history taking. Eur J Oral Sci 1996;104:191.

74. Zero DT. Etiology of dental erosion-extrinsic factors. Eur J Oral Sci 1996;104:162.

75. Schuetzel P. Etiology of dental erosion-intrinsic factors. Eur J Oral Sci 1996;104:178.

76. Smith BGN, Knight JK. An index for measuring the wear of teeth. Br Dent J 1984;156:435.

77. Jeffcoat MK, Wang IC, Reddy MS. Radiographic diagnosis in periodontics. Periodontol 2000 1995;7:54.

78. Patur B, Glickman I. Roentgenographic evaluation of alveolar bone changes in periodontal disease. Dent Clin North Am 1960;4:47.

79. Puckett J. A device for comparing roentgenograms of the same mouth. J Periodontol 1968;39:38.

80. Rosling B, Hollender L, Nyman S, Olsson G. A radiographic method for assessing changes in alveolar bone height following periodontal therapy. J Clin Periodontol 1975;2:211.

81. Richey B, Orban B. The crests of the interdental septa. J Periodontol 1953;24:75.

82. Hausmann E, Allen K, Clerehugh V. What alveolar crest level on a bite-wing radiograph represents bone loss? J Periodontal 1991;9:570.

83. Goaz PW, White SC. Oral radiology: Principles and interpretation. St Louis: Mosby, 1994:330.

84. Streckfus CF Parsell DE, Streckfus JE. Relationship between oral, alveolar bone loss and aging among African-American and Caucasian individuals. Gerontol 1999;45:110.

85. Vrotsos JA, Parashis AO, Theofanatos GD. Prevalence and distribution of bone defects in moderate and ad-

vanced adult periodontitis. J Clin Periodontol 1999; 26:44.

86. Bender IB, Seltzer S. Roentgenographic and direct observation of experimental lesions in bone. J Am Dent Assoc 1961;62:152.

87. Bender IB, Seltzer S. Roentgenographic and direct observation of experimental lesions in bone: II. J Am Dent Assoc 1961;62:708.

88. Ramadan ABE, Mitchell DF. A roentgenographic study of experimental bone destruction. Oral Surg 1962;15:934.

89. Theilade J. An evaluation of the reliability of radiographs in the measurement of bone loss in periodontal disease. J Periodontol 1960;31:143.

90. Chaytor DV. Clinical criteria for determining implant success: Bone. Int J Prosthodont 1993;6:145.

91. Gröndahl HG, Gröndahl K. Subtraction radiography for the diagnosis of periodontal bone lesions. Oral Surg. 1993;55:208

92. Gröndahl HG, Gröndahl K, Webber RL. A digital subtraction technique for dental radiography. Oral Surg 1983;55:96.

93. Reddy MS, Bruch JM, Jeffcoat MK. Contrast enhancement as an aid to interpretation in digital subtraction radiography. Oral Surg Oral Med Oral Pathol 1991;71:763.

94. Vandre RH, Webber RL. Future trends in dental radiology. Oral Surg Oral Med Oral Pathol 1995;80:471.

10

Phyllis L. Beemsterboer

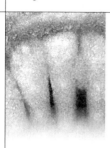

Treatment Planning for the Periodontal Patient

Chapter Objectives

1. Define the role of the dental hygienist in treatment planning.
2. Describe the goals and rationale for periodontal treatment planning.
3. Describe the phases of dental treatment.
4. Compare and contrast the periodontal disease case types.
5. Identify the considerations for sequencing dental hygiene treatment in Phase I and Phase IV therapy of periodontal treatment.
6. Determine overall prognoses and prognoses for individual teeth.
7. Define informed consent and describe its importance to treatment planning.

Key Terms

Diagnosis
Informed consent
Periodontal disease case types I, II, III, IV, and V

Phases I, II, III, and IV
Prognosis
Treatment plan
Treatment sequence

Treatment planning for the periodontal patient is a process that requires the assessment preventive, therapeutic, and evaluative skills of the dental hygienist and the dentist. Th treatment plan is the blueprint for management of the dental case and is an essenti aspect of successful therapy.[1] This plan includes all procedures performed to attain a maintain the long-term oral health of the patient and should involve all members of th health care team and the patient. This chapter describes current strategies and classific tion systems for planning the treatment of the periodontal patient and describes progn ses for periodontally involved teeth.

GOALS OF TREATMENT

The total treatment plan is the sequential outline of the essential services and procedures to be provided by the dental health care team for the patient to eliminate disease and restore the oral cavity to health and function. The dental hygiene **treatment plan** consists of services that are performed by the dental hygienist within the total treatment plan.[2] Treatment planning occurs after the assessment of all clinical data and reflects the **diagnosis** and **prognosis** of the patient. The treatment plan defines the methods and sequence of delivering appropriate treatment.[3, 4]

The goals of the treatment plan are the same, regardless of the sequence of treatment or the individual who is delivering the dental care. These goals are to eliminate and control etiologic and predisposing factors of disease, maintain health, and prevent recurrence of disease.[2, 5] Treatment planning provides an opportunity to explain problems and treatment goals to the patient in understandable terms.[6] Listening to the patient is crucial in the treatment planning process. The dental hygienist must utilize the verbal feedback from the patient to judge the patient's level of understanding. A true partnership between the patient and the dental team working toward mutual treatment goals has the greatest chance for success.

The treatment plan can be divided into various segments, or phases, for coordination of the total treatment of the patient. An individualized, well thought-out treatment plan must be established before the beginning of treatment and must be carefully monitored. The role of the dental hygienist may vary depending on the type of case, experience of the hygienist, requirements of the state dental practice act, practice setting, and philosophy of the periodontist or dentist.

PHASES OF TREATMENT

Carranza[1] divided the treatment plan into four main phases. Each phase suggested a particular group of procedures and included evaluation of patient response. The **treatment sequence** begins with a preliminary phase, incorporating immediate treatment needs; followed by **Phase I**, etiologic treatment; **Phase II**, surgical treatment; **Phase III**, restorative treatment; and **Phase IV**, maintenance treatment. The phases

of therapeutic periodontal procedures, along with the sequence of other needed dental procedures, are presented in the Sequence of Periodontal Procedures.

The purpose of the preliminary phase of treatment is to bring all emergency and other

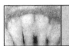

SEQUENCE OF PERIODONTAL PROCEDURES

Preliminary Phase
Treatment of emergencies
Dental or periapical
Periodontal
Other
Extraction of hopeless teeth and provisional replacement if needed (may be postponed to a more convenient time)

Phase I Therapy (etiotropic phase)
Plaque control
Diet control (for patients at high caries risk)
Removal of bacterial plaque and calculus, and root planing
Correction of restorative and prosthetic contributing factors
Removal of caries and restoration of teeth (temporary or final, depending on whether a definitive prognosis for the tooth has been arrived at and on the location of the caries)
Antimicrobial therapy (local or systemic)
Occlusal therapy
Minor orthodontic movement
Provisional splinting

Evaluation of Response to Phase I
 Rechecking gingival condition
  Pocket depth and gingival inflammation
  Plaque, calculus, caries

Phase II Therapy (surgical phase)
Periodontal surgery, including placement of implants
Root canal therapy

Phase III Therapy
Final restorations
Fixed and removable prosthodontics
Orthodontics

Evaluation of Response to Restorative Phase
 Periodontal examination

Phase IV Therapy (maintenance phase)
Periodic recall visits and examinations
Plaque and calculus removal
Gingival condition (pockets, inflammation)
Occlusion and tooth mobility
Other pathologic changes

Reprinted by permission from Carranza FA Jr.: The treatment plan. In Carranza FA Jr., Newman MG, eds. Clinical Periodontology, 8th ed. Philadelphia: W.B. Saunders, 1996.

critical situations under control. Dental and periodontal abscesses should be treated. Hopeless teeth should be removed and provisional restorations, such as temporary partial dentures, fabricated. Endodontic therapy can be performed to relieve pain even if their completion carries over to other phases of treatment, and oral lesions of any kind should be evaluated and treated or referred.

Phase I therapy describes the procedures that are designed to control or eliminate the etiologic factors of the disease process. Patient education and plaque control instruction occur at the beginning of this phase. Scaling and root debridement and planing are performed. Antimicrobial agents are used and/or recommended for home use. Other authors refer to this stage as initial therapy, nonsurgical therapy, cause-related therapy, or the hygienic phase of treatment.[7, 8]

Phase II therapy is the surgical phase of treatment. During this phase, procedures are undertaken to reduce the effects of disease. Regenerative techniques are performed to help restore periodontal tissues that have been lost due to disease.

Phase III therapy usually involves restorations and replacement of missing teeth. Procedures included in this phase are restorative dentistry, extensive orthodontics, and any needed occlusal therapy.

Phase IV therapy is the maintenance phase. Patients remain in this phase for a lifetime. Although this phase is often referred to as "recall," the accepted term is periodontal maintenance because the patient's periodontal health must be continuously monitored from this point. As described extensively in Chapter 15, the maintenance phase begins after phase I, but not necessarily before all phases of treatment have been completed. Patients with extensive surgical and restorative needs often have treatment extend over many months, even years. Periodontal maintenance occurs during the other phases of treatment because decline in the status of periodontal patients has been observed after 90 days. In their classic studies, Ramfjord and Ash showed the success of 3-month maintenance intervals with long-term periodontal maintenance.[7]

The interval between periodontal maintenance appointments is determined by the peri-odontal condition and the plaque control that the patient is able to attain and maintain. Most patients who have been treated for moderate to advanced periodontal disease require maintenance visits every 3 months.[9-11] Periodontal maintenance is described fully in Chapter 15.

ROLE OF THE DENTAL HYGIENIST

The dental hygienist is often responsible for treatment of the periodontal patient in the nonsurgical, or Phase I, and maintenance, or Phase IV, stages of periodontal treatment. Because of the complexity of periodontal treatment required to meet planned goals, a series of appointments is often required. The sequence of treatment depends on a number of factors, including the periodontal diagnosis and prognosis, the patient's systematic and periodontal condition, and the patient's preferences.

Disease classifications are useful for diagnosis, prognosis, and treatment planning because they help define the extent of disease and facilitate communication between members of the treatment team. Various periodontal classification systems have been used over the years and have been modified to reflect advances in knowledge and research.[1] A classification system is a method for comparing treatment approaches and results. Communicating about cases is greatly facilitated by the use of a system that is understood and used by a large number of dental professionals. The American Academy of Periodontology (AAP) classification was adopted in 1986 and modified in 1989. The system describes **periodontal case types I, II, III, IV, and V.** It is used routinely across the United States.[3] In some states, the dental and dental hygiene board examinations identify the patient required for the licensure examination by using the periodontal disease case type classification.

For treatment planning, identifying the peri-odontal disease case type is a first step in determining the extent of disease and assigning the appropriate treatment time and sequence. The case types are shown in Periodontal Disease Case Types and can be used for concise clinical reference. Notice that these case types refer to the extent of disease rather than the specific disease or condition being treated.

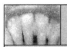

PERIODONTAL DISEASE CASE TYPES

Case Type I: Gingivitis
Inflammation of the gingiva
Presence of gingival hyperplasia and edema
Tissue retractability, gingival pockets
No bone loss

Case Type II: Slight Chronic Periodontitis
Gingival inflammation into the alveolar bone crest
Early bone loss
Pocket depths of 4 to 5 mm
Localized areas of moderate periodontitis

**Case Type III: Moderate Chronic or
Aggressive Periodontitis**
Increased destruction of periodontal structures
Moderate to severe bone loss
Pocket depths of 5 to 7 mm
Presence of tooth mobility
Localized areas of advanced periodontitis

**Case Type IV: Advanced Chronic or
Aggressive Periodontitis**
Severe destruction of periodontal structures
Increased tooth mobility
Pocket depths of 7 mm and greater
A number of teeth with guarded prognosis

**Case Type V: Refractory Chronic or
Aggressive Progressive Periodontitis**
Periodontitis characterized by rapid or slow bone
    and attachment loss; associated with
    inflammation and continued pocket formation
Resistance to normal therapy

Patient education to attain good plaque control and disease prevention is a critical element of treatment. It is often the responsibility of the dental hygienist and includes oral hygiene instruction and prevention education. Effective behavior change is difficult to achieve if the patient does not understand the relationship between oral condition and plaque control. Time spent providing the patient with plaque control and prevention instruction can make a significant difference in the overall success of periodontal treatment. The patient education process continues throughout the treatment sessions and during all phases of care. The most successful approach to patient education is to involve the patient as a partner in the process. For a further discussion of patient compliance and aspects of prevention education, see Chapters 11 and 15.

Patient education for plaque control must be initiated after the assessment and classifications are established. This component of dental hygiene care is often postponed or even ignored. The appropriate time to begin discussing the cause of periodontal disease, and its control by the patient, is as early as possible in the sequence of care, during Phase I rather than waiting for Phase IV.

Decisions about the number of appointments needed to provide appropriate dental hygiene care, the sequence of treatments and the required adjunct techniques, such as the use of local anesthetics, are based on the complexity of the case. There are many factors to consider in making these decisions, and they determine the degree of difficulty involved in providing periodontal debridement. The factors affecting the number and length of treatment visits required to provide nonsurgical therapy are presented in Considerations for Determining the Dental Hygiene Care Plan.

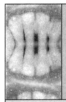

CONSIDERATIONS FOR DETERMINING THE DENTAL HYGIENE CARE PLAN

- Patient general health and tolerance of treatment
- Number of teeth present
- Amount of supragingival calculus
- Amount of subgingival calculus
- Probing pocket depths
  (Amount of attachment loss is less significant during treatment planning than when assessing the case or considering the prognosis)
- Furcations
- Alignment of teeth
- Margins of restorations
- Developmental anomalies
- Physical barriers to access
  (i.e., gagging or limited opening)
- Patient cooperation
- Patient sensitivity
  (requiring use of anesthesia or analgesia)

TREATMENT PLANNING FOR PERIODONTAL DISEASE CASE TYPES

Treatment plans can be estimated for periodontal patients with the periodontal disease case type classification system. These plans should be considered estimates, not templates for dental hygiene care. Every case must be considered individually, and treatment visits must be varied according to the degree of difficulty involved in treating the conditions present. A suggested outline of treatment plans by case type is shown. See Suggested Dental Hygiene Treatment Plans for Periodontal Disease Case Types.

The systemic and periodontal condition of the patient dictates how the dental hygienist sequences either a single session or a series of nonsurgical treatment sessions. The normal procedures for clinical assessment completed at every treatment session for every patient include a review of the medical history, monitoring of vital signs, extra- and intraoral examination, and review or re-examination of dental and periodontal charting.

The patient may have systemic conditions that alter the number and length of treatment appointments. For example, patients with chronic illnesses may tolerate shorter treatment appointments very well but may be exhausted after longer ones. Various medications can also complicate treatment, and they should be carefully noted and monitored. Patients with physical or mental disabilities can present challenges that require modification of treatment plans.[12]

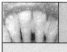

SUGGESTED DENTAL HYGIENE TREATMENT PLANS FOR PERIODONTAL DISEASE CASE TYPES

Type I: Gingivitis
Often completed in one treatment visit

1. Assessments
2. Patient education and plaque control instruction
3. Scaling and periodontal debridement
4. Establish appropriate maintenance interval
5. Re-evaluation at subsequent appointment or first maintenance visit

Type II: Slight Chronic Periodontitis
Often requires more than one treatment visit

1. Assessments
2. Patient education and plaque control instruction; probably more complex, requiring augmentation and reinforcement at subsequent visits
3. Scaling and periodontal debridement, probably requiring anesthetics and analgesics
4. Establish appropriate maintenance interval
5. Re-evaluation by dental hygienist and dentist

Type III: Moderate Chronic or Aggressive Periodontitis
Often treated by quadrants, requiring several treatment visits

1. Assessments, consider referral to periodontist
2. Patient education and plaque control instruction, probably more complex, requiring augmentation and reinforcement at subsequent visits
3. Scaling and periodontal debridement by quadrant, often requiring anesthetic use
4. Establish appropriate maintenance interval
5. Re-evaluation by dental hygienist and dentist

Type IV: Advanced Chronic or Aggressive Periodontitis
Often treated by quadrants, but may require therapy by sextants, over several treatment visits

1. Assessments, strongly consider referral to periodontist
2. Patient education and plaque control instruction, probably more complex, requiring augmentation and reinforcement at subsequent visits
3. Scaling and periodontal debridement by quadrant or sextant
4. Establish appropriate maintenance interval
5. Re-evaluation by dental hygienist and dentist

Type V: Refractory Chronic or Aggressive Periodontitis
May be treated in single or multiple treatment visits
Pocket depth is present, but often with little calculus or plaque

1. Assessments, usually will require referral to periodontist
2. Patient education and plaque control instruction
3. Scaling and periodontal debridement
4. More frequent recalls often required
5. Courses of antibiotics and microbiologic diagnostic monitoring may be required
6. Establish appropriate maintenance interval.
7. Re-evaluation by dental hygienist and dentist

Many conditions requiring modifications to treatment plans are presented in Chapter 17.

A common practice that is now considered outdated is referred to as "gross scaling." Gross scaling was an approach to removing calculus by scaling large deposits at the beginning of the periodontal treatment. Successive appointments then allowed the clinician to "fine" scale and remove the remaining deposits. This two-stage approach was developed when calculus was considered a mechanical irritant, before it was understood that periodontal disease is a bacterial infection. Partial debridement encourages localized healing around a tooth, possibly trapping bacteria at the base of the pocket, leaving unresolved infection and masking deeper infection.[13] The currently accepted technique is to completely scale a quadrant, sextant, or more teeth at a session. This practice often requires that local anesthesia be administered to permit treatment to be completed in comfort. Effective anesthesia allows the clinician to gain greater instrumentation access to the periodontal pockets. The immediate goal of instrumentation for each nonsurgical session is removal of all adherent bacterial plaque and calculus deposits. The dental hygienist judges the smoothness of the root surfaces as the indicator for effective and complete calculus and plaque removal. The long-term goal, restored oral health, is the true measure of successful therapy. This goal is evaluated through examination of tissue response to debridement and maintenance of clinical attachment.

A treatment planning option has been proposed that includes one or two appointments on consecutive days for debridement. The treatment is provided in conjunction with the aggressive use of antimicrobial agents for full-mouth disinfection and was tested on 40 patients with aggressive and severe forms of periodontal diseases. It called for complete scaling and root planing within 24 hours in 2 to 4 hour appointments, application of chlorhexidine to all niches where pathogens would likely remain after the thorough scaling, addition of twice daily chlorhexidine rinses to the oral hygiene routine, and spraying the tonsils with chlorhexidine daily. The disinfectant rinses and spray continued daily for two months. Results showed greater probe depth reductions in deeper pockets after 8 months when compared

to treatment provided by quadrant at two-week intervals with no additional use of disinfectant, essentially treatment that relied on traditional mechanical debridement.[14] In addition to probe depth improvements in the disinfection group, periodontal pathogens were reduced or eliminated in greater proportion when compared to the mechanical therapy group.[15] These data suggest that as our understanding and use of antimicrobial agents in periodontal therapy increases, treatment plans will evolve to maximize therapeutic results. More information and confirmation of these promising results will no doubt be forthcoming.

*I*NFORMED CONSENT

Any treatment plan should consider the wishes and preferences of the patient. The patient must be fully aware of the extent of the disease and the treatment options that are being considered.

Informed consent is the permission to proceed with treatment granted by the patient to the health care provider. Informed consent can be verbal or written. Verbal consent is often called implied consent and is used in routine clinical situations where little or no risk is apparent. Written or express consent is common practice in most periodontal practices where invasive and surgical care is rendered and the risk is greater. Each state has laws that address this issue. The patient should always be informed of the disease process present in the mouth, the treatment proposed, and the alternatives to that treatment.[16] This discussion would also include the consequences of providing no treatment or partial treatment. See Elements of an Informed Consent.

Because of the possibility of lawsuits, it is now common practice to ask patients to sign a consent form acknowledging in writing their understanding of the treatment options and possible outcomes. Thus, the informed consent can be the written document on which the treatment plan is listed and the signatures of all concerned parties are recorded. It is the basis of the legal relationship between the health care provider and the patient.[6] Communication is very important in the informed consent process. The patient must have the opportunity to

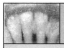

ELEMENTS OF AN INFORMED CONSENT

- Reason for the procedure
- Description of the procedure
- Benefits from the procedure
- Risks that could result from the procedure
- Prognosis with the procedure
- Prognosis if the procedure is not performed
- Other options or alternatives available

ask questions and understand the answers before signing any document or proceeding with any treatment option. The dental hygienist should also be careful not to promise a particular result or outcome.

Patients often become confused when faced with various treatment options. The written agreement clarifies for all parties the treatment plan. A written treatment plan is then truly the blueprint for care.

Documentation

Documentation is essential in all aspects of dental hygiene and periodontal care. After the patient fully understands the risks, benefits, and alternatives to treatment, has agreed, and signed a consent document, the dental hygienist must be equally careful in documenting treatment at every visit. These records are referred to as the chart notes or progress notes, and they reflect all aspects of treatment performed at a particular time. As an example, notes for a typical treatment visit would include review of health, oral examination, oral hygiene instruction, premedication taken, scaling and root planing, anesthetic used, patient response to treatment, post-operative instructions, and any other activities. Accurate documentation of progress notes at all visits is essential and must become as much a part of treatment as infection control practices. All entries in the patient's clinical chart should meet a high standard for completeness and clarity. Standards for chart documentation have been defined by Schoen.[17] See Elements of Acceptable Progress Notes.

PROGNOSIS

Prognosis is the prediction or forecast of the extent and duration of disease and its response to treatment. The dental prognosis is influenced by patient factors (general health, cooperation, type of disease) and evaluated by the clinician. Prognosis is a major consideration in treatment planning because treatment should be based on what intervention is expected to provide an optimal outcome.[7]

All information available from the subjective and objective assessment of each patient is applied to formulate the prognosis. In periodontal disease, the determination of the prognosis has two components: an overall case prognosis and an individual prognosis for each tooth.[1] The factors that are considered in making an overall prognosis for the person with periodontal disease are age; systemic health; type of periodontal disease; oral conditions, including inflamma-

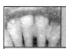

ELEMENTS OF ACCEPTABLE PROGRESS NOTES

Progress notes shall:
- Be legible, dated and signed by the provider.
- Be chronological in sequence.
- Include description of service, teeth or area, anesthetic, and any noteworthy occurrences.
- Include dates of broken and canceled appointments.
- Include summaries of telephone calls related to treatment or problems.
- Include notes of prescriptions, drugs, or materials dispensed.
- Include referrals and requests for radiographs, and results.
- Include the recall plan.
- Be corrected by drawing a line through the incorrect entry so it can still be read, followed by the correct entry, dated and signed.
- NOT be written in pencil, erased, or "whited-out."

Reprinted by permission from Schoen MH, Freed J, Gershen JA, Marcus M. Elements of acceptable progress notes. In Guidelines for Criteria and Standards of Acceptable General Dental Practice (Special Emphasis on Group Practice). J Dent, 1989;11:662–669.

tion and bone levels; and the attitude and perceptions of the patient. Many clinicians consider the attitude, perceptions, and cooperation of the patient the most critical factors in the long-term success of periodontal treatment.

The prognosis of the individual teeth is predicted first on the basis of the overall prognosis and then on the status of each tooth according to pocket depths, mobility, amount and location of furcation involvement, location of the mucogingival tissue, tooth morphology, bone levels, general condition of the tooth, and ability to modify etiologic factors.

Prognosis may be described as good, fair, guarded, or poor. A good prognosis suggests that a tooth or dentition will remain healthy and in function for an indefinite period of time. A fair prognosis suggests that conditions may worsen at some time in the future. A guarded prognosis indicates that efforts to save the tooth or teeth may not be successful. A poor or hopeless prognosis suggests that the condition may not be treatable, and the tooth or teeth may be lost in the near future. It is important to remember that the overall prognosis for the dentition may differ from that of the individual teeth. It is common to have a periodontal patient having one or more teeth with poor prognosis but an overall prognosis that is good. Successful therapy may include removal of some teeth in order to preserve the dentition. Prognoses are summarized in Elements for Determining Prognosis in Periodontal Disease.

Most often the prognosis is determined and the planned treatment is ideal, formulated in the best interests of the patient and intent upon preserving all teeth for as long as possible. Occasionally these plans are later changed or compromised because the patient views things differently. Sometimes patients choose to reject treatment altogether. The dental hygienist is dedicated to providing the best possible treatment and it is sometimes difficult to accept the choice of lesser treatment or loss of teeth. It is important to remember that all patients deserve to know the treatment options and how decisions may alter their oral health in the future. This knowledge is best related by discussion of prognosis for treatment, but the patient is the one who accepts the treatment or chooses to modify it.

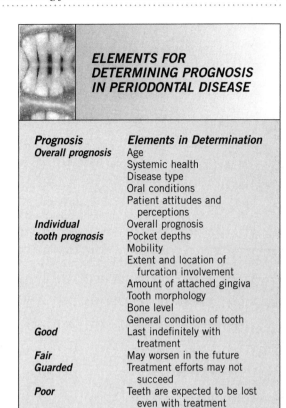

ELEMENTS FOR DETERMINING PROGNOSIS IN PERIODONTAL DISEASE

Prognosis	Elements in Determination
Overall prognosis	Age
	Systemic health
	Disease type
	Oral conditions
	Patient attitudes and perceptions
Individual tooth prognosis	Overall prognosis
	Pocket depths
	Mobility
	Extent and location of furcation involvement
	Amount of attached gingiva
	Tooth morphology
	Bone level
	General condition of tooth
Good	Last indefinitely with treatment
Fair	May worsen in the future
Guarded	Treatment efforts may not succeed
Poor	Teeth are expected to be lost even with treatment

TREATMENT PLANNING IN DENTAL HYGIENE

The dental hygiene treatment plan is an individualized approach to treatment for a specific patient that details the care to be provided by the dental hygienist. It is a portion of the total treatment plan of comprehensive care for the dental patient, sometimes called the dental hygiene care plan. The plan must be adapted to the needs of the patient and presented in an orderly sequence to allow for thoroughness in completing each procedure.[2] The time required for each treatment session depends on the oral condition and extent of care to be provided. Generally, 1-hour appointments are scheduled for each treatment visit, but this time frame is used only as a guideline. The philosophy and customs of the practice and the preferences of the dental hygienist and patient will influence this aspect of treatment planning.

Determining a treatment sequence is influenced by a number of factors including the location and extent of infection, the presence

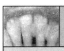

DENTAL HYGIENE TREATMENT PLAN PHASE I THERAPY: PERIODONTAL PRACTICE

Mrs. Johnson is a 34-year-old Hispanic woman with a history of slightly elevated blood pressure. She is not taking any medications, nor is she allergic to anything except pollen. Her family history is unremarkable, and she states that her periodontal condition is of great concern to her because she is a backup singer for a movie studio. She is also concerned about "getting cavities." The patient is new to the periodontal practice of Dr. Smith and has undergone a complete assessment. Mrs. Johnson has been diagnosed as AAP case type II with moderate amounts of calculus in all quadrants. The tissue in the lower right sextant is of concern to the periodontist and the patient because it is red and inflamed. The dental hygienist has been asked to create a treatment plan and to manage care before returning the patient to Dr. Smith for further evaluation.

Treatment 1
Review assessment findings and diagnosis by periodontist.
Take vital signs and baseline indices.
Begin plaque control instruction and fluoride recommendations.
Review treatment plan and treatment goals.
Scale and perform periodontal debridement of maxillary and mandibular right quadrants with anesthesia.

Treatment 2
Review assessment findings, diagnosis, and vital signs.
Evaluate previous scaling and root debridement results.
Continue plaque control instruction and comparative indices.
Scale and perform periodontal debridement of maxillary and mandibular left quadrants with anesthesia.

Treatment 3 (1-Month Evaluation)
Review assessment findings and diagnosis as well as vital signs.
Evaluate previous scaling and periodontal debridement results.
Retreat areas that did not respond to debridement.
Continue plaque control instruction and comparative indices.
Perform selective polishing.
Review treatment goals with patient.
Schedule with Dr. Smith for re-evaluation.
Establish recall interval.

---

of pain, or medical or physical limitations of the patient, to name just a few. All aspects of the patient's care must be considered in choosing which area to begin treatment.

The periodontal patient requires a follow-up visit to evaluate the response of the tissues to the scaling and debridement procedures. This appointment is often called the "tissue check," "re-evaluation," or "1-month evaluation." Tissue healing and the patient's progress toward effective plaque control can be observed and evaluated at this juncture. The appropriate interval for periodontal maintenance can then be determined by the dental hygienist. In many practices, the follow-up visit is the logical and convenient time for the periodontist or dentist to examine the patient and initiate the next step in the total treatment plan.

A term used by some dental hygienists is the "dental hygiene process of care."[18] This term is defined as an organized systematic group of activities that provides the framework for delivering quality dental hygiene care.[19] Using this definition, the components of dental hygiene care are divided into five categories: assessment, diagnosis, planning, implementation, and evaluation. The emphasis of treatment is on the process aspects, that actions are continuously moving toward maintaining or restoring dental health. In this system, diagnosis and prognosis fit into the second step, and treatment planning is in the third.

The sample dental hygiene treatment plans (Dental Hygiene Treatment Plan Phase I Therapy: Periodontal Practice and Phase IV Therapy: General Practice) provided are examples for determining care in particular cases. These sample treatment plans, presented by case type, are intended to show the individuality of each treatment plan in the application to clinical practice.

The diagnosis, prognosis, and treatment plan are based on the knowledge, clinical judgment, and evidence from research that the dental hygienist assimilates and applies to each case. This

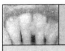

DENTAL HYGIENE TREATMENT PLAN PHASE IV THERAPY: GENERAL PRACTICE

Mr. Coffield is a 52-year-old white man who has recently completed treatment with a periodontist in the southern part of the state. He is new to the area and to the practice of Dr. Mills. He was referred to Dr. Mills by a colleague. Mr. Coffield is AAP case type III. He has a history of rheumatic fever and is interested in his general and dental health. He was not pleased about having periodontal surgery and performs a complicated regimen of oral cleaning twice a day in order to avoid further surgery. The dental hygienist is the first person in the office to see and treat Mr. Coffield.

Treatment 1
Take medical and dental history.
Evaluate need for premedication and consult with MD.
Reappoint for care.
Discuss possibility of referral to periodontist with Dr. Mills.

Treatment 2
Review medical and dental history.
Confirm antibiotic medication.
Review radiographs from previous dentist.
Take vital signs and baseline indices.
Assess plaque control status and fluoride needs.
Determine treatment plan and goals.
Provide appropriate home care instructions and education.
Scale and perform periodontal debridement of the full mouth in order to minimize the number of appointments requiring antibiotic premedication.
Schedule with Dr. Mills for examination and evaluation.

Treatment 3 (1-Month Evaluation)
Review medical history.
Confirm antibiotic premedication.
Evaluate previous scaling and periodontal debridement results.
Review home care.
Consider referral to a periodontist.
Establish recall interval.

information, cost considerations, and patient preferences comprise the decision-making process that takes place in periodontal therapy. Making rational treatment decisions is a process that is receiving increased attention from the dental research community because of the need and desire to assure high quality dental care.[20] The treatment plan is the guideline for the management of comprehensive care and is an essential part of successful therapy for every dental patient.

STUDY QUESTIONS

MULTIPLE CHOICE

1. Which phase of treatment describes the procedures designed to control or eliminate the etiologic factors of disease?

   a. Preliminary phase
   b. Phase I therapy
   c. Phase II therapy
   d. Phase III therapy
   e. Phase IV therapy

2. Which phase of treatment describes the procedures for restoration or replacement of teeth?

   a. Preliminary phase
   b. Phase I therapy
   c. Phase II therapy
   d. Phase III therapy
   e. Phase IV therapy

3. The goals of treatment planning are to eliminate and control factors of disease and to prevent recurrence of disease. The dental hygienist can use treatment planning as an opportunity to explain problems to patients in understandable terms.

   a. Both statements are TRUE.
   b. Both statements are FALSE.
   c. The first statement is TRUE, the second is FALSE.
   d. The first statement is FALSE, the second is TRUE.

4. All of the following factors influence the number and length of treatment visits for dental hygiene care EXCEPT one. Which one is the EXCEPTION?

   a. amount of calculus
   b. severity of periodontal pockets
   c. weight of patient
   d. willingness of patient to cooperate

5. The term describing the basis of the legal relationship between the health care provider and the patient is:

   a. prognosis
   b. treatment plan
   c. informed consent
   d. phase of therapy

6. All of the following factors influence the number and length of treatment visits for dental hygiene care EXCEPT one. Which one is the EXCEPTION?

   a. number of teeth present
   b. amount of supragingival calculus
   c. amount of subgingival calculus
   d. age of patient
   e. furcation involvement

7. An appropriate treatment plan includes consideration of the wishes of the patient. The dental hygienist decides on the treatment plan then informs the patient of the extent of disease.

   a. Both statements are TRUE.
   b. Both statements are FALSE.
   c. The first statement is TRUE, the second is FALSE.
   d. The first statement is FALSE, the second is TRUE.

8. The treatment plan is a guideline for the management of comprehensive care. The treatment plan is essential for every periodontal patient.

   a. Both statements are TRUE.
   b. Both statements are FALSE.
   c. The first statement is TRUE, the second is FALSE.
   d. The first statement is FALSE, the second is TRUE.

9. The phase of treatment that addresses any periodontal emergency is called the

   a. Preliminary phase.
   b. Phase I.
   c. Phase II.
   d. Phase III.
   e. Phase IV.

10. The elements of informed consent include all of the following factors EXCEPT one. Which one is the EXCEPTION?

    a. risks and benefits
    b. implied consent
    c. prognosis if treatment is performed
    d. prognosis if treatment is not performed

SHORT ANSWER

11. What are the two goals of treatment planning?

    _____

    _____

12. What factors might influence the role of the dental hygienist in treatment planning?

    _____

    _____

13. List the factors that are considered in making an overall prognosis for a periodontal patient.

    _____

    _____

14. What are the categories of prognosis?

_____

_____

15. List the variables that are related to making decisions about the degree of difficulty in providing periodontal debridement.

_____

_____

REFERENCES

1. Carranza FA Jr., Newman MG. Clinical Periodontology 8th ed. Philadelphia: WB Saunders, 1996.
2. Wilkins EM. Clinical Practice of the Dental Hygienist, 7th ed. Philadelphia: Lea & Febiger, 1994.
3. American Academy of Periodontology. Parameters of care. Chicago: American Academy of Periodontology, 1995.
4. Coleman GC. Dental treatment planning. In Principles of Oral Diagnosis. St. Louis: CV Mosby, 1993.
5. American Academy of Periodontology. Proceedings of the World Workshop in Periodontics. Chicago: American Academy of Periodontology, 1989.
6. Woodall IR, Wiles C. Formulating a treatment plan, case presentation and appointment plan. In Comprehensive Dental Hygiene Care, 4th ed. St. Louis: CV Mosby, 1993:371-390.
7. Ramfjord SP, Ash MM. Periodontology and Periodontics: Modern Theory and Practice. St. Louis: Ishiyaku EuroAmerica, 1989.
8. Schluger S, Yuodelis R, Page R, Johnson RH. Periodontal Disease, 2nd Ed. Philadelphia: Lea & Febiger, 1990.
9. Fedi P Jr. The Periodontic Syllabus, 2nd ed. Philadelphia: Lea & Febiger, 1989.
10. Knowles JW, Burgett FG, Nissle RR, Shick RA, Morrison EC, Ramfjord SP. Results of periodontal treatment related to pocket depth and attachment level: eight years. J Periodontol 1979;50:225-233.
11. DeVore CH, Beck FM, Horton JE. Plaque score changes based primarily on patient performance at specific time intervals. J Peridontol 1990;61:343-346.
12. Weikel D, McLeran H, Barnard S. Modifications of dental hygiene care for patients with special needs. In Comprehensive Dental Hygiene Care, 4th ed. St. Louis: CV Mosby, 1993:391-424.
13. O'Hehir TE. Gross scaling: an antiquated concept. Dent Hyg News 1993;7:19-20.
14. Mongardini C, van Steenberghe D, Dekeyser C, Quirymen M. One stage full- versus partial-mouth disinfection in the treatment of chronic adult or generalized early-onset periodontitis. I. Long-term clinical observations. J Periodontol 1999;70:632-645.
15. Quirymen M., Mongardini C, Pauwels M, Bollen CML, van Eldere J, van Steenberghe D. One stage full- versus partial-mouth disinfection in the treatment of chronic adult or generalized early-onset periodontitis. II. Long-term impact on microbial load. J Periodontol 1999;70:646-656.
16. Karch JD. Diagnosis and management of the periodontal patient. In Risk Management Series. Chicago: American Dental Association, 1986.
17. Schoen MA. A quality assessment system: the search for validity. J Dent Edu 1989; 53:658-61.
18. Mueller-Joseph L., Peterson M. Dental Hygiene Process: Diagnoses and Care Planning. Albany: Delmar Publishing, 1995.
19. Wilkins EM. Clinical Practice of the Dental Hygienist, 8th ed. Philadelphia: Lippincott Williams & Wilkins, 1999.
20. Matthews DC. Decision making in periodontics: a review of outcome measures. J Dent Educ 1994;58:641-649.

11

Dorothy A. Perry / Phyllis L. Beemsterboer

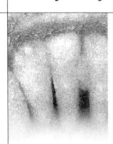

Plaque Control for the Periodontal Patient

*C*hapter *O*bjectives

1. List the goals for plaque control with the periodontal patient.
2. Describe the role of plaque as an etiologic agent in gingival and periodontal diseases.
3. Compare and contrast the mechanisms used for the mechanical and chemical removal of plaque.
4. Understand the role of motivation in compliance and non-compliance of patients in plaque control programs.

*K*ey *T*erms

Anticalculus agents
Bacterial plaque
Bass tooth brushing method
Charters tooth brushing method
Dental floss
Dr. Charles C. Bass
Interdental brushes
Patient motivation
Permeability
Plaque control

Powered tooth brushing
Roll tooth brushing method
Rubber-tip stimulators
Scrub tooth brushing method
Stillman tooth brushing method
Subgingival irrigation
Supragingival irrigation
Substantivity
Toothpicks
Toxicity

The most important and fundamental role of the dental hygienist in periodontal therapy is the education of the patient. Success in this role permits patients to become knowledgeable about their disease and make lifestyle changes that will help them lead healthier lives. It is essential to incorporate individualized **plaque control** into periodontal therapy because dental plaque is the causative agent of gingival and periodontal diseases. Conscientious, daily supragingival plaque removal inhibits the formation of subgingival plaque and the progression of these diseases. In combination with regular calculus removal, adequate plaque control removes a source of infection from the body and facilitates the lifelong maintenance of the natural teeth.

PLAQUE AS AN ETIOLOGIC AGENT

A number of classic studies provide evidence of the importance of supragingival plaque control. Löe and colleagues[1] showed the cause and effect relationship between the accumulation of **bacterial plaque** and the development of gingivitis in adults within 21 days. The gingivitis was reversible within a period of 7 days when proper plaque control was initiated. Supragingival plaque appeared to be responsible for the development of a subgingival flora associated with periodontal disease.[2] Thorough toothbrushing to remove supragingival plaque limited subgingival plaque growth in monkeys.[3] Further, adequate supragingival plaque control incorporated into periodontal maintenance programs limited periodontal attachment loss in adults.[4] Figure 11-1 shows the effects of plaque accumulation related to gingival inflammation.

GOALS OF PLAQUE CONTROL FOR THE PERIODONTAL PATIENT

The goals of plaque control are numerous. The dental hygienist must understand each goal to develop a successful plaque control program for every periodontal patient. The goals include maintenance of gingival and periodontal health, caries control, patient responsibility, managing the complexity of plaque control, and **patient motivation**.

Maintenance of Gingival and Periodontal Health

Gingival and periodontal health, once restored through therapeutic efforts, however complex, cannot be maintained without the participation and cooperation of the patient in performing daily supragingival plaque removal. An oral environment that is free of inflammation because of good plaque control rarely becomes reinfected.[5]

Caries Control

A good plaque control program provides all aspects of prevention for the patient. Proper oral hygiene to control gingival inflammation is important, but the prevention of dental caries is also significant for the periodontal patient (Figure 11-2). Root caries is a great threat to survival of the teeth when attachment loss and recession expose the roots to the oral environment. Teeth that could be maintained for years by treating the periodontal disease can be lost in weeks or months as a result of caries on the root surfaces or in furcation areas. For a full discussion of root caries, see Chapter 15.

Patient Responsibility

The plaque control program helps to place responsibility for long-term maintenance of the teeth in the hands of the patient. The dental hygienist and dentist play integral roles in therapy and maintenance, but the plaque control program places the responsibility for continued oral health directly on the daily participation of the patient. The dental hygienist has the opportunity to individualize the plaque control program, modify it over time, and present it as a way for the patient to control the long-range outcome of therapy.

Complexity of Plaque Control for the Periodontal Patient

Plaque control for periodontal patients usually involves far more than simple toothbrushing and dental flossing (Figure 11-3). Significant areas of attachment loss are often associated with disease, sometimes as a result of surgery to reduce probe depth. Attachment loss results in exposure of tortuous root anatomy that patients must learn to clean mechanically. This situation is often complicated by deep probing depths.

Periodontal plaque control requires the dental hygienist to use both knowledge and imagination to find the appropriate plaque control aids for each patient. Describing a favorite brushing technique and encouraging the use of floss will not suffice. The range of aids must be explored, including chemotherapeutic agents, to find a workable combination for the patient.

Often, some trial and error is required to address the periodontal patient's problems. Some aids work better for some people than others, some require more dexterity, and some require more patience. The dental hygienist may ask the patient to try a variety of devices and agents before agreement is reached on the

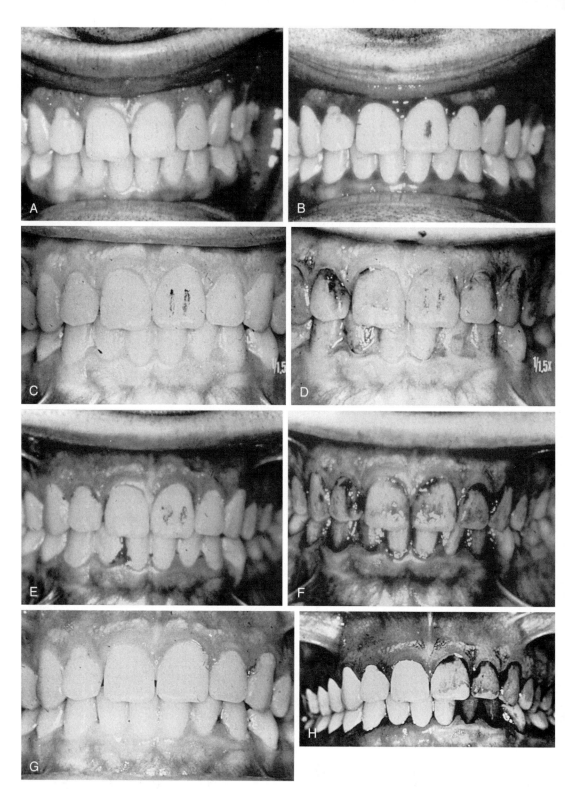

FIGURE 11-1. Experimental gingivitis in humans. **A.** Day 1: Healthy gingiva with pink tissue that conforms to the architecture of the teeth. **B.** Day 1: Healthy gingiva disclosed to show good plaque control (day numbers are marked on central incisor). **C.** Day 11. Gingiva after 11 days with no plaque control. Note the rolled margins and reddened marginal gingiva. **D.** Day 11: Disclosed plaque accumulation. **E.** Day 21: Heavy plaque accumulation and gingival swelling; the tissue bleeds upon gentle probing. **F.** Day 21: Disclosed plaque accumulation. **G.** Day 28: Plaque control was instituted on the right side of the mouth on day 21. Note the improved tissue health after seven days of plaque removal. Gingival redness has disappeared and the tissue conforms to the architecture of the teeth. **H.** Day 28: Disclosed dentition showing heavy plaque accumulation remains on the left side of the mouth.

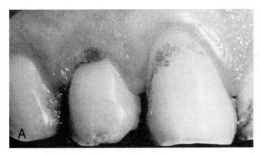
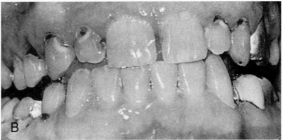

FIGURE 11–2. Root caries. **A.** A single lesion in an area of recession on the maxillary 1st bicuspid. The area on the cuspid is stained but not soft. **B.** Extensive root caries lesions. (Courtesy of W. Stephen Eakle DDS, UCSF School of Dentistry.)

best ones to adopt. For some patients, multiple sessions are needed to master techniques on their unique periodontal architecture.

The importance of developing an effective plaque control program is a primary responsibility of the dental hygienist. Dental hygiene treatment, however challenging technically, is not complete without it. With an appropriate plaque control program, the dental hygienist, as a teacher, transfers a significant portion of oral health care and control back to the periodontal patient.

Periodontal Patient Motivation

Perhaps the most challenging aspect of plaque control for the periodontal patient is motivation to initiate and continue a lifelong process of improved daily plaque control. Most of the patients have had poor plaque control that has contributed to the disease process. The habits of a lifetime are hard to change, and new oral hygiene procedures will likely require a greater investment in time, from 15 minutes to one-half hour per day. The dental hygienist must

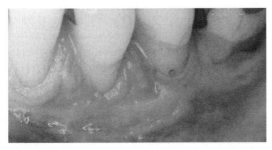

FIGURE 11–3. Significant attachment loss resulting from periodontal disease creates complex plaque control problems. Often, tooth brushing and flossing are not sufficient for plaque control. In this case additional interproximal cleaning devices and caries control measures are required.

educate, motivate, and encourage each patient to adopt the recommended procedures, then reinforce the behavior changes as time passes.

MECHANICAL PLAQUE REMOVAL

The most widely accepted prevention methods in periodontology involve personal and professional mechanical oral hygiene measures.[6] Over the centuries, the rationale for cleaning the teeth has changed from cosmetic intent to disease prevention.[7] However, the patient's concern about maintaining a pleasing appearance should not be underestimated. In today's health-conscious society, the cosmetic appeal of white teeth and fresh breath are powerful influences on the behavior of the public. There is ample evidence of this appeal in the quantity of cosmetic advertising that is seen.

Mechanical plaque removal incorporates chemotherapeutic agents as adjuncts to the physical removal of plaque. However, chemical agents alone are not sufficient to remove plaque and control disease. Standard tools are toothbrushes augmented by a variety of devices that permit access to hard-to-reach areas. The following section describes tooth brushing and other techniques for removing plaque.

Tooth Brushing

The toothbrush is the most widely accepted and adopted tool for cleaning the teeth. It is the modern version of the African twig or chew stick, a frayed branch used for mechanical cleansing. There is evidence of toothbrushes in China as early as 1000 AD, but the device did not receive wide distribution until the late 18th century. The first brushes were made of hog bristle, often with bone or ivory handles. The Victorians created elaborate handles, including many made of silver. Consequently, early toothbrushes were expensive and were often used by the entire family.[7]

In the 1930s, when nylon-bristle brushes were introduced, toothbrushes became affordable for everyone. The legacy of the Victorian era was that most brushes sold were stiff-bristled, like the old hog-bristled brushes, until the 1960s. Stiff-bristled brushes removed plaque, but were associated with trauma to the tooth structure and gingiva.[8] Because of the work of pioneers such as Arnim, Bass, and Barclay, soft-bristled toothbrushes used with a defined plaque removal technique have become the standard.[7]

Dr. Charles C. Bass[9] proposed the optimum characteristics of toothbrushes. He studied bristle stiffness, scratching of the gingiva in humans and animals, gingival puncturing, bristle trim, and the presentation of bristles on the brush head. His recommendations are summarized. See Characteristics of the Ideal Toothbrush.

A review of tooth brushing behavior suggests that most of the American population brushes once each day, with the frequency increasing to twice per day as people get older. In addition, people brush because they believe that they are reducing the incidence of decay. They are not necessarily aware of the beneficial gingival health effects of plaque removal by the toothbrush. Interestingly, most people spend less than 1 minute brushing, concentrate on the upper teeth and buccal surfaces, and brush less on the lingual surfaces and lower teeth.[10] An important point for dental hygienists is that effective brushers were most often taught brushing techniques in a dental office.[10] Awareness of the association between good plaque control through brushing and better gingival health may be increasing because of the extensive media advertising about gingivitis. However, the evidence reinforces the importance of teaching good brushing techniques to dental patients and emphasizing the reasons for doing the job well.

Since Bass's time, many brushes have been designed. Very complex bristle designs, many with handle modification, have been marketed. Manufacturers claim superiority in one aspect of cleaning or another but always related to plaque removal alone, rather than improvements in gingival health. Minor variations in plaque removal due to brush design have not been shown to lead to clinically significant differences in gingival health. One toothbrush may work better than another in the hands of the patient, but there is no evidence to demonstrate that one toothbrush design is superior to others.[11]

TOOTH BRUSHING METHODS

There are several specific tooth brushing techniques. The popularity of various techniques has waxed and waned over the 20th century. The **scrub** technique is probably the oldest. It merely applies a name to the typical uninstructed action of brushers. The **Charters** and **Stillman** techniques for gingival massage were popular in the 1930s, and the **roll** technique was most commonly recommended in the 1960s. **Bass** described what is probably the most popular method taught today, and his theories were popularized in the 1970s.

No one method of brushing has been found superior to the others.[12] The Charters and Stillman methods are primarily of historical interest because they are far less likely to remove plaque from the gingival sulcus area. The best method is the one that suits the individual's needs and abilities, and the responsibility of the dental hygienist is to instruct the patient as to how to perform the task thoroughly.

SCRUB

The scrub method is the simplest brushing technique, consisting of merely placing the bristles next to the teeth and moving them back and forth, or scrubbing. Nearly anyone, includ-

CHARACTERISTICS OF THE IDEAL TOOTHBRUSH	
Handle	Straight, 6 inches long, $7/16$ inches wide
Head	3 evenly spaced rows with 6 tufts each
Bristles	80 nylon bristles per tuft, 0.007 inches in diameter, $13/32$ inches long
Trim	Rounded finish

ing children, can become adept at this technique. However, people who brush vigorously may believe that they have done a thorough job, even if many areas of plaque have been missed. Extremely vigorous scrubbing, especially with a stiff-bristled brush, can lead to gingival trauma and recession.

ROLL

The roll technique is taught by explaining that the teeth should be brushed the way they grow, down on the upper teeth and up on the lower teeth. Bristles are placed next to the gingiva, then the handle of the toothbrush is turned to stroke the bristles across the sides of the teeth. This action is repeated five times in each location until all of the teeth are brushed. The technique requires a fair amount of concentration to apply the brush to each place along both arches of the teeth and sufficient dexterity to "roll" the brush on the buccal and lingual surfaces. In addition, the rolling strokes must be performed slowly so that the gingival one-third of the teeth will be adequately cleaned.[13]

CHARTERS

The Charters technique requires placement of the brush at a 45° angle to the tooth surface, with the bristle ends pointing away from the gingiva, but toward the interproximal surfaces of the teeth. The bristles rest on the gums. Pressure is applied to force the bristles between the teeth, and slight rotary movement is initiated. Then the brush is lifted from the gingiva and replaced in the same spot, repeating the massage three or four times. Essentially, the bristles are repeatedly pressed against the gingival margin, then lifted away in order to massage the gums and increase blood flow. The bristles are also pressed into the occlusal surfaces using a slight rotary motion so that they fit into the pits and fissures. Charters also recommended the use of metal picks or **toothpicks** for interproximal stimulation. **Dental floss** was to be used only to remove fibrous food caught between faulty contacts.[14]

Although the rationale for massage may be unproven, the effectiveness of the Charters method for plaque removal was validated by at least one clinical study. The study subjects were instructed to use the technique, and its effectiveness in removing all plaque was verified by a dental hygienist every day over the 6-week study period. In this case, the subjects used

interdental wood sticks, rather than metal picks, to ensure interdental cleaning.[15]

STILLMAN

Stillman also advocated toothbrush massage by describing a technique reputed to fill the gingival blood vessels with oxygenated blood. His technique required placement of the bristles pointing apically, but not at right angles to the gingiva, to minimize puncture. Pressure is placed on the bristles causing them to flex and the tissue to blanch. Then the pressure is released. The procedure is repeated for all teeth in all areas of the mouth while the brush is rinsed several times with a salt water and sodium bicarbonate solution.[16] This technique may result in plaque removal, although its effectiveness at plaque removal around the gingival margin is questionable.

BASS

Bass described his technique in relation to the goal of tooth brushing, which is plaque removal. He designed a method aimed at gingival and crevicular cleaning (Figure 11-4) and described it as "applying the ends of the bristles to the areas with firm pressure and moving the brush back and forth ('vibratory motion') with short strokes, thereby dislodging soft material by the digging action of the ends of the bristles wherever they can be applied."[17] The bristles of a soft, multitufted toothbrush are placed at a 45° angle to the long axis of the teeth. The vibratory motion is used to force the bristles into the sulci and between the teeth as effectively as possible. The lingual surfaces of the anterior teeth are brushed with the heel of the

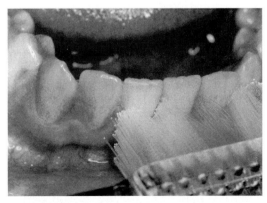

FIGURE 11-4. Toothbrush in place using the Bass technique with bristles placed at a 45° angle to the gingival margin, concentrating on the gingival third of the tooth.

toothbrush, and all other areas are brushed with the length of the brush head. The occlusal surfaces are brushed with controlled back-and-forth motions. The Bass technique has been described as "modified" by the addition of the rolling stroke. This modified stroke is supposed to lift debris away from the gingiva. In practice, clinicians and patients often start with a vibratory motion as described by Bass, but then modify it in unique ways, such as bigger strokes or circular strokes.

POWERED TOOTH BRUSHING

Powered, or electric, toothbrushes are popular and useful devices. Many people prefer **powered tooth brushing** or find it easier to use, particularly if they have any dexterity problems. Powered tooth brushes are as effective as manual brushing for reducing plaque, gingivitis, and bleeding.[18]

Powered toothbrushes have different types of actions. The head portion of the brush can be vibrating, oscillating, rotary, counter-rotary, or have a sonic vibration feature. All have been shown to be effective when used correctly.[19, 20, 21] Studies comparing powered toothbrushes to manual brushes over two- to four-month intervals have demonstrated greater reductions in inflammation and plaque for the powered brushes.[6] These studies are all relatively short-term clinical trials. It can only be assumed that long-term effectiveness is similar to manual brushing, because of these results and a record of success in clinical practice. There are no long-term studies evaluating the multiple parameters that would provide irrefutable evidence; however, it is clear that powered toothbrushes have a place in the armamentarium of the dental hygienist.

There is also a rotary electric toothbrush. It has shaped tips and can readily be applied to both the gingival margin and the interproximal areas. It is as effective in plaque removal and gingivitis reduction as conventional tooth brushing, flossing, and toothpick use for periodontal maintenance patients.[22]

RECOMMENDATIONS

The Bass technique of brushing is probably the technique that is most accepted by the dental profession today, whether for periodontal patients or for patients who have no periodontal disease. The vibratory, back-and-forth motion of

the bristles into the sulcus permits the greatest cleaning potential and applies the rationale for brushing to the mechanical action. The technique is adaptable enough so that even the complex architecture of severely periodontally damaged dentitions can be cleaned. In addition, patients can be taught to maneuver the brush around the proximal surfaces of abutment teeth, where long root surfaces and heavy plaque accumulation are common.

Strict adherence to one ideal brushing procedure is not recommended. The best brushing technique for the individual patient must be created with the knowledge of what works in ideal situations and what difficulties the individual patient faces. An individualized plaque control program often starts with a simple brushing method, such as the Bass method, with the toothbrush bristles aimed directly at the plaque on the gingival third of the teeth and into the sulcus. Then the technique should be modified by the dental hygienist to permit cleaning of all accessible areas of the teeth.

Powered toothbrushes are useful and can be reasonable substitutes for patients who have difficulty brushing or simply prefer powered toothbrushes. Periodontal patients have demonstrated marked decreases in plaque scores when their manual toothbrushes were replaced with powered toothbrushes. The improvements lasted over the three-year period of the study.[23] Powered toothbrushes should be considered for plaque control in periodontal patients and adopted, if appropriate, for the individualized plaque control program.

Interproximal Cleaning with Mechanical Aids

Toothbrushes do not clean interproximally in most cases. For this reason, interdental cleaning with at least one additional device is necessary for thorough plaque removal. Several studies have documented that the addition of daily flossing to a tooth brushing regimen leads to reductions in inflammation, plaque, and calculus deposits.[24, 25, 26]

Many interproximal cleaning aids are available. Some provide better access to long exposed root surfaces than others. Each should be evaluated for use in the individualized plaque control program.

DENTAL FLOSS

Dental floss is available in a variety of sizes and thicknesses. Waxed, unwaxed, round, flat, thick, thin, tape, red, green, shred-resistant, and fuzzy versions are available, to name a few. When properly used, it can clean the interproximal surfaces of the teeth, extending under the gingival margin, often to the junctional epithelium, where a toothbrush cannot reach. However, it is likely to miss plaque in root surface grooves and furcations.

Bass evaluated and was the first to define an optimum dental floss. His ideal characteristics included that it be made of nylon because of uniformity and strength of fibers, that it be unwaxed to prevent waxy buildup on tooth surfaces, and that it be thin and multifilamented, with few twists per inch.[27] Subsequent research has shown that there is little, if any, difference between the myriad types of floss in cleaning ability.[12] In addition, wax, as Bass first demonstrated, can be deposited on tooth surfaces in vitro, but in a study of wax deposition on teeth scheduled for extraction, no wax residue could be found.[28] This finding suggests that dental hygienists and patients should choose a particular floss based on personal preference and ease of use.

Proper flossing technique (Figure 11-5) requires that a piece of floss about 18 inches long be grasped firmly with both hands. A small portion is pinched off by the thumbs and forefingers for control. Then the floss is inserted into the proximal space by working it back and forth, slipped under the papilla by wrapping it around the tooth, and used with up-and-down strokes to clean the surface. After that, the floss must be wrapped around the adjacent tooth and the cleaning procedure repeated. After one or two interproximal surfaces are cleaned, the floss often becomes dirty or frayed. Then the patient must move along the piece of floss, grasping it in a different place, so that a fresh length of the strand can be used to clean the next surface. Dental floss is not reusable, so after all of the surfaces are cleaned, the floss strand is thrown away.

Floss Threaders. Dental floss can be used to clean under the pontics of fixed bridges, and around abutment teeth, when it is threaded under the soldered joints of fixed restorations. Threading is accomplished with a needle-like device called a floss threader or bridge threader. The floss is threaded through the eye of the device and then inserted under the contact area of the bridge. The floss is then used to clean around the abutment teeth, using standard back-and-forth motions, and under the pontic, with up-and-down or back-and-forth motions. The floss is pulled out to the side. This task can be difficult for patients to master.

FLOSS TOOLS OR AIDS

Many patients have a difficult time learning to floss correctly. It is difficult to hold the floss, gain access to the proximal surfaces, and clean the surfaces, particularly when the patients are looking at a reversed image in the mirror. In many cases, the hardest part is holding and manipulating the floss. Floss tools can help with this problem. There are two types of tools: those that are reusable and require the patient to wrap the floss around the device and single-use disposable tools with prestrung floss.

Reusable floss tools have C-shaped or U-shaped working ends. The floss is stretched across the device, and the plastic handle is inserted in the mouth, instead of the fingers, to manipulate the floss. The C-shaped ends often work better in the anterior areas, and the U-shaped ends work better in the posterior areas. Once the floss tool is threaded, it is inserted interproximally, and the cleaning procedure is the same as for finger flossing.

The advantage of floss tools is that they can improve access. However, there are some drawbacks. It can be difficult to wind the floss onto the handle so that it is taut. Floss usually must be threaded around buttons and grooves on the device. Sometimes winding the floss is as difficult as learning to floss with the fingers. In

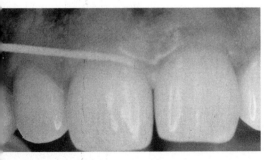

FIGURE 11-5. Dental floss must be wrapped around the tooth and slipped subgingivally for interproximal access. It cleans thoroughly between the teeth when no attachment loss is present.

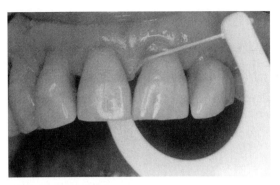

FIGURE 11–6. Disposable floss tools are convenient for some periodontal patients and make it possible to floss.

addition, when using floss on a cleaning tool, it is harder to move the floss to obtain a fresh piece when it becomes frayed or dirty. The patient must unwind and then rewind floss more than once, perhaps many times, to floss all of the teeth. Also there is no way to use the floss tool under a fixed bridge, so some other device is required to clean these areas. These disadvantages of the floss tool make it less attractive than it first appears. Its proper use is usually more time consuming than finger flossing.

Disposable floss tools (Figure 11-6) eliminate the problems of threading and winding floss onto a handle. The floss is stretched on the working end of the tool in the manufacturing process. The handles are small and may be hard to grasp, and it often takes more than one tool to floss all of the teeth. These tools work as well for patients as finger flossing.[29] They are convenient for travel and for use by children.

OTHER FLOSSING MATERIALS

Other materials can be used for flossing besides commercial dental floss. Black recommended passing a thread between the teeth.[7] Thread is inexpensive, but thin and easily broken. However, thicker materials, such as yarn or gauze, can be very useful. These materials can be used like dental floss to clean large interproximal spaces and around abutment teeth. They are thicker than floss, so they may clean large spaces faster and be easier to grasp. In addition, their texture may permit better access into developmental grooves.

INTERDENTAL BRUSHES

Interdental brushes facilitate the mechanical cleaning of proximal root surfaces, including access into the developmental grooves. They are useful devices for periodontal patients who have attachment loss, long exposed root surfaces, and complex root architecture to clean.

Interdental brush systems usually include a reusable handle and a disposable brush tip. The tip is inserted in the end of the handle, secured at a 90° angle to the handle, and used to brush interproximally in spaces that are large enough to permit access. An in-and-out brushing stroke is used, and the interproximal space should be cleaned from both the buccal and lingual aspects. Furcation areas may also be large and accessible enough to permit brushing with this device. The brush may be rinsed and reused in the same patient's mouth, but brush tips tend to wear out quickly. Often periodontal patients must replace the brush tips at least once each week with regular use, and some patients complain about the cost (Figure 11-7). Patients sometimes prefer interproximal brushes to floss[30] and it may not be necessary to floss in areas that are accessible to the interproximal brush.

In addition to the reusable handle system, there are disposable interproximal brushes. These are used with the same technique and discarded when the brush tips wear out. These disposable brushes add to the patient's cost, but are convenient for travel and use by children.

TOOTHPICKS

Toothpicks are a popular interdental cleaning aid. Many dental patients use them to remove large food particles wedged between the teeth, even if use is sporadic. They are a fixture in society and are available in many public areas,

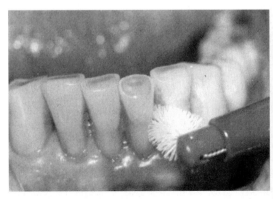

FIGURE 11–7. The interdental brush thoroughly cleans large interdental spaces and complex, exposed interproximal root surfaces.

especially restaurants. To take advantage of the popularity of this device, the dental hygienist must educate the patient to use toothpicks for plaque removal in an organized way, not just sporadic picking. Toothpicks are less effective than floss for interproximal cleaning, possibly because of difficult access on lingual surfaces. The use of a toothpick with a handle for access was shown in at least one clinical study to be as effective as dental flossing.[12]

Toothpick handles permit the mounting of one or two toothpick tips, several millimeters long, onto a handle. Some handles have curved or bent necks intended to improve access to the posterior teeth. The technique (Figure 11-8) is to affix the toothpick ends on the handle, then apply the tip to the gingival margin and trace around the necks of the teeth. The handle can permit the tip to slip into furcation areas, subgingival root surfaces, and developmental grooves to rub plaque off. The tip can also be directed subgingivally into periodontal pockets, where plaque can be dispersed. Some practitioners recommend soaking the tip before use to soften it so that it frays slightly and covers more surface area.

There are also specially designed triangular toothpicks made of a soft wood, such as balsa. These can be placed with the base of the triangle on the gingiva and pushed in and out of large proximal spaces. They provide good plaque removal on the buccal surfaces, but are difficult to apply to the lingual surfaces and the more posterior teeth. These devices are of less use to periodontal patients because of their access limitations. They cannot be used with handles to improve access.

Plastic Picks. A variety of plastic tooth-pick-like devices are available. These devices provide some combination of positive attributes, depending on the design. Instruction on their use should be predicated on educating the patient about plaque removal. They are used like toothpicks and may be convenient for patients to carry in a pocket or purse. They can be rinsed and reused rather than thrown away like wooden picks. This feature may be attractive to some individuals.

RUBBER-TIP STIMULATORS

Interdental stimulation, commonly called gingival massage, was a popular concept in plaque control until the 1970s. Massage was thought to increase keratinization, clean the surface of the gingiva, stimulate blood flow, and squeeze fluid from the gingival sulcus. Indeed, manipulation of the interdental tissues with tools, such as rubber-tip stimulators or toothpicks, increases keratinization of the epithelium in treated areas. However, the use of these instruments also results in plaque removal from the surfaces of the teeth.[12] As the current concept of plaque control evolved, the emphasis was placed on plaque removal rather than tissue effect, and it is understood that inflammation starts in the sulcus, not on the keratinized surface of the gingiva. This knowledge suggests that tools used to stimulate the interproximal tissue are useful because of their plaque-removing effects.

Rubber-tip stimulators are convenient, inexpensive devices that can be useful to periodontal patients. The tip is a conical piece of firm rubber or plastic that is several millimeters long. The tip is placed proximally, resting the side of the cone on the gingiva, and worked in a small circular motion. All interdental spaces should be cleaned from both the buccal and lingual surfaces. In addition to this technique, the rubber tip may be adapted and applied to the gingival margins of the teeth, traced along the gumline like a toothpick in a holder as described earlier (Figure 11-9).

RECOMMENDATIONS

The periodontal patient must be educated to perform total plaque control. Cleaning around all surfaces of all teeth must be the premise from which tools and techniques are recommended.

The dental hygienist often begins with tooth

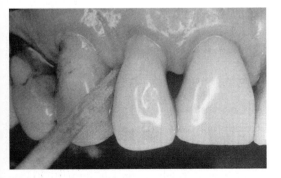

FIGURE 11-8. Toothpicks can also be used for plaque control to access complex root architecture and subgingival areas.

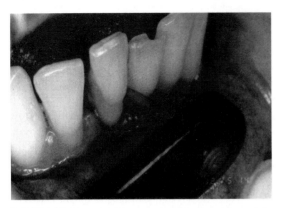

FIGURE 11–9. The rubber-tip stimulator can be used for interproximal plaque removal by periodontal patients, but the role of stimulation of the gingiva has not been identified.

brushing, which is a daily lifetime habit for most patients. Instruction may involve teaching a new technique or modifying an existing one to ensure maximal cleaning efficiency.

Interproximal cleaning must be emphasized from the beginning, but some experimentation may be required to find the best tool or combination of tools. In addition, the dental hygienist often teaches interproximal plaque control to periodontal patients before surgical treatment. When periodontal surgery is performed, the architecture is changed, sometimes dramatically, resulting in different needs for cleaning. The dental hygienist must assume that teaching plaque control to periodontal patients is a dynamic process that may require more than one tool and more than one instruction session.

For patients who have never flossed, refuse to floss, or are beginning interproximal cleaning, the rubber-tip stimulator can be useful. It is easy to use and inexpensive. Additionally, these stimulators are present on the handles of some toothbrushes, so the patient does not have to keep track of new devices or find them at the store. For these reasons, it can be a good tool to begin the process of educating the patient to clean the proximal surfaces.

Dental floss is a good tool for periodontal patients, but it is rarely the only interproximal aid needed. Even in cases of mild attachment loss, the exposed proximal root anatomy has developmental grooves that the floss glides over, leaving masses of attached plaque. The situation is more complicated with the maxillary molars, where furcations are present on the mesial and distal surfaces. Regular dental

flossing is also a difficult habit to acquire. Studies indicate that although approximately 40 percent of Americans report using floss, only 10 percent floss daily and another 10 percent floss once or twice a week.[10] Although floss is a significant oral hygiene tool, it is not the only tool, nor is it always the best tool for the periodontal patient.

Interproximal brushes in various sizes and configurations have the distinct advantage of cleaning the complex architecture on root surfaces. They can clean around abutment teeth and under fixed bridges. The brushes must be replaced often, so patients must have a source to buy replacements and must be committed to the expenditure. It is also difficult for some patients to load the brush onto the handle because it requires threading a thin wire into a small hole and securing it. Any physical impairment, such as arthritic finger joints, makes this process difficult. Also patients often must be reminded to wear their eyeglasses to see the operation better. Disposable interproximal brushes provide an alternative in these cases.

The importance of mechanical plaque control is to individualize the recommendations to meet the needs and abilities of each periodontal patient. A rote presentation of the dental hygienist's favorite tooth brushing technique and interproximal aid will not address the variety of needs and periodontal conditions seen in clinical practice. Individualization is the key to increased compliance and success in plaque control.

Irrigation

In the 1960s irrigation of the oral cavity as an adjunct to plaque control became popular with the marketing of pulsating jet irrigators. These devices force water between the teeth using a single jet of pulsed beads of water or multiple, fractionated jets of pulsed beads of water. The devices did not reduce plaque formation and had a minimal effect on gingivitis scores in a clinical study of 155 college-age women. However, they did reduce calculus formation.[31] In fact, another study reported that only 8.1 percent of stainable material was removed from the mouths of 10 experimental subjects by water jet irrigation alone. An additional 67.6 percent was removed by tooth brushing.[32]

More recent studies, reviewed by Ciancio,[33]

relating to water jet irrigation, have shown significant decreases in gingivitis when used in a regular plaque control regimen at home. Significant results were seen in studies of varying duration, from 6 weeks to 6 months. Improved gingival health was noted regardless of whether a chemical plaque control agent was used during the irrigation. Gingivitis reductions in the range of 25 percent were noted, and some studies showed comparable results to the beneficial effects of rinsing with the antimicrobial agent chlorhexidine. **Supragingival irrigation** with chlorhexidine showed some additional benefit. Plaque scores were not always reduced by irrigation, corroborating the results of the earlier work reported above. Cianco[33] suggested that although the mass of plaque may be minimally affected by irrigation, its toxicity may be altered, explaining the beneficial effects of oral supragingival irrigation.

The technique for supragingival irrigation (Figure 11-10) is to direct the irrigator tip between the teeth at right angles to the interdental papillae and hold it there for several seconds to permit flushing of the proximal surfaces. Then the tip is moved along the gingival margin to the next proximal area. The pressure setting on the irrigator may be gradually increased if the tissue condition permits.[34] This procedure should be performed in a bathroom while the individual leans over the sink to avoid creating a mess with dripping water. Oral irrigation is associated with bacteremia, occurring in as many as 50 percent of patients with periodontitis. However, the relationship of bacteremia

caused by oral irrigation to infective endocarditis is not known.[34] If there is any question, the patient's physician should be consulted about the use of daily home oral irrigation. Generally speaking, patients who need antibiotic coverage for dental treatment and those with acute conditions, such as pericoronitis, should not use supragingival irrigation.

RECOMMENDATIONS

The preponderance of data suggests that supragingival oral irrigation is an acceptable tool to be recommended by the dental hygienist in plaque control programs for periodontal patients because it reduces gingivitis. It is especially useful for patients who cannot or will not adopt mechanical devices for interproximal cleaning. In addition, as the evidence detailing the use of irrigation for the delivery of antimicrobial agents grows, irrigators may become more significant in periodontal plaque control. The use of oral irrigation as a delivery vehicle for chemical plaque control is covered in the next section.

CHEMICAL PLAQUE CONTROL

Chemical plaque control has increased in popularity and importance in recent years as studies have shown the positive effects of various medicaments on the oral environment. A variety of over-the-counter and prescription agents are available for dental patients. These agents have known, if variable, abilities to control the growth or regrowth of bacterial plaque. No longer are mouthwashes thought to be only cosmetic. Some of these agents can provide significant advantages to periodontal patients, who often have complex gingival architecture that is time consuming and difficult to clean solely with mechanical devices.

Chemical antiplaque agents should possess several properties.[35]

1. **Antiplaque action**. This activity can be bactericidal or bacteristatic (affecting the functioning of the cells to render them less virulent by affecting bacterial adhesion, growth, or metabolism).

2. **Substantivity**. This property is the ability of the substance to adhere to structures in the oral environment and be released

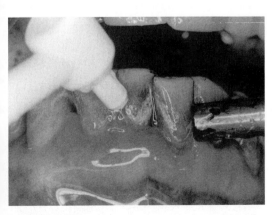

FIGURE 11-10. A water jet irrigator tip in place for supragingival irrigation. This tip is pointed at a 45° angle to the marginal gingiva (a high-volume suction tip appears on the right and was used to facilitate the photography).

slowly over time, enhancing the duration of effectiveness. The bacterial population in the mouth recovers rapidly from the assault of many antibacterial substances because they are rapidly cleared. Substantive agents, such as chlorhexidine digluconate, possess positively charged ions that adhere to the predominantly negatively charged tissues in the mouth for several hours. They remain in the mouth to exert a continued effect on plaque bacteria.

3. **Low toxicity and non-irritating**. Agents must be nontoxic to tissues because they must adhere for a substantial period. Low toxicity allows them to extend their effects on the bacterial population without damaging host tissues.

4. **Low permeability**. The oral mucosal tissue is easily permeated by chemicals. For this reason, users of drugs such as smokeless tobacco and cocaine ingest the drugs through this route. An effective antiplaque agent must have low permeability to allow its retention in the oral cavity.

Agents available on the market are primarily toothpastes and mouthwashes. Most are over-the-counter products, but some are prescription items. Generally, these products are for daily use in the home. However, irrigation of tissues in the dental office is being performed, and research on its effectiveness continues.

Chlorhexidine

The most effective antibacterial agent available today is chlorhexidine, sold by prescription in the United States as a mouthwash containing 0.12 percent of the active ingredient, chlorhexidine digluconate. This agent reduces plaque and gingivitis in humans.[36, 37] Extensive reviews of clinical studies of the effectiveness of chlorhexidine are presented in the Proceedings of the World Workshop in Clinical Periodontics in 1989[38] and again in 1996.[6] These indicated that plaque and gingivitis are reduced by 60 percent in short-term studies, and by 55 percent and 45 percent, respectively, in separate long-term studies. Chlorhexidine is highly substantive, not being cleared from the mouth for several hours. It acts by altering the bacterial cell wall and interfering with the adsorption of bacteria to

teeth. In addition, no changes in the composition of bacteria or the resistance of organisms to this substance has been shown.[39]

Chlorhexidine is now available as a gelatin chip with sustained release (see Chapter 7). In some parts of the world, it is also found in toothpastes and in a spray delivery system. However, the most common use in the U.S. is as a mouthrinse.

A number of side effects have been reported with the use of chlorhexidine mouthwash. Dark brown staining of the teeth (Figure 11–11) and increased supragingival calculus formation are common. Some patients experience a reversible desquamation of the oral tissue. In addition, poor taste and altered taste sensation are common. The mouthwash contains 11.6 percent alcohol, so patients who are sensitive about using products containing alcohol should be warned.[6, 38]

The dental hygienist should recommend the use of chlorhexidine as a mouth rinse, full strength (0.12 percent), twice per day for 30 seconds using 15 ml of the rinse. The concentration of chlorhexidine mouthwash available in the United States is 0.12 percent, less than the 0.2 percent formulations used in Europe. Research has verified that the 0.12 percent chlorhexidine rinse marketed in the United States is comparable to the European product that has been used for many years.[40] Long-term use does no harm other than the cosmetic inconvenience of staining and some reported taste alteration.

Chlorhexidine also reduces gingivitis when used in a 1:1 dilution with water (0.06 percent)

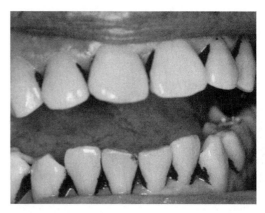

FIGURE 11–11. Chlorhexidine stain in a periodontal patient. The dark stain has accumulated in all of the proximal areas.

in an oral irrigator, for supragingival irrigation, once per day.[41] There are also specially designed tips that have been shown to permit subgingival access better than the standard tip used for supragingival irrigation.[34] Compared with rinsing with chlorhexidine according to the recommended regimen, delivery through the irrigation device enhanced the plaque and gingivitis reductions by a small amount. The researchers speculated that the use of the irrigator may enhance the penetration of the drug beneath the inflamed gingival margin. The side effects of staining and calculus formation occurred with both rinsing and irrigation.[42] The daily use of a chlorhexidine solution or water in a home irrigator for subgingival application appears to have a benefit for periodontal maintenance patients. However, the consensus report from the World Workshop in Periodontics in 1996 stated that professional subgingival irrigation has no clear substantial long-term benefits in the treatment of periodontal patients.[6] Additional research into various delivery methods is needed to confirm the short- and long-term effects of subgingival irrigation with antimicrobial agents.[43]

Periodontal patients who benefit from the use of chlorhexidine mouthwash are those who cannot or will not control supragingival plaque through mechanical means. In addition, refractory cases and patients who have had periodontal surgery may be helped by chemical plaque control. The dental hygienist, in conjunction with the dentist or periodontist, should recommend the use of chlorhexidine based on an assessment of the needs of the individual patient. Chlorhexidine at 0.12 percent strength has been tested extensively and has been accepted by the American Dental Association as effective for the control of gingivitis.[44]

Essential Oil Mouthwash (Phenolic Compounds)

Mouthwashes containing essential oils, thymol, eucalyptol, menthol, and methyl-salicylate reduce plaque and gingivitis by about 30 percent. These phenolic compounds probably work by altering the bacterial cell wall.[33] These products contain a substantial percentage of alcohol, up to 26.4 percent, have a strong flavor, and can cause staining. They are available over the counter, which can be advantageous for patients. They are also less costly than chlorhexidine mouthwash. One product has been on the market for many years and carries the American Dental Association seal verifying that 6-month studies show that it is effective in reducing gingivitis.[45] In addition, it is a popular product with many individuals. This product provides a reasonable alternative to chlorhexidine for patients who would benefit from chemical plaque control to augment their mechanical efforts. It has also been shown to be effective in helping patients who have undergone periodontal surgery to maintain plaque control during the healing phase.[46] However, there are reported side effects. Some patients report a burning sensation and bitter taste.[33]

Triclosan, another phenolic compound has recently become available in the U.S. The product is available without prescription and has shown promising results as an antiplaque and antigingivitis agent, especially when combined with other agents. Triclosan toothpastes with either zinc citrate or a copolymer of methoxyethylene and maleic acid as the active agent have been shown in numerous studies to reduce plaque and gingivitis. Research continues in this area to further evaluate the mode of delivery and long-term effects on periodontal disease.[6, 47]

Quaternary Ammonium Compounds

Cetylpyridinium chloride, a quaternary ammonium compound, is the active ingredient in two commonly available mouthwashes. In addition, some preparations contain the ingredient domiphen bromide. These products reduced gingivitis in a number of very short-term clinical studies. Their mechanism of action is probably the ability to increase bacterial cell wall permeability, decrease cell metabolism, and reduce cell attachment to tooth surfaces.[33] Quaternary ammonium compounds have not been accepted by the American Dental Association because their ability to reduce gingivitis has not been adequately documented in long-term or short-term studies.

Stannous Fluoride

Stannous fluoride has been used extensively in dentistry for its caries-inhibiting effects. Reports in the 1970s and 1980s strongly suggested the possibility that stannous fluoride possessed anti-plaque properties. As reviewed by Tinanoff,[48] stannous fluoride alters bacterial cell metabolism and cell adhesion properties in addition to reacting with tooth surfaces for caries prevention. Clinical studies have shown delayed microbial repopulation of periodontal pockets in some cases, but these data have not been confirmed. Stannous fluoride gel has shown antigingivitis effects in extremely inflamed tissue around abutment teeth and orthodontic bands. This substance does have anticaries activity and, when used on a daily basis, may have an additional benefit for periodontal health. The usual strength for daily home use is 0.4 percent stannous fluoride delivered in gel or toothpaste form. Some of the available products carry the American Dental Association seal for caries control. None has demonstrated antigingivitis effects of sufficient quantity or duration to carry an additional seal for gingivitis effects. Tooth staining (Figure 11-12) is a common side effect of this product, and some patients complain of poor taste. The value of stannous fluoride in reducing caries cannot be extrapolated to the prevention of gingivitis or periodontitis.[6] But the evidence does suggest a potential benefit warranting further investigation.

Sanguinarine

Sanguinarine is a plant alkaloid derived from the bloodroot plant and chemically termed benzophenathradine. It is available in toothpaste and oral rinse forms. Sanguinarine has shown some plaque and gingivitis reduction in short-term studies, but mixed results in long-term studies. Only one long-term study has shown significant clinical improvements in gingival health. That study included a regimen using both the paste and the rinse in orthodontic subjects. The mechanism of action of sanguinarine may be to alter bacterial cell wall structure to interfere with adhesion.[38] The product does not carry the American Dental Association seal and is not preferable to other agents.

THE PROBLEM OF DELIVERY TO THE SITE OF DISEASE

The most meticulous supragingival plaque control does not remove plaque in pockets deeper than a few millimeters.[49] Subgingival plaque control is a goal to be desired, but not easily achieved. It is accomplished by the dental hygienist during scaling and root planing, but the pathologic plaque bacteria begin to grow back quickly. The patient is also limited in achieving subgingival plaque control because mechanical oral hygiene devices may not reach into pocket depths or may be impossible to apply into pockets. For these reasons, the notion of lavage, flushing or irrigating the periodontal pockets to remove plaque, especially using an antimicrobial agent, is attractive. This procedure could place the antimicrobial agent directly into the site of infection rather than limiting it to supragingival areas.

Subgingival Irrigation

Subgingival irrigation has been evaluated in a variety of circumstances. It has been delivered by powered oral irrigation devices and by blunt needles and syringe systems (Figure 11-13). A number of agents and regimens have been tested. Results are promising, but inconclusive. Subgingival irrigation can be viewed as an office procedure performed by the dental hygienist at treatment visits, an at-home procedure performed daily by patients, or as a combination of the two.

According to Greenstein,[50] several aspects of irrigation must be considered. These include penetration of drugs into the pockets, relationship to scaling and root planing, and safety.

Irrigation with a syringe fitted with a blunt needle[51] and powered oral irrigation devices[50] have been shown to penetrate into periodontal pockets. Not all data show penetration to the base of deep pockets, but it appears that agents reach at least 3 mm subgingivally. Therefore, it

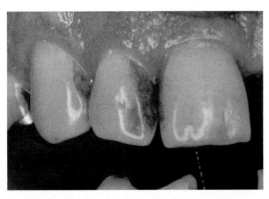

FIGURE 11-12. Stannous fluoride stain in this periodontal patient appears diffuse and less dark than chlorhexidine stain.

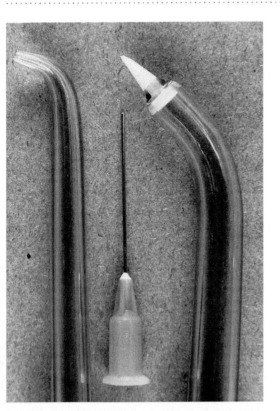

FIGURE 11–13. A selection of available irrigation tips. The cannula (center) should be used only for subgingival irrigation in the dental office.

is possible to deliver antimicrobial agents subgingivally, at least well into the pocket, if not to the base. When treated with antimicrobial subgingival irrigation, bacterial populations rebound quickly unless the treatment is preceded by scaling and root planing.[50] This observation suggests that scaling and debridement of pockets are essential for the maximum therapeutic effect of irrigation. Lastly, negative effects of subgingival irrigation, such as self-inflicted wounds, microbial infections in the tissues, and resistant strains, have not been reported. Subgingival irrigation appears to be a safe procedure.[50] However, there is no one agent that is recommended for subgingival irrigation. Chlorhexidine has been studied the most extensively, but it has neither United States Food and Drug Administration approval nor American Dental Association recommendation for use as an irrigant.[52]

OFFICE-APPLIED AGENTS

Antimicrobial agents can be applied by the dental hygienist in the office during or after scaling and root planing procedures. This procedure is commonly done with a disposable syringe fitted with a blunt needle or an irrigating pump device with a thin canula. It can also be accomplished by running an antimicrobial irrigant through the ultrasonic tip during scaling.[53] In a review of studies of irrigation after scaling and root planing, Shiloah and Hovious[52] affirmed that the scaling removed most of the attached and unattached bacterial plaque. They pointed out that many attempts to improve the results by altering the bacterial plaque immediately after scaling with a variety of antimicrobial agents did not yield significant results. Greenstein reached the same conclusion in describing the relationship between scaling and antimicrobial irrigation.[50] There is general agreement that routinely following scaling procedures with irrigation in the dental office is of questionable benefit, but is not harmful.[49, 50]

HOME-APPLIED AGENTS

In contrast to irrigation in the dental office, irrigation during maintenance intervals, performed at home by the patient, has demonstrated positive effects on gingival health. Irrigation using a powered irrigating device has been shown to reduce the number of bleeding sites and the amount of gingivitis over a 6-month period.[42] In this study, irrigation with water achieved almost as good a result as irrigation with dilute chlorhexidine, and both were better than conventional mechanical oral hygiene procedures.[42] Another study tested home irrigation with dilute iodine and found improved gingival health after 8 weeks compared with a no-irrigation control group.[54] This study also included lavage in the dental office after scaling and root planing, so it was not possible to determine the specific effects of home irrigation. However, the preponderance of evidence suggests that daily lavage has a greater effect than antimicrobial treatment immediately after scaling.

Home irrigation with or without antimicrobial agents has been shown to improve periodontal health by reducing gingivitis scores. It is a safe procedure and benefits patients with gingivitis and those on periodontal maintenance.[49] However, there is insufficient evidence to suggest that irrigation alters the pathogenic plaque or increases recall intervals.

Anticalculus Agents

A number of toothpastes are available that have **anticalculus agents** that are active ingredients.

They inhibit the formation of new supragingival calculus. These are commonly referred to as tartar control toothpastes. The active ingredients are the soluble pyrophosphates that inhibit amorphous calcium phosphate around the teeth from crystallizing into hydroxyapatite, the most common crystal in calculus. In addition, toothpastes containing zinc citrate retard calculus formation. Clinical studies show approximately 20 to 40 percent reductions in supragingival calculus formation when anticalculus toothpastes are used. A small percentage of patients experience sloughing of the epithelium with the use of these products, in which case the products should be discontinued.

One study of pyrophosphate-containing toothpaste reported a 25.9 percent reduction in supragingival calculus formation on six lower anterior teeth for a study population of 217 subjects over 2 months. In addition, the number of sites with calculus formation was 25.5 percent lower with the use of the pyrophosphate paste.[55] A similar study evaluating all measurable teeth, not just the mandibular anteriors, showed a 32.4 percent reduction in supragingival calculus formation and a 32.1 percent reduction in the number of sites of calculus after 6 months.[56]

Zinc citrate-containing dentifrice has also been evaluated in clinical studies. Its mechanisms of action are less well understood, but may be related to the plaque-inhibiting action of zinc or some inhibition of crystallization. One study of 187 subjects followed for 6 months compared zinc citrate with pyrophosphate-containing dentifrice and a regular fluoride toothpaste. The zinc citrate dentifrice reduced new supragingival calculus formation by 32.3 percent and the pyrophosphate paste reduced it by 21.4 percent compared with the control toothpaste.[57]

One study reported the relative effectiveness of three formulations of calculus control dentifrices: zinc citrate, pyrophosphate, and pyrophosphate with an additional ingredient. The calculus index for the six anterior teeth of 112 subjects decreased from 8.8, 8.9, and 9.2, respectively, to 3.1, 3.2, and 5.0, respectively at 6 months.[58] The subjects all had a dental prophylaxis after the initial examination, so the 6-month scores represented new calculus formation, not reduction of existing calculus. All

products showed significant reduction from baseline levels.

Although supragingival calculus reduction has desirable cosmetic benefits for many patients, the health benefits to periodontal patients have not been established. Plaque is the etiologic agent in periodontal diseases; supragingival calculus may only represent inconvenience to patients and hard work to the dental hygienist. For these reasons, it is important to control its rate of formation. Calculus is associated with plaque on its porous surface, and it can make plaque control more difficult to perform. However, reduction in calculus deposition rates should not be considered a substitute for the health benefits of good plaque control.

PATIENT MOTIVATION

Motivating and changing patient behavior to institute and continue appropriate oral hygiene procedures is a major challenge in dental hygiene practice. These knowledge and behavioral changes begin with education provided to patients by the dental hygienist. Many theories and strategies have been tried in practice. In the 1970s and 1980s multiple-appointment education sessions were recommended as a possible improvement on the traditional chairside teaching provided by the dental hygienist. Two studies compared variations on these teaching strategies. Five 30-minute sessions over 14 days were compared with two 60-minute presentations of the same oral hygiene educational materials. Subjects who participated in both groups had significantly reduced plaque during 48 months of maintenance care, suggesting that five lessons provided no more benefits than two.[59] In addition, three teaching sessions were compared with one session plus two reinforcement follow-up visits. Both strategies significantly reduced plaque over a 2-year observation period; no one method was superior.[60] It is interesting to note the results of another study of patients who received oral health education from dental hygienists. These patients retained more knowledge about self-care and were better motivated than those who had never visited a dental hygienist.[61]

Clearly, the teaching of oral hygiene to achieve plaque reduction can be done in a vari-

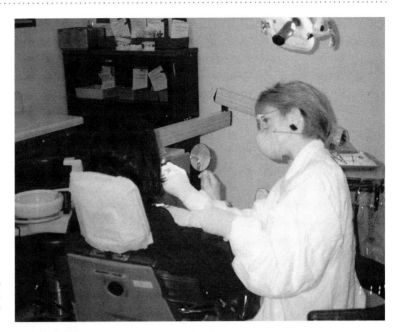

FIGURE 11–14. The dental hygienist teaching plaque control is critical to the success of periodontal therapy.

ety of ways. In addition, the dental hygienist has an important role in achieving these goals. You will determine your preferences and develop a successful style that is unique and knowledge-based so that your patients receive the maximum benefit from your professional care.

The Role of Reinforcement and Long-term Rapport

In a comparison of the Bass and roll brushing techniques, Gibson and Wade[62] expressed their disappointment at the poor performances of the subjects who were taught either technique. They emphasized the importance of the dental hygienist teaching and reinforcing good brushing techniques to promote changes in individuals' long-standing habits. Instruction given once

or twice in the experimental setting was not enough to achieve more than 50 percent plaque removal. This observation may well be true for plaque control in general.

No matter how great the potential for plaque removal with all of the techniques and devices described here, the dental hygienist plays a key role. Dental hygienists are educated to promote oral hygiene. Several studies have shown that the hygienist can provide these services at less cost than the dentist while maintaining a high quality of health care.[63] The responsibility of the dental hygienist to assess the individual periodontal patient's needs and educate, motivate, and customize the process is essential for successful periodontal therapy. The knowledge, patience, and time spent on this endeavor will help to restore periodontal patients to health and empower them to maintain it (Figure 11–14).

STUDY QUESTIONS

MULTIPLE CHOICE

1. The goals of a plaque control program for the periodontal patient include all of the following EXCEPT one. Which one is the EXCEPTION?

    a. maintenance of gingival and periodontal health
    b. caries control
    c. five lessons on plaque control
    d. patient responsibility
    e. patient motivation

2. Plaque control for periodontal patients includes tooth brushing and the use of dental floss.
   In areas where an interproximal brush can be used, it is not necessary to floss.

    a. Both statements are TRUE.
    b. Both statements are FALSE.
    c. The first statement is TRUE, and the second is FALSE.
    d. The first statement is FALSE, and the second is TRUE.

3. The tooth brushing method most modified and accepted by the dental profession for periodontal patients is the:

    a. Bass method
    b. Charters method
    c. Scrub method
    d. Stillman method

4. The percentage of Americans who floss on a daily basis is:

    a. about 6%
    b. about 10%
    c. about 25%
    d. about 50%

5. What is the name of the property of chemical anti-plaque agents allowing them to adhere to oral structures over time?

    a. toxicity
    b. antiplaque action
    c. permeability
    d. substantivity

6. Supragingival oral irrigation performed by patients at home on a daily basis can be expected to reduce gingivitis by about what amount?

    a. 10%
    b. 25%
    c. 50%
    d. 100%

7. Extensive tooth staining has been reported with which of the following products?

    a. chlorhexidine mouthrinse
    b. cosmetic mouthrinse
    c. quaternary ammonium mouthrinse
    d. sanguinarine mouthrinse

8. Subgingival irrigation of antimicrobial agents applied by the dental hygienist after scaling and root planing enhances tissue healing.
   Subgingival irrigation of antimicrobial agents applied by the dental hygienist after scaling and root planing has no demonstrated detrimental effects.

    a. Both statements are TRUE.
    b. Both statements are FALSE.
    c. The first statement is TRUE, and the second is FALSE.
    d. The first statement is FALSE, and the second is TRUE.

9. Phenolic compound mouthrinses work by altering bacterial cell walls.
   Phenolic compound mouthrinses reduce gingivitis approximately as much as quaternary ammonium products.

    a. Both statements are TRUE.
    b. Both statements are FALSE.
    c. The first statement is TRUE, and the second is FALSE.
    d. The first statement is FALSE, and the second is TRUE.

10. Clinical studies with anticalculus toothpastes have shown reduction in supragingival calculus in the range of:

    a. 5% to 10%
    b. 10% to 20%
    c. 20% to 40%
    d. 40% to 60%

SHORT ANSWER

11. Describe the main goals of plaque control.

    _____

    _____

12. What are the criteria for the selection of a specific brand of dental floss?

    _____

    _____

13. How does chlorhexidine work as an effective oral antibacterial agent?

    _____

    _____

14. What is the major challenge in establishing personal plaque control programs in dental hygiene practice?

_____

_____

15. Why is root caries a problem for the periodontal patient?

_____

_____

REFERENCES

1. Löe H, Theilade E, Jensen SE. Experimental gingivitis in man. J Periodontol 1965;36:177-187.
2. Kornman K. The role of antimicrobials in the prevention and treatment of periodontal disease. In American Academy of Periodontology: Perspectives on Oral Antimicrobial Therapeutics. Littleton, MA: PSG Publishing, 1987:37-46.
3. Waerhaug J. Effect of toothbrushing on subgingival plaque formation. J Periodontol 1981;52:30-34.
4. Axelsson P, Lindhe J. Effect of controlled oral hygiene procedures on caries and periodontal disease in adults. J Clin Periodontol 1978;5:133-151.
5. Caffesse RG. Maintenance therapy. Genco R, Goldman H, Cohen DW, eds. In Contemporary Periodontics. St. Louis: CV Mosby, 1990:483-492.
6. Hancock EB. Prevention. Ann Periodontol 1996;1:223-249.
7. Mandel ID. Why pick on teeth. J Am Dent Assoc 1990;121:129-132.
8. Niemi ML, Sandholm L, Ainamo J. Frequency of gingival lesions after standardized brushing as related to stiffness of toothbrush and abrasiveness of dentifrice. J Clin Periodontol 1984;11:254-261.
9. Bass CC. The optimum characteristics of toothbrushes for personal oral hygiene. Dent Items Interest 1948;70:697-719.
10. Gift HC. Current utilization patterns of oral hygiene practices: state-of-the-science review. In Löe H, Kleinman DV, eds. Dental Plaque Control Measures and Oral Hygiene Practices. Washington, DC: IRL Press, 1986:39-71.
11. Jepsen, S. The role of manual toothbrushes in effective plaque control: advantages and limitations. In: Lang, NP, Attstrom R, and Löe H, eds. Proceedings of the European Workshop on Mechanical Plaque Control. Carol Stream, IL: Quintessence Publishing Co. Inc., 1998:121-137.
12. Frandsen A. Mechanical oral hygiene practices: state-of-the-science review. In Löe H, Kleinman DV, eds. Dental Plaque Control Measures and Oral Hygiene Practices. Washington, DC: IRL Press, 1986:93-116.
13. Wilkins EM. Oral infections control: toothbrushes and toothbrushing. In Clinical Practice of the Dental Hygienist, 8th ed. Philadelphia: Lea & Febiger, 1999: 350-369.
14. Charters WJ. Eliminating mouth infections with the toothbrush and other stimulating instruments. Dent Digest 1932;38:130-136.
15. Lang NP, Cumming BR, Löe H. Toothbrushing frequency as it relates to plaque development and gingival health. J Periodontol 1973;44:396-405.
16. Stillman PR. A philosophy of treatment of periodontal disease. Dent Digest 1932;38:315-319.
17. Bass CC. An effective method of personal oral hygiene. J LA State Med Soc 1954;106:100-112.
18. Walsh M, Heckman B, Leggott P, Armitage G, Robertson PB. Comparison of manual and power toothbrushing, with and without adjunctive oral irrigation, for controlling plaque and gingivitis. J Clin Periodontol 1989;16:419-427.
19. Van der Weijden GA, Canser MM, Nijboer A, Timmerman MF, Van der Velden U. The plaque-removing efficacy of an oscillating/rotating toothbrush. J Clin Periodontol 1993;20:273-278.
20. Ciancio SG, Mather ML. A clinical comparison of two electric toothbrushes with different mechanical actions. Clin Preventive Dent 1990;12:216-219.
21. Van der Weijden GA, Timmerman MF, Nijboer A, Lie MA, Van der Velden U. A comparative study of electric toothbrushes for the effectiveness of plaque removal in relation to toothbrushing duration. J Clin Periodontol 1993;20:476-481.
22. Boyd RL, Murray P, Robertson PB. Effect on periodontal status of rotary electric toothbrushes vs. manual toothbrushes during peridontal maintenance: I. Clinical results. J Periodontol 1989;60:390-395.
23. Van der Weijden GA, Timmerman MF, Danser MM, van der Velden U. The role of electric toothbrushes: advantages and limitations. In Lang NP, Attstrom R, and Löe H, eds. Proceedings of the European Workshop on Mechanical Plaque Control. Carol Stream, IL: Quintessence Publishing Co. Inc., 1998:138-155.
24. Graves RC, Disney JA, Stamm JW. Comparative effectiveness of flossing and brushing in reducing interproximal bleeding. J Periodontol 1989;60:243-247.
25. Lang WP, Farghaly MM, Ronis DL. The relation of preventive dental behaviors to periodontal health status. J Clin Periodontol 1994;21:194-198.
26. Axelsson P, Lindhe J, and Nystrom B. On the prevention of caries and periodontol disease. Results of a 15 year longitudinal study in adults. J Clin Periodontol 1991;18:182-189.
27. Bass CC. The optimum characteristics of dental floss for personal oral hygiene. Dent Items Interest 1948;70:921-934.
28. Perry DA, Pattison GA. An investigation of wax residue on tooth surfaces after the use of waxed dental floss. Dent Hyg 1986;60:16-19.
29. Spolsky VS, Perry DA, Meng Z, Kissel P. Evaluating the efficacy of a new flossing aid. J Clin Periodontol 1993;20:490-497.
30. Christou V, Timmerman MF, Van der Velden U, Van der Weijden FA. Comparison of different approaches of interdental oral hygiene: interdental brushes versus dental floss. J Periodontol 1998;69:759-764.
31. Lobene RR. The effect of a pulsed water pressure cleansing device on oral health. J Periodontol 1969;40:667-670.
32. Fine DH, Baumhammers A. Effect of water pressure irrigation on stainable material on the teeth. J Periodontol 1970;41:468-472.
33. Ciancio SG. Powered oral irrigation and control of gingivitis. Biol Ther Dent 1990;5:21-24.
34. Wilkins EM. Clinical Practice of the Dental Hygienist, 7th ed. Philadelphia: Lea & Febiger, 1994:362.
35. Cummins D, Creeth JE. Delivery of antiplaque agents from dentifrices, gels, and mouthwashes. J Dent Res 1992;71:1439-1449.
36. Marsh PD. Microbiological aspects of the chemical con-

trol of plaque and gingivitis. J Dent Res 1992;71:1431–1438.

37. Jones CG. Chlorhexidine: Is it still the gold standard? Periodontology 2000 1997;15:55–62.

38. Ciancio SG. Non-surgical periodontal treatment. In Nevins M, Becker W, Kornman K, eds. Proceedings of the World Workshop in Clinical Periodontics. Chicago: American Academy of Periodontology, 1989:II-1–II-11.

39. Briner WW, Grassman E, Buckner RY, Rebitski GF, Sox TE, Setser RE, Ebert ML. Assessment of susceptibility of plaque bacteria to chlorhexidine after six months' oral use. J Periodont Res 1986;21(suppl 16):53–59.

40. Segreto VA, Collins EM, Beiswanger BB, de la Rosa M, Isaacs RL, Land NP, Mallatt ME, Meckel AH. A comparison of mouthrinses containing two concentrations of chlorhexidine. J Periodont Res 1986;21 (suppl 16):23–32.

41. Brownstein CN, Briggs SD, Schweitzer KL, Briner WW, Kornman K. Irrigation with chlorhexidine to resolve naturally occurring gingivitis. J Clin Periodontol 1990;17:588–593.

42. Flemmig TF, Newman MG, Doherty FM, Grossman E, Menkle AH, Bakdash MB. Supragingival irrigation with 0.06% chlorhexidine in naturally occurring gingivitis: I. 6 month clinical observation. J Periodontol 1990;61:112–117.

43. Vignarajah S, Newman HN, Bulman J. Pulsated jet subgingival irrigation with a 0.1% chlorhexidine simplified oral hygiene and chronic periodontitis. J Clin Periodontol 1989;16:365–370.

44. Council on Dental Therapeutics Accepts Peridex. J Am Dent Assoc 1988;117:516–517.

45. Council on Dental Therapeutics Accepts Listerine. J Am Dent Assoc 1988;117:515–516.

46. Zambon JJ, Ciancio SG, Mather ML, Charles CH. The effect of an antimicrobial mouthrinse on early healing of gingival flap surgery wounds. J Periodontol 1989;60:31–36.

47. Scheie AA. Modes of action of currently known chemical anti-plaque agents other than chlorhexidine. J Dent Res 1989;68:1609–1616.

48. Tinanoff N. Review of the antimicrobial action of stannous fluoride. J Clin Dent 1990;2:22–26.

49. Jolkovsky DL, Ciancio SC. Antimicrobial and other chemotherapeutic agents in periodontal therapy. In: FA Carranza and MG Newman, eds. Clinical Periodontology, 8th ed. WB Saunders Co, Philadelphia 1996;511–522.

50. Greenstein G. Subgingival irrigation: an adjunct to periodontal therapy. Current status and future directions. J Dent Hyg 1990;64:389–397.

51. Hardy JH, Newman HN, Strahan JD. Direct irrigation and subgingival plaque. J Clin Periodontol 1982;9:57–65.

52. Shiloah J, Hovious A. The role of subgingival irrigations in the treatment of periodontitis. J Periodontol 1993;6:835–843.

53. Nosal G, Scheidt MJ, O'Neal RO, Van Dyke TE. The penetration of lavage solution into the periodontal pocket during ultrasonic instrumentation. J Periodontol 1991;62:554–557.

54. Wolff LF, Bakdash MB, Pihlstrom BL, Bandt CL, Aeppli DM. The effect of professional and home subgingival irrigation and antimicrobial agents on gingivitis and early periodontitis. J Dent Hyg 1989;63:222–225.

55. Mallatt ME, Beiswanger BB, Stookey GK, Swancar JR, Hennon DK. Influence of soluble pyrophosphates on calculus formation in adults. J Dent Res 1985;64:1159–1162.

56. Zacheri WA, Pfeiffer HJ, Swancar JR. The effect of soluble pyrophosphates on dental calculus in adults. J Am Dent Assoc 1985;110:737–738.

57. Kazmierczak M, Mather M, Ciancio S, Fischman S, Cancro L. A clinical evaluation of anticalculus dentifrices. J Clin Preventive Dent 1990;12:13–17.

58. Kohut BE, Rubin MA, Baron HJ. The relative clinical effectiveness of three anticalculus dentifrices. J Clin Preventive Dent 1989;11:13–16.

59. Soderhölm G, Nöbreus N, Attström R, Egelberg J. Teaching plaque control: I. A five-visit versus a two-visit program. J Clin Periodontol 1982;9:203–213.

60. Soderhölm G, Egelberg J. Teaching plaque control: II. 30-minute versus 15-minute appointments in a three-visit program. J Clin Periodontol 1982;9:214–222.

61. Uitenbröek DG, Schaub RMH, Tromp JAH, Kant JH. Dental hygienists' influence on the patients' knowledge, motivation, self-care, and perception of change. Community Dent Oral Epidemiol 1989;17:87–90.

62. Gibson JA, Wade AB. Plaque removal by the Bass and roll brushing techniques. J Periodontol 1977;48:456–459.

63. Schou, L. Behavioral aspects of dental plaque control measures: an oral health promotion perspective. In Lang NP, Attstrom R, and Löe H, eds. Proceedings of the European Workshop on Mechanical Plaque Control. Carol Stream, IL: Quintessence Publishing Co. Inc., 1998; 287–289.

12

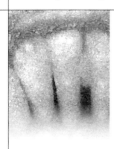

Dorothy A. Perry / Phyllis L. Beemsterboer

Nonsurgical Periodontal Therapy

*C*hapter *O*bjectives

1. Define nonsurgical periodontal therapy.
2. List the components of nonsurgical periodontal therapy.
3. Describe the short-term and long-term goals of nonsurgical periodontal therapy.
4. Identify the techniques and application for nonsurgical periodontal therapy procedures.
5. Describe the process of healing after periodontal debridement procedures, scaling, root planing, and gingival curettage.
6. Explain the limitations of calculus removal and the expectations for clinician proficiency.

*K*ey *T*erms

Coronal polishing
Dentinal hypersensitivity
Dentinal sensitivity
Gingival curettage
Hand instrumentation
Hydrodynamic theory of dentinal
  sensitivity
Irrigation
Nonsurgical periodontal therapy

Periodontal debridement
Powered instrumentation
Prophylaxis
Root planing
Scaling
Selective polishing
Sonic scaling
Specific plaque hypothesis
Ultrasonic scaling

Nonsurgical therapeutic techniques are employed by dental hygienists and dentists to treat gingival and periodontal diseases. The term nonsurgical therapy is often considered a misnomer because the procedures performed, primarily the application of sharp blades to cut tissues, are a form of surgery. However, in periodontology, the term "surgery" is usually reserved for more invasive cutting procedures (see Chapter 13). Other terms used to describe **nonsurgical periodontal therapy** include cause-related therapy,[1] Phase 1 therapy,[2] etiotropic phase,[2] and preparatory[3] or initial therapy.[2] All terms refer to the concepts described in this chapter (Figure 12-1).

219

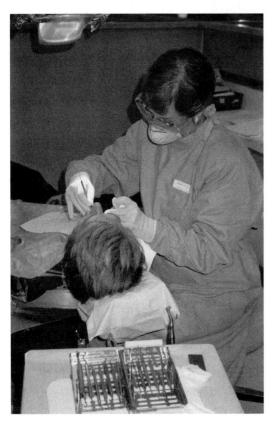

FIGURE 12–1. Dental hygienist performing nonsurgical therapy in the clinical setting.

In its broadest sense, nonsurgical therapy defines all of the procedures performed to treat gingival and periodontal diseases up to the time of re-evaluation, when the patient begins maintenance care, and the need for periodontal surgery to enhance results is determined. Nonsur-

gical therapy includes the procedures listed in Table 12-1.

The procedures described in this chapter include the technical procedures applied by dental hygienists and the instruments used during the treatment visit. These include the procedures and instruments required to debride the tooth surfaces of bacterial plaque and calculus, gingival curettage as needed, and supragingival plaque removal by selective application of polishing techniques.[4] Patient plaque control is a cornerstone of long-term successful therapy. Every patient must participate in treatment by adopting a regular and effective plaque removal regimen. Positive, long-term effects of periodontal therapy have been documented with plaque control and patient compliance (Figure 12-2).

DEFINITIONS OF NONSURGICAL PERIODONTAL THERAPIES

This chapter discusses the biologic basis and rationale for nonsurgical therapeutic procedures performed in the dental office. It describes **scaling** procedures, both **hand instrumentation and powered; root planing; gingival curettage**; and **coronal polishing**. Treatment often requires the use of pain control (Figure 12-3).

The definition of procedures must be clear and consistent. Specific definitions follow for commonly used terminology plus terms that

TABLE 12–1. Nonsurgical Periodontal Therapy Procedures

Technique	Application
Oral hygiene instruction for daily supragingival plaque control	Comprehensive, individualized, reinforced at each appointment
Calculus removal	Scaling and root planing techniques, considered part of periodontal debridement[4]
Subgingival plaque removal and identification of plaque-retentive factors	Instrumentation techniques and possibly antimicrobial chemotherapeutics, also considered part of periodontal debridement[4]; possible referral for treatment of plaque-retentive conditions
Gingival curettage	Instrumentation techniques to alter the environment of the pocket wall, if necessary
Occlusal evaluation	Identification of occlusal-related factors affecting the periodontium
Coronal polishing	Selective procedure for supragingival plaque and stain removal and cosmetic appearance

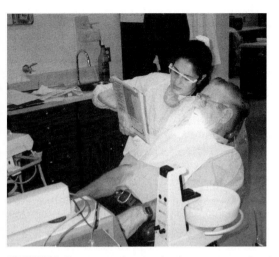

FIGURE 12–2. Patient education for the prevention of oral diseases is the most important role of the dental hygienist.

are achieving acceptance in the dental hygiene community.

Scaling

The American Academy of Periodontology (AAP) defines scaling as "instrumentation of the crown and root surfaces of the teeth to remove plaque, calculus, and stains from these surfaces."[5] However, others refer to subgingival scaling as the removal of subgingival calculus[6] or deposits.[7] Scaling is most commonly thought of as the removal of identifiable deposits of calculus. Associated plaque deposits are also removed during the procedure. The focus of the application of the instruments is to remove calculus, and success of treatment at the time

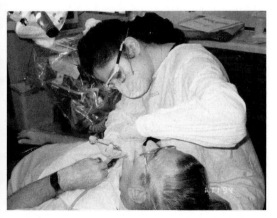

FIGURE 12–3. The dental hygienist has many patient treatment options available for nonsurgical periodontal therapy, including the use of pain control techniques.

of the therapy is determined by explorer evaluation of root smoothness.

Scaling may be accomplished with sharp hand instruments or with **sonic** or **ultrasonic scaling** instruments.

Root Planing

Root planing is defined by the AAP as "a treatment procedure designed to remove cementum or surface dentin that is rough, impregnated with calculus, or contaminated with toxins or microorganisms."[5] This procedure focuses not on identifiable deposits of calculus, but on the entire root surface associated with the periodontal pocket. The goal when root planing has traditionally been to remove the surface layer of cementum and/or dentin to create a glassy, hard surface. At that point, the dental hygienist could be confident that the treated pockets are free of deposits and contaminants on and embedded in the root surfaces. Root planing was thought to render root surfaces less prone to the re-establishment of the etiology of disease, bacterial plaque, than scaling alone. The difference between scaling and root planing is a matter of degree; root planing involves a specific effort to instrument every portion of the root surfaces, not simply identifiable calculus.

The goal of root planing, leaving the roots clean, has not changed, but the extent to which root tissue is scraped away to create a glassy, hard texture using this procedure is under scrutiny. There is no evidence that the root-planed teeth are easier to maintain or less likely to be associated with periodontal diseases than those that have been rendered simply free of calculus and plaque.

Root planing, like scaling, may be successfully performed by hand instrumentation or powered devices.

Periodontal Debridement

The term "**periodontal debridement**" has been proposed to replace the older notions of scaling and root planing. It includes supragingival debridement, subgingival debridement, and deplaquing, with a minimum of tooth structure removal.[4] This term incorporates the notion of removal of plaque, plaque retentive features, and calculus, both above and below the gingiva.

The goal of periodontal debridement is to restore the periodontium to health, not to produce glassy, hard root surfaces that are free of various deposits.

Prophylaxis

Prophylaxis, as defined by Wilkins,[3] is a preventive procedure to remove local irritants to the gingiva, including complete calculus removal followed by root planing. The procedure is also termed oral prophylaxis, dental prophylaxis, or simply, prophy. The purpose of the procedure is to assist the patient in the preservation of periodontal health. The role of root planing during prophylaxis is to render the surfaces smooth so they will be easier for the patient to clean and less likely to retain deposits. These assumptions are common,[3] but are not verified by research.[8]

Prophylaxis is basically a preventive and maintenance procedure for periodontal patients. It is usually accomplished during one appointment, and it has many facets. A comprehensive explanation of periodontal maintenance is found in Chapter 15.

Coronal Polishing

Coronal polishing is the use of polishing agents to remove stains from the teeth. It also removes supragingival plaque deposits. It is most commonly performed by rubber-cup application of polishing agents with a slow-speed handpiece. There are also air devices that polish teeth with a power-driven unit that sprays a slurry of surfaces. The polishing procedure is commonly referred to as an oral prophylaxis or a prophy, but this term is incorrect. Coronal polishing may have some esthetic value for patients and may help to motivate them to maintain a clean mouth, but it has no therapeutic value.

Stains on the teeth are generally considered harmless, so their removal is secondary to the therapeutic and preventive goals of the dental hygienist. Coronal polishing is now recommended to be performed selectively,[3] and it is no longer the ritual at the end of the dental hygiene appointment that it once was.

Selective coronal polishing, or simply **selective polishing**, is choosing the surfaces to polish on the basis of the presence of plaque and stain that cannot be removed with normal patient oral hygiene practices and that are of concern to the patient. The term selective polishing has been used since the mid 1970s when research on enamel and root surfaces after polishing revealed changes in the hard tissues. In a 30-second polishing with pumice, up to 4 microns of tooth substance may be removed; repeated frequently, as with a periodontal maintenance patient, it can have a significant effect on the tooth surface. Abrasives used with rotary polishing have been shown to scratch amalgam, composite resin, and gold restorative materials. Studies also demonstrated that plaque removal prior to the application of fluoride was not necessary because the presence of plaque does not alter the uptake of fluoride by tooth structure. Other concerns are bacteremia and heat generated by the power-driven prophylaxis angle. Wilkins, in her 4th edition of the *Clinical Practice of the Dental Hygienist* in 1976, introduced the selective polishing procedure approach and encouraged this modification in treatment.[9] She stressed the critical importance of presenting personal plaque control instruction over the polishing procedure during the patient appointment, a limited period of time. The teaching time to provide the patient with the knowledge to perform self-care is more valuable than a cosmetic procedure.

The application of selective polishing by dental hygienists has been met with reluctance, possibly because many patients expect to have the teeth polished and enjoy the clean and fresh feel and taste in the mouth after the procedure.

Gingival Curettage

Curettage has been defined by the AAP as "scraping or cleaning the walls of a cavity or surface by means of a curette."[5] It is a commonly misused term that has been applied to a variety of procedures, from removal of the pocket lining, termed closed curettage, to a surgical flap procedure, called open curettage. Specifically, curettage performed by the dental hygienist (legally permitted in some, but not all, states) is limited to closed curettage and has been defined as the removal of the inflamed soft tissue lateral to the pocket wall.[6] It is a specific attempt to remove all of the pocket lining epithelium with the curette blade or powered scaling tip placed against the soft tissue wall.

This type of curettage is separate from inadvertent curettage, which is partial, accidental, and incomplete removal of the pocket lining during scaling and root planing or periodontal debridement procedures. Subgingival curettage and flap, or open, curettage are surgical procedures. For further definition and description of these procedures, see Chapter 13.

GOALS OF NONSURGICAL PERIODONTAL THERAPY

The goals of nonsurgical periodontal therapy must be considered in terms of the immediate treatment goals at the time of the appointment and the long-term goals for the patient. At the time of treatment, during periodontal debridement procedures, the goal for the dental hygienist is to promote plaque control and to instrument the tooth surfaces until they are clean and smooth, touching all portions of the roots to disrupt plaque and remove calculus. This end point at the treatment appointment is probably best evaluated by explorer detection of a smooth surface.[8] Calculus removal may be considered a subgoal at the treatment appointment rather than its primary focus.[4] The immediate goal of treatment is not to render the roots glassy and hard through extensive planing away of tooth structure.

The long-term goal of treatment is to restore gingival health. For periodontal patients, this goal often requires multiple appointments with the dental hygienist. The restoration of gingival health is the sum of good plaque control, complete periodontal debridement, and sufficient time for healing to occur, several months for complete healing of both the epithelium and connective tissue.[8] The goals are summarized in Table 12–2.

RATIONALE FOR NONSURGICAL PERIODONTAL THERAPY

The rationale for nonsurgical periodontal therapy is to remove the etiologic agent of disease, bacterial plaque, and its associated factors. Clinical trials have consistently demonstrated that scaling and root planing reduces gingival inflammation, reduces probing depths, and results in gains of clinical attachment in most

TABLE 12–2. Goals of Nonsurgical Periodontal Therapy

Short term	Long term
Plaque control instruction and reinforcement	Appropriate daily oral hygiene procedures

Clean surfaces
  Calculus removal
  Plaque removal
	Compliance with plaque control and maintenance schedule

Evaluation:
  Plaque assessment
  Smooth surfaces
	Evaluation:
	  tissue health restored

periodontal patients.[10] There are also secondary influences on periodontal health that must be considered. Calculus, although not an etiologic agent in itself, is virtually always associated with plaque, and its removal is associated with improved periodontal health. This chapter discusses plaque and calculus removal performed by the dental hygienist because that is an important technical element of dental hygiene care. Chapter 11 discusses patient education and motivation for daily plaque control.

In addition, anatomic and iatrogenic plaque traps, such as overhanging restorations and malposed teeth, must be considered during nonsurgical therapy. Even though these features are primarily elaborate plaque control problems, the dental hygienist should recognize them, design specific plaque control measures, and refer the patient for further treatment. Replacement restorations or orthodontic movement of the teeth can simplify plaque control and help the patient to achieve periodontal health. These local factors are described in Chapter 5.

Several issues surround nonsurgical periodontal therapy. The following information is a summary of evidence supporting the provision of nonsurgical periodontal treatment. Information regarding plaque and calculus removal, the relative merit of smooth roots, removing the epithelial lining of pockets, and healing after nonsurgical treatment is presented.

Removal of Etiology

Dental hygienists remove the primary etiologic factor of periodontal disease, plaque, and its associated factors through scaling and root planing, cleaning and smoothing of the roots or, more broadly, periodontal debridement. These procedures are commonly considered demanding technical activities that require a large share of each therapeutic treatment appointment.

PLAQUE

Plaque is the primary causative agent in gingival and periodontal diseases. Animal studies provide strong evidence that these destructive diseases occur in the presence of microbes, but not in animals raised in germ-free environments. Although some periodontal destruction has been observed in germ-free (gnotobiotic) animal experiments, it tends to be localized and related to the impaction of foreign objects, such as hairs. The picture of inflammation and tissue destruction seen in conventionally raised animals with oral flora is vastly more widespread and severe.[8]

Bacteria live in the mouth and are present around diseased teeth. Convincing experimental evidence that plaque causes human gingival disease was presented by Löe and co-workers in 1965.[11] The researchers initiated extensive plaque control in a small group of dental students and brought them to a level of excellent periodontal health. Then the subjects refrained from oral hygiene procedures for 3 weeks. Within 10 to 21 days, every subject had gingivitis, which resolved in about 1 week when oral hygiene practices were resumed. In addition, the microbial composition of dental plaque changed from one of a Gram-positive flora to one dominated by Gram-negative organisms.

Animal studies, the landmark study on human experimental gingivitis, and much additional research shows that plaque removal is a goal of nonsurgical periodontal therapy. The dental hygienist cannot focus solely on calculus removal.

As the understanding of plaque as the pathologic agent has grown, various periodontal diseases have been associated with specific plaques. All plaques are no longer considered intrinsically bad. The **specific plaque hypothesis** was proposed by Loesche in the 1970s.[12] This information has helped to provide better therapy, including the use of appropriate antimicrobial agents to improve treatment results. An excellent example of the application of the specific plaque hypothesis to treatment is juvenile periodontitis. In the 1960s, this disease was recognized as different from typical periodon-

titis because the conventional therapy, which consisted of scaling and root planing in the localized affected areas of the anterior teeth and first molars, at best slowed the loss of these teeth. In the 1960s, a specific plaque bacterium, *Actinobacillus actinomycetemcomitans*, was associated with these lesions. Therefore, treatment aimed at the bacteria, conventional therapy plus the use of appropriate antibiotics, resulted in successful restoration of periodontal health with less tooth loss.

Periodontal diseases may have different bacterial origins, but similar symptoms. They will eventually be much better understood so that therapies directed toward the specific plaque in each individual can be used.[13] Greater understanding of the characteristics of individual plaques will lead to better therapies, probably including a greater use of antimicrobial agents, and dental hygienists will administer these treatments in the years to come.

Although more specific gingival and periodontal diseases are recognized, nonsurgical periodontal therapy focuses on total plaque removal. However, the current understanding is not limited to a nonspecific plaque theory, in which the amount of plaque rather than the quality of plaque is considered the causative agent in disease. Bacteria-specific tests and treatments have been developed and will be more widely used as the understanding of periodontal diseases increases. For a further description of how bacteria-specific diagnostic techniques be may applied in periodontal therapy, see Chapter 9.

It is possible to effectively remove all of the supragingival plaque. To do so, the patient employs oral hygiene procedures and the dental hygienist performs coronal polishing. However, subgingival plaque is not effectively altered by supragingival oral hygiene procedures, especially in deeper pockets of 5 mm or greater. Supragingival oral hygiene procedures have limited effects on symptoms associated with deeper pockets, such as bleeding on probing.[14]

Subgingival plaque removal is essential in nonsurgical therapy to disrupt the established colonies of bacteria and let a younger plaque develop that is less associated with pathology. Dental hygiene procedures with hand instruments and ultrasonic scalers adequately accomplish subgingival plaque removal. A study published in the 1980s compared plaque removal in pockets performed with hand instruments and ultrasonic tips. Both were effective in removing approximately 67 percent of the plaque in pockets deeper than 5 mm, and the ultrasonic instruments performed as well as the hand instruments.[15] However, laboratory methods to detect remaining plaque and calculus on instrumented root surfaces may overestimate the amount of deposit left behind. The AAP consensus report on nonsurgical periodontal therapy suggests that 11 percent plaque remaining on root surfaces after thorough instrumentation is more likely. Ultrasonic tips appear to be as effective as hand instruments in cleaning root surfaces.[16]

CALCULUS

Calculus is little more than calcified plaque. As plaque ages, the organic matrix and bacterial cells calcify. It adheres to tooth surfaces through pellicle attachment, mechanical locking, and intercrystalline forces. This material varies in crystal composition, type of attachment, and degree of difficulty in removal.[8] Although calculus is an inert substance, its role appears to be that of plaque retention, and its removal is associated with a return to periodontal health (Figure 12–4).[17]

The thoroughness of calculus removal by instrumentation has been studied and shows surprising results. Kepic and colleagues[18] showed residual calculus on most teeth after 45 to 60 minutes of treatment time per quadrant. Even when teeth were instrumented for as long as 39 minutes each, residual calculus was noted regularly in deeper pockets, and totally clean surfaces were achieved only in the 3 to 4 mm range.[19] The preponderance of evidence reviewed by Stutsman-Young[4] suggested that total calculus removal was not an achievable goal. Definitive instrumentation techniques leave some residual deposits on the teeth. However, these deposits, surely present in the subjects of long-term studies used to verify the effectiveness of periodontal treatment, do not appear to cause treatment to fail.[20]

The dental hygienist must endeavor to remove all calculus, yet must have reasonable expectations. Some residual calculus is likely to remain, especially in deeper pockets, but patients can probably tolerate some small amount. If the long-term goal of restoring periodontal health has not been achieved after conscientious nonsurgical therapy, the dental hygienist must suspect residual calculus (and plaque) and re-treat nonresponding areas. Areas in the periodontium that do not respond to therapy, even after re-treatment and evaluation, may benefit from long-term subgingival antimicrobial treatment or surgical intervention. For a description of surgical interventions in periodontal therapy, see Chapter 13.

Root Smoothness

Achieving root smoothness is important for evaluating short-term goals during treatment appointments. The dental hygienist must develop a tactile sense that permits detection of obvious calculus on the teeth. This sensitivity is useful in determining the amount of calculus present in the untreated patient, the existence of irritat-

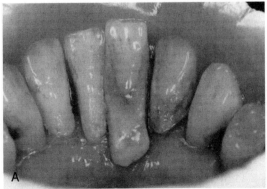 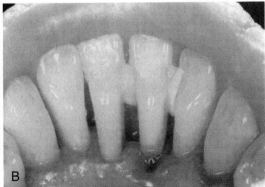

FIGURE 12–4. The effects of nonsurgical periodontal therapy. **A.** Pretreatment radiograph of a 45-year-old female with severe periodontal destruction and calculus accumulation. **B.** Periodontal healing 4 weeks after nonsurgical periodontal treatment. Note the temporary splint placed to limit mobility of teeth #24, 25 and 26.

ing factors such as overhangs, and the point at which thorough instrumentation (periodontal debridement) is finished at each appointment. Glassy, smooth root surfaces are not end points in treatment. After instrumentation, some roots feel smooth, whereas others have varying degrees of granular roughness. Experience suggests that the roots in an individual patient's mouth will all feel smooth to approximately the same degree after thorough instrumentation. This uniform smoothness should be identified. Most importantly, no surfaces should feel rough, as if calculus is still present. Plaque should be dislodged from all accessible surfaces.

Explorer-detectable root roughness may not be calculus, but merely the texture of the root. This roughness has never been shown to be harmful through quantifiable research. Armitage reviewed the reasons why dental hygienists and dentists attempt to smooth roots to a glassy, hard texture through root planing. These are: (1) Smooth surfaces are easier to clean; (2) smooth surfaces retard plaque formation; (3) rough surfaces mechanically irritate gingival tissues; and (4) smooth surfaces promote gingival healing.[8] He noted the following points:

1. Slightly rough root surfaces, those that are scaled and cleaned but not planed in a systematic way to remove cementum and leave glassy surfaces, do not accumulate plaque more rapidly than smoother surfaces. The appealing notion that rough surfaces would present more of a plaque control problem for patients is borne out by experience with obvious calculus or overhanging restorations. However, the roughness associated with calculus and poor restorations is far greater than the slightly granular texture of calculus-free root surfaces.

2. Studies evaluating plaque formation on rough root surfaces are equivocal. Early studies that used visual appraisal of deposits or colony counts on surfaces showed that smooth surfaces had less plaque formation. However, root texture was not measured. The only study that attempted to measure root texture with quantifiable Profilometer (Micrometrical Manufacturing, Ann Arbor, MI) readings found that the amount of root roughness did not affect plaque formation.

3. No experimental evidence indicates that rough root surfaces are mechanical irritants and would therefore delay healing.

4. Smooth root surfaces do not appear to promote better or faster healing than rough surfaces. In fact, in some studies, gingiva next to root surfaces that were notched for orientation of researchers after tooth extraction healed uneventfully in the mouth. This indicated that roughness itself had no effect on wound healing.

Because smooth surfaces are clinically associated with the restoration of gingival health, all clinicians believe that smooth root surfaces are good. The question is, do the root surfaces need to be glassy smooth? It appears that variation in smoothness is acceptable as long as calculus that makes surfaces feel rough and irregular has been removed and plaque disrupted.

Root roughness has been equated with incomplete instrumentation because of concerns that endotoxins (lipopolysaccarides) formed by plaque bacteria invade into the root structure. Removal of endotoxins would require the planing away of diseased cementum. This practice supports the old notion of "necrotic" root surfaces. Much has been learned about the penetration and removal of lipopolysaccaride endotoxins. Studies indicate that endotoxins do not penetrate deeply into cemental surfaces and that retained toxins are associated with missed calculus and plaque rather than diseased cementum.[4] Nyman and co-workers[21] compared the healing of quadrants after periodontal surgery. One side was treated with conventional root planing, the other with calculus carefully flicked off and the root surfaces polished before the tissue was sutured back in place. There was no difference in the healing of the differently treated areas; cementum removal through root planing did not improve healing beyond that achieved by calculus removal and polishing.

These data indicate that toxins are superficially located on root surfaces and relatively easily removed. Extensive root instrumentation is not required beyond the removal of calculus and plaque. Thus, the rationale for simple root planing, removing root roughness to achieve glassy smooth root surfaces, is no longer valid. However, the conscientious removal of calculus and plaque with minimum destruction of cementum, termed "periodontal debridement,"[4] is justified. The repeated removal of tooth structure during nonsurgical therapy appointments and subsequent maintenance visits is not a goal of therapy, and it may result in thinned and sensitive root surfaces. Dramatically thinned root surfaces are shown in Figure 12–5. This thinning is an example of overinstrumentation, or root planing without rationale.

Gingival Curettage

Gingival curettage, also called closed curettage or nonsurgical gingival curettage (truly a misnomer), has traditionally been performed to remove inflamed pocket lining for reasons distinct from periodontal debridement. Inflamed pocket lining is composed of thin, ulcerated strands of epithelium, with rete pegs extending into the underlying connective tissue and granulation tissue containing disorganized masses of cells.[2] It may also contain dislodged calculus and plaque bacteria. Removal of this tissue was traditionally assumed to enhance pocket reduction beyond the results achieved by scaling and root planing alone, providing faster healing and the formation of new connective tissue attachment to the root surfaces. This rationale has been seriously questioned in recent years.

No clinical studies have shown greater pocket reduction, more rapid healing, or greater new attachment after gingival curettage has been performed compared with scaling and root planing alone.[22, 23] In animal studies, gingival curettage promoted the formation of long junctional epithelium during healing, rather than new connective tissue attachment.[24] Clinical trials reviewed by Kalkwarf[22] indicated that tissue healed through long junctional epithelium rather than connective tissue attachment can be maintained successfully for years, suggesting that it is a satisfactory treatment result.

There appears to be little rationale for the regular use of gingival curettage in the treatment of chronic adult periodontitis. The suggested treatment indications for gingival curettage remain to be evaluated. They include attempts to form new attachment when conventional surgical techniques are not advisable, attempts to reduce non-responsive inflammation prior to other surgical efforts, and to treat persistent inflammation during periodontal maintenance, especially if pocket reduction surgery has been previously performed.[23]

It is important to note that 80 percent of dental hygiene programs in the United States teach the gingival curettage procedure. The following reasons are given: Curettage is a legally sanctioned duty in many states, it is performed by practitioners in the community, and it appears on the national board examination for dental hygiene.[25] Despite the controversies about increasing the treatment effectiveness of periodontal debridement, gingival curettage still has a place in this era of increased emphasis on nonsurgical therapies. Removal of disorganized granulation tissue and ulcerated epithelium of pocket linings remains appealing, even if data do not show faster healing. Elimination of bacteria and their products in tissues during the treatment of periodontal diseases keeps this

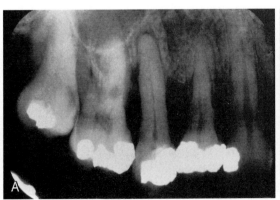
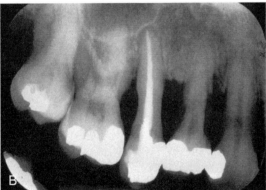

FIGURE 12–5. Radiographs of overinstrumentation of root surfaces. **A.** Pretreatment x-ray of periodontally involved posterior teeth. **B.** The same teeth 3 years later, after periodontal therapy and 11 maintenance visits. The roots have been planed to a substantially reduced dimension. This is an example of excessive root planing during the maintenance phase. (Courtesy of Thomas Bramanti, DDS, PhD.)

treatment modality viable, especially when surgical treatment is not possible. As knowledge regarding bacteria-specific periodontal diseases increases, there will be better delineation of the appropriate times to perform the procedure.

Gingival curettage is not intended to replace periodontal debridement or periodontal surgical techniques. For the dental hygienist, it is an adjunct treatment that has limited application for patients in whom nonsurgical therapeutic results must be maximized. The indications for gingival curettage are as follows[6]:

1. Inflamed anterior areas in which tissue redness and swelling persists after periodontal debridement. Every effort should be made to achieve maximum results through nonsurgical therapy in these areas. The anterior teeth generally are not amenable to surgical techniques for pocket reduction because of the negative esthetic consequences of making the teeth appear longer.
2. Attempts at pocket reduction in patients who need, but cannot tolerate, periodontal surgical procedures, such as medically compromised patients. Removal of disorganized and diseased tissue is appealing in these cases, even if evidence does not show faster healing.
3. Treatment of areas with recurrent inflammation during maintenance appointments, after active periodontal treatment has been completed. Removal of all possible sources of reinfection, including the pocket lining, is the goal. Residual calculus or other mechanical plaque traps are often the problem at these sites, so scrupulous attention to calculus and plaque removal in these areas remains the primary treatment.

Healing

Healing after scaling, root planing, and gingival curettage occurs as repair of existing tissues rather than regeneration of tissues lost in the periodontal disease process. When periodontal debridement is performed in most dentitions with infection, pocketing, bone loss, and inflamed periodontal tissues, the epithelium will heal, inflammation will be resolved, long junctional epithelial attachment may occur, and re-

cession will often result. In addition, subgingival bacterial plaque will re-form in the remaining deep pockets but, at least initially, will consist of different, less pathogenic bacteria than those associated with untreated periodontal pockets. The formation of new bone to replace bone that is lost, new connective tissue attachment to the root surface, and new cementum on the root are not predictable outcomes.

HEALING AFTER PERIODONTAL DEBRIDEMENT

Periodontal debridement causes some removal and disruption of the epithelial attachment to the tooth, junctional epithelium, and deeper connective tissue. The epithelial lining of the pocket wall is also often disrupted and partially removed (inadvertent curettage).

When the junctional epithelium has been injured or separated from the tooth surfaces, as it would be during periodontal debridement treatment, healing can be expected to take approximately 1 week. Animal studies show that hemidesmosomes begin to reattach from the apical end of the junctional epithelium and are present intact after 7 days. Normal turnover of cells in the junctional epithelium is about 5 days, so repair after disruption, not removal, of junctional epithelium occurring during periodontal debridement is probably similar to the normal course of events in tissue turnover. These cells originate at the apical end of the epithelial attachment and migrate toward the coronal end of the junctional epithelium.[26]

Inflammatory activity occurs in the underlying connective tissue during the disease process and is also one result of treatment. Connective tissue fibers are disrupted and lysed beneath the epithelium. Healing of inflamed connective tissue is complex, requiring many cells and mediators. It takes considerably longer than healing of epithelium, up to several months.[27] New connective tissue fiber attachment to the tooth surface is not an expected outcome, but the development of an elongated junctional epithelial attachment may result in reduced probe readings. Because of the fragile state of healing connective tissues, probing after treatment should be avoided for 3 to 4 weeks.[14]

HEALING AFTER GINGIVAL CURETTAGE

Healing of the epithelial lining of the pocket after periodontal debridement and gingival curettage can be expected to take 5 to 12 days. The epithelium proliferates apically from the cut edge of the oral epithelium and covers the exposed connective tissue. The junctional epithelium, which has been removed during the gingival curettage procedure, forms from these migrating cells and is histologically similar to the original junctional epithelium. The connective tissue response is complex and takes longer to resolve. Healing may result in a long junctional epithelial attachment, thus reducing probing depths, but is not thought to create new connective tissue attachment to the roots.[27] Probing of healing tissues after gingival curettage should also be avoided for at least 4 weeks.

REPOPULATION OF MICROORGANISMS AFTER THERAPY

Periodontal debridement is effective in reducing the volume of plaque bacteria in treated sites. The numbers of organisms are reduced dramatically and grow back in different proportions. The bacterial plaque shifts from predominantly Gram-negative flora to one that is Gram-positive, with many fewer motile forms, especially spirochetes. This new flora is similar to those found in periodontally healthy sites. Bacteria repopulate in a specific order, starting with *Streptococcus* and *Actinobacillus* species, followed by *Viellonella, Bacteroides, Porphyromonas, Prevotella*, and *Fusobacterium* species. *Capnocytophaga* species and spirochetes are the last to grow back. The cycle may take as long as 6 months to complete.[18] Repopulation can be expected to be variable because of a number of factors, most likely operator differences in complete removal of plaque and calculus.[17] Poor supragingival plaque control and invasive bacteria remaining in the tissues also may affect the repopulation process.[18]

CLINICAL RESPONSE

After thorough periodontal debridement procedures, clinical response that can be expected is a reduction of pocket depths, changes in attachment, recession, fewer bleeding sites, and less reddened tissue. Minimum amounts of new bone are generated after nonsurgical periodontal therapy. In contrast, extensive bone growth is seen after surgical interventions. Greenstein[14] reviewed the clinical results from a variety of studies clarifying the results of nonsurgical ther-

apy. Generally, shallower pockets are reduced less than deeper ones, and redness and bleeding are reduced dramatically. The greatest amount of healing is seen 3 to 6 weeks after nonsurgical periodontal therapy. However, changes continue to occur up to 12 months after treatment; then the situation stabilizes.[28]

Data suggest that in pockets with initial probe depths of 1 to 3 mm, there is little pocket reduction, attachment loss of up to 0.89 mm after 5 years, and possibly slight recession of less than 1 mm. Pockets with initial depths of 4 to 6 mm tended to be reduced in probe depth by about 1 mm through some combination of gain in attachment of about 0.5 mm and recession making up the rest of the difference. Results of these studies vary, with longer studies showing more recession.[14]

Deeper pockets of more than 7 mm showed the greatest pocket reduction, about 1.5 to 3 mm, made up of attachment gain of about 1 mm and the rest recession. In the studies reviewed, the number of bleeding sites was reduced by 50 percent or more, and gingival redness was reduced to near zero after nonsurgical therapy.[14]

Baderstein and associates[28] showed similar results and noted that differences can occur between clinicians. Figure 12–6 shows overall healing results were similar for all subjects, but that operator 2 generally achieved slightly less recession and possibly more gain in attachment. Generally, sites with deeper initial probe depths responded with greater improvements, with 2 mm or more reduction.

Attachment gain must be considered carefully. Attachment changes are computed by measuring the periodontal probe depths and then adding the distance to a fixed reference point on the tooth, usually the cementoenamel junction. Periodontal probes penetrate the epithelial attachment by 1 mm or more, especially in inflamed tissue.[8] What is considered attachment gain may simply be a more accurate reading of probing pocket depth following healing after treatment. The periodontal probe is less likely to penetrate healed junctional epithelium and intact connective tissue fibers after treatment is performed than when probing inflamed tissue. The re-evaluation probe depths, measured several weeks after treatment, probably reflect the histologic depth of pockets more accurately than the pretreatment probe depths.

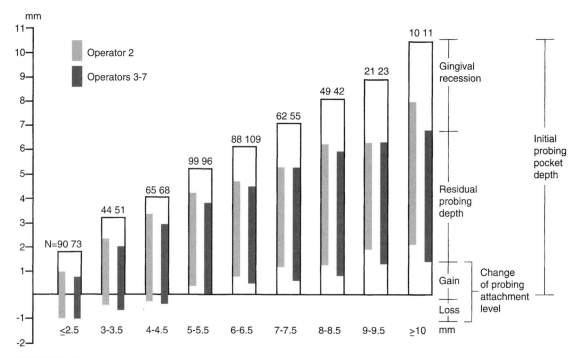

FIGURE 12–6. Average values for gingival recession, residual probing depth, and gain or loss of probing attachment at 24 months related to initial probing pocket depth. The mean values for operator 2 are compared with the mean values for other operators, showing slight differences in results. (Used with permission from Baderstein A, Nilueus R, Egelberg J. Effect of non-surgical periodontal therapy: IV. Operator variability. J Clin Periodontal 1985; 12:190–200. ©1985 Munksgaard International Publishers Ltd., Copenhagen, Denmark.)

The re-evaluation depths are important for monitoring the long-term results of treatment and determining whether more extensive periodontal therapy is needed. Results should not be evaluated less than 3 or 4 weeks after therapy.[14]

SENSITIVITY

Dentin, or root surface, sensitivity is commonly created or increased after periodontal treatment procedures. This is usually true following surgical procedures, but often after nonsurgical debridement as well. Patients commonly return for a second or third appointment for periodontal debridement and report sensitivity to cold or tooth brushing in previously treated areas. Most sensitivity is mild and resolves in a few weeks. However, in some cases, sensitivity is extreme and inhibits patients' plaque control efforts. This sensitivity can lead to poor therapeutic results and possibly to caries formation. The dental hygienist must be aware of the causes and treatments available for dentin sensitivity and develop strategies to deal with the problem.

Dentin or root sensitivity is often referred to as **dentinal hypersensitivity**, an extreme or unexpectedly elevated response. Periodontal

debridement results in the removal of some cementum and dentin because of the nature of the procedures performed, which expose some fresh dentin surfaces to the oral environment. Exposed dentin is sensitive, not necessarily hypersensitive, making "root sensitivity" a better descriptor of this condition.[29]

The **hydrodynamic theory of dentin sensitivity** is supported by a growing body of evidence. This theory is the accepted explanation for root sensitivity. Dentin can become sensitive when patent dentinal tubules are exposed to the oral environment. Tubules course directly to the pulp chamber of the tooth and are filled with fluid. The odontoblastic processes extend into the tubules at the pulpal ends. The hydrodynamic forces stimulate pain responses through these open tubules. Stimuli such as cold, sweet, acid (including plaque acids), drying, and scraping with a metal instrument cause a rapid and immediate flow of the tubule contents outward, stimulating the odontoblastic processes and causing pain. The A-delta nerve fibers coursing around the odontoblasts only react with pain, so these stimuli can only cause pain. Heat stimulation causes an inflow of fluid into the pulp chamber, also disturbing the nerve fibers. However, this pain reaction comes from C-fibers deeper in the pulp and can lead to a dull, aching pain in the jaw. Heat-stimulated pain is not considered dentin sensitivity, but a more serious indication of irreversible pulpal changes.[30]

No evidence of the incidence of sensitivity after periodontal therapy procedures is avail-able. However, it is a commonly reported problem.[31] Subgingival scaling procedures, including periodontal debridement, caused post-treatment sensitivity to cold blasts of air in half of the subjects in one study, beginning immediately after treatment and diminishing in 3 to 4 weeks.[32] Another case report of postscaling sensitivity over 3 years of maintenance therapy

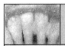

EVOLUTION OF PERIODONTAL INSTRUMENT

As early as the 10th century AD, scholars interested in oral health designed tooth scrapers and named them after themselves. Albucasis created a set of 14 scrapers, a few examples of which exist today. Pierre Fouchard, known as the "Father of Modern Dentistry," made many contributions to dentistry, including designing instruments that he named after himself. Other pioneers in periodontal therapy in the early 20th century designed and refined scaling instruments and continued the naming tradition. Each refinement was expected to improve the usefulness of the instruments and the results of therapy. Hirshfeld, Hartzell, McCall, Bunting, and Gracey are some of the dentists whose instrument designs have outlived them and are still in use today.

John McCall wrote complaining of the crudeness of periodontal instruments in the 1930s, and the fact that there seemed to be no philosophy as to the most efficient method of instrumentation. He believed that perfection of scaler designs and their use in treatment techniques were the basic requirements for success in periodontal therapy.[47] Another 20th century pioneer, John Riggs, is credited with developing instruments that were

designed for specific surfaces of the teeth and uses during treatment. Riggs' instruments were rustic by today's standards as they lacked contra-angled shanks. Hoe scalers and periodontal files were also introduced in the early 20th century, but the designs were not refined until C. M. Carr introduced sets that included 18 groups of eight hoes, divided into three classes according to length of shank. Thus, a full set of instruments consisted of 144 hoes and six sickle scalers. Carr's extensive set of working-end designs allowed scaling techniques to become more standardized, and probably served to encourage others to continue to refine scaler designs. McCall worked to improve the temper of metal scalers, thus making them stronger. Thomas Hartzell and Austin James refined the designs of Carr and McCall. Clinicians today continue to refine and improve instrument design with the same goal, that of improving therapeutic techniques and restoring periodontal health.[48]

Figure 12–7A is the complete set of Carr's hoes and sickles. Figure 12–7B is a detail of three hoes; each working-end design is the same, but the shanks vary in length to permit access into pockets of different depths.

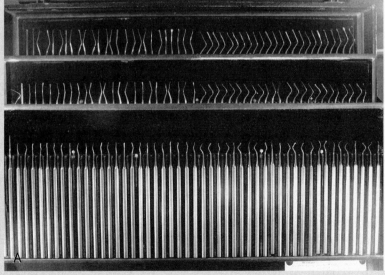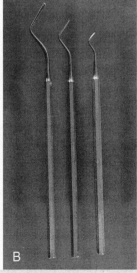

FIGURE 12–7.

resulted in the extraction of four lower anterior teeth. These teeth, viewed under scanning electron microscopy, showed odontoblastic processes protruding out of the dental tubules into the environment. The area was so sensitive that the patient could not tolerate the teeth in the mouth, even though the periodontal condition was stable.[33]

Not all scaled teeth become sensitive, probably because scaling creates a smear layer over the treated surfaces. This layer contains crystalline debris (mostly calcium and phosphorus), covers the dentin surface, and greatly reduces fluid flow.[34] Scaling removes the existing smear layer and creates a new one; this layer is fragile and can be removed through tooth brushing and possibly an acidic diet.[35]

The dental hygienist should plan a strategy for the treatment of sensitivity at the nonsurgical therapy appointment. Any sensitive areas should be identified with the patient's help and treatment initiated for those areas. If the patient reports more sensitive areas at subsequent appointments, the affected sites should be treated in the office, and the patient should be sent home with a product and information that may help.

Several chemicals have been used to treat sensitivity in the dental office. Perhaps the most commonly used preparations are fluorides. A 33.3 per cent paste of kaolin, glycerine, and sodium fluoride has been burnished into sensitive root surfaces for decades. This paste works because the burnishing action creates a smear layer, occluding tubules, rather than because of the precipitation of fluoride-rich crystals on the surface.[36] Calcium hydroxide in a water slurry has also been burnished onto sensitive surfaces and has provided immediate, if short-lived, relief.[37] Again, the burnishing may provide a protective smear layer. Cavity varnishes painted onto exposed surfaces can also provide relief.[37] Both potassium oxylate[38] and ferric oxylate[39] remove the smear layer and precipitate crystals, significantly occluding the dentinal tubules. These effects are relatively short-lived, lasting 1 to 2 weeks.[39]

To complicate the understanding of post-treatment root sensitivity, most roots go through a natural process of crystallization and occlusion of the patent dentinal tubules. This process occurs a few weeks after treatment and often diminishes or eliminates post-procedural

sensitivity. It is not clear how long a desensitizing agent works or needs to be applied. Informing the patient and providing some form of immediate relief after therapy are often indicated.

Patients can use a variety of toothpastes for desensitizing the teeth at home. Pastes containing potassium nitrate have some data to suggest that they work effectively.[40] Others containing strontium chloride have been available for many years and show evidence of efficacy.[41] A recent study showed that fluoride toothpastes may work as well as strontium chloride to provide relief.[42] These agents usually require regular use for several weeks. Once patients obtain relief, they are reluctant to give up the product. In the case of strontium chloride products, the dental hygienist must also consider the benefits of regular fluoride use and either recommend products that contain fluoride or find another avenue to apply fluoride, such as office treatments or daily use of a fluoride mouth rinse.

The dental hygienist must have a strategy for helping patients with post-therapy sensitivity. This strategy should include warning the patient prior to treatment about possible sensitivity, treating existing sensitive areas, using in-office therapies, and prescribing home treatments. Often the passage of time greatly reduces the problem, but these treatments can make the wait less painful and patients more comfortable.

PREDICTIVENESS OF RESULTS

Periodontal debridement is effective for the treatment of infectious periodontal diseases.[14] It reliably results in decreased probing depths and less bleeding, increases in attachment in deep pockets, and a generally healthier oral environment in almost all cases. These results can be relied on to occur, even in cases of advanced periodontitis. Baderstein and co-workers[43] reported that outcomes from scaling and root planing were not compromised by the severity of lesions 24 months after treatment, regardless of whether treatment was performed with hand or ultrasonic instruments. Sites with deep initial probing depths showed a high incidence of attachment gain. In another analysis, Claffey and associates[44] showed that even deep initial probing depths tended to gain attachment after nonsurgical periodontal therapy. Subjects with higher proportions of attachment gain after therapy had few sites that lost attachment. They also reported that sites with probing attachment loss after 24 months were more frequently associated with bleeding, plaque, suppuration, and residual probing depth than sites that did not lose attachment.[44] However, the predictability of any one clinical parameter has been shown to be low, so the need to record and consider attachment loss measurements was critical in evaluating the results.[45] At best, the predictability of attachment loss over 5 years was 30 percent for high plaque or bleeding scores, and residual probing depth of 7 mm or more was 50 percent predictive.[46] Probing depth that deepened by 1 mm or greater was predictive of attachment loss approximately 80 percent of the time.[46]

The dental hygienist should monitor patients carefully over time, evaluating probing depths and attachment loss. The fact that a pocket is deep does not mean that it cannot be stabilized through nonsurgical therapy. The presence of plaque and bleeding over time is a source of concern and should be addressed, but these events are not absolute signs of periodontal disease activity. Increases in probing depths or attachment loss are cause for concern, re-treatment, and possibly referral to a specialist for evaluation. All dental hygiene assessments should be used to evaluate the results of treatment, and re-treatment or referral should be planned accordingly.

TECHNIQUES

Hand Instrumentation

The use of hand scalers and curettes for instrumentation has a long tradition in periodontal therapy. For a brief discussion of instrument development, see The Evolution of Periodontal Instruments. Universal curettes and sickles are among the oldest instrument designs. These instruments have cutting edges on both sides of the blade. Sickles are machined to a pointed end, and universal curettes have rounded ends. Area-specific curettes were first designed in the 1930s by Clayton Gracey. Several variations exist today. Last to enter the marketplace were ultrasonic scaling instruments. These appeared in the 1960s and were a modification of an ultrasonic instrument designed to cut tooth structure. These instruments could not compete with high-speed drills, so they were modified for use as scalers. Many new instruments will no doubt be introduced in the future.

In addition to design differences between instruments, there are variations in materials. Most curette manufacturers use stainless steel. Carbon steel instruments are also available that hold a sharp cutting edge but they are more brittle than stainless steel. In addition, some manufacturers treat their stainless steel curettes and sickles cryogenically and claim longer-lasting sharpness of the cutting edges.

Periodontal instruments, such as scalers and curettes, have a long tradition of successful service in therapeutic settings. Variations in design and materials permit the dental hygienist to select instruments based on personal preferences and treatment needs.

This section describes commonly used periodontal instruments, but is not meant to be an inclusive list of the available options. Individual clinicians develop preferences for specific designs and materials.

UNIVERSAL CURETTES

Universal curettes are designed to adapt and instrument all surfaces of all teeth in the mouth. The curette blades have cutting edges on both sides and are usually double-ended. Thus, one universal curette can scale around all of the teeth in the dentition.

AREA-SPECIFIC CURETTES

Area-specific curettes have been available since the 1930s. The first ones, designed by Gracey, are still popular today (Figure 12–8). The blades of the Gracey curettes have one cutting edge and are usually double-ended. The curettes are numbered to identify the recommended locations. Gracey 1/2, 3/4, and 5/6 curettes are generally used in the anterior areas, possibly the bicuspids. Gracey 7/8 and 9/10 curettes are designed to instrument the buccal and lingual surfaces of the posterior teeth. The Gracey 11/12 curette has extra bends in the shank to allow it to adapt to the mesial surfaces of the posterior teeth. The Gracey 13/14 curette adapts to the distal surfaces of the posterior teeth. Two modifications of the Gracey curette design are the Gracey 15/16 and Gracey 17/18.

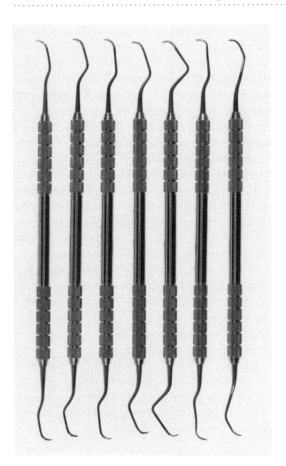

FIGURE 12–8. Gracey instruments as originally designed by Dr. Clayton Gracey in the 1930s.

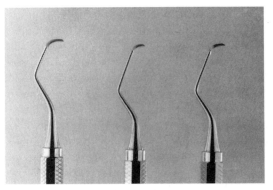

FIGURE 12–9. The Gracey 7/8 instrument in three popular versions (left to right): conventional design, shorter and thinner blade with an extended shank, and extended shank configuration.

two cutting edges on each blade and can be adapted under the gingiva no more than 1 or 2 mm to break off ledges of calculus. It is a useful instrument when ultrasonic or sonic scaling is not an option (Figure 12-10).

Hoes, Chisels, and Files. Hoes, chisels, and files are instruments designed for removing heavy calculus. The chisel is a push instrument, and the hoe and files are pull instruments. All are designed to crush and disrupt heavy deposits of calculus (Figure 12-11).

These are modifications of the current 11/12 and 13/14 designs that some clinicians believe provide better access to the mesial and distal surfaces of the posterior teeth.

Recent modifications of the Gracey design have provided area-specific instruments with extended shanks to reach into deeper pockets. Also, a modification of the length and thickness of the blade has resulted in the availability of an area-specific curette series with smaller blades that adapt well to the healthier tissues of maintenance patients. These options permit the dental hygienist to customize the instrumentation approach for specific situations (Figure 12-9).

SPECIAL INSTRUMENTS

Sickles. Sickle scalers are heavy calculus removers designed primarily to be used on supragingival calculus. The sickle design ends in a sharp point, making it unacceptable for deep scaling in periodontal pockets. The sickle has

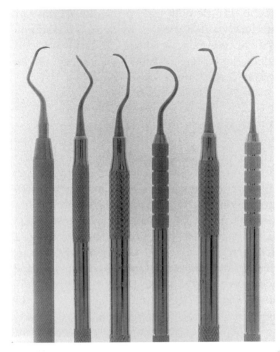

FIGURE 12–10. Sickle scalers come in a wide variety of shapes and shank designs. This variety makes the sickle adaptable to more areas of the mouth.

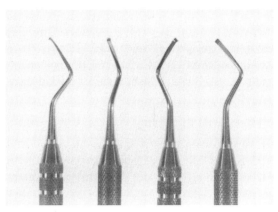

FIGURE 12–11. Files are used for removing tenacious calculus, particularly when ultrasonic instrumentation is not available.

EVA. EVA (EVA Prophylaxis System, Unitek Co., Monrovia, CA) is a motor-driven, oscillating system of files and points for removing overhanging margins and recontouring restorations. The files are triangular, and they move rapidly in and out. The tips are diamond-coated to permit rapid action. Care must be taken not to damage the papilla when the tip is placed proximally.

EXPECTATION OF COMPETENCY

The technical skill of the dental hygienist is the critical element in successful non-surgical periodontal therapy. Variations in instrument design provide the dental hygienist with choices. Few studies have compared how well hand instruments perform calculus removal. Many dental hygienists believe that area-specific curettes work better on all teeth or on teeth with attachment loss. Other clinicians believe that universal curettes are the only acceptable instruments. One study was initiated to compare conventional area-specific curettes with newly designed area-specific curettes with longer shanks, which are supposedly better able to scale in deep pockets.

Nagy and co-workers[49] evaluated 140 root surfaces instrumented by standard rigid Gracey curettes or longer-shank rigid Gracey curettes for 15 minutes per tooth. Probe depths were as great as 7 mm. Both types of curettes worked equally well. Mesial surfaces were clean to a deeper level than other surfaces, but that was true for both types of curettes. The knowledge and skill of the dental hygienist is most important. Types of instruments remain personal choices.

It is more difficult to render furcation areas calculus free than other surfaces. In a study of scaling efficiency on multirooted teeth, even experienced clinicians left calculus in furcations most of the time. Also, calculus was still present after flaps had been laid to permit access for scaling. Clinicians used a variety of hand and ultrasonic instruments in this study and spent 11.4 to 15.1 minutes scaling each tooth. From this work, two points were clarified: experienced clinicians removed more calculus, and complete calculus removal in molar furcation areas is difficult, if not impossible, to achieve.[50]

Sonic and Ultrasonic Instrumentation: Powered Scaling

Sonic and ultrasonic instrumentation of tooth surfaces has dramatically increased in popularity in recent years. This increase is the result of the re-examination of the role of root planing in nonsurgical therapy. For years, ultrasonic instruments were primarily recommended for heavy deposit removal. It was thought that their use had to be followed by hand instrumentation to completely remove necrotic root substance. As discussed earlier, this theory is not supportable.

Much research has been conducted to evaluate the effectiveness of sonic and ultrasonic instrumentation. This information is summarized here to emphasize the value of these often underused tools. It is important to understand how well both sonic and ultrasonic instruments, or powered scalers, work in achieving the short-term and long-term goals of nonsurgical periodontal therapy.

A number of questions must be addressed in assessing the usefulness of powered scalers. These questions include:

1. Do sonic and ultrasonic instruments work equally well?
2. Does powered scaling remove plaque from root surfaces?
3. Does powered scaling effectively remove calculus?
4. Does powered scaling leave root surfaces feeling clean and smooth, the short-term goal of therapy during the appointment?

5. Does powered scaling achieve the long-term goal of restoring periodontal health?
6. What happens to the endotoxin on the root surfaces?
7. Are the aerosols produced during powered scaling a cause for concern?
8. Are the new modified tips better than the standard designs?

ULTRASONIC OR SONIC?

Ultrasonic scaling devices generate vibrations in the range of 20,000 to 40,000 cycles per second. These are separate units that use magnetostrictive or piezoelectric systems to generate ultrahigh frequencies of scaling tip movement. Ultrasonic instruments work by a combination of mechanical, irrigation, cavitation, and acoustic streaming forces. Sonic scalers attach directly to the high-speed handpiece and generate vibrations of 2000 to 6000 cycles per second. The technique for using both sonic and ultrasonic instruments requires only that the tip be kept moving rapidly, touching the tooth surface to remove calculus. No lateral pressure is applied, because lateral force applied during powered instrumentation can cause severe root damage.[51]

Ultrasonic and sonic scalers have been compared in laboratory settings using extracted teeth. According to Jotikasthira and coworkers,[52] both ultrasonic and sonic scalers remove calculus effectively. They reported that sonic scalers were at least as effective as ultrasonic scalers for calculus removal, if not slightly better. In terms of root surface roughness and removal of tooth structure, ultrasonic instruments caused slightly less trauma to the roots than sonic instruments. However, all root damage was superficial and localized. Overall, the cemental surfaces were left smooth. In addition, the time required to achieve good results was similar for both types of powered scalers. No damage was seen in this study that would contraindicate the use of either type of scaler. Another extensive review of ultrasonic scalers suggested that both types of powered scalers produce excellent and similar results.[4]

PLAQUE REMOVAL

Ultrasonic instrumentation is remarkably efficient at removing plaque from root surfaces.[53] Cavitation, the inwardly collapsing bubbles of water that are produced as the stream touches the vibrating tip, appears to have an antimicrobial effect in lysing the bacterial walls and flushing debris away, out of the pockets.[4] The stream of fluid also reaches the bottom of the pocket, providing a flushing effect during treatment.[54]

ENDOTOXIN REMOVAL

In vitro studies verify that ultrasonic instrumentation is as effective as hand instrumentation in detoxifying root surfaces. Fibroblast attachment occurs equally on diseased root surfaces after either type of instrumentation.[55] Root surface cytotoxic materials, or lipopolysaccarides, are removed by ultrasonic scaling with overlapping, light strokes of approximately 50 g, which is about the same pressure as light probing. Root surfaces treated this way for 0.8 seconds/mm^2 show the same properties as control root surfaces from periodontally healthy teeth.[56] There was no remaining toxic material that could interfere with healing.

CALCULUS REMOVAL

Dragoo[57] showed that ultrasonic tips are effective in calculus removal. Using a curette efficiency index, where a score of 1 meant no calculus present and a score of 3 indicated gross amounts, he compared standard ultrasonic tips with newly designed thinner tips and hand curettes. The thinner ultrasonic tips were 16 percent to 27 percent more effective in calculus removal than hand curettes and 27 to 46 percent better than standard ultrasonic tips. All instruments reached to within approximately 1 mm of the apical extent of pockets, and the thin ultrasonic tips appeared to clean more efficiently in the deeper areas.

A number of clinical studies have evaluated calculus removal. A review by Suppipat[58] published in 1974 described several studies in which teeth were scaled, half by ultrasonic instrumentation and half by hand curettes. Evaluation by judges who were blind to the type of experimental treatment found no difference in post-treatment evaluations.[58]

ROOT SMOOTHNESS: SHORT-TERM GOALS

Root smoothness is the yardstick by which the dental hygienist determines the end point of each treatment appointment. It is a short-term goal. Explorer examination of root surfaces to determine the presence of calculus or root smoothness is a valuable tool for the dental hygienist. Some clinicians prefer to use the periodontal probe for this evaluation. Whatever instrument is used, if clicks and bumps of calculus are felt, the teeth should be instrumented until they are smooth. All of the surfaces in a specific patient should be instrumented to approximately the same degree of smoothness. If an area on a root surface feels rougher than other treated areas, missed or residual calculus must be suspected and the area treated again. All surfaces should be clean of plaque and free of calculus. These smooth surfaces do not require that the cementum be shaved off by further systematic instrumentation. All treated dentitions will feel smooth and calculus free after treatment, but root surfaces may not attain a glassy, hard-textured surface.

HEALING AFTER TREATMENT: LONG-TERM GOALS

Although laboratory and clinical evaluations of the efficiency of calculus removal are of interest, the important comparison between ultrasonic instrumentation and hand instrumentation is healing after therapy. These comparisons demonstrate the long-term goal of nonsurgical periodontal therapy, healing, and provide the basis for selecting a mode of therapy. Periodontal healing after treatment of moderate and advanced periodontitis was reported in studies by Baderstein and colleagues in the 1980s. These clinical studies evaluated patients with moderate and advanced periodontal disease. Half of the mouth was treated by hand instrumentation and the other half by ultrasonic instrumentation.[27, 59] These studies verified the equal ability of hand and ultrasonic instruments to achieve the long-term goals of therapy, no matter which type of instrument is used.

Baderstein and colleagues[59] evaluated 15 subjects with moderately advanced periodontitis over a period of 13 months. Plaque, bleeding, probing depth, and attachment loss were examined. Subjects were given oral hygiene instructions repeatedly during the first month of the study. Instrumentation was performed and subjects were evaluated at month 2 (1 month after treatment). Monthly clinical assessments were performed for 13 months, and teeth were reinstrumented 2 months and 6 months after the first treatment. The percentage of surfaces with plaque was reduced from 65 to 73 percent to about 12 percent after the oral hygiene instruction and remained at that level throughout the study. The percentage of bleeding surfaces ranged from 77 to 90 percent. This percentage was not substantially reduced by oral hygiene instruction alone, but was reduced by instrumentation. The percentage of bleeding surfaces was 36 to 41 percent at 2 months and was reduced to 8 to 16 percent by 6 months. The percentage then remained at the 6-month level. Mean probing depths were 4.1 to 4.5 mm at the beginning of the study. Oral hygiene alone reduced probing depths by 0.03 to 0.07 mm. One month after instrumentation, depths were reduced by 0.5 to 0.7 mm, and at 4 months, pockets were reduced by 1.3 to 1.7 mm. They remained at that level. Attachment loss also changed over the course of the study. Shallow pockets lost a little attachment, as expected, and deep pockets of 7 mm or more gained 1.1 to 1.5 mm in attachment. Quadrants were randomly assigned to hand instrumentation or ultrasonic instrumentation, and an examiner who was blind to the treatments evaluated all of the subjects. There was no difference between the results achieved by hand instrumentation and those achieved by ultrasonic instrumentation.

Baderstein and co-workers[27] also evaluated subjects with more advanced periodontal disease in a study of similar design. Subjects had probe depths of greater than 5 mm, and many depths of 8, 9, and 10 mm were included in the study. The same parameters were evaluated. First, oral hygiene instruction was given. Three months later, the teeth were instrumented, and then reinstrumented at 6 and 9 months. Subjects were evaluated monthly for 24 months.

Plaque was reduced significantly by the oral hygiene instruction, and the level remained stable throughout the study. Bleeding initially occurred at 84 to 90 percent of the surfaces. Little effect was seen with oral hygiene alone, and the percentage of bleeding sites was reduced to 14 to 18 percent at 12 months after instrumentation. Mean probing depths were 5.5 to 5.8 mm. They were reduced to 5.1 to 5.3 mm by oral hygiene and further reduced to 3.6 to 3.9 mm 12 months after the first instrumentation. Notable recession was seen over 12 months, 1.6 to 1.8 mm. The attachment loss pattern was similar to that of other studies: shallow pockets lost attachment slightly, and deeper pockets tended to gain. The treatment results did not differ between quadrants scaled with hand instruments and those scaled with ultrasonic instruments.

The decision to use ultrasonic instruments rather than or in addition to hand instrumentation when providing nonsurgical periodontal therapy should be based on the preference of the dental hygienist and the patient. Both treatments are effective and achieve the short- and long-term goals of periodontal debridement.

There is one major contraindication to treatment with ultrasonic scaling. The electromagnetic field generated in the handpiece can interfere with the functioning of some cardiac pacemakers.[60] Most pacemakers are shielded and are not affected by this field, but not all. The dental hygienist cannot determine which type of pacemaker the patient may be wearing. In fact, the patient may not know. To ensure that powered scaling will do no harm, ultrasonic instruments should not be used on patients with pacemakers. In addition, dentists and dental hygienists who wear pacemakers should not operate ultrasonic devices.[61] Sonic scalers do not create an electromagnetic field and may be used as a substitute.

AEROSOLS

Infection control is a constant and important part of dental hygiene practice. The application of universal infection control standards is an absolute requirement of the United States Occupational Health and Safety Administration. These requirements indicate that contaminated splatter and aerosol spray be minimized in dental and dental hygiene practice. Obviously, a rapidly moving, water-cooled device such as an ultrasonic tip will create substantial splatter and aerosol. Aerosols generated by subgingival powered scaling contain blood.[62] The prevention of disease transmission and use of barrier techniques during powered scaling procedures is therefore essential. It is necessary for dental hygienists or dentists to wear appropriate face masks and protective eyewear when using these devices.[63] High volume suction devices can significantly reduce the amount of aerosol contamination.[64, 65, 66]

Asking patients to rinse for 30 seconds with an antiseptic mouthwash before ultrasonic scaling reduced recoverable colony-forming bacterial units from aerosols by 94 percent. Rinsing

with a non-antiseptic mouthwash reduced the bacterial counts by 33 percent.[63] Preprocedural rinsing may help to reduce bacteria, but its effect on viruses is unknown. In addition, blood-borne contaminants inoculated into the aerosol and splatter by subgingival ultrasonic scaling are not likely to be affected by preprocedural rinsing. Until further questions are answered, preprocedural rinsing is not a required component of infection control. If it is adopted by individual dental hygienists or clinics, it must be used for every patient to meet the requirement of universal infection control, not selectively on patients who are known to be infectious.

NEW AND OLD DESIGNS FOR TIPS

The studies described earlier demonstrating long-term healing after nonsurgical periodontal therapy compared hand instruments with conventional ultrasonic insert designs that have been available for years. The results clearly indicated that standard ultrasonic tip designs worked as well as hand instruments.

Until the 1980s, all ultrasonic inserts and sonic tips were fairly thick and blunt. Some were curved in various dimensions. Many dental hygienists found them awkward to use subgingivally. Some dentists and dental hygienists began to sharpen and reshape the tips to make them more adaptable. Sharpening resulted in thinning the diameter of the tips rather than creating a cutting edge. These recontoured tips have been used successfully and safely.[4] Dragoo advocated their use exclusively and showed in laboratory experiments that thin, curved tips reached more deeply than traditional designs and clean more efficiently than hand curettes.[57] Piezoelectric tips have also been sharpened and reduced in dimension in an effort to make them more adaptable. These tips also work well after modification.[67] Thin and curved ultrasonic tips are now available commercially for use with various ultrasonic units. One study showed greater root surface removal and greater residual root surface roughness after the use of a diamond-coated ultrasonic insert.[68] Caution should be used with any insert during powered scaling. There are no long-term studies comparing treatment results with the various designs of tips. The dental hygienist should sample several designs and select those that are the most comfortable to use and seem to be the most efficient. Certainly, the thinner, curved tips should be considered because they adapt very well into deeper pockets and furcations.

CHEMICAL ADJUNCTS

Irrigation

Irrigation as an adjunct to nonsurgical periodontal therapy has become popular because the antibacterial goal of periodontal debridement is better understood. In this chapter, irrigation is the term used to refer to a lavage, or flushing, of pockets during or after periodontal debridement procedures. Scaling has a tremendous antimicrobial effect on pocket microflora. Whether instrumentation is performed with hand scalers or powered scalers, the bacterial population is vastly reduced through mechanical removal. For an antimicrobial agent delivered as an irrigant to have an additional effect, several requirements must be met.[69]

1. The agent must reach the site of disease activity, the base of the pockets.
2. Antimicrobial agents must be used at bacteriocidal concentrations.
3. Medicaments must be substantive, or present long enough to work.

Rinsing with an antimicrobial mouth rinse has negligible effects on subgingival flora. However, antimicrobial agents used as irrigants penetrate to the bottom of the periodontal pockets if applied with a syringe using a canula tip or with pulsed irrigation devices using a soft rubber tip or a canula.[70]

Antimicrobial agents are available that provide good antiseptic potential. Solutions used as irrigants reduce microbial populations. Effective products include 0.12 percent chlorhexidine, 0.4 percent stannous fluoride, and 0.05 percent povidone-iodine. However, irrigation without previous scaling permits calculus to interfere with the penetration of medicament and reduces microbe levels for a few days at most.[70]

Irrigation preceded by periodontal debridement suppressed microbial populations for 2 to 6 months, but it is not clear which treatment caused the long suppression. Scaling and root planing alone have tremendous antimicrobial effects in the periodontal pockets that last for weeks.[71] Even a substantive antimicrobial, such

as chlorhexidine, would have to be available in the pocket for many days to interfere with plaque regrowth. It would seem that periodontal debridement is the primary treatment and that irrigation is not reliable in augmenting its effects. Shiloah and Hovious[71] agreed that irrigation during nonsurgical therapy has limited effects, but point out one study that reported improved probing depths after 1 year when ultrasonic periodontal debridement was performed with 0.05 percent povidone-iodine as an irrigant. This evidence suggests that antimicrobial irrigation during a nonsurgical periodontal therapy appointment may be beneficial if performed under the right conditions. Certainly, research is needed to determine the adjunctive effects in hard-to-scale areas, such as furcations, deeper pockets, and nonresponding sites. Currently, although antimicrobial solutions are available and systems can deliver them to the infectious sites in the pockets, they do not appear to be present long enough to change the repopulation of the pockets. The exception to this may be tetracycline, which binds to root surfaces. It has shown advantage in increasing attachment levels in treated teeth over a six-month period.[72] Convincing evidence of improved healing based on repeated, well-controlled clinical trials, however, remains elusive. For this reason, irrigation during the nonsurgical therapy appointment is only possibly synergistic with periodontal debridement.[70] Therefore, irrigation is an elective part of therapy.

Calculus Softeners

Calculus softeners known as scaling gels have been marketed to help the dental hygienist to remove deposits from the teeth. These gels are placed into the periodontal pockets on top of the calculus and are designed to chelate minerals out so that scaling is easier. Little work has been done to evaluate these materials and the evidence supporting the use of those products is not strong. One study looked at the effects of the gel on tooth surfaces and restorative materials and found that it was safe to use.[73] No morphologic changes were seen on intact enamel or dentin after exposure times of up to 12 minutes. Many restorative materials appear to be unaffected by these short exposure times. Clinical evaluation is limited. Two studies showed that teeth were not rendered more sensitive after treatment with the gel and scaling than after scaling alone,[74, 75] and no damage to the tooth surfaces or gingiva was seen. However, no data support the ease of calculus removal or reduction in treatment time other than the opinions of the clinicians in one trial.[75] Nagy and co-workers concluded that the results of their double-blind clinical trial did not support the use of calculus softening gel as an adjunct to root instrumentation in periodontal therapy.[76] As attractive as is the notion of a chelating agent to soften calculus and make periodontal debridement easier, there is no evidence to support its use.

RECOMMENDATIONS

Greenstein[14] noted that meticulous root debridement coupled with compliance with maintenance regimens, both regular recalls and daily oral hygiene care, provides the dental hygienist and dentist with successful non-surgical periodontal care that is reliable and predictable. Dental hygienists can contribute to the periodontal health of the population by accepting this responsibility and ensuring that their clinical skills are excellent and that time is provided in the daily schedule to adequately perform nonsurgical periodontal therapy.

Ramfjord[20] defined the true measure of the quality of life for periodontal patients as the function and preservation of the teeth in an esthetic state with a minimum of sensitive teeth. The dental hygienist should endeavor to provide care with these goals in mind. Nonsurgical periodontal therapy reduces infection, preserves teeth, and improves health, function, and appearance. These are the goals of all periodontal therapy.

STUDY QUESTIONS

MULTIPLE CHOICE

1. The goal of periodontal instrumentation is to return the periodontium to a state of health.
   Periodontal health is achieved through periodontal therapy that creates glassy hard and smooth root surfaces at each treatment visit.

   a. Both statements are TRUE.
   b. Both statements are FALSE.
   c. The first statement is TRUE, the second is FALSE.
   d. The first statement is FALSE, the second is TRUE.

2. The term for removal of the inflamed soft tissue wall lining the periodontal pocket is:

   a. Gingival curettage
   b. Root scaling
   c. Selective polishing
   d. Root planing

3. The name of the prominent dental researcher who introduced the concept of the specific plaque hypothesis in the 1970s is

   a. Carranza
   b. Löe
   c. Loesche
   d. Ramfjord

4. Complete calculus removal using hand instruments or powered instruments is a goal for the dental hygienist BECAUSE removal of calculus is essential to the restoration of periodontal health.

   a. Both the statement and the reason are correct and related.
   b. Both the statement and the reason are correct but NOT related.
   c. The statement is correct, but the reason is NOT.
   d. The statement is NOT correct, but the reason is correct.
   e. Neither the statement NOR the reason is correct.

5. Experimental evidence indicates that rough root surfaces are mechanical irritants BECAUSE they delay healing.

   a. Both the statement and the reason are correct and related.
   b. Both the statement and the reason are correct but NOT related.
   c. The statement is correct, but the reason is NOT.
   d. The statement is NOT correct, but the reason is correct.
   e. Neither the statement NOR the reason is correct.

6. Periodontal debridement is an effective therapy consisting of removal of local irritants.
   It results in decreased probing depths and increased clinical attachment, particularly in deeper pockets.

   a. Both statements are TRUE.
   b. Both statements are FALSE.
   c. The first statement is TRUE, the second is FALSE.
   d. The first statement is FALSE, the second is TRUE.

7. The profile of dental plaque changes after periodontal debridement.
   It becomes a mixed flora of mostly gram-negative species.

   a. Both statements are TRUE.
   b. Both statements are FALSE.
   c. The first statement is TRUE, the second is FALSE.
   d. The first statement is FALSE, the second is TRUE.

8. The periodontium can be accurately probed about how long after nonsurgical periodontal therapy?

   a. 4 to 6 days
   b. 4 to 6 weeks
   c. 1 to 2 days
   d. 1 to 2 weeks

9. Powered scalers appear to be about equal in their abilities to remove plaque and calculus BECAUSE they all operate effectively at the same frequency.

   a. Both the statement and the reason are correct and related.
   b. Both the statement and the reason are correct but NOT related.
   c. The statement is correct, but the reason is NOT.
   d. The statement is NOT correct, but the reason is correct.
   e. Neither the statement NOR the reason is correct.

10. The cornerstone of long-term and short-term goals of periodontal therapy is:

    a. complete calculus removal
    b. effective plaque control
    c. ultrasonic scaling
    d. universal infection control

SHORT ANSWER

11. Describe the difference between scaling and root planing.

    _____

    _____

12. Compare the short- and long-term goals of nonsurgical therapy.

_____

_____

13. According to the hydrodynamic theory, what causes dentin to become sensitive?

_____

_____

14. List the products that can be used to provide relief of dental sensitivity after non-surgical periodontal therapy.

_____

_____

15. Is ultrasonic instrumentation as effective as hand instrumentation in detoxifying root surfaces?

_____

_____

REFERENCES

1. Lindhe J. Textbook of Clinical Periodontology. Philadelphia: WB Saunders; 1983:327-352.
2. Carranza FA. The treatment plan. In FA Carranza and MG Newman, eds. Clinical Periodontology, 8th ed. WB Saunders; 1996:399-400.
3. Wilkins EM. Clinical Practice of the Dental Hygienist. Philadelphia: Lea & Febiger; 1989:292
4. Stutsman-Young N, O'Hehir TE, Woodall I. Periodontal debridement. In Comprehensive Dental Hygiene Care, 4th ed. St. Louis: Mosby-Year Book, 1993:553-570.
5. Ad hoc Committee to Revise the Glossary of Periodontic Terms. Glossary of Periodontal Terms, 3rd ed. Chicago: American Academy of Periodontology, 1992.
6. Carranza FA Jr, Perry DA. Clinical Periodontology for the Dental Hygienist. Philadelphia: WB Saunders, 1986:222.
7. Allen DL, McFall WT Jr, Jenzano J. Periodontics for the Dental Hygienist. Philadelphia: Lea & Febiger, 1987:280.
8. Armitage GC. Biologic Basis of Periodontal Maintenance Therapy. Berkeley: Praxis, 1980:33-115.
9. Wilkins EM. Clinical Practice of the Dental Hygienist, 4th ed. Lea and Febiger, St Louis; 1976:214.
10. Cobb CM. Non-surgical pocket therapy: mechanical. Ann Periodontol 1996;1:443-490.
11. Löe H, Theilade E, Jensen SB. Experimental gingivitis in man. J Periodontol 1965;36:177-187.
12. Loesche WJ. The bacterial etiology of periodontal disease: the specific plaque hypothesis. In Clark JW, ed. Clinical Dentistry. Philadelphia: JB Lippincott, 1987:1-11.
13. Sanz M, Newman MG, Nissengard R. Periodontal microbiology. In Carranza FA, Glickman's Clinical Periodontology. Philadelphia: WB Saunders, 7th ed. 1990:342-372.
14. Greenstein G. Periodontal response to mechanical nonsurgical therapy: a review. J Periodontal 1992;63:118-130.
15. Thornton S, Garnick J. Comparison of ultrasonic to hand instruments in the removal of subgingival plaque. J Periodontol 1982;53:34-37.
16. Ciancio S. Non-surgical periodontal treatment. In Nevins M, Becker W, Kornman K, eds. Proceedings of the World Workshop in Clinical Periodontics. Chicago: American Academy of Periodontology, 1989:II-1-II-20.
17. Rawlinson A, Walsh TF. Rationale and techniques of non-surgical pocket management in periodontal therapy. Br Dent J 1993;174:161-166.
18. Kepic TJ, O'Leary TJ, Kafrawy AH. Total calculus removal: an attainable objective? J Periodontol 1990; 61:16-20.
19. Stambaugh RV, Dragoo M, Smith DM, Carasali L. The limits of subgingival scaling. Int J Periodont Res Dent 1981;1:30-41.
20. Ramfjord SP. Long-term assessment of periodontal surgery versus curettage or scaling and root planing. Int J Technol Assess Health Care 1990;6:392-402.
21. Nyman R, Westfelt E, Sarhed G, Karring T. Role of "diseased" root cementum in healing following treatment of periodontal disease: a clinical study. J Clin Periodontol 1988;15:464-468.
22. Kalkwarf KL. Tissue attachment. In Nevins M, Becker W, Kornman K, eds. Proceedings of the World Workshop in Clinical Periodontics. Chicago: American Academy of Periodontology, 1989:V-1-V-21.
23. Carranza FA. Gingival curettage. In FA Carranza and MG Newman eds. Clinical Periodontology, 8th ed. WB Saunders, Philadelphia; 1996:584-592.
24. Yukna RA. A clinical and histological study of healing following the excisional new attachment procedure in rhesus monkeys. J Periodontol 1976;47:701-709.
25. DeVore CH, Hicks MJ, Whitacre HL, Clancy-Schertel M. Non-surgical gingival curettage in dental hygiene curricula. J Dent Educ 1993;57:762-765.
26. Robertson PB, Buchanan SA. Would healing after periodontal therapy. In Genco RJ, Goldman HM, Cohen DW, eds. Contemporary Periodontics. St. Louis: CV Mosby; 1990:382-393.
27. Baderstein A, Nilveus R, Egelberg J. Effect of non-surgical periodontal therapy: II. Severely advanced periodontitis. J Clin Periodontol 1984;11:63-76.
28. Baderstein A, Nilveus R, Egelberg J. Effect of non-surgical periodontal therapy: IV. Operator variability. J Clin Periodontol 1985;12:190-200.
29. Newbrun E. Dentinal sensitivity. In Wei S, ed. Clinical Uses of Fluorides. Philadelphia: Lea & Febiger, 1985:93-102.
30. Brannstrom M, Linden LA, Astrom A. The hydrodynamics of the dental tubule and of pulp fluid; a discussion of its significance in relation to dentinal sensitivity. Caries Res 1967;1:310-317.
31. Cuenin MF, Scheidt MJ, O'Neal RB, Strong SL, Pashley DH, Horner JA, Van Dyke TE. An in vivo study of dentin sensitivity: the relation of dentin sensitivity and the patency of dentin tubules. J Periodontol 1991;62:668-673.
32. Fischer C, Wennberg A, Fischer RG, Attstrom R. Clinical evaluation of pulp and dentine sensitivity after supragingival and subgingival scaling. Endodontic Dent Traumatol 1991;7:259-263.
33. Haugen E, Johansen JR. Tooth hypersensitivity after periodontal treatment: a case report including SEM studies. J Clin Periodontol 1988;15:399-401.
34. Pashley DH, Galloway SE. The effects of oxalate treatment on the smear layer of ground surfaces of human dentine. Arch Oral Biol 1985;30:731-737.
35. Absi EG, Addy M, Adams D. Dentine hypersensitivity:

the effect of toothbrushing and dietary compounds on dentine in vitro: an SEM study. J Oral Rehabil 1992;19:101–110.

36. Pashley DH, Leibach JG, Horner JA. The effects of burnishing NaF/kaolin/glycerin paste on dentin permeability. J Periodontol 1987;58:19–23.

37. Zaimoglu A, Ayden AK. An evaluation of smear layer with various desensitizing agents after tooth preparation. J Prosthet Dent 1992;68:450–457.

38. Kerns DG, Scheidt MJ, Pashley DH, Horner JA, Strong SL, Van Dyke TE. Dentinal tubule occlusion and root hypersensitivity. J Periodontol 1991;62:421–428.

39. Dragolich WE, Pashley DH, Brennan WA, O'Neal RB, Horner JA, Van Dyke TE. An in vitro study of dentinal tubule occlusion by ferric oxalate. J Periodontol 1993;64:1045–1051.

40. Tarbet WJ, Silverman G, Fratarcangelo PA, Kanapka JA. Home treatment for dentinal hypersensitivity: a comparative study. J Am Dent Assoc 1982;105:227–230.

41. Carranza FA. General principles of periodontal surgery. In FA Carranza and MG Newman, eds. Clinical Periodontology, 8th ed. WB Saunders, Philadelphia, 1996: 569–578.

42. Pearce NX, Addy M, Newcombe RG. Dentine hypersensitivity: a clinical trial to compare 2 strontium desensitizing toothpastes with a conventional fluoride toothpaste. J Periodontol 1994;65:113–119.

43. Baderstein A, Nilveus R, Egelberg J. Effect of non-surgical periodontal therapy: VIII. Probing attachment changes related to clinical characteristics. J Clin Periodontol 1987;14:425–432.

44. Claffey N, Loos B, Gantes B, Martin M, Egelberg J. Probing depth at re-evaluation following initial periodontal therapy to indicate the initial response to treatment. J Clin Periodontol 1989;16:229–233.

45. Baderstein A, Nilveus R, Egelberg J. Effect of non-surgical periodontal therapy: VII. Bleeding, suppuration, and probing depth in sites with probing attachment loss. J Clin Periodontol 1985;12:432–440.

46. Baderstein A, Nilveus R, Egelberg J. Scores of plaque, bleeding, suppuration and probing depth to predict probing attachment loss: 5 years of observation following nonsurgical periodontal therapy. J Clin Periodontol 1990;17:102–107.

47. McCall JO. The evolution of the scaler and its influence on development of periodontia. J Periodontol 1939;10:69–81.

48. Fales MH. History of periodontology and the role of the dental hygienist. In DA Perry, PL Beemsterboer, and EJ Taggant, eds. Periodontology for the Dental Hygienist. WB Saunders, Philadelphia, 1996:1–18.

49. Nagy RJ, Otomo-Corgel J, Stambaugh R. The effectiveness of scaling and root planing with curets designed for deep pockets. J Periodontol 1992;63:954–959.

50. Fleischer HC, Mellonig JT, Brayer WK, Gray JL, Barnett JD. Scaling and root planing efficacy in multirooted teeth. J Periodontol 1989;60:402–409.

51. Flemmig TF, Petersilka GJ, Mehl A, Hickel R, and Klaiber B. Working parameter of a magnetostrictive ultrasonic scaler influencing root substance removal in vitro. J Periodontol 1998;69:547–553.

52. Jotikasthira NE, Lie T, Leknes KN. Comparative in vitro studies of sonic, ultrasonic and reciprocating scaling instruments. J Clin Periodontol 1992;19:560–569.

53. Brieninger DR, O'Leary TJ, Blumenshine RVH. Comparative effectiveness of ultrasonic and hand scaling for the removal of subgingival plaque and calculus. J Periodontol 1987;58:9–18.

54. Nosal G, Scheidt MJ, O'Neal R, Van Dyke TE. The penetration of lavage solution into the periodontal pocket during ultrasonic instrumentation. J Periodontol 1991;62:554–557.

55. Checchi L, Pelliccioni GA. Hand versus ultrasonic instrumentation in the removal of endotoxins from root surfaces in vitro. J Periodontol 1988;59:398–402.

56. Smart GJ, Wilson M, Davies EH, Kieser JB. The assessment of ultrasonic root surface debridement by determination of residual endotoxin levels. J Clin Periodontol 1990;17:174–178.

57. Dragoo MR. A clinical evaluation of hand and ultrasonic instruments on subgingival debridement: Part 1. With unmodified and modified ultrasonic inserts. Int J Periodontics Restorative Dent 1992;12:310–323.

58. Suppipat N. Ultrasonics in periodontics. J Clin Periodontol 1974;1:206–213.

59. Baderstein A, Nilveus R, Egelberg J. Effect of nonsurgical periodontal therapy: I. Moderately advanced periodontitis. J Clin Periodontol 1981;8:57–72.

60. Adams D, Fulford N, Beechy J, MacCarthy J, Stephens M. The cardiac pacemaker and ultrasonic scalers. Br Dent J 1982;152:171–174.

61. Council on Dental Materials and Equipment. Status report on professional scaling and stain-removal devices. J Am Dent Assoc 1985;111:801–802.

62. Barnes JB, Harrel SK, and Rivera-Hidalgo F. Blood contamination of the aerosols produced by in vivo use of ultrasonic scalers. J Periodontol 1998;69:434–438.

63. Fine DH, Mendieta C, Barnett ML, Furgang D, Meyers R, Olshan A, Vincent J. Efficacy of preprocedural rinsing with an antiseptic in reducing viable bacteria in dental aerosols. J Periodontol 1992;63:821–824.

64. Harrel SK, Barnes JB, and Rivera-Hidalgo F. Reduction of aerosols produced by ultrasonic scalers. J Periodontol 1996;67:28–32.

65. King TB, Muzzin KB, Berry CW, and Anders LM. The effectiveness of an aerosol reduction device for ultrasonic scalers. J Periodontol 1997;68:45–59.

66. Rivera-Hidalgo F, Barnes JB, and Harrel SK. Aerosol and splatter production by focused spray and standard ultrasonic inserts. J Periodontol 1999;70:473–477.

67. Checchi L, Pelliccioni Ga, D'Achille C. Sharpening of ultrasonic scalers. J Clin Periodontol 1991;18:505–507.

68. Lavespere JE, Yukna RA, Rice DA, and LeBlanc DM. Root surface removal with diamond-coated ultrasonic instruments: an in vitro and SEM study. J Periodontol 1996;67:1281–1287.

69. Greenstein G. Subgingival irrigation: an adjunct to periodontol therapy. Current status and future directions. J Dent Hyg 1990;64:389–397.

70. Greenstein G. Effects of subgingival irrigation on periodontal status. J Periodontol 1988;58:827–836.

71. Shiloah J, Hovious A. The role of subgingival irrigations in the treatment of periodontitis. J Periodontol 1993;64:835–843.

72. Christersson LA, Norderyd OM, Puchalsky CS. Topical application of tetracycline -HCL in human periodontitis. J Clin Periodontol 1993;47:88–95.

73. Barkmeier WW, Jabro MH, Latta MA. Scanning electron microscopic analysis of the local effects of a periodontal scaling gel on selected surfaces. J Clin Dent 1992;3:39–42.

74. Jabro MH, Barkmeier WW, Latta MA. A clinical evaluation of the effects of a periodontal scaling gel. J Clin Dent 1992;3:42–46.

75. Smith SR, Foyle DM, Daniels J. An evaluation of a pre-scaling gel (Sofscale) on the ease of supragingival calculus removal. J Clin Periodontol 1994;21:562–564.

76. Nagy RJ, Endow JP, Inouye AE, and Otomo-Corgel J. The effects of a single course of a calculus-softening scaling and root planing gel: a scanning electron microscopic study. J Periodontol 1998;69:806–811.

13

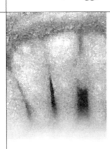

Edward J. Taggart / Dorothy A. Perry

Periodontal Surgery

Chapter Objectives

1. Describe the rationale for periodontal surgical treatment.
2. Identify the role of the dental hygienist in the surgical treatment of periodontal diseases.
3. Recognize the clinical conditions that are most likely to benefit from periodontal surgery.
4. List and define the types of periodontal surgery.

Key Terms

Access to root surfaces
Excisional periodontal surgery
Guided tissue regeneration
Horizontal bone loss
Incisional periodontal surgery
Infrabony pockets
Intrabony pockets
Mucogingival surgery
Osseous defects
Osseous surgery

Periodontal pack
Periodontal flap surgery
Pocket elimination surgery
Pocket reduction surgery
Postoperative instructions
Postoperative procedures
Regeneration surgery
Suprabony pockets
Vertical bone loss

Periodontal surgery has been used since early in the 20th century to help dentists to control the progression of periodontal disease. Although advances in root instrumentation techniques and antibiotic therapy have improved the available treatment modalities for periodontal infections, periodontal surgery will continue to be a necessary procedure in the foreseeable future. It is important for the dental hygienist to understand the indications for and contraindications to basic periodontal surgical procedures and to advise patients of the potential therapies available. In many situations, the dental hygienist is the best therapist to discuss the options for periodontal surgery and alert the dentist to the possible need for surgical intervention.

RATIONALE FOR PERIODONTAL SURGERY

Periodontal surgery is indicated to control the progress of periodontal destruction and attachment loss when more conservative non-surgical treatment is not sufficient. The definition of nonsurgical treatment in dentistry is perhaps a misnomer. Surgery is often defined as the practice of treating diseases by instrumentation or manual operations. By this definition, almost all dental procedures would be defined as surgery. Dentists often limit the definition of surgery to cutting procedures with sharp instruments, especially scalpels or knives. Even by this definition, most periodontal therapy qualifies as surgery because sharp scalers and curettes cut both hard and soft tissues in the periodontal environment. Scaling and root planing result in intentional cutting of the root surfaces and inadvertent cutting of the surrounding soft tissues. However, they are considered part of non-surgical periodontal therapy. This chapter limits the definition of periodontal surgery to techniques that intentionally cut into soft tissues to control disease or change the size and shape of tissues.

Periodontal educators have identified a number of goals for periodontal surgery.[1] These goals are defined in Goals for Periodontal Surgery.

All of these goals are valid reasons for recommending periodontal surgery. Tissue regeneration and dental implant surgeries have been developed in recent years to supplement the other established procedures. These newer procedures more predictably regenerate periodontal tissues that are lost to disease and permit the placement of secure prostheses to replace missing teeth.

GOALS FOR PERIODONTAL SURGERY

Pocket reduction
Drainage of periodontal abscesses
Correction of a mucogingival defect
Esthetic improvement
Providing access for restorative dental procedures
Regeneration of tissue lost because of disease
Placement of dental implants

Adapted with permission from Ramfjord SP and Ash MN. Periodontology and Periodontics. Philadelphia: WB Saunders, 1979.

Advantages of Periodontal Surgery

The major benefit and indication for periodontal surgery as an adjunct to periodontal treatment is to gain **access to the root surface** for scaling and root planing. It also improves access for patient plaque control. Periodontal surgery results in better access to furcations, complex root surfaces, and **infrabony pockets** (those apical to the crest of bone), areas that are the most difficult to treat by scaling and root planing. Improving access for plaque control by the patient may require removing tissues or bony forms that block the patient from adequately removing as much plaque as necessary to control the disease. Other advantages of periodontal surgery include improved access to periodontal abscesses to obtain drainage and the ability to expose root surfaces for restorative dentistry. In addition, numerous new techniques are being used to improve patient esthetics by altering the position of the gingival margin.

Disadvantages of Periodontal Surgery

There are a number of disadvantages and contraindications to periodontal surgery. These include the health status or age of the patient as well as specific limitations for each of the periodontal surgical procedures. From the patient's perspective, the disadvantages of surgery are usually limited to time, cost, esthetics, and discomfort.

The dental hygienist is in the unique position to discuss all of these concerns with the patient before periodontal surgery is performed. The hygienist is often involved with ongoing maintenance procedures and is well known to the patient or has developed a good rapport with the patient while performing nonsurgical periodontal procedures. By being involved in the patient's decision-making process, the hygienist contributes to the patient's understanding and acceptance of the proposed surgical procedure. This contribution may be helpful to the patient in maintaining the teeth.

GENERAL CONSIDERATIONS FOR PERIODONTAL SURGERY

Several things must be considered when prescribing periodontal surgical therapy. The periodontist usually makes a final decision to proceed with periodontal surgery after sufficient time is allowed for healing after the non-surgical procedures, at least four weeks. The amount of pocket reduction that is observed after these procedures indicates the extent of surgical procedures still required. The patient's concerns and fears must also be considered and the patient fully informed of all factors related to the surgical treatment plan, including what to expect during the procedure and healing process. In prescribing periodontal surgery, the periodontist carefully considers probing pocket depth, the amount of bone loss, the importance of the tooth to function and esthetics, and the patient's level of plaque control, age, and health.[2]

Probing Pocket Depth

A periodontal pocket is a deepened gingival sulcus with a root surface infected with plaque, covered by an ulcerated epithelial surface and having underlying inflamed connective tissue. The pocket is bound coronally by the gingival margin, on one side by the root surface, on the other side by the epithelial surface, and at the base by the junctional epithelium. Studies have shown that scaling and root planing are effective in controlling periodontal disease to probing depths of about 4 mm.[3] Pockets deeper than 5 mm are difficult to instrument and therefore often remain infected even after the best dental hygiene care. Pockets with probing depths greater than 9 mm suggest extreme loss of attachment, which makes the long-term prognosis for retaining the affected teeth poor. Therefore, periodontal surgery is most successful when treating periodontal pockets with probing depths of 5 to 9 mm.

It is important to remember that probing pocket depth is not always equal to clinical attachment loss. The probing depth is the measurement from the crest of the gingival margin to the base of the pocket. The deeper the probing depth, the more difficult is the complete removal of calculus. Therefore, the indication for periodontal surgery is stronger. Attachment loss, rather than probing depth, is measured from the cementoenamel junction to the base of the pocket. If the gingival margin is on the root surface, as when there has been recession, the attachment loss is greater than the probing depth. If the gingival margin is on the enamel surface of the crown, as in gingival hypertrophy, then the attachment loss is less than the probing depth. Attachment loss represents bone destruction, which in turn affects the long-term prognosis of the tooth. The concepts of probing depth and clinical attachment loss are discussed in Chapter 9.

Although surgery may be needed to treat pockets deeper than 5 mm, not all of these pockets require surgery. The 5 mm guideline is only the first step in identifying patients who may be helped by periodontal surgery. Patients with moderate pocket depths of 5 to 6 mm may be monitored with a "wait and see" approach to determine whether nonsurgical periodontal therapy and careful maintenance are adequate. If there is no progression of the periodontal disease in these cases, then periodontal surgery is not necessary.

It is not always safe to wait and see. If the periodontal disease progresses and more attachment loss results, the prognosis for a tooth may become worse. Also, probing measurements are inexact. Measurements may differ by as much as 1 mm because of variations in probing technique. Therefore, to be sure that the disease is progressing, a 2 mm increase in probing depth (and thus bone loss) must be observed over time. If surgery is postponed, the dentist (and patient) must be willing to risk this 2 mm bone loss.[4]

Bone Loss

The base of the periodontal pocket is not at the level of the crest of the alveolar bone. There is usually 1 to 2 mm of connective tissue attachment between the probing depth and the alveolar bone.[5] This area is termed the biologic width and must be considered when estimating the amount of attachment remaining on a periodontally involved tooth.

Bone loss caused by periodontal disease results in **osseous defects.** These may occur in either a horizontal dimension, where the bone resorbs equally on the mesial and distal surfaces of the teeth (Figure 13-1), or a vertical dimen-

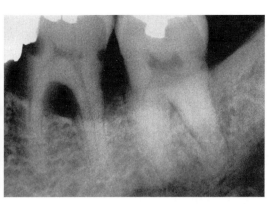

FIGURE 13–1. Horizontal bone loss around the mandibular molars. Obvious furcation involvement of the first molar and cervical caries is seen at the mesial and distal cementoenamel junction of the first molar. (Courtesy of UCSF Division of Periodontology.)

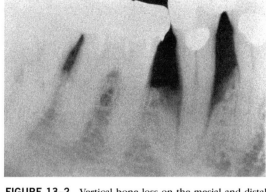

FIGURE 13–2. Vertical bone loss on the mesial and distal surfaces of the mandibular second premolar. Although there has been some horizontal bone loss on the adjacent teeth, the bone level is reduced on the premolar, resulting in infrabony pockets.

sion, where the resorption is unequal (Figure 13-2). Pockets that are coronal to **horizontal bone loss** are often called **suprabony**, whereas those that extend apically beyond the crest of the bone are called **infrabony pockets**.

Vertical bone loss may also occur in a variety of configurations that are usually described by the number of bony walls remaining. When the walls of the osseous defect are within the bone housing, they may be termed intrabony defects (Figure 13-3).

The amount of bone remaining around a tooth is an important consideration in the decision to perform periodontal surgery. Large amounts of bone supporting a tooth may allow the clinician to take a wait-and-see approach to postpone or avoid periodontal surgery. However, if the amount of bone is already reduced, delaying periodontal surgery may radically de-

crease the prognosis for the tooth (Figure 13-4).

Periodontal surgery that includes modification of the bone level or shape is called **osseous surgery**. The amount of bone remaining is important in determining whether periodontal surgery will be beneficial. If too much bone has been lost through disease or so much bone must be removed during surgery that the tooth will be weakened, osseous surgery becomes a less attractive option for treatment. Other procedures, such as grafting or regeneration techniques, may be required. Generally, osseous surgery is indicated when at least half of the bone remains to support the tooth (Figure 13-5).

Value of the Tooth

Not all teeth have equal value when periodontal surgery is considered for a patient. Some peri-

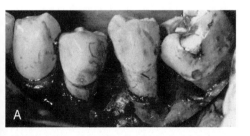

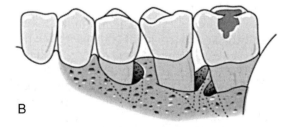

FIGURE 13–3. Intrabony defects. **A.** A two-wall defect on the distal aspect of the first premolar, a one-wall defect on the distal aspect of the second premolar, and a three-wall defect on the mesial aspect of the first molar are evident in this photograph. **B.** The diagram shows the remaining walls of bone around the periodontal pockets. The two-wall defect on the first premolar shows bone destroyed on the distal root surface and the buccal alveolar process. Two bony walls remain. The one-wall defect on the second premolar shows bone destroyed on the distal root surface and both the buccal and the lingual alveolar process. One wall remains. The three-wall defect on the mesial aspect of the molar shows bone destroyed on the root surface, but the alveolar process remains. Three walls of bone also remain.

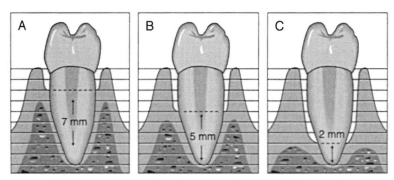

FIGURE 13–4. Prognosis based on amount of bone loss. **A.** When some bone loss is present, it may be safe to postpone surgery, to take a wait and see approach. An additional bone loss of 2 mm may not alter the prognosis of the tooth. **B.** When half of the bone has been lost, an additional 2-mm loss can seriously jeopardize the tooth; therefore, surgery is highly recommended. **C.** With advanced bone loss, surgery may be performed in an effort to save the tooth, but the prognosis is poor.

odontally involved teeth cannot be saved, and others are not worth making heroic attempts to treat. Third molars, for example, may not be in good positions for mastication, and they may be extracted without altering the patient's chewing pattern. An abutment tooth for a functioning fixed bridge, however, can be important to the patient, and often every attempt to salvage a particular tooth through periodontal surgery is strongly indicated.

Personal Plaque Control of the Patient

The progression of periodontal disease may increase after periodontal surgery if plaque is not adequately controlled.[6] Therefore, every patient should have the best possible supragingival plaque control established before surgical therapy is initiated. If plaque control is poor, surgical intervention should be postponed or abandoned because it will not prevent the recurrence of periodontal infection and the possible loss of teeth.

Age and Health of the Patient

Patients who are in poor health are not good candidates for periodontal surgery. However, the periodontal disease may contribute to the poor general physical condition, and the periodontist may decide, in concert with the patient's physician, that periodontal surgery is appropriate. Older patients usually heal as well as younger patients after periodontal surgery, so age in itself is not a contraindication to surgery. The patient's age is a significant factor when considering the progress of the periodontal disease. Patients with pocket depths exceeding 5 mm and half of their supporting bone lost who are relatively young (younger than 30 years of age) have an aggressive form of periodontal disease, such as early-onset periodontitis. Surgery is strongly indicated to control this infec-

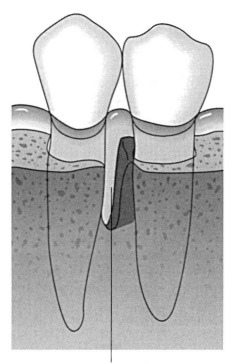

Infrabony pocket

FIGURE 13–5. Bone loss during periodontal surgery. The shaded portion shows bone that would need to be removed during surgery to eliminate the bony defect. However, this bone removal would substantially weaken the adjacent tooth, which is a consideration in planning the surgery.

tion. Older patients (older than 60 years of age) with the same clinical conditions, however, usually have a more slowly progressing disease. Surgery may be less critical for these patients. It is important to remember that the human life span is increasing. Periodontal surgery, if strongly indicated, should not be denied a patient just because of advanced age. The quality of life of older patients may be significantly improved by controlling periodontal disease and retaining the dentition.

Patient Preference

Some patients are reluctant to have periodontal surgery, no matter how strong the indications may be. It is important for the patient to know all of the ramifications of delaying recommended periodontal surgery and the possible effects on the long-range prognosis of the teeth. All patients must be appraised of the alternatives, risks, and benefits of every dental procedure before deciding whether to undergo periodontal surgery. The architecture of gingival tissues resulting after periodontal surgery is more conducive to plaque control and maintenance. Patients who decide not to have surgery must be willing to undergo more frequent periodontal maintenance procedures and perform more complex subgingival plaque control in an effort to slow the progress of their disease.

TYPES OF PERIODONTAL SURGERY

Many methods of classifying periodontal surgery have been described. One approach is to name the procedure for the clinician who first described it, for example, the Widman flap. Another approach is to describe how the procedure is performed, as with gingivectomy, which means to remove the gingiva. A convenient classification of periodontal surgical procedures into five basic categories was proposed by Lang and Löe.[7]

1. Procedures for **pocket reduction** or **elimination**.
2. Procedures for **access to the root surface**.
3. Procedures for treatment of **osseous defects**.

4. Procedures for correcting mucogingival defects.
5. Procedures for new attachment.

Procedures for Pocket Reduction or Elimination

The goal of these procedures is to reduce periodontal pocket depth by removing soft tissues to a level at which plaque control and maintenance procedures are effective, usually not exceeding 3 to 4 mm in depth. Methods for pocket reduction include **excisional** (gingivectomy) and **incisional** (flap) **periodontal surgery**.

EXCISIONAL PERIODONTAL SURGERY

Excisional periodontal surgery removes the excess tissue from the wall of the periodontal pocket. It is useful for the rapid reduction of gingival pockets. The most basic excisional surgical procedures are termed gingivectomy, meaning excision of the gingiva; or gingivoplasty, meaning surgical reshaping of the gingival tissues. In practice, both procedures are often performed in combination. Gingivectomy is a reasonably simple surgical procedure and is usually the first consideration for pocket reduction. However, contraindications to gingivectomy are numerous, and there are relatively few instances in which gingivectomy is the sole therapy required. It is often performed with a special set of surgical instruments, although standard scalpel blades and electrosurgical devices may also be used. Recently, dental laser equipment has become popular for gingivectomy.

Indications. The presence of deep periodontal pockets with fibrous tissue is the major indication for gingivectomy. Drug-induced gingival hyperplasia is ideally treated by this form of excisional surgery. This condition is often caused by antiseizure medication, such as phenytoin; calcium channel blockers, such as nifedipine; or immunosuppressive drugs, such as cyclosporine. Other indications include familial gingival hyperplasia and localized crown lengthening for restorative dentistry. Periodontal scaling and root planing, complemented by adequate plaque control procedures, should be completed 3 to 6 weeks before the surgery to allow tissues to heal. Often, the need for gingivectomy cannot be determined until tissue shrinkage after scaling and root planing has occurred. Edematous, friable, and hemorrhagic tissues are not easily incised and therefore require adequate healing time after scaling and root planing and before surgery.

Procedure. During gingivectomy, the surgeon marks the bottom of the pockets with a periodontal probe or forceps. The gingiva is excised with knives at a 45° angle to the gingival surface, keeping the incision within the keratinized gingiva. This practice results in a thin tissue margin at the dentogingival junction. After removal of the majority of the gingival tissues, the underlying exposed connective tissue is refined and trimmed with knives, burs, or other instruments. Exposed root surfaces are carefully examined for residual calculus and roughness, and they are cleaned and smoothed as necessary with curettes. Bleeding after surgery is controlled with saline-dampened gauze pads, and the surgical area is packed with a periodontal dressing to reduce postoperative discomfort and protect the sensitive underlying connective tissue. Healing is usually uneventful, and the gingival epithelium is reestablished 2 weeks after surgery (Figure 13-6).

Contraindications. There are many contraindications to excisional surgery. For this reason, it is not the most common technique for periodontal pocket reduction. If the gingival resection leaves a wide wound, healing is relatively slow while the epithelium grows in from the edges of the wound, and there is significant postoperative discomfort. The anatomy of the surrounding area may prevent incising the tissues at the proper angle, or minimal width of attached gingiva may prevent keeping the incision within the keratinized tissue. The inability to access infrabony pockets, those below the crest of the alveolar bone and a common

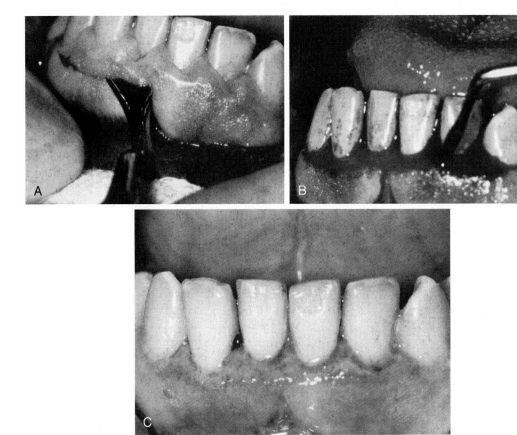

FIGURE 13–6. Gingivectomy procedure, excisional periodontal surgery. **A.** The gingivectomy incision through the keratinized tissue to the root surfaces of the teeth. **B.** The exposed connective tissue is trimmed with a periodontal knife to smooth and shape it to a physiologic form. **C.** Healing of the gingivectomy wound after 1 week. Tissue is beginning to epithelialize by growing in from the margins of the wound.

finding in periodontitis, is perhaps the major contraindication. Gingivectomy also exposes the root surfaces of the teeth, resulting in possibly unacceptable esthetics, and may leave the teeth sensitive to heat and cold and susceptible to root caries (Figure 13-7).

INCISIONAL PERIODONTAL SURGERY

Incisional surgery, commonly called **periodontal flap surgery** or simply, flap surgery, is the procedure of choice when excisional periodontal surgery cannot be performed for pocket reduction. This procedure is called flap surgery because the tissues are pushed away from the underlying tooth roots and alveolar bone, much like the flap of an envelope. Flap surgery includes a variety of techniques for pocket depth reduction. Depending on the clinical circumstances and the preference of the surgeon, the alveolar bone may be resected or modified during the surgical procedure. Flap surgery has fewer contraindications than gingivectomy, so incisional procedures are by far the more common type of surgery performed by periodontists. The usual incisional technique for pocket reduction with flap surgery is called the apically

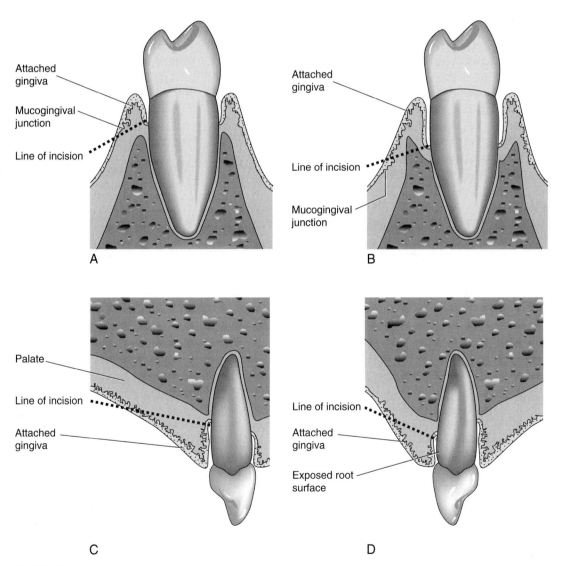

FIGURE 13–7. Contraindications to excisional surgery. **A.** The incision cannot be made entirely through the keratinized gingiva. **B.** Infrabony pockets interfere with the correct line of incision. **C.** Incision would leave a wide wound as indicated on the palatal surface. **D.** Removal of gingiva can expose long root surfaces that may be unsightly to the patient, sensitive to cold, and susceptible to root caries.

positioned flap because the flap is sutured at a more apical location on the tooth roots to reduce pocket depth.

Indications. Deepened periodontal pockets, which are contraindicated for gingivectomy, are the primary indication for incisional surgery. Suprabony pockets are often best treated by flap surgery. However, flap surgery also allows access to infrabony pockets, so the procedure is often combined with other osseous surgery procedures to treat existing bony defects.

Procedure. Pockets are probed to determine their depths, and the bony contours are "sounded" by pushing the periodontal probe through the tissues until the crest of the alveolar bone is detected. The surgeon uses this information to design the incision around the necks of the teeth to retain as much tissue as possible while allowing for pocket reduction. In thick tissues, this incision may be several millimeters away from the root surfaces. Flaps of gingiva are created that are pushed away from the alveolar bone and teeth, usually on the buccal and lingual surfaces, with a periosteal elevator. In this way, the infected epithelium, connective tissue, and granulation tissues can be removed with curettes, scalers, and ultrasonic instruments. The roots are examined for residual calculus and cleaned and smoothed as necessary. The flaps are then readapted at a more apical level to reduce the pockets. At this stage, the surgeon may reduce the bony ledges or may further elevate the flaps past the mucogingival junction to position it for proper adaptation. The surgical wound is closed by suturing the flaps together in the interproximal papillae and closely adapting them around the root surfaces. A periodontal dressing may be applied to help adapt the gingiva to the alveolar bone and assist with pocket reduction by applying pressure to the healing flap (Figure 13-8).

Contraindications. There are few contraindications to periodontal flap surgery beyond those that preclude any periodontal surgical intervention. The gingival tissues must be wide and thick enough to allow proper incision. Often, the incision must be modified to preserve as much tissue as possible. Like excisional surgery, apically positioning the gingival flaps exposes the root surfaces. The positioning may have to be altered or compromised for esthetics

or in caries-prone patients. Fluoride mouth rinses should be recommended for periodontal surgery patients to reduce the potential for root caries.

Special modifications of pocket reduction surgery include combinations of incisional and excisional techniques, such as distal wedge surgery and internal beveled gingivectomy. These techniques are indicated in specific areas, such as the palatal tuberosity region, or where tissues are thick and are not easily managed by one method alone (Figure 13-9).

Procedures for Gaining Access to the Root Surface

The goal of surgical procedures for accessing the root surfaces is to create conditions for reattachment of the gingival tissues to the root. These access procedures include the modified Widman flap,[8] the excisional new attachment procedure,[9] and open-flap curettage.[10] Most of these procedures are similar and differ only in the detail of the techniques. The modified Widman flap, for example, uses three incisions to separate the pocket lining from the tooth in a controlled manner, whereas the excisional new attachment procedure usually does not involve elevating the flap past the mucogingival junction. The goal of all of these procedures is the same: To gain access to the root surface of the teeth roots for plaque and calculus removal, including scaling and root planing. Pocket reduction by apical positioning is not the goal of access flap procedures.

Indications. Access flap procedures are used to treat periodontal pockets in esthetically sensitive areas or where pocket reduction is not desired or indicated. Many periodontists perform access flap procedures instead of pocket reduction procedures because there are few long-term data to show that reducing the pocket depths through surgery extends the life of the teeth.[11]

Procedure. Access flap techniques are similar to pocket reduction flap techniques except that attention is mainly directed at cleaning the root surfaces and preserving as much gingival tissue as possible. Incisions are made through the crest of the gingiva, and the gingival tissues are reflected only far enough to allow the clinician to see the root surfaces and the crest of

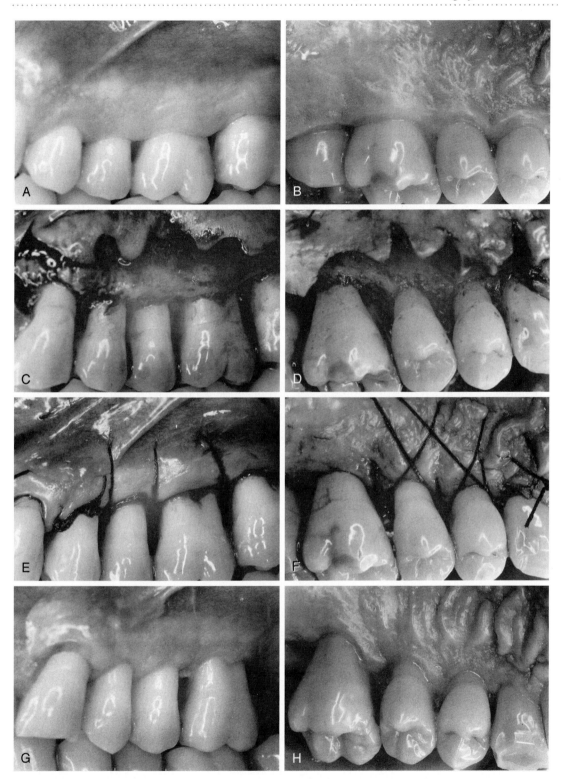

FIGURE 13–8. Apically positioned flap surgery for pocket reduction. **A.** Preoperative appearance of the buccal surface. The probe depths were 6 to 8 mm. **B.** Preoperative appearance of the palatal surface. **C.** Flaps reflected on the buccal surface. **D.** Flap reflected on the palatal surface. **E.** Flaps sutured apically, buccal view. **F.** Flaps sutured apically, palatal view. **G.** Tissues after 6 months of healing, buccal surface. The second molar has been extracted. **H.** Tissues after 6 months of healing, palatal surface. (Courtesy of Philip R. Melnick, DMD.)

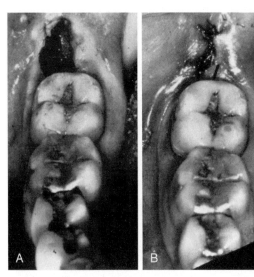

FIGURE 13–9. The distal wedge modification of flap surgery. **A.** A wedge of tissue beneath the separated flaps is removed on the distal aspect of a mandibular second molar. **B.** Flaps sutured to reduce pocket depth.

the alveolar bone. After complete debridement is performed, the gingival flaps are readapted to recover the roots. Although some pocket depth reduction usually occurs through shrinkage after access flap surgery, the major goal is reattachment of the connective tissues to the root surface during healing or creation of a long junctional epithelium resulting in increased attachment for the teeth. (Figure 13–10 also appears in the color supplement).

Contraindications. There are no specific contraindications to access flap procedures. However, the patient should understand that pocket depths may continue to be greater than 3 or 4 mm after therapy.

Procedures for the Treatment of Osseous Defects

Periodontitis, by definition, involves loss of the connective tissue attachment to the root surface of the tooth, with loss of alveolar bone. Often, this bone loss creates osseous defects around teeth that make healing unpredictable and result in gingival architecture that is difficult for the patient to maintain with acceptable plaque control and difficult for the hygienist to maintain with periodic scaling and root planing. During osseous surgical procedures, after reflecting the mucogingival flaps, the periodontist

sculpts the alveolar bone with chisels or specially designed dental burs to remove these osseous defects or allow for apical positioning of the flaps. If alveolar bone is removed that contains periodontal fibers that support the tooth, the procedure is termed ostectomy. If only bony ledges or nonsupporting bone is removed, the procedure is termed osteoplasty.[12] As with other surgical procedures, the two procedures are usually performed together to create a bone form that allows the gingival tissues to follow a positive gingival architecture, one that recreates the anatomic shape of periodontal health and is free from ledges and craters of bone (Figure 13–11).

Indications. Several changes to the bony architecture that result from periodontal infections benefit from reshaping the bone with osseous surgery. A primary indication is periodontal pockets that extend below the level of the osseous crest, or infrabony pockets. Also, thick bony ledges are sometimes encountered during pocket reduction surgery that prevent the gingival flap from being adapted at a more apical level. Reverse alveolar bony architecture, a type of bone loss in which the interproximal bone is apical to the facial and lingual bone (the reverse of the configuration in health), permits periodontal pockets to reform during healing. Correcting this bony deformity is another important indication for osseous surgery (Figure 13–12).

Procedure. After the mucoperiosteal flaps are elevated, bony ledges and craters are modified with burs and chisels to create a positive alveolar form that allows the overlying gingiva to follow a more physiologic contour. If possible, the walls of bony craters are removed with minimal loss of bony attachment. Ledges are thinned and interproximal bony regions fluted to a form that is more generally found in periodontal health.

Contraindications. Many osseous defects do not lend themselves to osseous recontouring. Either the bony defect is too deep to allow removal of the osseous walls or removing bone from one tooth will weaken the adjacent teeth to such an extent that all of them have a reduced long-term prognosis. Areas of severe bone loss are often best treated by reducing

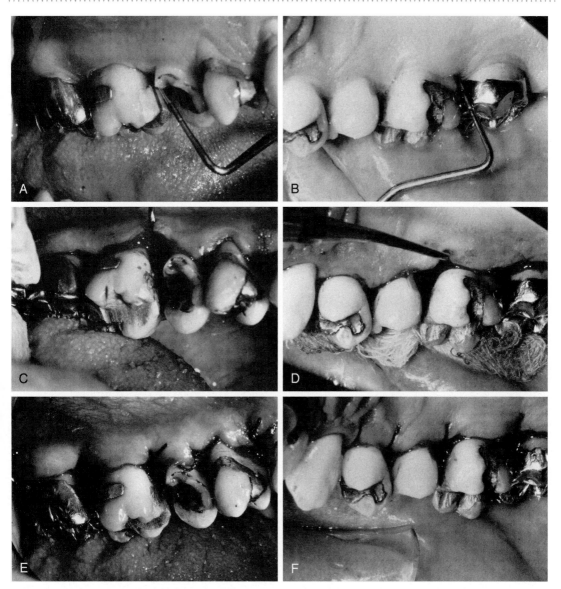

FIGURE 13–10. The modified Widman flap procedure as an example of an access flap. (See color figure.) **A.** Buccal view of the maxillary posterior quadrant. A probe is in place showing a 6-mm pocket on the mesial buccal aspect of the first molar. A fractured buccal cusp is seen on the second premolar. **B.** Palatal view of the same area with a probe in place showing a 7-mm pocket on the distal palatal surface of the first molar. **C.** Buccal view of the access flap, with minimal retraction, exposing the root surfaces for debridement. **D.** Palatal view of the same area, showing access to the root surfaces. **E.** Buccal view after debridement, with flaps approximated with interrupted sutures. Flaps are not apically repositioned. The surgical knots are all on the same side, the buccal side. **F.** Palatal view of the sutured flaps.

Illustration continued on following page

pocket depths and performing frequent maintenance care.

Procedures for Correcting Mucogingival Defects

Periodontal disease often causes deformities in the oral tissues because of the recession of the marginal gingiva and the development of fissures and clefts. Studies show that patients with poor plaque control often have recession associated with inflammation and calculus formation and that recession is a common finding among patients with periodontal disease.[13] Recession can lead to extension of the periodontal pocket beyond the mucogingival junction so that no attached gingiva exists on the tooth

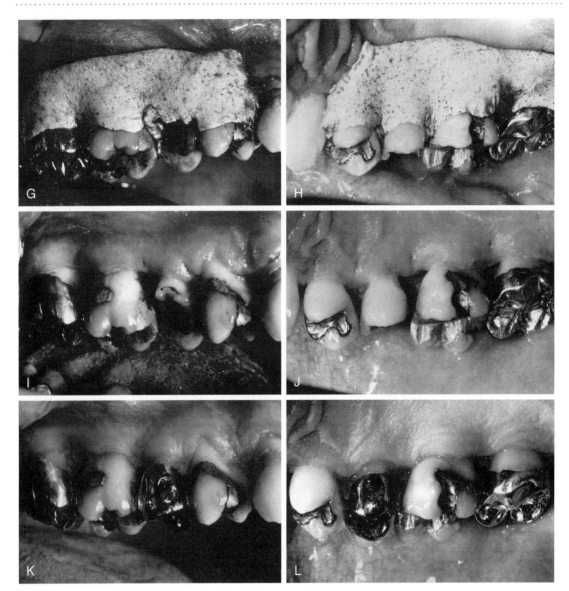

FIGURE 13–10 *Continued.* **G.** Buccal view of a periodontal pack applied over the wound to adapt the flaps to the root surfaces. **H.** Palatal view with a periodontal pack in place. **I.** Buccal view of the surgery area 1 week later, after removal of the sutures and pack. Accumulated plaque and food debris have been removed at the postoperative visit. **J.** Palatal view of healing after 1 week. There are tracks on the gingiva from the sutures, and the interdental papillary areas have not yet regenerated. **K.** Buccal view of the healed surgery site after 3 months. The contour of the interdental papillae is improved, and the second premolar has been restored with a full gold crown. **L.** Palatal view of healing after 3 months shows that the interproximal papillae are not fully recontoured. The healing process can take a year or longer. The patient should undergo supportive periodontal therapy, including 3-month recall scalings and the use of interproximal home care devices, such as the interproximal brush. (Courtesy of James F. Coggan, DDS.)

surface. These areas are called mucogingival defects and have been implicated in the spread of periodontal diseases into deeper tissues, although this role remains controversial. Chapter 9 further describes mucogingival defects.

Mucogingival defects may develop after orthodontic treatment, when the root surface of the tooth is moved through the alveolar bone.

Forceful toothbrushing with a stiff brush used incorrectly has also been implicated, but in these cases, the tissues are healthy and plaque control is often better than average. In addition, some patients appear naturally prone to gingival recession, with no other apparent cause detected.

Mucogingival surgery includes a variety of

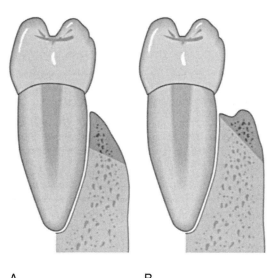

A   B

FIGURE 13–11. Osseous recontouring. **A.** Ostectomy is the removal of supporting bone from the tooth root. The shaded area represents the bone removed. **B.** Osteoplasty is the removal of nonsupporting bone from around the tooth. The shaded area represents the bone removed.

plastic surgery–type procedures to either augment the thickness of keratinized gingival tissues or increase the zone of attached gingiva. Although some authors suggest that a wide band of keratinized tissue is required to prevent further recession and the progression of periodontal disease, this belief is supported by little scientific evidence.[14] However, when plaque control is marginal or when a subgingival crown or filling is planned, most clinicians believe that a broad band of keratinized tissue may help to reduce subsequent inflammation and prevent further recession. Areas of recession are treated by either pedicle grafts or free mucosal grafts, although in recent years, connective tissue grafts have been increasingly used.[15]

Indications. Areas of recession that significantly reduce the width of the keratinized gingiva or have progressed beyond the mucogingival junction should be considered for tissue grafting procedures. Although there is no absolute minimal width of attached gingival tissue, the most often quoted ideal width is 3 mm, particularly if dental restorations will involve manipulation of the gingival tissues.[16] When gingival tissues are thin or receded, mucogingival procedures are sometimes performed before orthodontic tooth movement, although this approach is controversial. Other indications for surgical intervention to control mucogingival problems are broad labial or lingual frenum attachments near the gingival margin that may result in unsightly diastemata, and shallow vestibular depth that must be deepened to improve the fit and retention of removable dental prostheses.

Procedure. The procedures differ depending on the specific mucogingival procedure being considered. The most common procedures are lateral pedicle gingival graft, free autogenous gingival graft, and subgingival connective tissue graft. All of these procedures re-

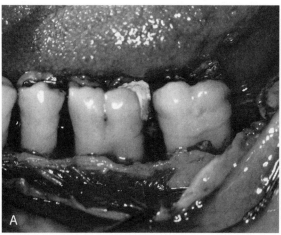
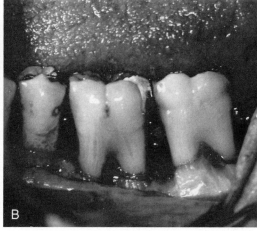

FIGURE 13–12. Reverse bony architecture. **A.** The flap is reflected, showing interproximal bone destroyed to a level apical to the buccal and lingual alveolar processes, reverse bony architecture. **B.** Bone reshaped by osseous surgery to achieve physiologic bone contours, recreating the normal anatomic configuration, which is also termed positive alveolar form or architecture. (Courtesy of Walter W. Fuller, DDS.)

quire access to adequate sites for donor graft tissue before the procedure can be performed. An important consideration in all of these procedures is preparation of the recipient site for the graft. During the surgery, all inflamed tissues should be trimmed from the recipient area, and the root surface to be covered should be root planed free of plaque, calculus, and cementum altered by bacterial endotoxins. Some clinicians have recommended conditioning the root surface with citric acid to denature endotoxins, but this practice has not been well supported by clinical studies. The selection of donor tissue to cover the recipient site is a major consideration. Lateral pedicle grafts, or the sliding of gingival tissue from an adjacent tooth or papilla, have been suggested as the best technique to attempt to cover exposed root surfaces because these grafts bring their blood supply with them. Limitations to pedicle grafts depend largely on the availability of an adequate source of donor tissue adjacent to the area that needs augmentation. The donor pedicle is sharply dissected from the underlying periosteal bed, rotated to the recipient site, and carefully sutured in place.

Free gingival grafts have donor sites located somewhere in the mouth away from the site that requires grafting. The most common site for donor tissue is the palate, but edentulous areas are also used. The recipient site is prepared in a similar manner to the pedicle graft site, and a donor graft of keratinized epithelium with some underlying connective tissue is removed by surgical excision. The graft is sutured in place and held with firm pressure until the initial blood clot forms to stabilize the graft. It is particularly important that the grafted tissue be immobile for the first week after surgery to allow for the establishment of circulation to the grafted tissue. Healing is usually uneventful, with the primary discomfort coming from the donor site where the epithelium has been removed. Postsurgical hemorrhage is a potential problem at the donor site because the epithelium and underlying connective tissue have been removed and no primary wound closure is possible. It must therefore heal by epithelial growth from the edges of the wound (Figure 13-13).

Most recently, grafting of subepithelial connective tissue has become the procedure of choice when root coverage is the objective of mucogingival surgery.[17] Histologic studies of healing free gingival grafts showed that most of the transplanted epithelium in free grafts was lost and that the genetics of the underlying connective tissue determined the potential for keratinization of healing tissue. Therefore, transplanting only the subepithelial connective tissue rather than the connective tissue and its covering epithelium has many advantages. The donor site wound can be primarily closed by suturing the epithelium in place, greatly reducing postoperative discomfort and bleeding. The tissue color and texture of the healed recipient site are more similar to preoperative appearance when the migrating epithelium comes from adjacent to the wound site rather than grafted palatal tissue.

Contraindications. Lack of adequate donor tissue is the major contraindication to mucogingival grafting surgery. Although this situation is less of a problem with connective tissue grafting than with either lateral pedicle grafts or free gingival grafts, there are still situations in which minimal or limited tissue is available. Often, this situation can be circumvented by a combination of procedures, such as first grafting tissue for width followed by a second procedure to provide root coverage.

Procedures for Regeneration of the Periodontium

Regeneration surgery procedures include a variety of surgical techniques that attempt to restore the periodontal tissues lost through disease. By definition, periodontal regeneration is the formation of new alveolar bone, new cementum, and new periodontal ligament on a tooth root surface that was previously diseased.[18] Current techniques include bone grafting and **guided tissue regeneration**. Technically, all types of periodontal treatment, including scaling and root planing, have the potential to yield periodontal regeneration. There is some regeneration of connective tissue and epithelium; however, it is not predictable. This category of surgery is reserved for procedures that increase the predictability of the growth of new tissues of the attachment apparatus.

PERIODONTAL BONE GRAFTING

Transplanting bone to restore that lost from periodontal disease has been attempted for

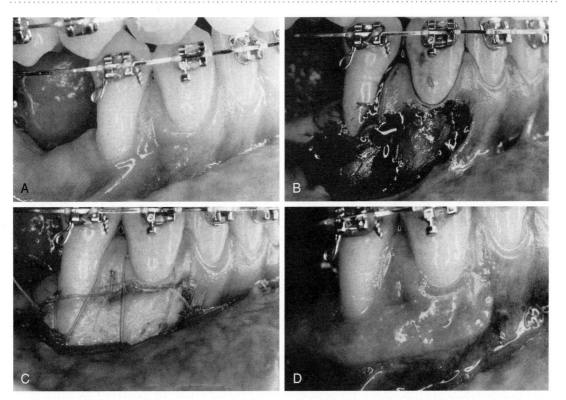

FIGURE 13–13. Free gingival graft to correct a mucogingival defect on orthodontically treated mandibular cuspid and premolar. **A.** Preoperative buccal view of a mucogingival defect. There is a possible contribution of the frenum on the mesial surface of the premolar **B.** A graft bed prepared to expose the connective tissue surface. **C.** A graft of palatal keratinized epithelium sutured in place. **D.** The healed tissue graft. Palatal tissue grafts, when healed, appear lighter than the surrounding gingiva because of the thickness of the palatal tissue. (Courtesy of Philip R. Melnick, DMD.)

many years. Only in the last 20 years has it been a reasonably predictable procedure, and it still has limited success. The classification of periodontal bone grafts is based on the source of graft material.

AUTOGRAFTS

Autografts are created from donor bone from the patient's own body. Bone may be taken from intraoral sites, such as tori, the maxillary tuberosity, or bone removed during osteoplasty. Bone may also come from extraoral sites, such as the iliac crest of the hip or the sternum. Extraoral autogenous bone marrow grafts form large amounts of bone, but problems with obtaining the graft and the possibility of root resorption with fresh bone marrow grafts make them less useful. Intraoral grafts are limited by the small amount of donor material. They have also shown limited osteogenic potential in clinical studies.[19] Still, most surgeons attempt to use as much autogenous bone as possible in an attempt to make bone grafting as biocompatible as possible.

ALLOGRAFTS

Allografts are created from bone that comes from another person. Cadaver bone, obtained from bone banks accredited by the American Association of Tissue Banks, is the most common source of bone allografts used in periodontics. The best clinical results have been obtained with bone that has been freeze-dried and demineralized with hydrochloric acid. The acid decalcification appears to unmask bone morphogenic protein, which some authorities suggest increases the osteogenic potential of the graft. Importantly, acid demineralization appears to reduce the risk of disease transmission from the deceased bone donor to the periodontal patient.[20]

ALLOPLASTS

Alloplastic grafts use a variety of synthetic bone minerals. They may be made of hydroxyapatite mineral or ceramics, such as plaster of Paris and tricalcium phosphate. The most successful material appears to be porous hydroxyapatite, although histologic evidence suggests that it functions as a nonirritating filler rather than promoting new bone formation.[21]

XENOGRAFTS

Xenografts are created from bone taken from another species, such as bovine (cow) or porcine (pig). Tissues from non-human species have strong antigenic reactions with human graft recipients. Until recently, the most successful use of these materials has been as fillers for large osseous defects, using graft material with all organic tissue chemically removed.

A unique approach to periodontal regeneration has been the introduction of a xenograph of enamel matrix graft material derived from the enamel organ of the pig. The graft material contains amelogenin, a protein expressed by Hertwig epithelial sheath during tooth development that stimulates growth of the roots of teeth. Amelogenin is found in man and other mammals. Purified amelogenin has been demonstrated to produce new cementum attached to dentin in animal experiments and to stimulate bone growth.[22] Subsequent application of this material to periodontal defects has demonstrated that this enamel matrix protein results in regeneration of bone. The substance has been shown to produce more bone growth in humans than standard periodontal surgical debridement.[23] Although no study has demonstrated that this material is superior to other regeneration materials such as freeze-dried decalcified bone allograft, it is much easier to use and does not require the use of a barrier membrane as required in guided tissue regeneration[24] (see the following section).

Another novel approach to bone grafting using genetically engineered synthetic collagen has recently been introduced. The material is an anorganic (all organic tissue removed) bovine xenograft that has been coated with a laboratory synthesized human peptide. The peptide is related to the biologically active locus of human type I collagen, which is the area of the cell that stimulates cell differentiation. This increases the potential for bone to grow and provides scaffolding for cell attachment. This effect increases the predictability of bone growth and periodontal regeneration.[25] Controlled clinical trials of this material demonstrated that this grafting material is superior to freeze-dried decalcified bone allografts and anorganic bone xenografts without the peptide.[26]

Clearly, the advent of genetic engineering of human tissues and cell cultural cloning techniques will define the future of periodontal wound healing. It is anticipated that great strides will be made in graft techniques in the near future. More predictable, simpler, and less invasive periodontal regeneration procedures will be possible with improvements in biotechnology.

Indications. Bone grafting can be attempted in infrabony defects that show a potential for regeneration. These are usually defects with sufficient osseous walls to promote healing, ideally three-wall defects. Furcation defects, particularly those of grade II (not through-and-through), are often good candidates for bone regeneration with osseous grafts.

Procedure. As with all periodontal procedures, meticulous root debridement of the surgical site is imperative. Full-thickness mucoperiosteal flaps are elevated and all granulation tissues removed with curettes. The bone graft material is prepared according to the distributor's instructions or harvested from the donor site and inserted into the defects. The best results appear to be obtained with primary closure of the flaps over the wound site (Figure 13-14).

Contraindications. There are no specific contraindications to bone fill procedures. The most predictable bone fills occur in clinical cases that have a maximum number of bony walls, improving the chances of success. Some authors believe that root surface demineralization with citric acid may increase success by detoxifying the root surface and exposing collagen fibrils in the cementum.[27] Others have suggested that root surface conditioning with fibronectin, a molecule that promotes connective tissue growth, increases regeneration. Although promising, these procedures have not shown significant improvement in clinical trials.[28]

GUIDED TISSUE REGENERATION

Another development in periodontics in the last decade has been the concept of guided tissue regeneration, or healing by selected cell repopulation. There had been speculation for many years that if the right cells were allowed to grow (and the wrong cells inhibited) in a healing periodontal wound site, the potential

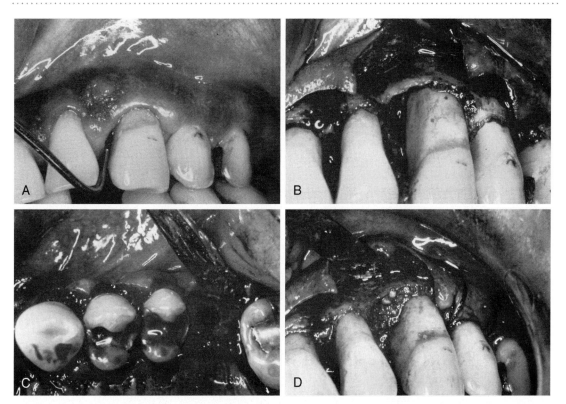

FIGURE 13–14. Bone graft surgery. **A.** Preoperative facial view of a 9-mm pocket on the mesial aspect of the maxillary cuspid. **B.** The flap is reflected, showing a three-wall intrabony defect on the mesial aspect. Calculus and a roughened root surface are seen in the deep pocket. **C.** Autograft bone harvested from the site of the missing first molar. **D.** Autograph bone transplanted to the cuspid bony defect.

Illustration continued on following page

for regeneration, or growth of a new attachment apparatus, would exist.[29] In a series of well-controlled experiments, researchers have produced new periodontal ligament, alveolar bone, and cementum on previously diseased root surfaces by selectively excluding gingival epithelial cells and fibroblasts. This technique permits the primary healing cells to proliferate from the alveolar bone and periodontal ligament, rather than from the growth of epithelium from the gingiva.[30] By placing a barrier membrane that excludes epithelial cells between the periodontal flap and the alveolar bone, only cells from the periodontal ligament space and the medullary bone are allowed to repopulate the site of lost tissue. This approach selectively causes a new attachment apparatus to grow. A number of materials have been suggested for these barriers, including expanded polytetrafluoroethylene membranes (ePTFE) and polylactic acid with citric acid ester membranes.

Indications. Infrabony defects and furcations appear to be the best candidates for guided tissue regeneration. In general, osseous lesions that are likely to respond well to other forms of bone fill or grafting are the most promising sites for guided tissue regeneration. In some cases, the results are remarkable.

Procedure. Flaps are reflected and, after adequate debridement of the intraosseous lesion, a membrane is placed over the opening in the bone or furcation and fastened to the tooth by suture or other stabilizing methods. The epithelium is closed over the membrane, and the wound is allowed to heal for a period of 30 to 60 days. When non-resorbable ePTFE material is used, the membrane must be removed surgically. The polylactic acid material resorbs through hydrolysis within 6 to 12 months (Figure 13–15).[31]

Contraindications. Guided tissue regeneration is the most predictable method for regenerating lost periodontal tissues. However, clini-

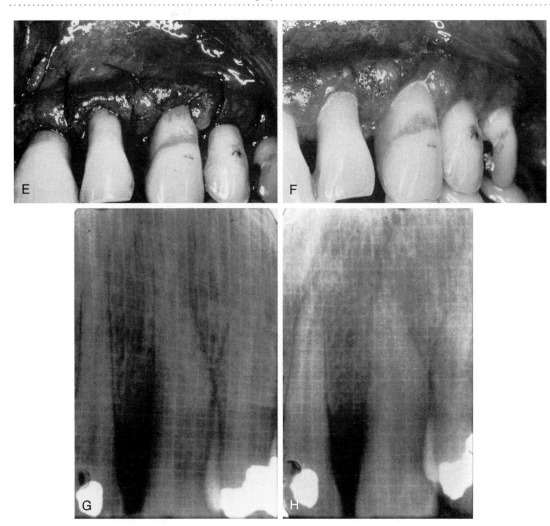

FIGURE 13–14 *Continued.* **E.** The flap is closely opposed with interrupted sutures to promote healing. **F.** Facial view of the healed tissues after 1 month. **G.** Preoperative bone level. **H.** Bone level 1 year postoperatively. There is a substantial increase in bone support for the tooth. (Courtesy of Philip R. Melnick, DMD.)

cal experience suggests that only the most favorable anatomic periodontal defects produce predictable results. Wide class III furcations and infrabony defects with fewer than two walls have met with limited success. The second surgical procedure required for removal of the ePTFE material is considered a disadvantage by some. However, many clinicians prefer it to the resorbable material because ePTFE has better handling properties.

PROCEDURES IMMEDIATELY AFTER PERIODONTAL SURGERY

A number of procedures are required to complete the periodontal surgery. These procedures include closing the wound with the placement of sutures, possibly covering the surgical wound with a protective dressing called a periodontal pack, and providing the patient with postoperative instructions.

Sutures

Sutures are required to close periodontal surgical wounds and to secure grafts in position. Periodontal surgeons generally use braided black silk sutures, which are easy to see and have good working properties. However, many other types of suture materials are available. Some periodontists prefer resorbable sutures, which have less potential for bacterial adher-

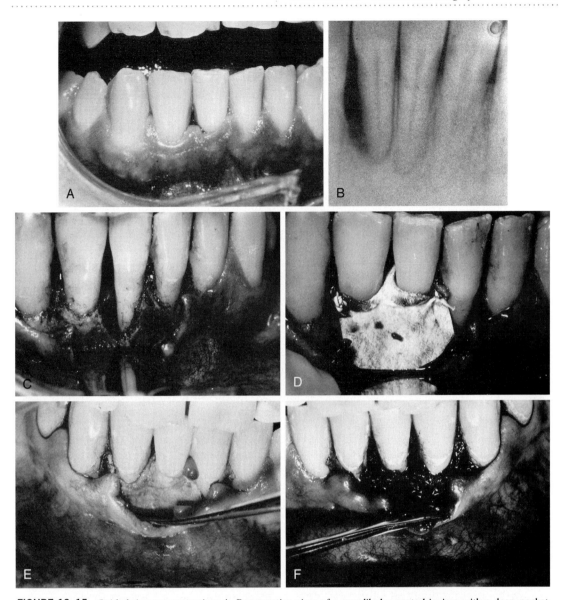

FIGURE 13–15. Guided tissue regeneration. **A.** Preoperative view of a mandibular central incisor with a deep pocket. **B.** Preoperative radiograph showing that the bony defect extends nearly to the apex of the central incisor. **C.** Flap exposing a large two-wall intrabony defect. **D.** Barrier membrane of expanded polytetrafluoroethylene material sutured over the defect. Flaps will be positioned over this membrane to keep the epithelium from growing into the bony defect. **E.** Membrane surgically exposed after 60 days of healing. **F.** Osteoid tissue that formed is visible after membrane removal. Flaps will be repositioned and sutured for final healing. (Courtesy of Gregory J. Conte, DMD, MS.)

ence. Others use sutures made of synthetic fibers.

Whatever type of suture material is placed, the sutures must be removed in 7 to 14 days. In most cases, that is enough time for wound healing to progress to a point at which sutures are no longer needed. If sutures remain in the tissues much longer than 14 days, they permit bacterial plaque to enter the wound site and produce healing complications. An infection re-

sulting from sutures that are retained too long is often called a "stitch abscess." This infection appears as a painful red, swollen area. Extreme inflammation slows healing and reduces the effects of periodontal surgery. Some synthetic fiber sutures, however, are designed to remain in place for as long as a month and are often selected for guided tissue regeneration procedures for exactly this reason. Although resorbable sutures are designed to dissolve in tissue fluids, they do not always dissolve in saliva and may require removal.

Many techniques are used for suturing periodontal flaps and grafts, ranging from simple stitches, termed interrupted sutures, to complex sling sutures that use the teeth for an anchor, or mattress sutures that allow flaps to be placed in a variety of positions.

Dental hygienists should know the basic rules that guide suture techniques.

1. It is best to tie the suture knots for any type or style of suture on the buccal surface. This placement allows for simple removal because the knot is easy to see and grasp with an instrument when the suture is cut. Thus, it is possible to avoid pulling the knot through the tissues during removal. If a periodontal pack or dressing is used, the lingual pack can be removed first, the sutures cut on the lingual surface, and the buccal pack removed. If any of the knots are caught in the buccal dressing, the sutures will pull out easily and not tear the tissue.
2. At least 2 or 3 mm of suture "tail" should be left beyond the knot. This tail allows the suture to be easily found at the postoperative appointment and gives the dentist or dental hygienist something to hold onto when cutting the suture for removal.
3. The location and number of sutures placed must be documented in the chart. This information aids in locating and removing all of the sutures to avoid traumatizing the healing wound at the postoperative appointment. It also prevents missing a suture and permitting a stitch abscess to develop.

Periodontal Pack

A **periodontal pack** or dressing is sometimes placed over the sutures to hold the flaps tightly to the teeth and underlying bone when pocket reduction surgery has been performed. It is also used after excisional surgery, such as gingivectomy, to protect the surgical wound from the oral environment and increase patient comfort during the first week of healing. Although many patients believe that a periodontal pack makes the surgical site more comfortable, some find the pack a nuisance and prefer not to have the dressing placed.

Several types of periodontal packs are available, but the most common type consists of a paste mixture that sets chemically to a firm, rubbery consistency. A light-cured product is available that allows the working and setting times to be more precisely controlled. Whatever dressing is selected, it is mixed according to the manufacturer's instructions and placed in a thin ribbon around the necks of the teeth in the area of surgery. To facilitate retention of the pack, it should be compressed into the interproximal spaces for a mechanical lock and the material should not extend coronal to the height of contour of the teeth. Bleeding must be controlled before a periodontal pack is placed because it will not control bleeding. Further, the periodontal pack does not prevent plaque formation. In fact, it prevents plaque control in the region of the surgery. The use of the periodontal pack is shown in Figure 13–10, G and H. (They also appear in the color supplement.)

Postoperative Instructions and Procedures

After periodontal surgery, **postoperative procedures** include a prescription for an analgesic and possibly an antibiotic. Many periodontists recommend the use of a disinfectant rinse twice a day to help with plaque control. A chlorhexidine or essential oil mouthwash may be used to freshen the mouth and inhibit plaque during primary healing in the first week or two after surgery.[32]

A number of suggestions and **postoperative instructions** should be given to the patient to ease postoperative discomfort and promote healing. They include the following recommendations:

1. Physical activity should be limited to allow the patient to rest and let the area of surgery heal.
2. Bleeding is usually limited, but if the wound area begins to seep blood after the patient leaves the office, it can usually be controlled with light finger pressure on a gauze sponge in the area of surgery. The patient should be instructed not to rinse because rinsing prolongs the bleeding.
3. A soft diet is usually recommended for the first several days to avoid disturbing

the area of surgery or the periodontal pack, if present. The patient should be urged to eat a nutritious, well-balanced diet to promote healing.

4. Any prescriptions for medications that may have been given should be reviewed with the patient.

5. The patient should be warned that portions of the periodontal pack may chip off before the postoperative appointment. Usually, the pack has done its job of tightly adapting the tissues to the teeth in the first several hours of healing, and little damage is done if the pack comes off after the first postoperative day.

6. The patient should be warned that some surgical procedures, particularly osseous surgery, commonly cause swelling. The patient should be told to use an ice pack for short intervals for the first few hours after surgery.

7. The patient should avoid smoking, which may cause the wound to heal more slowly.

8. Home care plaque control instructions should be reviewed carefully with the patient. Often, plaque control is more difficult during healing, but good plaque removal leads to better healing. Soft toothbrushes, the use of warm water during cleaning, and gentle interproximal cleaning can all be recommended. The unaffected teeth should be cleaned normally. The patient should be shown how to clean the area of surgery and encouraged to clean once a day, twice if possible. Often, an antiseptic mouthwash is recommended to help with plaque control and freshen the mouth.

9. The patient must be given a list of postoperative instructions that should be reviewed before the patient is dismissed. It is important that the instruction sheet include the telephone number to use if problems arise. The patient should be urged to contact the office if there are any problems or questions. A postoperative visit should be scheduled for about 7 days after the surgery. A sample postoperative instruction sheet is shown in Instructions Following Periodontal Surgery.

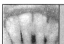

INSTRUCTIONS FOLLOWING PERIODONTAL SURGERY

Activity: Limit your activities to those requiring minimal exertion for the next few days.

Rinsing: Do not rinse your mouth for 24 hours.

Bleeding: Some slight bleeding may occur during the first 4 or 5 hours after the operation. This bleeding is not unusual. If bleeding continues, apply firm pressure for 20 minutes with a piece of gauze. Repeat as necessary. Do not remove the gauze during this period. Do not rinse with water to stop the bleeding. If bleeding persists, call the office.

Discomfort: Some discomfort is to be expected when the anesthesia wears off. If you have been given a prescription, fill it and take the medication as directed. If discomfort persists, call the office.

Eating: Limit yourself to a soft diet immediately after surgery. Avoid chewing in the area of surgery. Do not drink very hot beverages the first day. You may return to your regular diet as soon as you feel comfortable. Highly seasoned or spicy foods may irritate the area of surgery.

Dressing: A dressing material may have been placed around your teeth. It will become hard within about 2 hours and should not be disturbed. Although the dressing may remain in place until your next appointment, small parts may chip off. If a large portion of the dressing comes off, call the office for instructions.

Swelling: Swelling is expected after some procedures. You may use an ice pack on the outside of your face, 15 minutes on and 15 minutes off, for the next 4 hours. If you have excessive swelling in your neck or under your chin, call the office.

Smoking: Do not smoke. Smoking may interfere with the healing process and produce poor results.

Home care: If a surgical dressing is present, brush the top of the dressing lightly with a soft toothbrush. If no dressing is present, gently use a soft toothbrush to clean the area of surgery for the first few days. You may rinse gently with a medicated mouthwash if it was prescribed or warm salt water starting the day after surgery.

IF YOU HAVE ANY QUESTIONS OR CONCERNS, CALL THE OFFICE. Telephone number:

POSTOPERATIVE TREATMENT

The patient is usually scheduled for a postoperative visit 1 week after periodontal surgery.

At this appointment, the patient is examined, the periodontal pack and sutures are removed, and the surgical site is gently cleaned with a cotton swab that has been moistened with warm saline or a disinfectant mouthwash. Rarely, the surgeon may repack the area for an additional week. A surgical site with the periodontal pack, sutures, and accumulated plaque removed after 1 week is shown in Figure 13-10 I and J. (They also appear in the color supplement.)

Home care instructions for plaque control should be reviewed at this time. The tissue may still be tender from the surgery, so the patient must be instructed to gently clean the area with a soft toothbrush that has been made even softer by soaking in warm water. Because considerable tissue shrinkage and larger spaces between teeth may occur after periodontal surgery, interproximal brushes may be indicated. They should also be used gently. Dental floss should be used carefully during the first few weeks after surgery to avoid damaging the healing junctional epithelium and connective tissue attachment in the surgical area.

The importance of postsurgical plaque control cannot be overemphasized. Poor plaque control after periodontal surgery is the principal reason for slow healing and failure of the surgical treatment. Many clinicians recommend scheduling the patient for several postoperative visits for evaluation of plaque control during the healing phase.

Teeth in the area of surgery often become mobile as a result of swelling in the periodontal ligament space. The patient should be told that this swelling is normal and that the teeth usually become firm as the tissues heal. Sometimes the dentist may suggest a postsurgical splint to control mobility during the healing process.

Tooth sensitivity, especially to cold, is a common problem after periodontal surgery. Patients should be warned to expect a certain amount of sensitivity. Patients may reduce sensitivity during plaque control procedures by brushing the teeth with warm water for the first several weeks. Sensitivity is caused by exposure of the root surfaces to the oral environment from apically positioned periodontal flaps, shrinkage of the gingiva during healing, and root planing with cementum removal during the surgical procedure. Dentinal tubules are exposed to the oral environment, and hydrodynamic forces may cause pain. The use of home fluoride gels or rinses for the first month after periodontal surgery may alleviate sensitivity. In addition, topical desensitizing office treatments with potassium oxylate or ferric oxylate may help. Desensitizing toothpastes used at home, particularly those containing potassium nitrate, may be effective in controlling postsurgical sensitivity. In most cases, this sensitivity is greatly reduced after a month or two.[32]

The area of surgery should not be probed for at least 1 month to allow the junctional epithelium to heal and the gingival connective tissue fibers to mature. After 1 month, the region may be gently probed, but healing of the connective tissue fibers is not complete, so tissues are fragile. Connective tissues continue to heal and remodel for several months.

Periodontal maintenance should be continued at appropriate intervals during the surgical phase of periodontal treatment. Usually, periodontal debridement at intervals of 3 months or less should be continued until all planned surgical procedures are completed and the tissues have healed completely. At that time, a careful assessment of the patient's periodontal health can be made, and recall intervals can be gradually increased, if appropriate.

HEALING AFTER PERIODONTAL SURGERY

Healing of the periodontal surgical wound begins shortly after the procedure is completed. A blood clot forms at the surgical site, protecting the wound and allowing the tissue to begin to heal. The blood clot acts as a matrix and scaffolding for healing cells to migrate into the wound area. However, it is essential that the blood clot be as thin as possible because the inflammatory cells associated with wound healing are also required to remove the fibrin clot to complete healing. Firm pressure is placed on the flap margins after the flaps are sutured to minimize the thickness of the forming clot. The blood clot also provides stability to the wound by binding the displaced flaps to the underlying bone.

The epithelial cells are the first to heal. After an initial "stunning effect" of about 24 hours, they begin to divide and grow from the wound margins. Epithelial cells migrate about 0.5 to 1.0 mm/day, so that in 5 to 7 days, the gingival surface of the wound is covered. Epithelial healing is the point at which the wound is sufficiently protected so that the sutures and pack may be removed. The epithelial cells continue to grow for the next 2 weeks, mainly by thickening the epithelial layer, until normal anatomy is restored. In studies of the healing of periodontal surgical wounds, the junctional epithelium returned to its presurgical appearance in 10 to 12 days.[33]

Beneath the fibrin blood clot, the healing wound exhibits all of the classic signs of inflammation, including migrating lymphocytes and macrophages that help to eliminate bacteria and debris in the surgical site. As healing progresses, these inflammatory cells begin to digest the fibrin itself. Connective tissue healing begins after the epithelium has begun to heal and has laid down its basal lamina. Fibroblasts from the connective tissue adjacent to the surgical area begin to divide, proliferate, and migrate into the wound area. Capillaries from the adjacent tissues begin to grow into the site and result in the development of a capillary-rich and heavily cellular healing granulation tissue. The fibroblasts begin to lay down an extracellular matrix of collagen fibers that mature and remodel over the next 2 to 4 weeks. By 2 weeks after surgery, the wound strength approaches presurgical levels. The clinical appearance of an access flap procedure after 1 week is shown in Figure 13-10 I and J. Healing after 3 months is shown in Figure 13-10 K and L. (Also shown in color supplement.)

Osseous healing does not begin until late in the healing process. Approximately 1 month after osseous surgery, the wound site is populated with osteoblast cells. At this stage, there is active formation of uncalcified bone matrix called osteoid. This active tissue may be an effective autogenous grafting material. For this reason, healing tooth extraction sites, 1 or 2 months after tooth removal, are often chosen as a source of donor bone for periodontal bone graft surgery. Calcification continues to increase during the next 6 months. The alveolar bone requires 4 to 6 months to completely heal and remodel. Radiographs of bone regeneration surgical sites usually show significant increases in bone density 6 months to 1 year after surgery, as seen in Figure 13-14 G and H. (Also shown in color supplement.)

Gingivectomy wounds require slightly more time to heal than flap procedures because the epithelial cells must migrate relatively long distances from the wound margins. This type of healing is termed healing by secondary intention because the large area of fibrin clot must be completely replaced with epithelium, resulting in scar formation. Fortunately, in the oral cavity, scar tissue and gingival tissue both have the same types of cells and collagen fibers. Therefore, healed gingivectomy wounds have the same color and consistency as normal gingiva.

Free gingival grafts must obtain their nutrients from the underlying recipient site by diffusion for the 2 weeks after surgery. The grafted epithelium usually degenerates, and revascularization of the graft begins with anastomosis of the capillaries from the recipient site in 4 to 5 days. After 1 week, the gingival graft areas appear highly inflamed, with a white film of necrotic epithelium. Patients should be warned that this appearance represents the expected healing response and that the gingiva will begin to take on a more normal appearance in the ensuing weeks.

Bone grafting procedures usually take more time for healing than other osseous procedures. The bone graft material may need to be resorbed before new bone can be formed. Osteogenesis appears to be ongoing about 3 weeks after the graft is placed and new periodontal ligament, cementum, and alveolar bone are well formed and functioning in about 3 months.

Healing of the dentogingival junction to a root that was previously exposed to periodontal disease occurs in two ways. In one manner, a long junctional epithelium may develop that is tightly adapted to the root surface apical to the area of the former pocket. In the other manner, a new connective tissue attachment develops, with new periodontal ligament fibers inserting into reformed cementum and alveolar bone. This process is correctly termed regeneration. The purpose of guided tissue regeneration is to encourage new connective tissue attachment and delay growth of oral epithelium into the healing area next to the tooth. In most cases, both types of dentogingival healing occur. Long epithelial attachments form coronally, and new connective tissue attachments form only at the most apical levels of the pocket (Figure 13-16). (For a further discussion on regeneration and

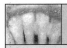

SCARRING OF THE ORAL SOFT TISSUES

It is of interest that despite extensive surgical interventions during periodontal surgery, including incisions made entirely through the gingiva and periosteum to the bone, there is little visible scarring. After periodontal surgery, the gingiva heals with a normal clinical appearance. Refer to Figure 13–10, K and L (also appears in the color supplement) for an illustration of normal healing. Among oral tissues, this general lack of visible scarring is unique to the gingiva. Scarring is occasionally seen in the attached gingiva but is much more commonly found in other areas such as the lip or mucosa. Endodontic surgery such as apioectomy, the removal of the apex of the root and surrounding infected tissue to permit healing of endodontic infections in bone, results in a thin white scar in the alveolar mucosa apical to the gingiva. It is differences in the connective tissue underlying the epithelium that account for this clinical finding.

Healing occurs as *regeneration* of tissues or *repair* of tissues. Regeneration is the process that completely restores injured tissue so that it is indistinguishable in function and appearance from the original. In the periodontium, a wound that only penetrates the epithelium will heal through regeneration. In this type of wound, epithelial cells migrate from the margins of the wound, and the new tissue is identical to uninjured epithelium. Repair is healing that occurs through the formation of a connective tissue *scar*.[34] It occurs in the periodontium when wounds penetrate into connective tissue or deeper. Scarring is a normal process that is indicative of the loss of mature tissues' ability to regenerate like embryonic tissues.[35]

Healing by repair after an injury is a process to restore tissues to functional integrity. It consists of a series of events that occur in an overlapping manner. These are the early wound healing or inflammatory phase, the remodeling phase, and the late phase of contraction and scarring.[35]

In the early phase after injury, the body forms a blood clot with a fibrin matrix. With skin wounds, the matrix is called a scab. This matrix permits the growth of cells into the wound area. Three or four days after the injury, the inflammatory cells, fibroblasts, and immature blood vessels form a highly vascular granulation tissue throughout the matrix. Healing is the gradual replacement of the matrix with functional tissues. The granulation tissue will eventually remodel and establish the healed scar.[35] During the first few days of healing, the fibroblasts also secrete substances that are hydrophilic (attract water), and thus the healing injury appears edematous.[34]

The remodeling phase of healing is the gradual change of the fibrin matrix and granulation tissue to dense, organized collagen. It begins with matrix formation and continues long after the wound appears healed clinically, perhaps for months. Re-epithelialization, or closure of the surface of the wound, occurs separately but at the same time as the inflammatory and remodeling phases of healing. It does not require a vital granulation tissue to migrate upon.[35]

The late phase of healing represents wound contraction and scar formation. As time progresses during healing, the collagen organizes along stress lines, gradually increasing the strength of the healing tissue. As collagen increases, much of the vascularization disappears and the wound appears as a pale white scar.[34] Wound contraction is a phenomenon by which the cells decrease the wound area, by drawing together the margins. It occurs independently of epithelial regeneration. Contraction forces are extremely strong and can result in major distortion of tissue, including enough force to bend bone.[35] Often the result is that even a large wound may contract 90% or more, resulting in a small white line scar.

In the gingival tissues, the collagen is thick and very dense under the attached gingiva. During the latter stages of wound healing, when collagen is organizing into scar tissue, contraction does not occur in this area to the extent that it can in mucosa, where the connective tissue is mostly elastic tissue and has less collagen. Epithelium regenerates over the connective tissue matrix, leaving a healed lesion that is indistinguishable clinically from the original gingival tissue. All the elements of wound healing do occur, and the remodeling of the collagen can be seen histologically. The denseness of the underlying collagen and the limited contraction of the wound in the gingiva result in a thin, avascular scar, but the scar tissue is clinically indistinguishable from adjacent normal gingiva. The figure below is an unusual example of scarring of the attached gingiva.

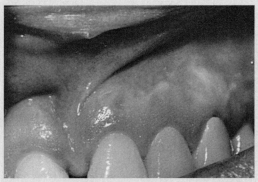

A scar in the attached gingiva resulting from endodontic surgery. The wound margins were not closely adapted together after surgery, causing migration of collagen cells and significant wound contraction, resulting in a visible scar, (Courtesy of David W. Rising, DMD.) Typically, there is no visible scarring after periodontal surgery. For an example of healing attached gingiva see Figure 13–10 **J, K**, and **L**.

scar tissue formation, see Scarring of the Oral Soft Tissues.)

THE ROLE OF THE DENTAL HYGIENIST IN PERIODONTAL SURGERY

The dental hygienist has a significant role in the overall treatment of the periodontal patient, including the surgical phase of therapy. The dental hygienist may be the most appropriate member of the dental team to discuss the advantages and disadvantages of surgical treatment with the patient. The periodontist or dentist is legally charged with the responsibility of informing the patient of the risks, benefits, and alternatives to periodontal surgery. However, the dental hygienist may act as the patient's advocate by asking questions and helping to provide the answers to concerns that the patient is unable to articulate.

The dental hygienist also plays a central role in the postsurgical treatment of the periodontal patient. Postoperative care, including suture and dressing removal, postsurgical plaque removal, follow-up wound care, and home care instructions, is often provided by the dental hygienist. The success of periodontal surgery depends primarily on long-term plaque control by the patient. This plaque control is particularly critical after surgical treatment, when tissues may be tender and specialized methods of interdental plaque control are needed.

In many periodontal offices, the dental hygienist has an important place in the surgical

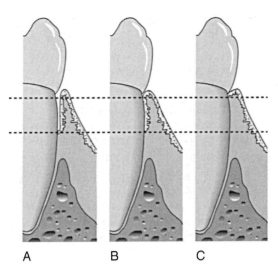

FIGURE 13–16. Healing of the periodontal tissues to the root surface after periodontal surgery. **A.** Preoperative periodontal pocket. **B.** Healing by long junctional epithelium is the more common result. **C.** Healing by new connective tissue attachment is possible, but likely only in the most apical regions of the pockets.

team. The dental hygienist provides presurgical plaque control, scaling, and root planing therapy; observes and assists during the surgical treatment (and, incidentally, notes the success or failure of specific instrumentation techniques for plaque and calculus removal in deep pockets); and often provides the bulk of postsurgical treatment and follow-up care. A comprehensive understanding of the goals, indications, specific surgical procedures, contraindications, and course of events for these procedures is mandatory to fulfill the obligation of complete, informed care of the periodontal patient.

STUDY QUESTIONS

MULTIPLE CHOICE

1. The types of periodontal surgery in which the periodontist shapes the alveolar bone with chisels or burs to remove bony defects are called procedures for:

   a. Pocket reduction or elimination
   b. Access to the root surface
   c. Treatment of osseous defects
   d. Correcting mucogingival defects
   e. Creating new attachment

2. The types of periodontal surgery that increase the predictability for growth of new tissues of the periodontal apparatus are called procedures for:

   a. Pocket reduction or elimination
   b. Access to the root surface
   c. Treatment of osseous defects
   d. Correcting mucogingival defects
   e. Creating new attachment

3. Periodontal surgery is most successful when pocket depths are between 5 mm and 9 mm deep because indications for periodontal surgery are more affected by measurements of clinical attachment loss than by those of pocket depths.

   a. Both the statement and the reason are correct and related.
   b. Both the statement and the reason are correct but NOT related.
   c. The statement is correct, but the reason is NOT.
   d. The statement is NOT correct, but the reason is correct.
   e. NEITHER the statement NOR the reason is correct.

4. Drug-induced gingival hyperplasia is most likely best treated surgically by gingivectomy.
   Gingivectomy is an incisional form of periodontal surgery.

   a. Both statements are TRUE.
   b. Both statements are FALSE.
   c. The first statement is TRUE and the second is FALSE.
   d. The first statement is FALSE and the second is TRUE.

5. The periodontist usually considers cost and time to be major disadvantages of periodontal surgery.
   The patient usually considers cost, time, discomfort, and esthetics to be the major disadvantages of periodontal surgery.

   a. Both statements are TRUE.
   b. Both statements are FALSE.
   c. The first statement is TRUE and the second is FALSE.
   d. The first statement is FALSE and the second is TRUE.

6. Regenerative periodontal surgical procedures:

   a. Selectively encourage the growth of cells of the attachment apparatus
   b. Selectively encourage the growth of the cells of the epithelium of the closely approximated flaps
   c. Selectively discourage the growth of cells of the attachment apparatus
   d. Selectively discourage the growth of the cells of the epithelium on the surface of the excisional wound

7. The most common oral site for donor tissue for free gingival graft procedures is the:

   a. Palate
   b. Buccal mucosa
   c. Lingual mucosa
   d. Tongue

8. What is the term for a periodontal bone graft that is made from bovine or porcine bone material?

   a. Allograft
   b. Alloplast
   c. Autograft
   d. Xenograft

9. Age is an important consideration in recommending periodontal surgery because the prognosis of successful treatment of disease is reduced as patients age.

   a. Both the statement and the reason are correct and related.
   b. Both the statement and the reason are correct but NOT related.
   c. The statement is correct, but the reason is NOT.
   d. The statement is NOT correct, but the reason is correct.
   e. NEITHER the statement NOR the reason is correct.

10. The following forms of periodontal surgery are examples of incisional surgery EXCEPT one. Which one is the EXCEPTION?

    a. Regeneration surgery
    b. Gingivoplasty
    c. Mucogingival surgery
    d. Pocket reduction surgery

SHORT ANSWER

11. What is the primary reason for performing periodontal surgery?

_____

_____

12. List the factors that must be considered before periodontal surgery.

_____

_____

13. Describe the concept of guided tissue regeneration.

_____

_____

14. What is an apically positioned flap?

_____

_____

15. Describe the role of the dental hygienist in periodontal surgery.

_____

_____

REFERENCES

1. Ramfjord SP, Ash MM. Periodontology and Periodontics, Philadelphia: WB Saunders, 1979:498.
2. Green E, Parr RW, Taggart, EJ. Surgery in Periodontal Maintenance Therapy. San Francisco; Praxis, 1984:8-22.
3. Stambaugh RV, Dragoo M, Smith DV, Carasali L. The limits of subgingival scaling. Int J Periodontics Restorative Dent 1981;1:31-41.
4. Green E, Parr RW, Taggart EJ. Surgery in periodontal maintenance therapy. San Francisco: Praxis, 1984.
5. Maynard JG, Wilson RDK. Physiologic dimensions of the periodontium significant to the restorative dentist. J Periodontol 1979;50:170-174.
6. Lindhe J, Westfelt E, Nyman S, Socransky SS, Heijl L, Brathall G. Healing following surgical/non-surgical treatment of periodontal disease: a clinical study. J Clin Periodontal 1982;9:115-128.
7. Lang NP, Löe H. Clinical management of periodontal diseases. Periodontology 2000 1993;2:128-139.
8. Ramfjord SP, Nissle RR. The modified Widman flap. J Periodontol 1974;45:601-608.
9. Yukna RA. Longitudinal evaluation of the exisional new attachment procedures in humans. J Periodontol 1978;49:142-144.
10. Smith DH, Ammons WF, Van Belle Ga. Longitudinal study of periodontal status comparing osseous re-

11. contouring with flap curettage. J Periodontol 1980: 51:367-375.
11. Moskow B. Longevity: a critical factor in evaluating the effectiveness of periodontal therapy. J Clin Periodontol 1987;14:237-244.
12. Friedman N. Periodontal osseous surgery: osteoplasty and ostectomy. J Periodontol 1955;6:257-269.
13. Joshipura KJ, Kent RL, DePaola PF. Gingival recession: intra-oral distribution and associated factors. J Periodontol 1994;65:864-871.
14. Wennstrom JL. Lack of association between width of attached gingiva and development of soft tissue recession: a five-year longitudinal study. J Clin Periodontol 1983;10:206-221.
15. Langer B, Calagna LJ. The subepithelial connective tissue graft: a new approach to the enhancement of anterior cosmetics. Int J Periodontics Restorative Dent 1982;2:23-33.
16. Maynard JG, Wilson RDK. Physiologic dimensions of the periodontium significant to the restorative dentist. J Periodontol 1979;50:170-174.
17. Cabrera PO. Connective tissue grafting: an option in reconstructive periodontal surgery. J Am Dent Assoc 1994;125:729-737.
18. Mellonig JT. Periodontal regenerative surgery. In Periodontal Disease Management. Chicago: American Academy of Periodontology, 1994;385-397.
19. Ellegaard B, Low H. New attachment of periodontal tissues after treatment of intrabony pockets. J Periodontol 1971;42:648-652.
20. Mellonig J, Prewett A, Moyer M. HIV inactivation in a bone allograft. J Periodontol 1992;63:979-983.
21. American Academy of Periodontology. Periodontal regeneration: Report of the Research, Science and Therapy Committee. Chicago: American Academy of Periodontology, 1993:5.
22. Hammarstrom L. Enamel matrix, cementum development and regeneration. J Clin Perio 1997;24:658-668.
23. Sculean a, Donos N, Blaes, A, Lauermann M, Reich E, Brecx M. Comparison of enamel matrix proteins and bioabsorbable membranes in the treatment of intrabony periodontal defects. A split-mouth study. J Periodontol 1999;70:255-262.
24. Mellonig J. Enamel matrix derivative for periodontal reconstruction surgery: technique and clinical and histologic case report. Int J Periodont Rest Dent 1999; 19:9-19.
25. Bhatnagar RS, Qian JJ, Wedrychowska A, Sadeghi M, Wu YM, Smith N. Design of biomimetic habitats for tissue engineering with P-15, a synthetic peptide analogue of collagen. Tissue Engin 1999;5:53-65.
26. Yukna RA, Callan DP, Krauser JT, Evans GH, Aichelnamm-Reidy ME, Moore K, Cruz, R, Scott JB. Multicenter clinical evaluation of combination anorganic bovine-derived hydroxyapatite matrix (ABM) cell binding peptide (P-15) as a bone replacement graft material in human periodontal osseous defects. 6-month results. J Periodontol 1998;69:655-663.
27. Garrett JS, Crigger M, Egelberg J. Effects of citric acid on diseased root surfaces. J Periodontal Res 1978; 13:155-163.
28. Caffesse RG, Kerry GJ, Chaves ES, McLean TN, Morrison EC, Lopatin DE, Caffesse ER, Stults DL. Clinical evaluation of the use of citric acid and autologous fibronectin in periodontal surgery. J Periodontol 1988;59:565-569.
29. Melcher AH. On the repair potential of periodontal tissues. J Periodontol 1976;47:256-260.
30. Gottlow J, Nyman S, Karring T, Wennstrom J. New attachment formation in the human periodontium by guided tissue regeneration: case reports. J Clin periodontol 1986;13:604-616.

31. Laurell L, Falk H, Fornell J, Johard G, Gottlow J. Clinical use of a bioresorbable matrix barrier in guided tissue regeneration therapy: case series. J Periodontol 1994;65:967-975.

32. Carranza FA. General principles of periodontal surgery. In FA Carranza and MG Newman, eds. Clinical Periodontology, 8th ed. Philadelphia: WB Saunders, 1996:569-578.

33. Takata T, Nikai H, Ijuhin N, Okamoto H. Ultrastructure of regenerated junctional epithelium after surgery of rat molar gingiva. J Periodontol 1986;57:776-783.

34. Wound healing. In E Rubin and JL Faber, eds. Pathology. Philadelphia: JP Lippincott, 1988; 77-89.

35. Bertolami CN, Messadi DV. Complications associated with wound healing. In Kaban LB, Pogrel MA, Perrott DH, eds. In Complications in Oral and Maxillofacial Surgery, Philadelphia: WB Saunders, 1997:41-53.

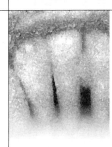

14

Dorothy A. Perry

Dental Implants

Chapter Objectives

1. Describe the types of dental implants used in dentistry and explain the role of these prosthetic devices in the attainment of periodontal health and function.
2. Provide the long-term success rates for restoring edentulous and partially edentulous mouths with implants.
3. Briefly describe the types of materials used in implant therapy.
4. Discuss the set of criteria that are applied to judge success of implants both biologically and functionally.
5. List the appropriate techniques and instruments required for maintenance of implants.
6. Describe the maintenance procedures and home care instructions appropriate for patients with implants.

Key Terms

Abutment
Dental implant
Failing implant
Maintenance
Osseointegration

Peri-implantitis
Superstructure
Titanium
Titanium oxide surface
Transosteal implant

Artificial replacements for natural teeth have been an elusive goal for more than 1500 years. Implant attempts have been reported in ancient Egypt and Central America. Modern attempts to place artificial teeth into the jaws with plates or screws were, until recently, considered experimental and not well accepted by the dental community because of low rates of success, less than 50 percent retained for five years.[1]

In 1982, a new type of implant was introduced to the United States that had documented long-term survival rates of 90 percent or greater. It was referred to as the osseointegrated implant and was invented and reported by Brånemark and co-workers in Sweden,[2] who had conducted extensive studies since 1952.[3] This information has spread throughout the dental community and has resulted in an exponential growth in the use of dental implants as a viable treatment modality.[3] Implants are now used in edentulous mouths to support dentures, as **abutments** in partially edentulous mouths to support fixed bridgework, and as single tooth replacements. Many patients can benefit from implants as long as they meet certain requirements for rehabilitation.[4, 5, 6]

Dental implants provide firm, fixed anchors in the jaw that permit dentists to address some of the failings of dentures. Dentures rest on the mucosa so that the underlying bone continues to remodel and resorb. This process results in the need for occasional relining or the construction of new prostheses, and facial changes continue to occur as a result of this gradual bone loss. In addition to the changes in patient appearance and the expense of continued dental treatment when no teeth are present, the retention and function of conventional dentures are a common problem as suggested by the multimillion dollar market for denture adhesives.[7] Dentures can now be supported by implants so that pressure diffuses through the bone, resulting in enhanced function and greatly reducing the extent of bone remodeling caused by loading forces (the forces caused by functioning of the restored teeth or dentures). The presence of stable bone structure under dentures minimizes the facial changes associated with edentulism.[7] Dentures can be held in place over implants with a variety of locking mechanisms, screws, and clips.

In addition to improving denture success, the use of implants as abutments to support fixed bridgework permits patients to have successfully restored dentitions without removable partial dentures. As fixed bridge abutments, implants can improve function, eliminate unsightly clasps, and keep the teeth in the patient's mouth at night rather than in a glass. Single tooth implant replacements permit dentists to replace lost teeth without the preparation of healthy adjacent teeth to place conventional fixed bridgework (Figure 14–1).

The success rate of osseointegrated implants is supported by more than 20 years of animal research and 10 years of follow-up studies in humans.[7] Long-term success rates for restoring completely edentulous mouths with implants and prostheses range from 94 percent to 97

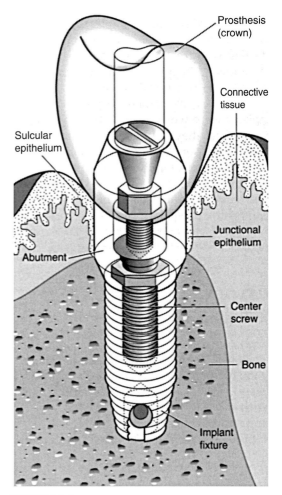

FIGURE 14–1. Implant: prosthesis, abutment, and fixture.

percent. Single tooth replacements have equally high success rates. A recent study reported prospective longitudinal data for placing implants in molar positions, those areas with lower documented success rates. When cases are carefully selected, the success rate for mandibular molar implants is 91.5 percent after six years, and 82.9 percent for maxillary molars.[8]

There continues to be enormous potential for the use of implant therapy. According to the 1985 National Institute for Dental Research Survey of Employed US Adults and Seniors, 42 percent of American adults older than 65 years of age and an average of 4 percent of those 35 to 64 years years of age were completely edentulous. People older than 65 years old have lost an average of 10 of their 28 teeth, and people aged 55 to 65 years have lost an average of nine teeth.[9] These statistics suggest a substantial market for implants in dental health care.

Studies report significant patient satisfaction with implant-restored dentitions. A survey of 61 patients with multiple implants in place for 3 months to 14 years showed great patient satisfaction with treatment. Of these patients, 98 percent were happier with their dental health than previously, when they had traditional dentures. Further, 97 percent responded that the implants were worth the trouble, and 89 percent said that they would undergo the extensive implant procedures again. The main reasons patients reported for choosing implant therapy were improved eating ability and alleviation of problems with dentures.[10] The success of osseointegrated implants has given dentistry a potent new treatment to restore appearance, comfort, and function to dental patients.

HISTORY

Definition of Osseointegration

Brånemark and co-workers created the term **osseointegration,** meaning "direct structural and functional connection between ordered, living bone and the surface of a load-carrying implant." This condition has also been termed "functional ankylosis."[3] It is achieved by the use of specific materials, most widely **titanium,** and careful surgical technique. When fibers or cells are permitted to grow between the implant and the bone, it is referred to as fibroosseous integration. This situation may not be as stable an anchor for restoration[11] and is not widely accepted.[3]

The most studied implants, and those with the longest documented success rates, are made of pure titanium. The outer layers of titanium implants oxidize into a stable inert titanium oxide that is nonreactive with the living tissues around it. When the implant is placed in the jaw and osseointegration occurs, the bone approaches the **titanium oxide surface** to within 20 nm. The microscopic space remaining between the bone and the implant is filled with glycosaminoglycans and proteoglycans, but there is no conclusive evidence of bonded union.[3] Achieving this intimate contact between bone and implant increases the stability and long-term clinical success of the implant.[11]

Biomaterials

Pure titanium implants oxidize on the outer layer to form a hard, brittle, and stable titanium oxide surface. This surface has the characteristics of a stable ceramic material and is unlike corrosive iron oxides, such as rust. This stable surface characteristic permits close adaptation of bone to the implant surface. Other materials, such as hydroxyapatite and aluminum oxide, also have these properties.[11] There are many biologically compatible materials that can be used for implants. The most widely used are titanium and its alloys, about which there is the most data in clinical studies. Other metals such as tantalum, and alloys such as cobalt/chromium/molybdenum have been studied. Precious metals such as gold and platinum are less compatible. Other materials such as aluminum oxide ceramics (alumina and sapphire), ceramics, carbon, carbon-silicon compounds, and hydroxyapatite have been used. Hydroxyapatite is used widely as a surface coating on other materials,[3] and these coatings provide for more rapid bone apposition. These coatings have been found not to be stable, however, and can be partially or totally removed from the implants.[12]

Titanium implants are available with plasmasprayed surfaces, which are thin, pebbly coatings of titanium on a surface of pure titanium. These sprayed implants have more surface area and are believed to permit faster bone adaptation and greater surface area for bonding.[11] In addition to surface materials, implants are available in various shapes, such as screws, blades, and hollow cylinders with vents. Research is being conducted to evaluate the various types of implants and determine which types provide the best long-term success rates for implant patients (Figure 14–2).

Tissue Interface

The supracrestal gingival tissues that surround titanium dental implants are analogous to normal gingiva. A basement lamina and hemidesmosomes are present in the epithelial cells intimately contacting the osseointegrated implant. The main differences occur at the interface between the gingival tissues and surrounding bone because periodontal ligament, true epithelial attachment, and dentogingival fibers do not form.

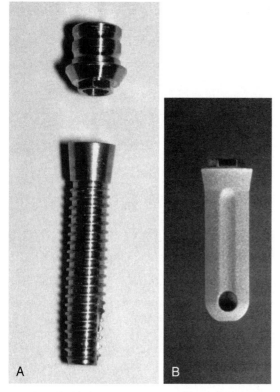

FIGURE 14–2. A. Titanium implant with abutment. **B.** Hydroxyapatite-coated implant.

The sulcular epithelium is nonkeratinized, similar to the sulci next to teeth. The cells at the base of the sulcus form a junctional epithelium[3, 11] that adheres to the implant surface. The junctional epithelium attaches to the implant through a basal lamina and hemidesmosomes. The interface is often referred to as the "biologic seal" and is thought to prevent ingress of bacteria and toxins to the osseointegrated implant surface.[13] Data show the mean sulcus depth in healthy implants that are in place for 1 year to be 2.78 mm,[11] with a range of depths of 1.3 to 3.8 mm.[14]

The connective tissue lying above the bone and beneath the junctional epithelium in the peri-implant tissue touches the titanium surface directly. The fibers run parallel, rather than perpendicular, to the titanium surface, and there are no insertions of fibrils into the implant. In a roughened plasma-sprayed implant surface, collagen fibers may run perpendicular to the implant, suggesting the potential for fiber insertion.[11]

It has been suggested that the fibro-osteal or fibro-osseous integration permits a peri-implant ligament to grow between the implant and bone. This ligament may reduce the occlusal stress transmitted to the bone, thereby increasing the long-term success of the implant. Documentation for this theory is lacking.[4]

The microbiota associated with healthy implant sites and that associated with healthy periodontal sites are similar. In addition, implants placed in mouths with remaining natural teeth have a microbial population similar to that of the existing teeth. Failed implant sites also have a microbial population that resembles that of sites with periodontal disease.[15] The microbiota of **failing implants** is qualitatively similar to that of chronic periodontitis and refractory or recurrent forms of periodontitis, but the levels of some pathogens have been shown to differ.[16]

Subgingival sites in healthy implants are populated by high percentages of coccoid cells and nonmotile rods. Few spirochetes have been found.[17] In one study evaluating suspected periodontal pathogens located around clinically healthy implants, the suspected periodontal pathogens *Actinobacillus actinomycetemcomitans, Porphyromonas gingivalis,* and *Prevotella intermedius* were cultured from around implants in patients with minimal plaque who had not had maintenance visits for 6 months or longer. *P. intermedius* was identified in 7 of 37 implant sites in 19 patients, *A. actinomycetemcomitans* was found in one, and *P. gingivalis* was found in none.[18] This finding suggests the importance of regular maintenance visits for all implant patients to help prevent the formation of potentially pathogenic bacterial plaques.

Types of Implants

Several types of implants are available. They are mentioned briefly here, but the focus of this chapter is the osseointegrated implants known as endosseous implants.

ENDOSSEOUS TYPE

Endosseous implants are titanium implants of various shapes that are placed within the bone. The first endosseous implant described, and the one with the most reported long-term success, was the Brånemark pure titanium implant with a screw shape. The titanium surface oxidizes into a thin, nonreactive titanium oxide layer to which the bone adheres (Figure 14–3).[19]

Titanium alloy implants are also commonly

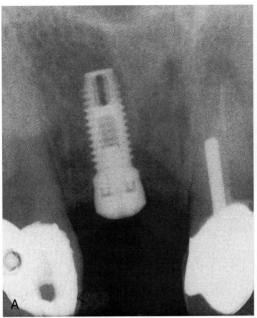
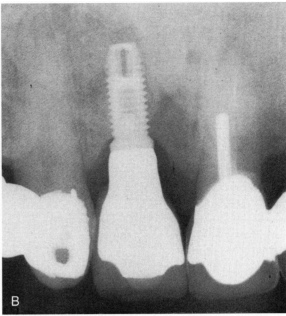

FIGURE 14–3. Endosseous implant replacing tooth #8. **A.** The implant in place. **B.** The crown attached to the implant. (Courtesy of Frederick C. Finzen, DDS.)

used. Alloys of titanium exhibit increased strength and resist surface scratching.

In addition, endosseous implants are available that are flame sprayed with a plasma of titanium that forms a thin protective titanium oxide layer. This material is resistant to chemical attack and permits bonding to bone. Some suggest that bonding is more rapid than with non-sprayed surfaces. However, the plasma-sprayed surface is irregular, permitting a larger surface area for bone ingrowth than smooth titanium. The long-term success with plasma-sprayed implants may be similar to that with pure titanium types.[19]

Calcium phosphate ceramic materials, such as hydroxyapatite and tricalcium phosphate, resemble inorganic material in the human skeleton. Coating the surface of a titanium implant with such materials may make it reactive with bone, allowing bone formation on the implant surface, rather than close bonding, as with pure titanium with an oxidized surface. The biochemical bond is stronger than either the bone or ceramic alone. However, the strength of the bond is dependent on the interface of the metal and the coating.[3]

Aluminum oxide–coated titanium implants, or single-crystal sapphire implants, have many of the characteristics of pure titanium implants.

Research is being conducted to evaluate the long-term success of this type of implant.

SUBPERIOSTEAL TYPE

Subperiosoteal implants consist of a cast framework that is placed over the bone and under the periosteum. They typically have projections through the oral mucosa to permit anchoring of removable dentures.[14, 20]

TRANSOSTEAL TYPE

Transosteal implants are anchors placed all the way through the mandible. They are commonly referred to as staple implants. These implants also provide anchors for removable lower dentures (Figure 14-4).[14, 20]

Prosthetic Restoration

The placement of prosthetic restorations on implants is known as loading. Options include the construction and permanent placement of large, fixed prostheses that replace many teeth; the crown of a single tooth; bridgework with natural tooth abutments; and the placement of overdentures. Fixed prostheses are screwed or cemented onto the implants and can be retrieved by the dentist. Overdentures may rest on bars or domes or may be held in place with

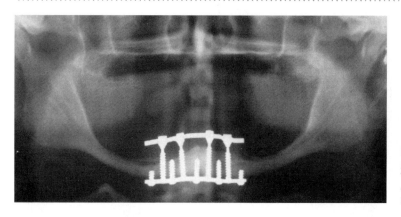

FIGURE 14–4. Panographic radiograph of transosteal (staple) implant. The metal extends through the mandible. (Courtesy of Frederick C. Finzen, DDS.)

clips or screws. Figure 14–5 shows a variety of implant prostheses.

SUCCESS OF IMPLANTS

The clinical success of implants is influenced by many factors. These include the quality and quantity of the bone in which the implant resides, the systemic health of the patient, and the extent of occlusal forces. Albrektsson and Sennerby[1] defined successful implants as meeting a set of goals rather than in terms of simple survival rates. They recommended five criteria for success which indicate osseointegration, patient comfort, function, and implant survival. These are:

1. An individual, unattached implant must be immobile when tested clinically.
2. A radiograph must not show any evidence of peri-implant radiolucency.
3. Vertical bone loss must be less than 0.2 mm annually after the implant's first year of service.
4. There must be no pain, infection, neuropathy, paresthesia, or violation of the mandibular canal.
5. In this context, success rates of 85 percent at the end of a 5-year observation period and 80 percent at the end of a 10-year period are the minimum criteria for success.

With the use of these criteria in a multicenter study of 8139 implants after 5 to 8 years, the success rates for osseointegrated pure titanium implants were greater than 90 percent for those placed in the mandible and greater than 80 percent for those placed in the maxilla.

Others have suggested the use of additional clinical criteria to judge the success of implants. Langer[22] recommended considering the following factors:

1. Mucosal health as determined by clinical parameters such as lack of redness, bleeding on probing, or suppuration.
2. No significant or progressive loss of supporting bone.
3. No persistent infection.
4. Functioning of the implant with no patient discomfort.
5. No increased mobility when the prosthesis is removed.
6. A prosthetically useful implant.

These criteria also emphasize the importance of the implant to the patient, with its comfort and utility being the ultimate measures of success. Therefore, in addition to the number of years that they are present in the mouths of patients, implants should enhance the quality of the individual's life, and not lead to persistent infection or complications.

Cochran[12] adapted a set of criteria for success from the literature that includes both biologic and service-to-patient markers. The following criteria emphasize that success is measured on a continuum, rather than with distinct parameters, with the goal being improved health and function.

1. Less than 1 mm mobility in any direction.
2. No radiolucency.
3. Bone loss not greater than 1/3 of the implant.
4. Provide functional service for five years in 75 percent of cases.
5. Absence of persistent and/or irreversible

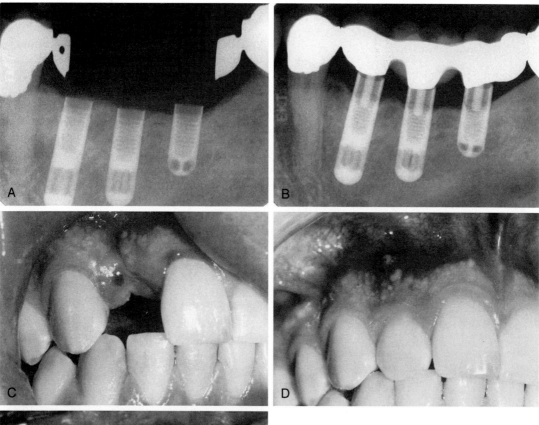

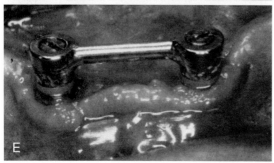

FIGURE 14–5. Implant restorations. **A.** Three implants supporting a bridge attached to the remaining permanent teeth. (Courtesy of Dr. Dennis Davis.) **B.** Bridge in place. (Courtesy of Dr. Dennis Davis.) **C.** Clinical appearance of a missing lateral incisor. (Courtesy of Frederick D. Finzen, DDS.) **D.** Single tooth implant with crown replacing the missing lateral incisor. (Courtesy of Frederick C. Finzen, DDS.) **E.** Bar attached to two implants on the anterior mandible. The overdenture clips onto the bar and provides the patient with better function.

signs/symptoms such as pain, infection, neuropathies, paresthesia, violation of mandibular canal.

6. Clinically immobile.
7. No peri-implant radiolucency.
8. Bone loss less than 0.2 mm annually after the first year of service.
9. Eighty-five percent success after 5 years, 80 percent success after 10 years.
10. Implant design allows restoration satisfactory to patient and dentist.
11. Implant still in mouth.
12. Absence of continuous marginal bone loss.
13. Minimal marginal bone loss.
14. Absence of persistent soft tissue complications.
15. Surgical retrievability.
16. Probing depth less than 4 to 5 mm, bone loss less than 4 mm.
17. No mechanical failure (i.e., fracture).
18. Bone loss does not reach apical ⅓ of implant.
19. Non-standardized radiographs demonstrate less than 50% of implant has bone loss.

Success in implant therapy is not simple to define. The important message to the dental hygienist is to be knowledgeable about implants, educate the patients, and provide the services needed to help maximize the life of each implant and restoration.

AMERICAN DENTAL ASSOCIATION APPROVAL OF IMPLANTS

The American Dental Association provides an acceptance program for endosseous implants through its Council on Dental Materials, Instruments and Devices.[4] The existence of this program indicates the complex and usually multidisciplinary nature of implant therapy. Accepted implants have shown success for a minimum of 5 years in clinical trials of 50 or more patients. Provisionally accepted implants have demonstrated success for a period of 3 years.

IMPLANT SURGERY

The success of implant therapy is dependent on many factors, including compliance and acceptability of the patient, surgical technique, and quality of the restorative dentistry. One extremely significant factor is the surgical procedure performed to place the implant or implants into the bone. Slow, careful osteotomy (drilling into the bone) is required to minimize heat production and ensure an initially stable implant.

Two-step Procedure

Implants usually require two surgical procedures done several months apart. First, the implant is placed in the jaw, covered with gingiva, and allowed to heal so that osseointegration may occur. After a period of about 3 months in the case of mandibular implants and 6 months in the case of maxillary implants, the implant is surgically exposed and can be loaded. The differences in healing time are related to the fact that the maxilla has less dense bone, and therefore, the surgical wound and osseointegration take longer to heal.[21] The term "loading" refers to the placement of the implant in function by attaching abutments and fixed or removable prostheses.[21, 22]

One-step Procedure

One-step implant surgery is the less common technique of placing implants through the gingiva so that a second surgery to place abutments is not required. Like two-step surgery, where implants are initially placed subgingivally and later uncovered, the placement of abutments and functional loading of the exposed implants should not occur until at least 3 months after surgery.[21, 23]

Success of Implant Surgery

The success of implant surgery is dependent on several factors. The bone must be healthy[21] and must not be overheated during preparation of the implant site in order to minimize bone cell death.[6] If a layer of necrotic bone is left behind, a fibrous layer may form around the implant, resulting in fibro-osteal integration, which is not associated with long-term success.[11] The surgical site must be precisely sized so that the implant fits closely to the bony walls. Incision sites and sutures should be located away from the embedded implant to help to prevent bacterial seepage into the healing site. Keratinized tissue is the preferred gingiva around implants because it limits gingival movement that could disrupt good tissue and bone interface,[11] simplifies oral hygiene, and permits better cosmetic results.[6] The use of multiple implants requires precise placement of parallel implants to allow prostheses to be attached with screws.[21]

The addition of loading forces, the abutments and restorations placed on the implants, is best delayed 3 to 6 months to permit healing. If the implant is placed in use immediately, a fibrous capsule develops, reducing the chances of long-term success.[11]

Bone Management

A single implant will not support a large load. Multiple implants are placed in large edentulous areas to distribute the load and increase the chances for successful long-term osseointegration. Adequate bulk of bone must also be available at each implant site to permit successful implant osseointegration. An implant that is placed in too small an area of bone will fail.[11]

CONTRIBUTION OF DENTAL HYGIENE TO THE FIELD OF IMPLANTOLOGY

There is general agreement that **maintenance** procedures are necessary to prevent the onset of infections around implants, called **peri-implantitis.**[24] There is no cementum or fiber insertion on the endosteal implant, so the maintenance of the seal between the epithelium and the underlying bone is critical. If lost, the infection can extend directly to the bone.[25] Regular removal of plaque and calculus deposits, through good home care and maintenance care, plays a significant role, but one that is hard to quantify.

Specific maintenance routines and time frames have not been established, but they include assessment of patient status, personalized home care instructions, plaque and calculus removal, and the use of antimicrobial agents.[5, 9] Successful maintenance routines have been reported in the literature and are a popular topic for presentations at professional meetings.

MAINTENANCE OF DENTAL IMPLANTS

Maintenance is a critical aspect of long-term success for implant patients,[5, 26] even with patients who have implant-retained overdentures and no natural teeth present.[27] Research is beginning to identify the most appropriate methods and materials to maximize successful maintenance care. Evidence is growing as to which materials are the least damaging to potentially fragile implant surfaces and tissue interfaces and how often maintenance procedures should be performed.

Appropriate Instruments for Implants

Laboratory studies have shown that plastic curettes cause no significant changes to implant abutment surfaces.[28, 29] Conventional steel curettes are not recommended for implant maintenance because they roughen the implant abutment surfaces, making the surface less biocompatible with surrounding tissues.[13, 30, 31] It is important to avoid roughening the surface because plaque and calculus are more likely to adhere to exposed rough implant surfaces, leading to inflammatory tissue response and possible extension of the pocket to osseous structures.[25] Roughened surfaces may also be more difficult for patients to clean at home (Figure 14–6).

In addition, laboratory evaluations of curette-treated titanium implants suggest that less attachment of fibroblasts occurs after surfaces are rendered rough by curetting with steel instruments than when plastic or titanium-coated curettes are used.[32] The effect of roughening on the biologic seal is not fully understood, but it appears to be, at least, a mechanical inducement for plaque and calculus formation.

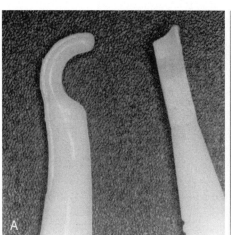
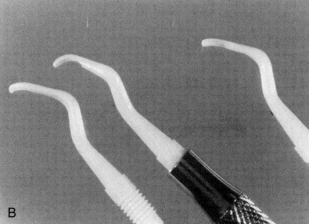

FIGURE 14–6. Calculus removal must be performed with plastic instruments to protect the implants. **A.** Plastic instruments designed to clean the 3- or 4-mm-diameter round implants. Plastic instruments sometimes feel awkward to use because they adapt differently than scalers and curettes. **B.** Plastic instruments are also available in more familiar curette shapes.

Maintenance Procedures

Maintenance procedures for implant patients include plaque assessment, oral hygiene instructions, and removal of subgingival and supragingival accumulations of plaque and calculus (Figure 14-7). These procedures must be performed without damage to the implants.[25, 30] Other than avoiding the use of metal curettes, laboratory studies of various agents used on implants provide insight, but not clearly consistent results, as to what materials are acceptable for use in the dental office and for home care. Gantes and Nilveus[30] reported results from a laboratory study that showed that steel sonic scaler tips and rubber-cup polishing with coarse prophylaxis paste removed ridges on titanium cores after use for as little as 15 seconds. Removal of these ridges caused a potentially significant alteration of titanium surfaces in patients' mouths. In addition, air-powder polishing with baking soda slurry at 70 pounds per square inch left substantial impact marks on titanium in the laboratory. Others have reported laboratory data simulating the effects of 15 years of maintenance on various implant surfaces by a variety of instruments. The results are summarized in Table 14-1.

The authors concluded that the effects of the various modalities, as evaluated by scanning electron microscopy, indicate that chlorhexidine rinsing and the use of various brushing techniques caused limited damage to implant surfaces. Among common office procedures, the use of rubber-cup polishing and medium-grit prophylaxis paste produced the least abrasion. Sonic scaling and ultrasonic scaling caused more abrasion and should be avoided.[11] The use of air-abrasive systems, or air-powder polishing, remains controversial. Recent laboratory studies reported that plaque removal with the air-abrasive system and plastic curettes was less damaging to implants than metal curettes, ultrasonics, or diamond polishing devices.[24, 28] Others reported slight changes and recommended its use with caution based on laboratory data only.[29, 33]

Until the time that sufficient data provide assurance that minor changes on titanium implant surfaces have no effect on gingival health and long-term success of implants, it is advisable to rely on maintenance instruments that minimize surface changes. These include the use of plastic curettes, rubber-cup polishing with a minimal abrasive, such as tin-oxide slurry, and home care implements. The use of metal curettes, titanium curettes, ultrasonics, and air-abrasive systems should be avoided.[25]

Maintenance Intervals

The goal of maintenance therapy for the dental implant patient is to facilitate the stable condition created by active treatment.[34] Implant patients should be considered periodontal maintenance patients rather than prophylaxis patients who are not susceptible to periodontal disease.[25] This treatment involves providing periodic assessment and prophylactic treatment of the periodontal structures with the goal of early detection and treatment of abnormalities or disease.

Recall appointments should be scheduled every 3 or 4 months for routine implant maintenance.[25] Recall intervals should not be extended beyond 6 months, even with the most compliant patients.[35] Recall should be more frequent than every 3 months if this interval is not adequate to reach treatment goals.

Assessments

Gentle probing with plastic periodontal probes aids in assessment.[34, 36] This assessment is more meaningful when the implant prosthesis is not present. Performing this procedure is controversial because it may permit penetration of the epithelial attachment by a sharp instrument, possibly damaging the biologic seal. In addition, because it is difficult to maneuver the probe around large, fixed restorations called **superstructures,** the recorded probe depths may be inaccurate and meaningless. Occasionally, fixed prostheses are removed by the dentist to permit

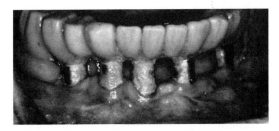

FIGURE 14-7. Multiple mandibular implants with superstructure in place showing accumulations of plaque and calculus.

TABLE 14–1. Effects of Various Cleaning Agents on Implant Materials

		Surface Changes		
Modality	Time Applied (estimating 6 months' wear)	Aluminum Oxide	Titanium (2 types)	Hydroxyapatite (coated)
Titanium scaler	480 strokes	Some	Some	Some
Ultrasonic	8 minutes	NS	Significant	Significant
Sonic	8 minutes	NS	Significant	Some
Air-powder polisher	8 minutes and 8 seconds per surface	Some	Some	Significant
Rubber cup and medium paste	8 minutes, light press	NS	NS	Some
Chlorhexidine rinses	45 hours and 38 minutes	NS	NS	NS
Interproximal brush	5475 strokes	NS	NS	NS
Motorized interproximal brush	91 minutes	NS	NS	NS
Reciprocal electric toothbrush	91 minutes	Some	Some	NS

NS = not significant.
Used with permission. Data from Thomson-Neal D, Evans GH, Meffert RM. Effects of various prophylactic treatments on titanium, sapphire, and hydroxyapatite-coated implants: An SEM study. Int J Periodontics Restorative Dent 1989;9:301–311.

more thorough evaluation of the implant area. Probing with a plastic probe should be considered at that time. In patients with removable prostheses, access for probing is easier and may be performed at each recall interval. Probe depths should be recorded conventionally, with six readings per implant.

The question is, how necessary is probing of implants? Meffert's review pointed out that probing depths for implants are consistently deeper than natural teeth, the histologic probe depth is greater, and the probe ends up closer to bone than when probing natural teeth. The depths found are not relevant because there is no connective tissue attachment, so the information adds little to the clinical examination of the implant. In the case of healthy surrounding gingival tissues, the Meffert study does not recommend taking and recording probing depths at maintenance appointments.[25]

The tone, color, consistency, and bleeding tendency of the tissues should be assessed[34, 35] and are probably more important than probe depths when evaluating the amount of inflammation present. In addition, percussion may be performed to elicit a sound. A strong metallic ringing indicates osseointegration.[34]

Radiographs should be taken regularly to evaluate the bone around the implant. Wilson[34] recommended taking periapical x-rays of the implant area 6 months, 12 months, and 3 years after placement of the prosthesis, then every 3 years unless problems arise. Others recommend taking radiographs every 3 months for the first year, then taking follow-up x-rays every year[35] or every 2 years,[36] or the use of standardized radiographs. Patients sometimes object to frequent radiographs, so the dental hygienist must be prepared to educate the implant patient about the importance of identifying early changes in the bone. Recognizing these changes permits timely treatment to preserve and extend the life of the implant.

Table 14-2 lists the recommended assessments for the dental hygienist to perform in patients with implants. These procedures should be performed in addition to regular assessments of the remaining natural dentition. These recall assessments should be performed every 3 months. They may be performed slightly less frequently in compliant patients with well-maintained implants, but recall intervals should not exceed 6 months.

Treatment

Treatment for implant patients at recall visits consists of a review of oral hygiene procedures,

TABLE 14–2. Assessments for Implant Maintenance Care

Procedure	Comment
Remove superstructure	May not occur at every visit with fixed superstructures
Evaluate tissue for tone, color, consistency, size, and texture	Look for signs of tissue inflammation
Check for mobility	May not be possible with splinted implants
Probe implant sulcus depth if inflammation is present	Use plastic probes only, six measurements per implant
Evaluate plaque for quantity and location	Customize home care advice
Evaluate calculus for quantity and location	Assure complete removal
Radiograph implant area	Done at frequent intervals as determined by the dentist
Record assessments	Reference data for other appointments

removal of subgingival plaque and calculus, removal of supragingival calculus and stain, and care of the remaining teeth and any prosthetic devices. In addition, the dentist should remove fixed prostheses periodically for cleaning and screw replacement. See Implant Maintenance Treatment Procedures.

A variety of refinements can be added to the basic treatment list. Swabbing chlorhexidine around the implant sulcus after therapy helps to control plaque growth for several hours. A reciprocating polisher with plastic tips can be used to polish the implant surface.[36]

Home Care Instructions for Implant Patients

It is essential that implant patients adopt good plaque control on a daily basis. Customized home care instructions must be provided to each implant patient and reinforced regularly. Most implant patients have lost teeth because of plaque accumulation and periodontal disease. Therefore, these patients are susceptible to oral infection and probably have not cleaned their teeth conscientiously or consistently in the past. Implant cleaning is difficult, regardless of whether the prosthesis is removable. Removable overdentures must be taken out daily for soaking and cleaning, and the plaque on the implant abutments must be removed with toothbrushes, floss, toothpicks, or other devices. Rinsing or swabbing the implants with chlorhexidine as an antimicrobial agent is commonly recommended.[25]

The presence of a fixed superstructure compounds the difficulties encountered in cleaning dental implants. Patients must learn to maneu-

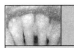

IMPLANT MAINTENANCE TREATMENT PROCEDURES

Home care instruction emphasizing missed plaque	Patient can demonstrate procedures and practice before professional cleaning
Remove subgingival calculus on implant	Gentle instrumentation with plastic curettes is accepted
Remove supragingival calculus and stain on implant	Use plastic curettes to flick off calculus and stains or polish off with rubber cup and fine paste, tin oxide, or toothpaste
Clean superstructure	Devices such as ultrasonic scalers and air-powder polishers may be used, avoiding the implants
Clean any remaining natural teeth	Use any acceptable procedure for scaling and root planing natural teeth
Caries and sensitivity control	Apply appropriate agents to natural teeth: fluorides for caries prevention and agents for control of dentinal sensitivity
Establish recall interval	Customize recall interval based on needs of the individual, every 3 months as a general rule

ver around large restorations to reach implant abutments that are merely 4 mm in diameter.

Soft toothbrushes, interproximal brushes, floss, tufted floss, yarn, gauze folded into a ribbon, single-tufted toothbrushes, wooden interdental cleaners, plastic interdental cleaners, rubber-tip stimulators, power-assisted interproximal brushes, power-assisted toothbrushes, antimicrobial rinses, imagination, and determination are used to clean dental implants. Figure 14-8 is an example of a difficult plaque control situation.

The regular use of home irrigators has not been fully explored, but appears promising. Daily home oral irrigation with 0.06 percent chlorhexidine using a subgingival tip and daily home rinsing with 0.12 percent chlorhexidine have been compared. Both reduced clinical signs of inflammation after a three-month trial. The irrigation group showed greater improvements on indices of gingivitis and bleeding, less staining, and more plaque removal than the rinsing group, but both groups improved significantly from baseline measures on bleeding and measures of gingival inflammation.[37] Others have reported safe use of oral irrigating devices.[36] Use of oral irrigators, particularly when delivering chlorhexidine, may be of significant benefit to implant patients, particularly those who like to use irrigators. They may be of considerable benefit to patients who must clean around large prostheses and find hand operated devices difficult to manage.

Conservative use of these devices can be recommended. Patients should be instructed to use low pressure and direct the stream across the implant sulcus. It is not known if directing pressure into the sulcus can damage the biological seal.

Patient motivation is a crucial element of dental hygiene care for the implant patient. Motivation involves encouraging the patient to attend regular maintenance visits and to comply with oral hygiene protocols. Wilson[34] reported that as many as 45 percent of periodontal patients do not return for regular maintenance visits. He emphasized the importance of informing implant patients of the significance of regular visits and good home care for the long-term success of the implants. In addition, reducing barriers to compliance and simplifying home care routines may help to increase patient acceptance of these responsibilities.

THE FAILING IMPLANT

Not all implant therapy succeeds. Although many implants have documented survival rates of more than a decade, these rates are not 100 percent. Between 5 and 15 percent of implants fail over time based on success rate estimates.[2] In clinical terms, after a period of function, data have shown bone loss exceeding 4 mm in 5 percent to 15 percent of implants, and probing depths exceeding 5 mm in 5 percent to 20

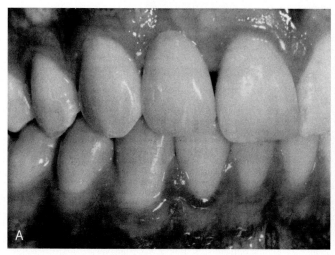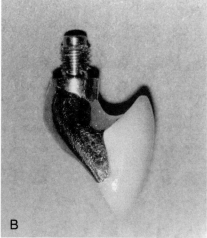

FIGURE 14–8. Home care for the patient with implants can be a challenge because implants are not always lined up precisely with the natural teeth in the arch. Home care must be individualized according to the plaque control needs of the patient. **A.** Single tooth implant replacing the maxillary lateral incisor. **B.** The implant crown, outside the mouth, showing its unusual design and emphasizing the difficulty of plaque control. (Courtesy of Frederick C. Finzen, DDS.)

percent of implants.[38] Most dental hygienists will encounter a failing or failed implant.

Recognition of Implant Failure

A failing implant is characterized by evidence of pocketing, bleeding on probing, exudate, and progression of bone loss. It may also exhibit mobility, a dull sound on percussion, and radiographic peri-implant radiolucency (Figure 14–9).[6] The disease is called peri-implantitis.[25, 38]

Treatment

When an implant fails, there is no recourse but to remove it. If an implant is in the process of failing, also called an ailing implant, exhibiting some or all of the characteristics associated with failure, some steps can be taken. Anti-infective therapy must be undertaken, including removal of plaque and calculus, use of both local and systemic antimicrobial therapy, and improved patient home care. Occlusal adjust-

ments can be made if excessive forces are considered a contributing factor. In addition, surgical techniques modified from periodontal surgical techniques for natural teeth can be employed to treat bone defects.[38]

The useful life of an implant may be extended through a variety of measures. However, the current consensus is that mobile implants are clear failures and should be removed.[6, 38]

IMPLANT THERAPY

Implant therapy is an exciting and growing part of dental care. Implants improve the quality of life for many patients. The dental hygienist plays a significant role in implant maintenance and patient motivation.

Implant therapy is not for everyone. Many factors must be considered by the informed patient before treatment is performed. For example, specific stresses are associated with surgery, and patients must be compliant with main-

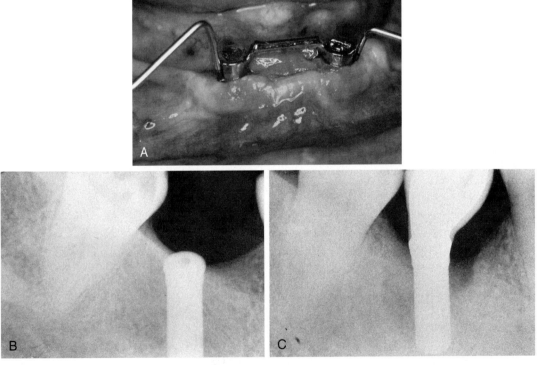

FIGURE 14–9. Clinical and radiographic appearance of failing implants. **A.** Failing implants supporting a bar that stabilizes a lower denture. Periodontal probes are inserted along the sides of the implants, indicating a lack of osseointegration. **B.** Single tooth implant 1 year after placement. Osseointegration appears favorable. **C.** The same implant 2 years after placement. The implant has the prosthesis in place, and radiographic evidence of bone loss is extensive. (Courtesy of Dr. Sasha Jovanovic.)

tenance requirements. Situations that interfere with compliance must be considered, such as psychological disorders or drug use.[9] Before the decision has been made to undergo implant therapy, the patient must fully understand that temporary discomforts, such as pain and swelling, speech problems, or gingivitis, may occur during treatment. Long-term problems can also occur. Mouth surgery always has the potential for problems with bleeding, infection, nerve damage, and other local tissue reactions. Implantology is a complex science in which success depends on a number of factors, including biomaterials, biomechanics, dental and medical evaluation, surgical requirements, healing, prosthodontics, and maintenance care.[9] Proper case selection is considered crucial to the success of treatment.[25, 38]

In well-informed patients, properly performed implant procedures can result in improved comfort and quality of life. Dental hygienists are likely to see many patients with implants in the coming years and must be ready to assume an important role in the education, maintenance, and support of implant patients.

STUDY QUESTIONS

MULTIPLE CHOICE

1. The dental implants with the longest success rates are made of:

   a. Aluminum oxide
   b. Hydroxyapatite
   c. Tin oxide
   d. Titanium

2. In which type of implant is a cast framework placed over the bone and under the periosteum?

   a. Endosseous
   b. Endodontic
   c. Subperiosteal
   d. Transosteal

3. According to the American Dental Association, Council on Dental Materials, accepted implants have demonstrated success in clinical trials of at least 50 patients for a minimum of:

   a. 1 year
   b. 3 year
   c. 5 years
   d. 10 years

4. The term "loading" refers to which aspect of implant therapy?

   a. Placement of the implant into the bone
   b. Placement of abutments and restorations on implants for function
   c. Size of the implant
   d. Bulk of the bone at the implant site

5. Which modality is clearly acceptable for cleaning of implant abutments?

   a. Air-powder polishing
   b. Rubber-cup polishing
   c. Sonic scaling
   d. Ultrasonic scaling

6. Implant patients should be considered periodontal maintenance patients and scheduled for assessment and treatment with the dental hygienist at what interval?

   a. Monthly
   b. Every three months
   c. Every six months
   d. Every twelve months

7. The microbiota of failing implants is similar in quality to that of adult periodontitis and recurrent forms of periodontal disease. The quantity of the pathogenic microbes differs around failing implants.

   a. Both statements are TRUE.
   b. Both statements are FALSE.
   c. The first statement is TRUE, the second is FALSE.
   d. The first statement is FALSE, the second is TRUE.

8. What percentage of implants can be expected to fail over time?

   a. 5 percent to 15 percent
   b. 20 percent to 25 percent
   c. 42 percent
   d. 50 percent

9. All of the following oral hygiene tools can be used safely for home care of the dental implant EXCEPT one. Which one is the EXCEPTION?

   a. Brushes, such as interproximal and single-tufted
   b. Floss, yarn, and gauze
   c. Power-assisted brushes
   d. Metal periodontal probes

10. Implants can be used intraorally as:

    a. Abutments for fixed bridgework
    b. Single tooth replacements
    c. Supports for full dentures
    d. All of the above

SHORT ANSWER

11. Define osseointegration.

    _____

    _____

12. List the main factors on which the success of implant therapy is dependent.

    _____

    _____

13. Why is it important to use plastic curettes when removing calculus from implant abutment surfaces?

    _____

    _____

14. What are the symptoms of a failing dental implant?

    _____

    _____

15. What are the two critical elements of patient compliance for the implant patient?

_____

_____

REFERENCES

1. Albrektsson T, Sennerby L. State of the art in oral implants. J Clin Periodontal 1991;18:474–481.
2. Albrektsson T, Dahl E, Enbom L, Engevall S, Engquist B, Eriksson AR, Feldmann G, Freiberg N, Glantz P-O, Kjellman O, Kristersson L, Kvint S, Köndell P-A, Palmquist J, Werndahl L, Astrand P. Osseointegrated oral implants. J Periodontol 1988;59:287–296.
3. Bernard GW, Carranza FA, Jovanovic SA. Biologic aspects of dental implants. In FA Carranza and MG Newman, eds. Clinical Periodontology, 8th ed. Philadelphia: WB Saunders, 1996:685–689.
4. Donovan TE, Chee WWL. ADA acceptance program for endosseous implants. J Calif Dent Assoc 1992;50:60–62.
5. Jovanovic SA. Clinical aspects of dental implants. In FA Carranza and MG Newman, eds. Clinical Periodontology, 8th ed. Philadelphia: WB Saunders, 1996:690–697.
6. Meffert RM, Langer B, Fritz ME. Dental implants: a review. J Periodontol 1992;63:859–870.
7. Fenton A. The role of dental implants in the future. J Am Dent Assoc 1992;123:37–42.
8. Becker W, Becker EB, Alsuwyed A, Al-Mubarak S. Long-term evaluation of 282 implants in maxillary and mandibular molar positions: a prospective study. J Periodontol 1999;70:896–901.
9. National Institutes of Health. National Institutes of Health consensus development conference statement: dental implants. J Am Dent Assoc 1988;117:509–513.
10. Grogono AL, Lancaster DM, Finger, IM. Dental implants: a survey of patients' attitudes. J Prosthet Dent 1989;62:573–576.
11. Listgarten MA, Lang NP, Schroeder HE, Schroeder A. Periodontal tissues and their counterparts around endosseous implants. Clin Oral Implant Res 1991;2:1–19.
12. Cochran D. Implant therapy I. Ann Periodontol 1996;1:707–790.
13. Thomson-Neal D, Evans GH, Meffert RM. Effects of various prophylactic treatments on titanium, sapphire, and hydroxyapatite-coated implants: an SEM study. Int J Periodontics Restorative Dent 1989;9:301–311.
14. Reiche O, Garg AK. Hygienic maintenance: vital aspects for the success of dental implants. Implant Soc 1990;1:5–14.
15. Klinge B. Implants in relation to natural teeth. J Clin Periodontol 1991;18:482–487.
16. Listgarten MA, Lai C-H. Comparative microbiological characteristics of failing implants and periodontally diseased teeth. J Periodontol 1999;70:431–437.
17. Köndell PA, Söder P-Ö, Landt H, Frithiof L, Anneroth G, Engström P-E, Olsson A-L. Gingival fluid and tissues around successful titanium and ceramic implants. Acta Odontol Scand 1991;49:169–173.
18. Ong ES-M, Newman HN, Wilson M, Bulman JS. The occurrence of periodontitis-related microorganisms in relation to titanium implants. J Periodontol 1992;63:200–205.
19. Weinlander M. Bone growth around dental implants. Dent Clin North Am 1991;35:585–601.
20. Wilkins EM. The patient with oral rehabilitation and implants. In Clinical Practice of the Dental Hygienist, 8th ed. Philadelphia: Lippincott Williams and Wilkins, 1999:411–424.
21. Han TJ. Surgical aspects of dental implants. In FA Carranza and MG Newman, eds. Clinical Periodontology, 8th ed, Philadelphia: WB Saunders, 1996:697–705.
22. Langer B. Dental implants used for periodontal patients. J Am Dent Assoc 1990;121:505–508.
23. Bader DA, Schroeder A, Sutter F, Lang N. The new concept of ITI hollow-cylinder and hollow-screw implants: Part 1. Int J Oral Maxillofac Implants 1988; 3:161–181.
24. Augthun M, Tinschert J, Huber A. In vitro studies on the effect of cleaning methods on different implant surfaces. J Periodontol 1998;69:857–864.
25. Meffert RM. Periodontal aspects of dental implantology. In CE Misch, ed. Contemporary Implant Dentistry, 2nd ed. St Louis, Mosby; 1999:647–660.
26. Meffert RM, Sevor J. Dental implant maintenance. San Antonio, TX: University of Texas Health Sciences Center, Department of Periodontics.
27. Den Dunnen ACL, Slagter AP, de Baat C, Kalk W. Professional hygiene care, adjustments and complications of mandibular implant-retained overdentures: a three-year retrospective study. J Prosthet Dent 1998;78(4):387–390.
28. Brookshire FVG, Nagy WW, Dhuru VB, Siebert GJ, Chada S. The qualitative effects of various types of hygiene instrumentation on commercially pure titanium and titanium alloy implant abutments; and in vitro scanning electron microscope study. J Prosthet Dent 1997;78:286–94.
29. Meschenmoser A, d'Hoedt B, Meyle J, Elbner G, Korn D, Hammerle H, Schulte W. Effects of various hygiene procedures on the surface characteristics of titanium abutments. J Periodontol 1996;67:229–235.
30. Gantes BG, Nilveus R. The effects of different hygiene instruments on titanium surfaces: SEM observations. Int J Periodontics Restorative Dent 1991;11:225–239.
31. Fox SC, Moriarty JD, Kusy RP. The effects of scaling a titanium implant surface with metal and plastic instruments: an in vivo study. J Periodontol 1990;61:485–490.
32. Dmytryk JJ, Fox SC, Moriarty JD. The effects of scaling titanium implant surfaces with metal and plastic instruments on cell attachment. J Periodontol 1990;61:491–496.
33. Chairay J-P, Boulekbache H, Jean A, Soyer A, Bouchard P. Scanning electron microscopic evaluation of the effects of an air-abrasive system on dental implants: a comparative in vitro study between machined and plasma-sprayed titanium surfaces. J Periodontol 1997;68:1215–1222.
34. Wilson TG. Maintaining periodontal treatment. J Am Dent Assoc 1990;121:491–494.
35. Muzzin KMB, Johnson R, Carr P, Daffron P. The dental hygienist's role in the maintenance of osseointegrated dental implants. J Dent Hyg 1988;62:448–453.
36. Koumjian JH, Kerner J, Smith RA. Hygiene maintenance of dental implants. J Calif Dent Assoc 1990;19:29–33.
37. Felo A, Shibly O, Ciancio SG, Lauciello FR, Ho A. Effects of subgingival chlorhexidine irrigation on peri-implant maintenance. J Am Dent 1997;10:107–110.
38. Jovanovic S. Diagnosis and treatment of peri-implant disease. In FA Carranza and MG Newman, eds. Clinical Periodontology, 8th ed. Philadelphia: WB Saunders, 1996:706–716.

15

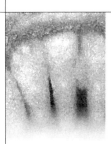

Mari-Anne L. Low

Periodontal Maintenance and Prevention

*C*hapter *O*bjectives

1. Explain the effectiveness of periodontal therapy in the prevention of disease, disease progression, and tooth loss.
2. Explain the critical importance of periodontal maintenance and the determinants of a successful maintenance program.
3. State the five major objectives of periodontal maintenance.
4. Recognize the importance of patient compliance with periodontal maintenance, and describe strategies to improve compliance with recommended maintenance intervals and oral hygiene regimens.
5. List the principal aims and components of the maintenance appointment.
6. Recognize the signs of recurrent periodontitis, and assess the potential contributing factors.
7. State the cause of root surface caries, and describe therapeutic approaches to prevent their development.
8. Explain the theories, causes, and management of dentin hypersensitivity.
9. Recognize the role of the dental hygienist in providing periodontal treatment.

*K*ey *T*erms

Compliance
Dentin hypersensitivity
Fluoride therapy
Gingival recession

Periodontal maintenance
Recall
Recurrent periodontitis
Root caries

Preventing recurrent disease and maintaining health are of fundamental importance for the success of periodontal therapy. Chronic gingival inflammation can resolve if the local etiologic factors are removed during the active phase of periodontal treatment. However, the long-term stability of results and the prevention of recurring disease require regular supervision in an effective periodontal maintenance program. **Periodontal maintenance** is "the continuing periodic assessment and prophylactic treatment of the periodontal structures that permit early detection and treatment of new or recurring abnormalities or disease."[1] Commonly referred to as **recall** maintenance, periodontal maintenance therapy or supportive periodontal therapy, the current terminology is periodontal maintenance, which more accurately describes the long-term maintenance phase of periodontal treatment.[2] The terms are used interchangeably in this book.

The overall goal of dentistry is to attain and maintain healthy and functional dentition for a lifetime. Within this context, the primary objective of periodontal maintenance is to preserve the stable state achieved during the active phase of successful periodontal therapy. This chapter focuses on issues that are relevant to maintenance, including: (1) The effectiveness of periodontal therapy in arresting the progression of periodontitis and preventing tooth loss; (2) the objectives of periodontal maintenance; (3) the importance of patient **compliance** with recommended recall schedules and plaque control regimens; (4) the components of the maintenance appointment; (5) the recurrence of periodontal disease; (6) the significance of caries in the periodontal maintenance population and the appropriate use of fluorides in caries prevention; and (7) the hypersensitivity of dentin after periodontal therapy and recommended treatment.

Providing preventive, educational, and therapeutic services for maintenance care is a challenging task. As a primary care provider in the treatment of periodontal disease, the dental hygienist retains significant responsibility for the maintenance patient after active periodontal treatment. Periodontal maintenance emphasizes the important link between preventive oral health care and dental hygiene care toward achieving optimum oral health. As the public becomes increasingly aware of the importance of oral health, the role of the dental hygienist in providing maintenance care will continue to grow.

SEQUENCE OF PERIODONTAL THERAPY

Periodontal maintenance plays a critical role within the spectrum of periodontal therapy. Periodontal therapy consists of a series of four phases of treatment: (1) the initial, or hygienic phase; (2) the re-evaluation phase; (3) the surgical phase; and (4) the maintenance phase (Figure 15-1). The initial phase consists of oral hygiene instruction and supragingival and subgingival debridement of bacterial plaque and calculus. During the re-evaluation phase, a second assessment of the periodontal condition is performed to determine the results of initial therapy and decide whether additional periodontal intervention is required. Immediately after re-evaluation, the maintenance program is initiated to ensure the stability of results attained in the initial phase. During this period, corrective surgical and restorative procedures are performed as indicated. The aim of the surgical phase is to provide reconstructive or surgical therapy to further improve the periodontal condition.

EFFECTIVENESS OF PERIODONTAL THERAPY

The major objective of periodontal therapy is to arrest the progression of periodontal disease by eliminating or reducing the local microbial etiologic factors. Overwhelming evidence shows the effectiveness of periodontal therapy in preventing disease, slowing the progression of disease, and minimizing tooth loss caused by periodontal sequelae. Many longitudinal studies show that periodontal therapy is effective in maintaining teeth in a state of health, function, and comfort for many years.[3] In contrast, untreated periodontal disease progresses, with a continual loss of the periodontium over time.[4] Ultimately, this chronic destruction is responsible for tooth mortality. Further, the stability of results obtained through active periodontal therapy requires a regular maintenance program. A 30-year case report (see the accompanying A 30-Year Case Report) shows the efficacy of early recognition and treatment followed by maintenance therapy and meticulous oral hygiene in arresting the progression of periodontal disease.

Prevention of Disease

Successful prevention of gingivitis and periodontitis begins with good personal oral hygiene and periodic professional maintenance

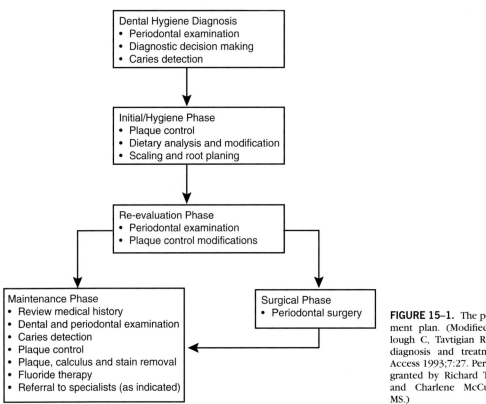

FIGURE 15–1. The periodontal treatment plan. (Modified from McCullough C, Tavtigian R. Perio trends: diagnosis and treatment planning. Access 1993;7:27. Permission for use granted by Richard Tavtigian, DDS, and Charlene McCullough, RDH, MS.)

A 30-YEAR CASE REPORT

The Mayre Heflebower story described by Seibert (1980) is a case report documented over a period of 30 years to show the value of preventive oral health care. Despite limited professional maintenance care, the success of periodontal therapy and daily oral hygiene in maintaining a comfortable and functional dentition for life is demonstrated in this documentation of a patient's periodontal history.

After the diagnosis of gingivitis with localized areas of periodontitis in 1947, the patient underwent nonsurgical periodontal therapy, including scaling, root planing, and curettage. In addition, she was provided with information and training in the control of microbial plaque and inflammation. This information ultimately became the basis of her self-maintenance program. Annual professional maintenance visits consisted of a complete oral soft and hard tissue examination, minor scaling of her mandibular anterior teeth, and a dental prophylaxis.

Success in arresting the progression of disease was apparent 26 years after the initial periodontal therapy as evidenced by the clinical health of the periodontal tissues and by comparison of the radiographs taken in 1949 and 1973 (accompanying Figures A, B, and C). No further measurable alveolar bone loss was detected at the time of her death in 1977 at age 77. The patient's success in maintaining a lifetime of optimal periodontal health underlines the importance of periodontal maintenance care.

The patient's benefit from preventive oral health care is documented in clinical and histologic data. This case provides an opportunity for dental health professionals to study the important contribution of prevention and maintenance.

From Seibert JS. The Mayre Heflebower Story. Philadelphia: University of Pennsylvania, 1980.

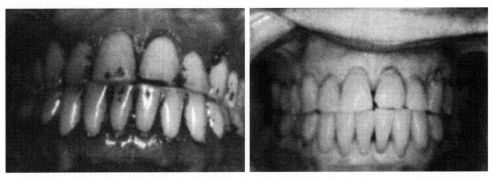

FIGURE A. Response to periodontal and maintenance therapy. Left. Before treatment, note the distribution of supragingival plaque stained with disclosing solution and the amount of gingival recession on the facial surface of the mandibular incisors. Right. After treatment and 20 years of maintenance therapy, the gingival tissues appear stable and healthy. (From Seibert JS. The Mayre Heflebower Story. Philadelphia: University of Pennsylvania, 1980.)

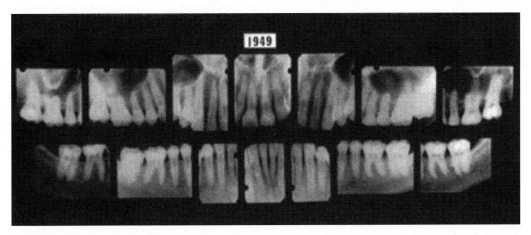

FIGURE B. Full mouth radiographs taken in 1949 after the initial periodontal therapy for the original diagnosis of gingivitis with localized areas of periodontitis in 1947. (From Seibert JS. The Mayre Heflebower Story. Philadelphia: University of Pennsylvania, 1980.)

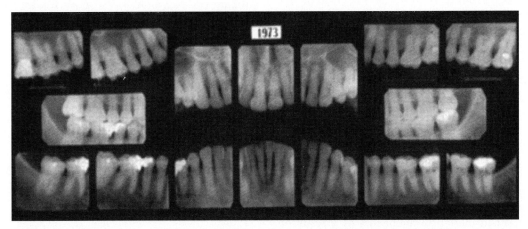

FIGURE C. Full mouth radiographs taken in 1973 after 26 years of maintenance therapy that primarily consisted of meticulous daily plaque control and annual maintenance care. Note the preservation of alveolar bone height compared with the radiographs in Figure B. (From Seibert JS. The Mayre Heflebower Story. Philadelphia: University of Pennsylvania, 1980.)

care to minimize or eliminate the etiologic factors that lead to the pathogenic state. As an oral health educator and clinician, the dental hygienist is an essential provider of preventive services in the initial phase of periodontal therapy and during periodontal maintenance care. Hence, the dental hygienist must recognize the benefits of periodontal therapy, maintenance care, and effective plaque control to appropriately select treatment modalities and to educate patients about the prevention of gingival and periodontal diseases.

Epidemiologic and clinical studies have provided strong evidence to correlate poor personal oral hygiene care and the presence of gingivitis.[5-8] A landmark study by Löe and coworkers[7, 8] described heavy plaque accumulation and generalized mild gingivitis in patients with a normally healthy periodontium after 9 to 21 days without any personal oral hygiene.[7, 8] The observed experimental gingivitis was reversed when daily plaque control procedures were reinstituted. These results provide the foundation on which plaque control is based. To encourage the patient to maintain a clean and healthy oral environment, the dental hygienist should emphasize the significance of personal oral hygiene and review appropriate plaque control techniques during each maintenance visit.

Gingivitis is associated with the occurrence of periodontal disease. Both human and laboratory animal studies have shown that gingivitis does not always proceed to periodontitis; however, periodontitis is always preceded by gingivitis.[4] Therefore, recognition and control of gingivitis are vital to the goals of maintenance therapy.

Both effective personal oral hygiene and professional maintenance therapy are critical to the prevention of periodontal disease. Despite its benefit in resolving gingivitis, daily plaque control alone has a limited effect on periodontal disease. Evidence suggests that supragingival plaque control alone can reduce inflammation associated with gingivitis; however, improvement in probing depths and clinical attachment is minimal in patients with periodontitis.[9] This limited clinical improvement may be a result of the unpredictable effect of supragingival plaque control in altering the subgingival microflora in pocket depths greater than 5 mm.[9] However, scaling and root planing has a significant effect on subgingival flora and probing depths.[10-16] This observation reinforces the importance of professional subgingival mechanical instrumentation at regular intervals in conjunction with personal oral hygiene to maintain periodontal health.

Prevention of Disease Progression

The periodontal response after effective nonsurgical and surgical therapy favors the re-establishment and maintenance of periodontal health. Numerous studies show that removing supragingival and subgingival bacterial deposits can resolve inflammation and halt disease progression.[9] In addition, significant advances in understanding the complex causes of periodontal disease and a wider selection of therapeutic modalities have contributed to successful periodontal treatment.

Commonly, several forms of therapy are combined to disrupt the pathogenesis of periodontal disease. Current periodontal therapies and the clinical benefits provided are shown in Table 15–1.

Research has verified the effect of periodontal therapies on clinical parameters such as bleeding on probing, loss of clinical attachment, and changes in gingival color and form. For example, two longitudinal studies evaluated the effects of four types of periodontal therapy—coronal scaling, root planing, modified Widman surgery, and flap surgery with osseous resection—on the prevalence of bleeding on probing and suppuration.[17, 18] Both studies confirmed all four therapies, followed by mainte-

TABLE 15–1. Available Periodontal Therapies and Potential Clinical Benefits

Periodontal Therapies	Clinical Benefits
• Non-surgical periodontal therapy—scaling and root planing • Periodontal surgery • Subgingival irrigation with antimicrobial medications • Subgingival sustained-release drug delivery systems • Systemic antimicrobial therapy	• Resolution of inflammation • Elimination of infection • Reduction of pocket depths • Arrested disease progression • Prevention of tooth loss • Enhanced patient comfort • Healthy gingival appearance

nance care at 3-month intervals, reduced the prevalence of these disease indicators. However, coronal scaling was less effective in sites with greater than 5 mm pocket depth. It may be that areas with increased probing depths continued to exhibit greater inflammation because adequate debridement was more difficult without surgical intervention. Maintenance care at 3-month intervals promoted the long-term results of all therapies.

Nonsurgical periodontal therapy, also called Phase I therapy or the hygienic phase, is recognized as an effective treatment to arrest or retard the progression of early periodontal disease. The American Academy of Periodontology defines nonsurgical periodontal treatment as the phase of periodontal therapy that includes plaque control, plaque removal, supragingival and subgingival scaling, root planing, and the use of chemical adjuncts.[19] Several longitudinal studies confirmed the effectiveness of nonsurgical periodontal therapy for early intervention of periodontal disease if followed by regular maintenance visits.[9] Research conducted in a patient group with moderate to advanced periodontal disease has demonstrated the short-term effects of initial periodontal therapy.[16] Treatment included oral hygiene instruction, scaling and root planing, and elimination of plaque retentive factors. Three to five months after therapy, the probing pocket depths were reduced and the probing attachment levels improved. These results show effective pocket depth reduction and increased clinical attachment levels in study subjects with moderate to advanced periodontitis.

Regular periodontal maintenance is critical to the success of both nonsurgical and surgical periodontal therapy. Numerous long-term studies have established the effectiveness of frequent maintenance care to halt or significantly reduce the rate of disease progression.[20] For example, studies comparing patients who received maintenance care three to six times per year with patients who received only one maintenance visit per year clearly showed the arrest of disease progression.[21-23] Patients who underwent maintenance care visits only once per year showed increased plaque and gingival indices, probing depths, and loss of clinical attachment. Thus, the benefits achieved by active periodontal therapy must be maintained by frequent maintenance care to prevent further deterioration of the periodontium.

Prevention of Tooth Loss

Many long-term studies have shown the effectiveness of periodontal therapy and maintenance care in reducing the number of teeth extracted because of end-stage periodontal destruction.[24] Several researchers have documented tooth loss in longitudinal studies of individuals either receiving or not receiving periodontal treatment, including maintenance therapy.[25-27] Tooth mortality rates in treated individuals ranged from 0.6 to 2.2 teeth lost over 10 years. By comparison, individuals with untreated periodontitis lost five to six teeth over 10 years.[28, 29] The tooth mortality rate in patients who received periodontal treatment and periodic maintenance was lower than that in those who received no periodontal treatment.[24, 27]

EFFECTIVENESS OF PERIODONTAL MAINTENANCE

Long-term success of periodontal and maintenance therapy has been documented in both prospective and retrospective studies.[9, 30] These studies show that both surgical and nonsurgical periodontal therapy are effective in halting the destructive disease if routine professional maintenance is obtained. Maintenance care must begin soon after active therapy and occur at 3- to 4-month intervals. Conversely, periodontal therapy without comprehensive maintenance care results in higher rates of loss of attachment than expected without treatment.[30] In fact, alveolar bone loss and tooth mortality rates in unmaintained individuals have been reported to be twice that observed in patients receiving maintenance therapy.[27, 31] Further, regular plaque control by the patient, in addition to proper maintenance care by the clinician, is necessary to maintain the results of periodontal therapy.[16] Poor oral hygiene permits an environment for opportunistic reinfection by putative periodontopathic microbes, possibly resulting in disease progression.

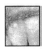

TABLE 15–2. Determinants of Successful Periodontal Maintenance

Factors	Rationale
• Collaboration between periodontist, dentist, and dental hygienist is established. • Partnership between patient and oral health care team is created. • Patient accepts responsibility for oral health. • Maintenance of periodontal health is influenced by patient's overall condition.	• Assures all oral care providers understand the patient's goals, treatment plan, and prognosis. • Facilitates a positive relationship and favorable outcome. • Success relies on patient's commitment to achieve and maintain oral health. • Factors to be considered include the nature and severity of periodontal disease, systemic health, mental health, and host response to therapy.

Determinants of Successful Periodontal Maintenance

The success of periodontal treatment relies on surgical and non-surgical procedures for thorough root debridement and long-term maintenance through periodic professional therapy and daily personal oral hygiene.[19] Several integrated factors contribute to the success of periodontal maintenance, as listed in Table 15–2.

OBJECTIVES OF PERIODONTAL MAINTENANCE

The overall objective of periodontal maintenance is to prevent the development of new or recurrent periodontal disease through supervised care and to preserve a functional and comfortable dentition for life. Specifically, there are five underlying objectives: (1) Preservation of clinical attachment levels, (2) maintenance of alveolar bone height, (3) control of inflammation, (4) evaluation and reinforcement of personal oral hygiene, and (5) maintenance of optimal oral health.[32]

Preservation of Clinical Attachment Levels

Monitoring the gain or loss of clinical attachment levels and probing depths is valuable in assessing periodontal health. A gain of clinical attachment level and improved probe depth measurements are common findings after active periodontal therapy. However, long-term results are highly dependent on patient compliance with maintenance care and the frequency of maintenance visits.[20] For poorly maintained patients with insufficient plaque control, clinical inflammatory parameters soon resemble those observed before treatment, and deeper probe depths, indicating the continued loss of attachment and alveolar bone, are common.[20]

Reductions in probe depths after periodontal therapy result from healing at the epithelial attachment and reduction of gingival swelling.[12, 33] Therefore, increasing probe depths are the most valuable and practical measurements to predict probing attachment loss in maintenance patients. They are more predictable than increased plaque scores, bleeding sites, or amounts of suppuration.[34]

Evaluation of the stability of periodontal health requires thorough documentation of probe depths and clinical attachment levels. These measurements are instrumental in monitoring the patients' periodontal status during the maintenance phase. However, there are no national guidelines recommending the frequency of these comprehensive evaluations. Suggestions include evaluation at annual or biannual intervals or at every maintenance visit.[35] Despite this lack of standardization, every recall appointment must include a periodontal evaluation, regardless of whether it is a comprehensive or a monitoring assessment. The monitoring examination has been described as a "directed" assessment in which all sites are evaluated for inflammatory changes, with problem sites recorded.[36] Thus, comparisons with baseline data can be made and significant changes identified.

Maintenance of Alveolar Bone Height

Periodontal disease is characterized by the progression of gingival inflammation into deeper periodontal structures, resulting in the loss of alveolar bone support for the teeth. A primary goal of periodontal maintenance is to preserve the alveolar bone height to prevent tooth loss. Periodic radiographic examinations are required to compare bone changes over time. Radiographs provide important data that can be used to evaluate the long-term stability of alveolar bone height during maintenance therapy. However, radiographic records of alveolar crestal height reflect only historical bone loss, not active bone destruction. They are a necessary record of therapy, but not a substitute for monitoring clinical parameters.

Control of Inflammation

Maintenance of satisfactory periodontal health requires control of inflammation and prevention of recurrent disease. Toward this end, personal oral hygiene is one of the most important aspects of periodontal maintenance. Studies of supervised maintenance programs that focused on refinement of personal oral hygiene skills showed that improved gingival and periodontal conditions were achieved in compliant subjects.[37] In contrast, Lindhe and colleagues[38] showed that maintenance patients with imperfect plaque control continued to exhibit loss of periodontal attachment. However, these patients did not receive subgingival instrumentation, only supragingival scaling. Others have shown that patients with imperfect plaque control could maintain clinical attachment levels as long as regular professional subgingival instrumentation was performed.[39] Poor oral hygiene alone, resulting in marginal gingival inflammation in maintenance patients, may not lead to increased periodontal destruction.[32, 39] However, these studies show that routine professional care, including disruption of the subgingival microbial ecosystem, plays a vital role in conjunction with daily oral home care to maintain a stable periodontium.

Evaluation and Reinforcement of Personal Oral Hygiene

Daily personal oral hygiene and professional maintenance care are the cornerstone of preventive periodontics. Each maintenance visit must include an evaluation of the patient's oral home care and reinstruction on proper plaque control techniques as needed. It has been shown that in patients who had 2 years of professionally monitored plaque control emphasizing meticulous oral hygiene, the subgingival microbiota changed to one associated with health.[38] Although perfect supragingival plaque control is an unrealistic goal for most patients,

the amount of plaque can be reduced to levels tolerated by the body. This change can prevent the re-establishment of gingivitis or reinfection by opportunistic periodontal pathogens. With the use of behavioral modification and motivational techniques, the dental hygienist plays a role in plaque control education that is equally as important and demanding as the more technical aspects of maintenance therapy.

Maintenance of Optimal Oral Health

An essential component of the maintenance program is the evaluation of the overall health of each patient. Updating the patient's medical record is imperative to identify any systemic conditions that may complicate or contraindicate dental and dental hygiene care. In addition to the periodontal examination, assessment of oral soft tissues, restorations, caries, hypersensitive dentin, occlusion, and dental prostheses must be performed each time the patient is seen for a maintenance visit. All of these assessments are part of the preventive and therapeutic services provided by the dental hygienist during maintenance therapy. Each is indispensable to help patients to achieve optimal oral health.

COMPLIANCE WITH PERIODONTAL MAINTENANCE

The overall success of periodontal therapy depends significantly on patient compliance with recommended recall schedules and oral hygiene regimens. Many studies show that patients who comply with maintenance recommendations have better periodontal health and overall prognoses than patients who forgo maintenance care.[40] Periodontal patients must be made aware that continued maintenance care and personal plaque control are essential elements of successful treatment. Failure to comply with these regimens can lead to further periodontal destruction and possibly to tooth loss. In essence, periodontal disease can be arrested and controlled, but not cured. Compliance requirements seem demanding, but for most individuals, the benefits of compliance far outweigh the risks of periodontal disease and tooth loss.

Compliance with Recommended Maintenance Intervals

Numerous studies show that periodontal health is maintained in individuals who comply with suggested maintenance intervals, regardless of the type of surgical or nonsurgical therapy administered.[9] In contrast, patients who do not comply or who comply erratically have increased periodontal deterioration.[41] Typically, patients who comply erratically show an increased loss of periodontal attachment,[42] require more corrective surgical procedures,[43] and tend to lose more teeth.[26]

Large variations are seen in data describing patient compliance with recommended maintenance therapy. In private periodontal practices, 16 to 95 percent of patients complied with 3-month maintenance intervals.[43, 44] University-based studies reported relatively low percentages of maintenance schedule compliance, ranging from 11 to 45 percent.[45-47] These discrepancies, like compliance, may have many causes and are not easily explained. However, it appears that obtaining patient cooperation is a major challenge for dental hygienists.

The reasons why patients do not comply with maintenance schedules are complex because each individual has different needs and experiences. (See Reasons for Non-compliance with Maintenance Schedules.) In general, noncompliance is seen more commonly in patients who perceive chronic diseases not to be life threatening.[48] Further, personality differences may exist between compliant and noncompliant patients. Personality attributes associated with compliance include self-confidence and positive self-image, whereas noncompliant patients may be more critical and child-like and may experience more stress.[49]

Compliance with Recommended Oral Hygiene Regimens

Bacterial plaque is the primary etiologic agent of gingivitis and periodontal disease,[8, 50] and it is well-established that meticulous oral hygiene can prevent both dental caries and periodontal disease.[21, 51] Adequate plaque control is a major determinant of successful periodontal therapy. Daily mechanical plaque control, including the use of a variety of cleaning aids, is the responsibility of the patient. However, the dental hygienist is responsible for educating patients and motivating patients to perform these tasks. Despite all of this information and instruction, compliance with plaque control regimens is often temporary.

Reported rates of compliance with suggested oral hygiene procedures vary, but are often disappointing. A survey of patients in a private dental practice showed approximately equal proportions of patients claiming to be highly, moderately, and poorly compliant.[52] Other findings suggest that at most 51 percent of patients claim high compliance, 38 percent report moderate compliance, and 11 percent are noncompliant 30 days after oral hygiene instruction.[53] Patient compliance with the use of interproximal cleaning devices appears no better, with less than 50 percent compliance.[54]

Suggested reasons for poor compliance with plaque control measures do not include negative attitudes toward dental care or physical or mental handicaps. Rather, periodontal patients report that oral hygiene procedures are cumbersome and time consuming. Improved plaque control may be achieved in these patients by introducing an electric toothbrush, which the patients perceive as faster and simpler than manual brushing.[55] Compliance with suggested oral hygiene regimens may also be directly related to the number of plaque control aids recommended at the maintenance visit. When more plaque control aids are recommended, decreased compliance is observed.[56]

Strategies to Improve Patient Compliance

Improving patient compliance with scheduled maintenance therapy and oral hygiene regimens

---

REASONS FOR NON-COMPLIANCE WITH MAINTENANCE SCHEDULES[40, 48]

- Fear
- Economic concerns
- Socioeconomic level
- Influence from family and friends
- Perceived indifference from the dental hygienist
- Failure to understand the significance of periodontal maintenance

is a challenging task for the dental hygienist. However, for most patients, better, if not ideal, compliance can be achieved.[48] Strategies to increase compliance involve increasing the patient's knowledge. The importance of periodontal maintenance, the benefits of preventive therapy, an appreciation of improved oral health, and the dental hygienist's commitment to maintaining a caring attitude and providing the highest quality professional services should be emphasized. Recommendations to improve compliance are listed in Table 15-3.[48]

Research suggests that the highest patient drop-out rate occurs during the first year of maintenance therapy. Thirty-five percent of the patients who received periodontal therapy thought that treatment was complete after the initial phase, before maintenance even began.[40] Therefore, special attention should be given to patients at the initiation of treatment and again at the commencement of periodontal maintenance to emphasize the importance of compliance and establish a positive long-term relationship.

Economic considerations are a common source of concern about suggested maintenance intervals. Socioeconomic status, educational level, and perception of oral health may affect a patient's attitude toward purchasing oral health care services. The cost of mainte-

nance appointments is often a primary determinant of patient compliance. A survey of noncompliant maintenance patients in a private periodontal practice showed that many were concerned about the long-term expense of treatment.[40] This concern may reflect a lack of appreciation for the cost-effectiveness of maintenance care. Because chronic periodontal disease is often asymptomatic, it can progress unnoticed. Subsequent re-treatment can be much more expensive than maintenance. The dental hygienist can correct these misconceptions and help the patient to understand the preventive and cost-effective aspects of maintenance care.

The popularity of healthy lifestyles and physical fitness has skyrocketed in recent years, and health concerns have become a part of mainstream American life. The promotion of physical and mental health and well-being focuses on prevention. This requires individuals to make decisions leading to healthier lifestyles. The promotion of oral health is a part of this trend. The media, federal and state governments, employers, health professionals, family, and friends greatly influence an individual's attitude toward health. Because oral health is often a reflection of systemic health, the dental hygienist is in an excellent position to encourage patients to maintain both their oral and physical health. As new evidence emerges suggesting a link be-

 TABLE 15–3. Recommendations to Improve Patient Compliance

Step	Rationale
1. Simplify	Speaking at the patient's level of understanding enhances communication efforts; patients tend to remember what is told to them first; the simpler the required behavior, the more likely it is that the patient will comply.
2. Accommodate	Recommendations should be tailored to the patient's needs and lifestyle; satisfied patients tend to comply more than dissatisfied patients.
3. Remind patients of appointments	Patients must recognize the importance of frequent supportive therapy to maintain periodontal health.
4. Keep records of compliance	Noting the patient's history of compliance with recommended maintenance schedules and plaque control regimens provides legal documentation as well as a guideline for behavior modification.
5. Inform	Written specifications of the recommended regimens can be reminders for patients.
6. Provide positive reinforcement	Positive feedback enhances compliance more than a negative approach.
7. Identify potential noncompliers	If noncompliance is suspected in a patient, the consequences of failure to comply should be discussed before therapy is initiated.

Used with permission from Wilson TG: Compliance: A review of the literature with possible applications to periodontics. J. Periodontol 1987;58:709.

tween periodontal and systemic diseases, patients' awareness of oral health as an essential component of overall well-being will increase. Moreover, evidence suggests that health-related behavior, including compliance, is often dictated by the individual's beliefs about health.[57] Hence, an appreciation of oral health is likely to improve compliance and ultimately help achieve success in periodontal maintenance.

As a health professional, the dental hygienist is obligated to continually educate and motivate patients to comply with recommendations for good oral health. The establishment of a partnership between the patient and the dental hygienist is essential to facilitate this learning relationship. Dental hygienists have sometimes been perceived as indifferent to patient concerns.[48] Maintaining a caring attitude and good rapport encourages patients to ask questions and express their fears and concerns regarding therapy. Dental hygienists should take advantage of opportunities to teach and provide a better understanding of maintenance therapy; this understanding, in turn, promotes patient compliance.

THE MAINTENANCE APPOINTMENT

Regular professional maintenance visits are the cornerstone of periodontal maintenance. The principal aims of the maintenance appointment are to: (1) Evaluate the stability of results after active therapy; (2) thoroughly remove bacterial plaque accumulations on the tooth surface; (3) eliminate all factors that favor the persistence of pathogenic bacteria; and (4) evaluate and reinforce plaque control. To achieve these objectives, the maintenance visit consists of a medical history update, a complete periodontal and dental examination, a radiographic examination if needed, a review of personal oral hygiene, and removal of supragingival and subgingival plaque and calculus (see the accompanying The Periodontal Maintenance Appointment).[41] On average, the maintenance appointment lasts 1 hour and generally provides sufficient time for thorough and proper care.[41] However, the length of the appointment can be adjusted depending on the needs of the patient. The next section describes the components of a periodontal maintenance appointment, com-

monly referred to as a "maintenance visit" or "periodontal recall."

COMPONENTS OF THE MAINTENANCE VISIT

Medical and Dental History Update

Before seeing the patient, the dental hygienist should review the patient's chart to determine the patient's medical history, dental history, need for premedication, record of compliance, and any special circumstances that may affect the dental hygiene care plan. The time necessary for this review is brief, but it is important to be familiar with each patient's background and needs.

The periodontal maintenance appointment must begin with a verbal and written update of the patient's medical history, dental history, current medications, and vital signs. Changes in health conditions may require modifications of the dental hygiene care plan. In addition, a review of the patient's dental history and specific dental concerns may alert the dental hygienist to conditions that require special attention.

Oral and Dental Examination

A thorough extraoral and intraoral examination of the soft tissues to detect pathologic conditions must be a routine component of each maintenance visit. If an abnormality is identified, the dental hygienist's responsibilities include providing detailed documentation and obtaining an evaluation by the dentist.

A complete dental examination that includes caries detection, restorative assessment, and prosthesis evaluation is performed during each maintenance appointment. Recognition of conditions that may be detrimental to the patient's periodontal health is an indispensable skill and an important responsibility of the dental hygienist. Factors that may cause adverse periodontal conditions include defective restorations, overhanging margins, open contacts, overcontoured crowns, and poorly fitting removable prostheses. Any oral conditions that appear to deviate from normal should be brought to the attention of both the patient and the dentist. In addition, even excellent restora-

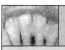

THE PERIODONTAL MAINTENANCE APPOINTMENT

Assessment Procedures
Medical and dental history update

- Review chart before seating patient
- Identify recent illnesses, current health status and medications, and other pertinent information
- Determine vital signs

Oral and dental examination

- Examine extraoral and intraoral soft tissues for pathologic conditions
- Detect caries, assess restorations, and evaluate prostheses

Periodontal evaluations

- Measure probing pocket depths
- Measure gingival recession
- Record specific sites of bleeding on probing
- Assess tooth mobility
- Classify furcations
- Evaluate sites of mucogingival involvement

Radiographic examination

- Obtain and review necessary radiographs

Plaque control evaluation

- Assess quantity and location of existing plaque
- Educate, motivate, and reinforce plaque control

Therapeutic Procedures
Oral hygiene instruction

- Review tooth brushing and interdental cleaning techniques

- Reinforce importance of daily oral hygiene care

Periodontal debridement

- Remove plaque and calculus deposits from supragingival and subgingival tooth surfaces

Polishing

- Selectively polish teeth with prophylaxis paste
- Floss interproximal areas

Fluoride therapy

- Apply topical fluoride preparations as necessary

Sensitivity therapy

- Apply topical antisensitivity preparations as needed
- Recommend and dispense toothpaste for sensitive teeth as needed

Referrals
Dental specialists

- Refer patient to periodontist for further periodontal evaluation and treatment
- Refer patient to appropriate dentist to address additional dental needs

Maintenance Intervals
- Establish appropriate interval for periodontal maintenance on an individual basis

---

tions and prostheses may cause plaque retention and problems with oral hygiene. These special problems can be identified and the patient taught techniques to clean such areas.

Periodontal Evaluation

Before any therapy is performed, assessment of the patient's current periodontal status is mandatory. The clinical parameters that are evaluated include probing pocket depths, clinical attachment loss, gingival recession, bleeding on probing, suppuration, tooth mobility, furcations, and mucogingival involvement.

PROBING POCKET DEPTHS

Periodontal probing is a valuable tool for the assessment of periodontal health. Evaluation of probing depths serves to complement the initial visual assessment of the gingival tissues. The periodontal probe is used to measure the normal sulcus and periodontal pocket depths from the base of the sulcus to the gingival margin.[58] Six measurements are taken for each tooth from the distobuccal, buccal, mesiobuccal, distolingual, lingual, and mesiolingual surfaces. To permit changes to be followed over time, a complete periodontal charting is performed at least once a year. Measurements that

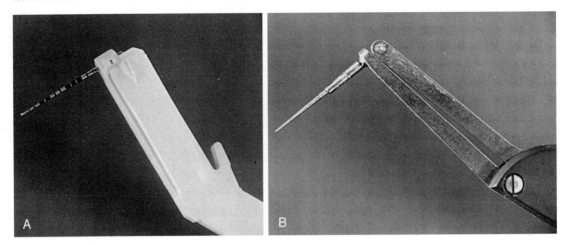

FIGURE 15–2. Examples of pressure-controlled probes.

deviate from this baseline record at maintenance intervals are entered on the patient's chart.

Research shows that clinical attachment changes are represented more accurately in measurements of attachment loss.[59] This measurement provides a better indication of the extent of periodontal destruction than simple probing depths. Determination of attachment loss is made from a fixed reference point on the tooth surface, such as the cementoenamel junction or the margin of a restoration to the base of the pocket. For a complete discussion of measuring attachment loss, see Chapter 9. This procedure is time consuming, but important to include in practice.

Reproducible and accurate measurements of probing depths and attachment loss are essential to monitoring patients' periodontal health during maintenance visits. Instruments to improve the evaluation of probing depths and attachment loss are now increasingly available. Since probing force can greatly influence probing measurements, both mechanical and electronic controlled force periodontal probes have been developed in an attempt to minimize this variable (Figure 15-2). Advantages of electronic probes include a constant probing force, electronic measurements to 0.1 mm, and computerized data storage.[60] Research indicates that controlled force probes underestimate probing depths compared to conventional manual probes, while the evidence for reproducibility is inconsistent.[61] Despite these drawbacks, the electronic data recording and computerized data storage may eliminate errors in recording probing depths when utilizing an assistant, increase the efficiency of obtaining measurements, and facilitate comparison of changes in pocket depths and attachment loss over time.[60] It is anticipated that electronic probes measuring probing depth and attachment loss will become more practical, cost-effective, and widely used in periodontal therapy with continued improvement in the design and technology of these instruments.

GINGIVAL RECESSION

Gingival recession is apparent when the root surface is clinically exposed as a result of apical migration of the junctional epithelium and loss of marginal gingiva (Figure 15-3). It represents increased attachment loss, but is not equivalent to the measurement of loss of attachment. Recession is measured from the cementoenamel junction to the gingival margin, and in conjunction with probing depths in this area, it provides an estimate of total attachment loss. The exposed root surfaces in the areas of recession are of special concern due to increased risk for **dentin hypersensitivity** and carious lesions. The dental hygienist must carefully assess all areas of recession for these conditions.

BLEEDING ON PROBING AND SUPPURATION

During the probing examination, noting the specific sites that elicit bleeding on gentle probing is important in the evaluation of periodontal health. Bleeding on probing is a reliable indicator of pocket inflammation and is a good, but not perfect, predictor of active disease.[62, 63] In

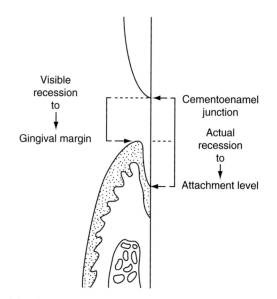

FIGURE 15–3. Gingival recession. The left side shows the visible recession measured from the cementoenamel junction to the gingival margin. The right side shows the actual recession measured from the cementoenamel junction to the base of the sulcus. (Used with permission from Wilkins EM. The gingiva. In Clinical Practice of the Dental Hygienist, 8th ed. Philadelphia: Lippincott/Williams and Wilkins, 1999: 197. Copyright 1999, Lippincott/Williams and Wilkins.)

Visible recession to Gingival margin

Cementoenamel junction

Actual recession to Attachment level

contrast, the absence of bleeding on probing indicates periodontal health in patients who are undergoing maintenance care.[64] Suppuration is the formation of pus that is visible at the entrance of the pocket when light pressure is placed on the external gingival surface. It is also referred to as exudate or purulent exudate. Pus is an accumulation of inflammatory cells and serum proteins. The amount and rate of suppuration are related to the severity of inflammation and indicate that the site requires treatment. Sites with bleeding or suppuration show some or all of the characteristic signs of inflammation: redness, swelling, heat, and pain. These sites must be treated during the maintenance visit or the patient rescheduled for further treatment. Further, a record of sites that showed bleeding on probing at previous visits helps to identify consistent problem areas that require further therapeutic intervention.

TOOTH MOBILITY

Tooth mobility must be routinely evaluated during maintenance visits because increasing mobility may signify a pathologic condition. Causes of mobility include inflammation of the periodontal ligament, loss of periodontal support, and trauma from occlusion.[65]

FURCATIONS

A furcation is characterized by a loss of clinical attachment and supporting bone of a multirooted tooth beyond the division of the roots. This situation complicates maintenance therapy. The status of furcations is evaluated with a periodontal probe or a curved probe (Nabers 1N or 2N) and recorded at every maintenance appointment. Successful long-term maintenance of furcations is possible;[66] however, frequent maintenance visits and conscientious daily home care in the furcation area are required. Instrumentation of these areas by the dental hygienist and daily plaque removal by the patient are technically demanding tasks. The dental hygienist must spend more time treating the furcation areas, because they are less accessible to debridement techniques, and teaching the patient home care techniques. Additionally, the patient must make special efforts to clean these areas.

MUCOGINGIVAL INVOLVEMENT

Extension of the pocket beyond the mucogingival junction and into the alveolar mucosa represents mucogingival involvement.[67] Although the attached gingiva is absent, maintenance of periodontal health and attachment is possible if adequate plaque control is achieved.[68] In comparison, gingival inflammation and further recession may occur if personal and professional oral hygiene care are neglected. Therefore, charting of mucogingival involvement and instruction in careful plaque control for these areas are necessary steps at all maintenance appointments.

Radiographic Examination

The need for radiographic examination during the maintenance program varies with each patient. The frequency of radiographs varies based on age, risk for disease, and signs and symptoms.[69] Indications for radiographs include caries activity, increased periodontal destruction, and suspected pathology.[70] It has been suggested that a full mouth series of radiographs should be taken every 2 to 4 years during maintenance care for comparison with previous films. This practice permits the detection of changes in alveolar bone height, repair of osseous defects, signs of trauma from occlusion, periapical pathology, and caries.[71] Vertical posterior bitewing radiographs are often preferred in periodontics to provide both caries detection and a better image of alveolar bone levels. These films may be taken annually.[72]

Evaluation of Plaque Control

After the periodontal examination is completed, a plaque evaluation is necessary to determine the patient's effectiveness in maintaining a clean oral environment. Bacterial plaque accumulations are easily seen when disclosing agents are used. The use of disclosing agents serves two purposes. First, a plaque score can be calculated, which can be recorded in the patient's chart and compared at subsequent maintenance visits to help motivate patients to comply with home care regimens. Second, the patient can be shown existing plaque as an educational tool to demonstrate improvements in oral hygiene techniques. At the very least, a written description in the chart of the amount and location of plaque is necessary.

Therapeutic Procedures

The extent of therapy performed at the maintenance visit depends on the information gathered during the assessment phase of the appointment. Personalized oral hygiene instruction must be provided. In addition, with the goal of total plaque and calculus removal in mind, meticulous instrumentation must be performed to remove subgingival and supragingival accumulations of calculus and plaque. Rubber-cup polishing may be necessary to remove extrinsic stains. Fluoride therapy and treatment for tooth sensitivity may be required as an adjunct to the periodontal maintenance visit.

ORAL HYGIENE INSTRUCTION

Oral hygiene instruction is an essential component of every preventive maintenance program. Both toothbrushing and interdental cleaning techniques should be emphasized to reinforce the importance of disrupting bacterial plaque accumulations on all surfaces of the teeth every day. Wide variation exists in the ability of each patient to maintain optimal oral cleanliness, so each oral hygiene regimen must be unique. As discussed previously, behavioral modification techniques are often necessary to improve compliance. Ongoing positive reinforcement and encouragement, often involving several maintenance appointments, can motivate patients to maintain improved oral hygiene.

Patients who have continued gingival inflammation despite compliance and plaque control efforts during maintenance care may benefit from the use of chemotherapeutic agents, such as chlorhexidine. A 0.12 percent chlorhexidine gluconate solution is both safe and effective to decrease the accumulation of supragingival bacterial plaque and prevent gingivitis.[73] Because the side effects include tooth staining and increased supragingival calculus formation, the long-term use of chlorhexidine may be impractical.[30] However, the superior quality of this chemotherapeutic agent for substantivity over phenolic and plant alkaloid mouthwashes[74] justifies its use for some patients with increased periodontal problems.

PERIODONTAL DEBRIDEMENT

Thorough removal of plaque and calculus deposits is achieved through scaling and root planing. After active therapy, the periodontal tissues generally exhibit increased health characterized by tight adaptation around teeth and more shallow probing depths; however, residual pockets may complicate the scaling procedures.[39] Effective removal of subgingival deposits in pocket depths of 3 mm or less is possible;[41] however, complete debridement of subgingival surfaces in pocket depths of 5 mm or greater is less reliable.[75] In areas with deeper pockets and/or furcation involvement that cannot be maintained in health, surgical therapy may be required. Because subgingival instrumentation is technically demanding, sufficient time must be allotted to perform thorough debridement. Often, areas with increased probing depths or bleeding on probing should be addressed first in order to permit efficient use of time during the maintenance appointment.[41] Selective use of local anesthesia may be necessary.

POLISHING

Historically, polishing the teeth with the rubber cup and prophy paste has followed scaling, root planing, and other periodontal procedures to completely remove acquired pellicle, bacterial plaque, and stains from the clinical crowns of the teeth, providing smooth and shiny tooth surfaces.[76] An improved understanding of the minimal therapeutic benefits and increased possible detrimental effects of polishing has changed the use of this once routine procedure (Table 15–4). Complete removal of pellicle and bacterial plaque provides a positive esthetic experience of a clean mouth that may motivate the patient to maintain good oral hygiene habits. However, the therapeutic value of polishing is limited, as pellicle begins to form within minutes and plaque accumulates within 1 to 2 hours later.[77] Similarly, the removal of stains is merely a cosmetic procedure, since extrinsic stain is not considered an etiological factor in gingivitis or periodontal disease.

Today selective polishing has become the standard of care for oral healthcare professionals. This view requires dental hygienists to be prudent in providing polishing procedures for their patients. Complete plaque removal can be achieved during the maintenance visit, with a toothbrush and prophy paste or toothpaste, a rubber cup and tin oxide slurry, or toothpaste at a very slow speed.[78] Esthetically displeasing stains should be removed during the maintenance appointment. The majority of these stains can be removed with careful instrumentation using either well-sharpened curets or

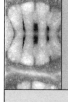

INDICATIONS AND PRECAUTIONS FOR SELECTIVE POLISHING[78]

- Explain to the patient the rationale for selective polishing.
- Do not apply selective stain removal techniques to cementum or dentin. If necessary in rare instances, extreme caution must be exercised.
- Use selective stain removal procedures only in areas visible when the patient smiles or talks.
- Use the least abrasive polishing agent necessary to achieve stain removal.
- Use the slowest speed and as little pressure as possible.
- Use personal and patient protective equipment, high-volume evacuation, and techniques to contain aerosols inside the mouth.
- Do not use motor- or air-driven instruments for patients with respiratory problems, xerostomia, communicable diseases that can be transmitted by aerosols, or for patients who are susceptible to bacteremia; do not use in areas of dental caries, thinned enamel or cementum (amelogenesis imperfecta, exposed roots, newly planed root surfaces), newly erupted teeth, primary teeth, demineralized (white spot) areas, titanium implants, or restorations.

From Nunn PF. "Selective Polishing"—Time for a change? Access 1977;11:38–42. Used with permission.

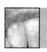

TABLE 15–4. Possible Detriments of Tooth Polishing[78]

Effect on Tooth Structure	Effect on Gingival Tissues
• Loss of tooth structure (e.g., enamel, dentin, cementum) • Increased tooth hypersensitivity on exposed cemental or dentinal surfaces • Increased roughness on tooth surface due to knicks and grooves caused by abrasives • Loss of fluoride-rich enamel layer increases risk for dental caries • Pulpal damage from heat generated with use of rubber cup and abrasive • Damage to composite and metallic restorations	• Removal of sulcular epithelium from crest of marginal free gingiva • Discomfort of tissues prevents adequate plaque control • Microorganisms enter tissues and proceed into the bloodstream resulting in bacteremia • Possible delayed tissue healing due to a negative response to abrasive particles forced into the sulcus

Used with permission from Nunn PF. "Selective Polishing—Time for a change?" Access 1997;11:38–42.

power-driven instruments.[78] (See Indications and Precautions for Selective Polishing.)

Many patients equate polishing to "cleaning the teeth" and expect this procedure at the conclusion of the maintenance appointment. Despite patients' expectations, the dental hygienist is ultimately responsible for providing the appropriate care to attain and maintain optimum oral health. Hence, a critical role of the dental hygienist is to educate patients on its minimal therapeutic benefits and the rationale for selective polishing.

FLUORIDE THERAPY

Frequently, a consequence of periodontal therapy is exposed root surfaces. This situation increases the risk of **root caries** and the development of dentin hypersensitivity. The cariostatic benefits of fluoride in the inhibition of demineralization and the enhancement of remineralization warrant professional application of topical fluoride preparations. Although the effectiveness of **fluoride therapy** for dentin hypersensitivity is uncertain, application of a concentrated sodium fluoride paste has been recommended[79] and may provide some relief of pain. Dentin hypersensitivity is discussed later in this chapter.

Recommendations and Referrals

At the conclusion of the maintenance appointment, a recommendation is made for the recall interval. This interval must be based on the patient's individual needs and on assessments made during the maintenance visit. In addition, an outline of the maintenance program helps each patient to understand and anticipate the requirements of a periodontal maintenance program. Recommendations and referrals to appropriate specialists for additional periodontal therapy or other specific dental needs should be made at this time.

Establishing Intervals for Periodontal Maintenance

Successful management of periodontal disease during the maintenance phase requires periodic professional care. Research supports the need for frequent maintenance therapy and oral hygiene instruction to prevent periodontal disease as well as dental caries.[21, 22] At the end of each periodontal maintenance appointment, the dentition is completely free of bacterial plaque and calculus. This condition facilitates the patient's efforts to maintain a clean oral environment. In addition, the maintenance appointment provides continued opportunities to reinforce plaque control and motivate patients to establish good oral hygiene habits.

There are no absolute rules regarding the appropriate intervals for periodontal maintenance. The maintenance period is determined by the individual needs of each patient. Information gathered during the assessment phase of the maintenance appointment provides the basis for determining the interval until the next maintenance visit. (See Factors for Determining

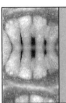

FACTORS FOR DETERMINING THE INTERVAL BETWEEN PERIODONTAL MAINTENANCE VISTS

- Probing depths
- Bleeding on probing
- Effectiveness of patient plaque control
- Age
- Medical history
- Dental history
- Periodontal history
- History of compliance with maintenance
- Compliance with oral home care regimen

the Interval Between Periodontal Maintenance Visits.) Clinical findings show the patient's current periodontal status. If the degree of inflammation is high, more frequent maintenance visits are warranted.

In general, the first maintenance visit, consisting of debridement and plaque control instructions, not probing, occurs 2 to 4 weeks after periodontal surgery. After this initial monitoring, the interval may be lengthened to 3 months.[32] Several studies suggest that 2- to 4-month intervals are adequate to maintain the stability of results and prevent progression of disease. These recommendations for scheduled maintenance visits should be considered only as guidelines because the value of maintenance is derived from the customized nature of the program.

RECURRENCE OF PERIODONTAL DISEASE

Periodontal disease can recur. In fact, **recurrent periodontitis** seems to be common, although no prevalence data are available.[80]

Several factors may contribute to the failure of maintenance of periodontal health. These include insufficient patient plaque control, incomplete removal of bacterial plaque and calculus during therapy, the presence of faulty restorations or prostheses that favor the reestablishment of disease, lack of patient compliance with recommended maintenance procedures, and systemic conditions that negatively affect the oral cavity.[71] The underlying factor in each case of treatment failure is the re-establishment of the pathologic subgingival flora, which results in continued pocket inflammation. In general, disease recurrence is localized to one or a few sites, although a generalized recurrence may also develop.[32]

Some patients do not respond to treatment even though optimal plaque control and thorough root debridement are performed. This condition, called "aggressive periodontitis," affects approximately 10 percent of the adult periodontitis population.[81] It is not known why these individuals do not respond favorably to conventional periodontal treatment regimens.

Recognition of the signs of recurrent periodontitis is a primary responsibility of every dental hygienist who provides maintenance care. While evaluating the periodontal status of the patient, the hygienist must recognize the following signs of failure: (1) increasing probing pocket depths (indicative of clinical attachment loss), (2) recurrent bleeding on probing, (3) chronic gingival inflammation, (4) gradual increases in radiographic bone loss, and (5) gradual increases in tooth mobility (Table 15-5).[71]

Re-treatment of areas with recurrent disease is accomplished with the same goal as initial periodontal therapy, which is to achieve and maintain stable periodontal health. The re-treatment phase usually begins with scaling and root planing of the reinfected sites[32] to debride the subgingival environment of all bacterial plaque and calculus. Four to six weeks after re-treatment, a complete periodontal re-evaluation is necessary to determine the results, prognosis, and treatment recommendations. If residual calculus remains and inflammation persists, surgi-

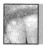

TABLE 15–5. Symptoms and Causes of Recurrence of Disease

Symptom	Possible Causes
Increased inflammation	Poor oral hygiene
	Subgingival calculus
	Inadequate restorations
	Deteriorating or poorly designed prostheses
	Systemic disease modifying host response to plaque
Recession	Toothbrush abrasion
	Inadequate keratinized gingiva
	Frenum pull
	Orthodontic therapy
Increased mobility with no change in pocket depth and no radiographic change	Occlusal trauma caused by lateral occlusal interference
	Bruxism
	High restorations
	Poorly designed or worn-out prostheses
	Poor crown-to-root ratio
Increased pocket depth with no radiographic change	Poor oral hygiene
	Infrequent recall
	Subgingival calculus
	Poorly fitting partial denture
	Mesial inclination into edentulous space
	Failure of new attachment surgery
	Cracked teeth
	Grooves in teeth
	New periodontal disease
Increased pocket depth with increased radiographic bone loss	Poor oral hygiene
	Subgingival calculus
	Infrequent recall visits
	Inadequate or deteriorating restorations
	Poorly designed prostheses
	Inadequate surgery
	Systemic disease modifying host response to plaque
	Cracked teeth
	Grooves in teeth
	New periodontal disease

Used with permission from Merin RL. Maintenance care. In Carranza FA. Glickman's Clinical Periodontology, 7th ed. Philadelphia: WB Saunders, 1990:973.

cal therapy may be necessary to provide access to eliminate the infection, reduce periodontal pockets, or repair the periodontium. Other treatment options for disease control include microbiologic monitoring and antibiotic therapy. Referral to a periodontist should be considered as these needs arise.

ROOT CARIES IN THE PERIODONTAL MAINTENANCE POPULATION

Root surface caries are a fundamental concern in the periodontal population because loss of periodontal attachment often results in exposed, susceptible root surfaces. Root caries is a soft, progressive lesion of the root surface that involves bacterial plaque and microbial invasion.[82] Teeth that might be maintained for years can be lost quickly to root caries. The carious lesion usually begins on the cemental surfaces of the root, at or near the cementoenamel junction, and proceeds to invade the underlying and peripheral dentin.[83] *Actinomyces viscosus* is the predominant organism present in bacterial plaque samples covering carious root surfaces.[84] Although their specific roles are unknown, a variety of microbial organisms are associated with root caries, with some different microbes than those typically found in lesions on smooth surfaces.[85]

For root caries to exist, an exposed root surface is a prerequisite. Various related conditions are listed in Predisposing Conditions for Root Surface Exposure. In periodontal health, the cemental root surface is covered by gingival tissues and functions as a major component of the periodontal attachment apparatus (Figure 15-4). However, in periodontal disease and other conditions that lead to gingival recession, the cementum becomes exposed as the junctional epithelium migrates apically and the gingival margin recedes. As a result, the loss of periodontal attachment and the subsequent exposure of cementum to the oral environment increase the risk for development of root caries. Additionally, root caries may exist in periodontal pockets, especially around crown restorations.

Prevalence of Root Caries

Root caries has received increased attention within the last two decades because of reduc-

tions in adult tooth loss. Variations in study designs make comparisons of prevalence data complex. Despite these variations, evidence confirms that a large proportion of adults have root caries.[86, 87] A survey during 1988-1991 found that 25 percent of adults in the United States had at least one decayed or filled root surface.[88] The root caries prevalence increased markedly with age, ranging from 7 percent to 56 percent, with men having more root caries than women (Figure 15-5). Certainly, the significance of root caries will increase as the United States population ages and people retain their teeth for longer periods.

Reports of the prevalence of root caries among specific periodontal populations also vary. One study of individuals with untreated moderate to severe periodontal disease reported that 58 percent of subjects exhibited some root caries.[89] Maintenance patients treated for 1 year after active therapy for advanced periodontal disease showed a 45 percent prevalence rate.[90] It cannot be assumed that periodontal disease causes root surface caries. However, it is the loss of gingival attachment, as a result of periodontal disease, that leads to an increased risk of root caries.

Risk Indicators of Root Caries

Generally, root caries is believed to be a multifactorial disease with many risk factors (Table 15-6). Although it may not cause root caries, periodontal disease is associated with root caries because it causes attachment loss (Figure 15-6). Loss of gingival attachment is considered

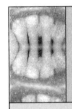

PREDISPOSING CONDITIONS FOR ROOT SURFACE EXPOSURE

1. Periodontal disease
2. Periodontal surgery
3. Malocclusion
4. Orthodontic treatment
5. Mechanical trauma (e.g., toothbrush abrasion)

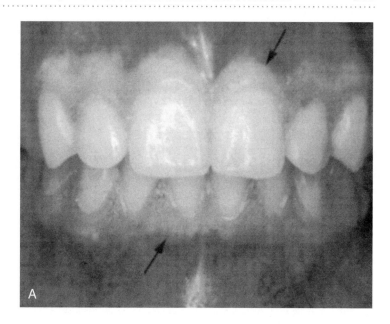

Recession   Position of Gingiva

FIGURE 15–4. The position of the gingiva in periodontal health and disease. **A.** Attached gingiva in a healthy periodontium covers the cemental surface, preventing root caries development. Arrows indicate the mucogingival junction. **B.** Visible and hidden gingival recession exposes the cementum to increase the risk of root caries development. (Modified from Carranza FA, Saglie FR. The gingiva. In Carranza FA, ed. Glickman's Clinical Periodontology, 7th ed. Philadelphia: WB Saunders, 1990: 15, 120.)

a significant risk factor along with age, number of teeth, presence of coronal caries, level of oral hygiene, water fluoridation, and years of education.[89] Incidence data from one study of seniors suggested that periodontal pockets greater than 3 mm deep and existing teeth with root caries were good predictors of risk.[91]

XEROSTOMIA

The protective role of saliva in the oral cavity is well documented. These protective functions include antimicrobial activity, control of pH, and removal of food debris from the oral cavity. Without these protective functions, the adverse effects of xerostomia, or dry mouth, may lead to difficulties with speaking, eating, swallowing, and wearing dentures. Additionally, xerostomic individuals have an increased risk of *Candida* infections, dental caries, and periodontal disease.[88]

Xerostomia is a relatively common finding that may be related to numerous conditions, including systemic disease (e.g., diabetes, Sjögren's syndrome, immunocompromised states), head and neck radiation therapy, drug therapy, dehydration, stress, and anxiety.[92] Several medications that cause xerostomia are listed (See Medications Associated with Causing Xerostomia.) Individuals with xerostomia complain of changes in both the quantity and quality of

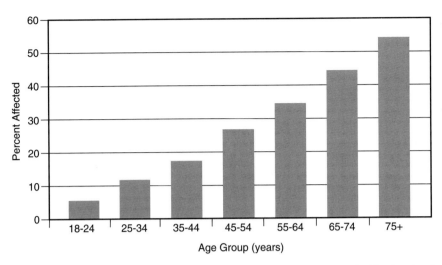

FIGURE 15–5. Prevalence of root caries. Survey of United States adults from the Third National Health and Nutrition Examination Survey (NHANESS III-Phase I): 1988-1991. (Winn DM, Brunelle JA, Selwitz RH, Kaste LM, Oldakowski RJ, Kingman A, Brown LJ. Coronal and root caries in the dentition of adults in the United States, 1988-1991. J Dent Res 1996;75(Spec Iss):642-651. Reprinted with permission from the Journal of Dental Research.)

the saliva, which may or may not be related to decreased salivary gland function.

An important role of the dental hygienist is to recognize the signs and symptoms of xerostomia (Table 15-7). The oral mucosa of a xerostomic patient may appear red, dry, and sticky. Angular cheilitis, characterized by cracking at the corner of the mouth, and infections may also be present. The saliva may appear to be stringy or foamy with little or no pooled saliva in the floor of the mouth.[93] Dental caries in individuals with xerostomia are often located at the cervical margins or incisal edges of the teeth. Both primary and recurrent caries may also arise at the margin of existing restorations.

Therapeutic management of xerostomia involves use of salivary substitutes or salivary stimulants. Temporary relief of symptoms may be achieved using water, glycerin preparations, or artificial saliva as salivary substitutes. Stimulation of natural salivary flow, using sugarless candy and chewing gum or medications, is useful for individuals with some remaining functional salivary glands (i.e., head and neck radiation therapy patients).

Prevention of dental caries is extremely important in xerostomic individuals as a result

MEDICATIONS ASSOCIATED WITH CAUSING XEROSTOMIA

- Antiacne drugs
- Antianxiety agents
- Antihypertensive drugs
- Antihistamines
- Antidepressants
- Muscle relaxants
- Antipsychotics
- Decongestants
- Antiparkinsonism drugs
- Diuretics
- Anti-inflammatory analgesics
- Antinauseants (motion sickness medications)

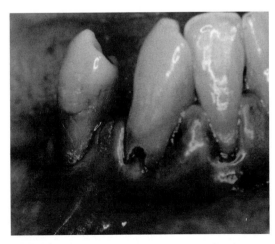

FIGURE 15–6. Root caries lesion in a periodontal patient.

TABLE 15–6. Potential Risk Factors for Root Caries

Risk Factor	Group of Interest	Relative Risk
Age	Older individuals	Increased
Fluoride	Consumers of fluoridated water	Decreased
Coronal caries	High number of coronal caries	Increased
Root caries	High number of root caries	Increased
Oral hygiene	Presence of plaque and calculus	Increased
Loss of attachment	Presence of gingival recession	Increased
Number of teeth	High retention of teeth	Decreased
Pockets > 3 mm	High number of increased pocket depths	Increased
Recent illness	Compromised systemic health	Increased
Tobacco use	Cigarette smokers and users of smokeless tobacco	Increased
Level of education	High level of education	Decreased
Level of anxiety	High level of anxiety	Increased
Social integration	High social integration	Decreased
Sugar consumption	High intake of sugared foods	Increased

Used with permission from Beck J. The epidemiology of root surface caries. J Dent Res 1990;69:1219, 1220.

of their reduced salivary flow. Strategies for minimizing the risk of caries include frequent dental visits, topical fluorides, and diet control.[93] Recommendations for topical fluorides in xerostomic individuals are listed in Table 15–8. The topical fluoride regimen of choice depends on the patient's preference and compliance.

Clinical Detection of Root Caries

An examination for caries during the maintenance appointment is important because of the increased vulnerability of the root surfaces in the periodontal maintenance population. Clinically, early root caries appears as multiple discolored areas that are tan or brown. (See Clinical Characteristics of Root Caries.) In advanced stages, these lesions coalesce and form ill-defined areas that may progress apically and may also encircle the root.[83] Active lesions feel soft and appear shallow (less than 2 mm deep), and usually are covered with bacterial plaque.[85] In contrast, arrested root caries is characterized

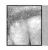

TABLE 15–7. Signs and Symptoms of Xerostomia

Signs	Symptoms
■ Dry and sticky mucosa	■ Difficult with eating
■ Stringy or foamy saliva	■ Difficulty with swallowing
■ Little or no pooled saliva in the floor of the mouth	■ Difficulty with speaking
■ Difficult to express saliva from major salivary glands	■ Difficulty with wearing dentures
■ Caries at the cervical margin, incisal edge, or margins of restorations	■ Burning sensation associated with oral candidiasis
■ Erythematous mucosa	■ Changes in taste
■ Angular cheilitis	■ Difficulty with eating spicy or acidic foods

Used with permission from Greenspan D. Xerostomia: diagnosis and management. Oncology 1996;10:7–11.

CLINICAL CHARACTERISTICS OF ROOT CARIES

Color	Active caries: Tan or brown Arrested caries: Dark brown or black
Distribution	Early caries: Multiple discolored areas Advanced caries: Ill-defined area of coalesced lesions
Texture	Active caries: Soft Arrested caries: Hard
Depth	Active caries: Shallow (less than 2 mm deep)
Presence of Plaque	Often
Pain/Discomfort	Rare

	Fluoride Rinses (0.5% sodium fluoride)	Fluoride Gels
Mode of Application:	Swish in mouth. Expectorate upon completion.	Apply with toothbrush or use custom-made plastic tray. Expectorate upon completion.
Frequency of Use:	Once or twice daily	Once or twice daily
Length of Use:	1 minute	2 to 3 minutes

TABLE 15–8. Topical Fluoride Treatment for Xerostomic Patients

Used with permission from Greenspan D. Xerostomia: diagnosis and management. Oncology 1996;10:7–11.

by a dark brown to black discoloration and a hard texture. This texture is most likely the result of a remineralized surface layer and a mineralization front advancing into demineralized dentin.[83] Because root caries can develop on any root surface, both clinical and radiographic examinations are essential for caries assessment. Unlike coronal caries, root caries does not generally produce any pain or discomfort.[94]

PREVENTION AND CONTROL OF ROOT CARIES

The prevention of root caries in the periodontal maintenance population is not a trivial matter because of the high prevalence and incidence rates. However, root surface lesions are not inevitable in high-risk populations. The dental hygienist is in a key position to educate patients about the risks and prevention of root caries. The principal strategies to prevent the development of root caries involve attempts to (1) increase the resistance of teeth through fluoride therapy; (2) reduce the number of microorganisms through effective plaque control; (3) modify the substrate by selecting noncariogenic foods; and (4) decrease the time the substrate is in the oral cavity by limiting the frequency of intake.[95] These strategies are based on the four etiologic factors that are involved in the caries process, as shown in Figure 15–7.

Fluoride Therapy

Systemic and topical fluoride therapies are significant components of any caries prevention program to increase the resistance of teeth against carious attack.

Fluoride Therapy. Fluoride works by inhibiting demineralization of the tooth surface, enhancing remineralization, and inhibiting bacterial activity. Evidence now indicates the primary anti-caries benefits of fluoride are achieved through its topical application rather than from systemic intake.[96] This is in contrast to the previous belief that fluoride incorporation in tooth mineral during development of the teeth was the major caries-inhibitory effect of fluoride.

Generally, a multiple fluoride approach is most effective in the inhibition of root caries. This approach includes the use of fluoride at home, in the dental office, and in the commu-

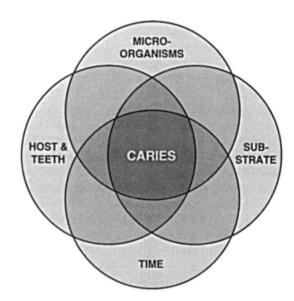

FIGURE 15–7. The etiology of dental caries. Four etiologic factors—cariogenic microflora, host, substrate, and time—must act concurrently for caries to develop. (Used with permission from Newbrun E. Current concepts of caries etiology. In Cariology, 3rd ed. Carol Stream, IL: Quintessence, 1989:29.)

nity. Common fluoride delivery systems to control root caries include dentifrices, mouthrinses, topical solutions and gels, and communal water supplies. When devising a therapeutic fluoride program for the periodontal patient, the dental hygienist must tailor recommendations to the individual's needs and environment.

Limited clinical data are available on the ability of conventional fluoride systems to prevent and reverse root caries. The benefits of daily, high-concentration fluoride application in solution or gel form have been explored primarily in individuals receiving therapeutic head and neck radiation. Combination fluoride therapy in these severely xerostomic patients consists of a series of professionally applied fluoride solutions or gels and daily home use of a 1.1 percent sodium fluoride gel or a fluoride rinse.[97] This fluoride treatment program is effective in controlling root caries, but it may be more than is needed by periodontal maintenance patients.

Water Fluoridation. Fluoride in drinking water reduces dental caries, but it is not sufficient to provide complete protection against cariogenic bacteria. The primary mechanism of action of fluoridated water is through topical delivery.[96] Systemic ingestion of fluoride plays a very limited role in caries prevention.

The benefits of fluoride in preventing root caries are well documented in studies of communities with nonfluoridated and fluoridated water supplies. For example, lifelong consumption of optimally fluoridated water effectively decreased the prevalence of root caries in adults.[98] Water fluoridation at five times the optimal level decreased the prevalence of root caries in lifelong adult residents of one community.[99] In addition, exposure to fluoridated water for 30 to 40 years reduced the incidence of root caries in the older adult population.[100] Clearly, community water fluoride levels are an important consideration in the prevention of root caries.

Fluoride Rinses. The use of home fluoride rinses by individuals who are at risk for root caries has been the subject of little controlled clinical research. One clinical trial has evaluated the effect of a daily fluoride rinse on root caries in an unsupervised home fluoride program.[101] After 3 years of use of a 0.05 percent sodium fluoride rinse, a 16 percent decline in the inci-

dence of root caries in older adults was observed. The rationale for unsupervised home use of fluoride rinses is based on self-application of high-frequency/low-concentration or low-frequency/high-concentration fluoride agents to prevent the development of root caries and arrest the progression of existing lesions. The fluoride rinse systems currently approved for use are 0.2 percent sodium fluoride used once per week, 0.05 percent sodium fluoride used daily, and 0.2 percent acidulated phosphate-fluoride used daily.[97] These fluoride rinses can be obtained either over the counter or by prescription, depending on the fluoride content. Although the cariostatic efficacy of these regimens has been clearly documented in school-based programs, there is little clinical evidence to support any particular recommendations for the prevention of root caries. Despite limited data, the regular use of daily fluoride rinses is frequently recommended by some dental practitioners for all patients undergoing periodontal maintenance because of the anticaries potential of this treatment.

Fluoride Solutions and Gels. High-concentration topical fluoride solutions and gels can be useful adjuncts to a caries prevention program. They are available in both professionally applied and self-applied formulations. However, the cariostatic benefits of these fluoride delivery systems for the periodontal population is not well established. The clinical data to support the efficacy of topical fluoride solutions or gels in the prevention of root caries is found in studies of patients receiving head and neck radiation therapy. Evidence from animal studies is strong and, combined with the limited clinical data, supports this therapy for periodontal patients.

Professional topical fluoride gels and solutions provide concentrated fluoride application at recall appointments to prevent dental caries. Currently, topical fluoride solutions or gels are approved for use in the United States in three regimens: 1.23 percent acidulated phosphate-fluoride, 2 percent neutral sodium fluoride, and 8 percent stannous fluoride. The two most commonly used office fluorides, 1.23 percent acidulated phosphate fluoride and 2 percent neutral sodium fluoride, are compared in Table 15–9. Usually, the topical fluoride solution or gel is applied semiannually at the maintenance visit. Since fluoride solutions may impede healing of

TABLE 15–9. Comparison of Office Fluorides

	1.23% APF (acidulated phosphate fluoride)	2.0% NaF (neutral sodium fluoride)
Fluoride Uptake	Rapid; 12,000 ppm after 1 minute	Slow; requires 4 minute application to exceed 1,000 ppm
Fluoride Strength	12,300 ppm	9,040 ppm
pH	3.0–4.0	7.0
Recommended Application Time	4 minutes	4 minutes
Recommended Application Method	Applicator tray provides maximum coverage and minimizes ingestion potential. May also be applied with swab.	Applicator tray provides maximum coverage and minimizes ingestion potential. May also be applied with swab.
Application Frequency	Twice annually	Twice annually
Flavor Acceptance	Varies with brand. Usually well tolerated with slight tart taste due to low pH.	Very well accepted with no aftertaste
Possible Adverse Effects	Possible etching or dulling of porcelain or composite resin	None reported
Contraindications	Hypersensitivity to fluoride or other ingredients. Not for use for children under age 3.	Hypersensitivity to fluoride or other ingredients. Not for use for children under age 3.
Patient Selection	Agent of choice for most caries-prone patients.	Agent of choice for patients: 1. with esthetic restorations (porcelain or composite). 2. with reduced saliva flow caused by radiation, chemotherapy, or medication. 3. who cannot tolerate acidic fluorides.

Modified with permission from Oral-B Laboratories. A complete caries prevention program includes both office and home fluorides. ETR 3262, 1997.

periodontal tissues, fluoride application should be avoided after extensive scaling, root planing, or surgical procedures.[102] Four minutes of direct application to the teeth with cotton, pellets, or a gel and tray system is recommended. Animal studies have shown that periodic application of each form of fluoride, including a 0.4 percent stannous fluoride formulation with 0.3 percent acidulated phosphate-fluoride, is effective in reducing root caries.[103] However, a significantly greater decrease was observed with the 2 percent sodium fluoride and 1.23 percent acidulated phosphate-fluoride systems. This observation suggests that standard, office-applied, gel and tray systems may be best used for in-office programs designed to prevent root caries.

Topical fluoride application at home provides additional protection against the development of root caries. The three gel formulations currently available for use are 0.5 percent acidulated phosphate-fluoride, 1.1 percent sodium fluoride, and 0.4 percent stannous fluoride.

Two commonly used home fluoride gels, 0.4 percent stannous fluoride and 1.1 percent sodium fluoride, are compared in Table 15–10. After thorough plaque control by the patient, the fluoride gel is applied daily, either by direct brushing onto the tooth surface for 1 minute or with the use of disposable or custom-made trays for 4 minutes. Clinical research is somewhat limited in evaluating these products for the prevention of root caries. Both 1.1 percent sodium fluoride and 0.4 percent stannous fluoride reduced root caries in patients undergoing head and neck radiation therapy.[104] Also, 0.4 percent stannous fluoride gel significantly reduced root caries in an animal model.[105] These data support the notion that daily topical fluoride gels are beneficial in controlling root caries. However, further work is necessary to identify more precisely the benefits of daily use of fluoride gels for the prevention of root caries in the periodontal maintenance population.

Fluoride Dentifrices. A wealth of research

TABLE 15–10. Comparison of Home Fluoride Gels

	0.4% SnF$_2$ (stannous fluoride)	1.1% NaF (neutral sodium fluoride)
Fluoride Strength	1,000 ppm	5,000 ppm
pH	2.8–5.0	7.0
Staining Potential	May produce extrinsic stains	None
Recommended Application Method	Apply with brush onto tooth surface after thorough plaque control for 1 minute (usually at bedtime). May use disposable or custom-made applicator tray for 4 minutes.	Apply with brush onto tooth surface after thorough plaque control for 1 minute (usually at bedtime). May use disposable or custom-made applicator tray for 4 minutes.
Application Frequency	Daily	Daily
Flavor Acceptance	Good (some brands slightly metallic in flavor)	Good
Possible Adverse Effects	May produce extrinsic stains	High concentration fluoride products should be kept out of reach of children.
Contraindications	Not for use for children under age 6	Not for use for children under age 6
Patient Selection	Agent of choice for patients when both caries control and plaque reduction are primary objectives.	Agent of choice for patients: 1. with esthetic restorations (porcelain or composite). 2. who cannot tolerate acidic fluorides (xerostomic and bulemic patients, patients with soft tissue irritation associated with radiation, chemotherapy or systemic disease).

Modified with permission from Oral-B Laboratories. A complete caries prevention program includes both office and home fluorides. ETR 3262, 1997.

since 1945 supports the ability of fluoride in dentifrices to control dental caries in children and adolescents. Over the past twenty years, the prevalence of dental caries in children in the United States has declined.[96] This decline is due in part to the universal use of fluoride dentifrice. Fluoride-containing dentifrices currently accepted for use by the American Dental Association consist of either a 0.24 percent sodium fluoride or a 0.76 percent sodium monofluorophosphate formulation. Recommendations for the use of fluoride dentifices by patients who are at moderate to high risk for caries entail brushing once or more per day with a fluoride-containing toothpaste.[106]

Less is known about the specific value of fluoride dentifrices in the prevention of root caries in adults. One longitudinal study of non-institutionalized adults compared 0.24 percent sodium fluoride dentifrice with a placebo in the prevention of root caries.[107] After 1 year, the data showed a significant decline in the incidence of both coronal and root caries in the group that used fluoride-containing toothpaste. Another study found that a sodium fluoride den-

tifrice reduced root caries by more than 65 percent.[94] Additional supporting evidence is documented in animal studies.[105] Further clinical research will no doubt confirm fluoride dentifrices as an important part of the daily plaque control regimen for periodontal maintenance patients.

In summary, the anti-caries activity of fluoride is well documented in both laboratory and clinical studies. Despite a lack of clinical research to clearly outline a fluoride therapy program for the periodontal maintenance population at risk for root caries, Table 15–11 summarizes the fluoride agents with the most potential to become a part of a recommended fluoride regimen based on current knowledge. Evidence supports the use of combination fluoride therapy to inhibit the development of dental caries.[108] However, the most effective combination of fluoride dentifrices with mouth rinses or topical gel applications has not been determined. The dental hygienist must tailor fluoride therapy to the needs of the patient. All maintenance patients should use a fluoride toothpaste in combination with other office- and home-

TABLE 15–11. Fluoride Therapy for Prevention of Root Caries

Preparation	Frequency of Use	Procedure
Systemic Fluorides Fluoridated Drinking Water 0.6 ppm–1.2 ppm	Lifetime	Routine daily consumption of fluoridated community water supply.
Topical Fluorides Fluoride Mouthrinse 0.05% NaF (250 ppm)	Daily	Rinse with 1 teaspoonful for 1 minute and expectorate after plaque control regimen at bedtime.

Fluoride Solutions or Gels
Professional Application
   2% NaF (9040 ppm) or
   1.23% APF (12,300 ppm)
	Semiannual	Direct application with cotton applicator or gel and tray technique for 4 minutes after thorough debridement. Expectorate.

Self-Application
   1.1% NaF (5000 ppm) or
   0.4% SnF_2 (900 ppm)
	Daily	Direct application with toothbrush for 1 minute or gel and tray technique for 4 minutes after plaque control regimen at bedtime. Expectorate.

Fluoride Dentifrices
   0.24% NaF (1100 ppm)
   or 0.76% MFP
	1 or 2 times daily	Apply with a soft toothbrush; brush all surfaces thoroughly with a sulcular toothbrushing technique. Expectorate.

NaF = neutral sodium fluoride; APF = acidulated phosphate fluoride; SnF_2 = stannous fluoride; MFP = sodium monofluorophosphate.

applied agents prescribed according to susceptibility and caries incidence.

Oral Hygiene

Overwhelming evidence shows that oral microorganisms are one of the primary etiologic agents for all dental caries, although the specific bacteria present may vary among the types of carious lesions.[85] The amount of cariogenic bacteria associated with root caries must be minimized through meticulous personal plaque control. Epidemiologic studies have not confirmed a consistent relationship between dental plaque scores and the prevalence of dental caries.[109] For example, oral cleanliness cannot be equated with decreased caries formation.[110] However, minimizing the amount of plaque is important in controlling periodontal disease and probably also has a beneficial effect on root caries.

Diet Modification

Diet plays a major role in the development of dental caries. For example, a sucrose-rich diet highly favors caries formation. Dietary carbohydrates such as glucose, sucrose, fructose, or cooked starch provide the substrate for cariogenic bacteria to produce organic acids. These acids promote demineralization of the tooth structure. Nutritional analysis to evaluate dietary habits and recommendations for diet modification are essential elements for caries-prone individuals. The dietary recommendations for periodontal patients described here apply to all individuals who are at risk for dental caries.

The dental hygienist plays a major role in assessing the dietary habits of patients who are at risk for dental caries and can provide suggestions for less cariogenic foods and beverages. Besides providing nutrition education and counseling, the dental hygienist can motivate and encourage patients to maintain a balanced diet to promote their overall oral and systemic health. Patients must accept responsibility for modifying their dietary habits and must be committed to the caries prevention program.

Nutritional Counseling. Effective techniques to obtain a patient's dietary record include a 24-hour recall and/or a detailed food diary kept for four consecutive days. Together the dental hygienist and patient can evaluate the diet history and set nutritional goals. Simple, well-defined, and concise nutritional guidelines should be tailored to each patient's needs (See Nutritional Counseling for the Periodontal Patient). Except for the restriction of a few foods and eating practices, a caries-preventive diet is based upon the same recommendations for a normal healthy, balanced diet.[109] Thus, the goal is to obtain all the necessary nutrients to maintain health and resistance to disease. Your patients can help identify substitutes that are appealing and satisfying. They will be more receptive to diet modifications if they understand the role of diet and actively participate in diet planning. Continued evaluation, modification, and positive reinforcement of the patient's dietary habits during the maintenance phase may enhance patient acceptance of and compliance with the personalized dietary program.

As part of the total preventive nature of maintenance therapy, dietary analysis and modification of dietary habits are in the best interest of periodontal patients for maintenance of optimal oral and systemic health. Dietary analysis and nutrition counseling will reduce the risks of coronal and root caries. In addition, periodontal maintenance patients will benefit because inadequate nutrient intake may exacerbate inflammation of the gingival tissues by decreasing resistance to disease.[111]

DENTIN HYPERSENSITIVITY IN THE PERIODONTAL MAINTENANCE POPULATION

Understanding the theories, causes, and management of dentin hypersensitivity is important for every dental hygienist because it is such a common occurrence in periodontal patients. Dentin hypersensitivity is characterized by sharp, intermittent pain of short duration or by dull, chronic pain. It can affect any number of teeth, and its occurrence is difficult to predict on susceptible surfaces. Pain is caused by various stimuli, such as cold, heat, sweet or sour foods, toothbrushes, or toothpicks. It is estimated that one in seven adult patients has dentinal hypersensitivity[112] and that nearly 40 million Americans experience hypersensitivity at some point.[113]

The terms "dentin sensitivity" and "dentin hypersensitivity" are often used interchangeably to describe the pain evoked on stimulation of exposed dentinal surfaces. Technically, the term sensitivity simply denotes a normal response to stimulation of newly exposed dentin, whereas hypersensitivity refers to excessive sensitivity. Hypersensitivity is the more common term.

Theories of Dentinal Pain Transmission

The hydrodynamic theory is the most commonly accepted explanation of hypersensitivity of the dentinal surface to external stimuli.[114] Stimulation of open dentinal tubules at the root surface is believed to cause fluid movement

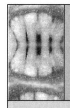

NUTRITIONAL COUNSELING FOR THE PERIODONTAL PATIENT

1. Recommend eating a healthy, balanced diet including a variety of foods.
2. Advise to avoid caries-producing foods, snacks, and beverages (i.e., foods with high sucrose content).
3. Encourage limiting consumption of sucrose-containing foods to mealtime and restricting between meal sugary snacks.
4. Suggest a list of foods and beverages to include and avoid in the diet
   • Include fresh fruits and vegetables, non-cariogenic sweeteners
   • Avoid candy, sugar-containing sodas, dried fruits
5. Develop a personalized meal plan tailored to the patient's lifestyle, financial resources, cultural preferences, and religious customs.

within the tubules. This movement transmits a signal to the nerves in the pulp chamber. The resulting sensation is pain. Closing off the exposed dentinal tubules would likely prevent fluid movement and inhibit pain transmission.[115] This principle is the basis of all treatments used today for dentinal hypersensitivity.

Factors Contributing to the Development of Dentin Hypersensitivity

Mechanical, chemical, thermal, or bacterial stimuli can cause tooth pain. Common mechanical causes are toothbrushing, touching with fingers or other objects, and drying. Chemical stimuli are usually acidic or sweet substances. Patients occasionally report dentin hypersensitivity with the use of tartar-control toothpastes containing pyrophosphates.[116] Acids from bacterial plaque can cause pain, and periodontal patients commonly report that hot and cold stimuli induce pain.[117]

Exposure of the root surfaces or loss of enamel is necessary for dentin hypersensitivity to occur. Periodontal maintenance patients commonly have exposed root surfaces because of histories of periodontal attachment loss and often surgery. Research has shown a direct relationship between increased hypersensitivity and the extent of root surface exposure in patients after periodontal surgery.[118] However, not all exposed dentin is painful or the result of periodontal treatment. Gingival recession is observed in normal aging, with malpositioned teeth, and as a result of improper tooth brushing techniques. Whatever the cause, various factors affect the nature of hypersensitivity, including patient age, the rate of exposure, and the effect of naturally occurring or environmental desensitizing mechanisms.[113] Some patients with minor gingival recession complain of hypersensitivity, while others with major recession experience no pain.

Root hypersensitivity after periodontal treatment is common. Often, scaling and root planing elicits dentin hypersensitivity. This effect is not surprising because scaling and root planing removes cementum covering the root surface, exposing the dentinal tubules. Pain may not occur immediately because a smear layer of microcrystalline debris initially covers the dentinal surface.[115] However, after approximately 7 days, the smear layer dissolves and hypersensitivity can occur.[115] Periodontal surgery also often exposes the dentinal tubules leading to hypersensitivity.

Individual variation in the extent and resolution of hypersensitivity occurs after periodontal treatment. Toothbrushing habits, intake of acidic foods, and rate of plaque development all affect hypersensitivity.[110] Fortunately, stimulated hypersensitivity resulting from scaling and root planing often decreases about 2 weeks after treatment.[119] Spontaneous remission of hypersensitivity is thought to occur 20 to 45 percent of the time without therapeutic measures.[120] Theories about the decrease in hypersensitivity include possible occlusion of the dentinal tubules by newly formed calculus, formation of reparative dentin within the pulp chamber of the tooth,[121] and precipitation of intratubular crystals from salivary minerals.[122]

Management of Dentin Hypersensitivity

Patients undergoing periodontal maintenance often experience pain when eating or drinking hot or cold foods and when the root surfaces are touched by scaling instruments. The dental hygienist must respond to these needs, explain the condition, and provide a therapeutic regimen. In addition, it is important to avoid aggravating the problem during maintenance visits by not drying hypersensitive surfaces with air or planing them unnecessarily.

Desensitizing agents are categorized into two types, chemical and physical, and are available for home use or in-office application (Table 15–12). Generally, these treatments provide some reduction of hypersensitivity, but results vary in degree of pain relief and duration of results. In-office therapy to treat dentinal hypersensitivity is successful in 20 to 40 percent of hypersensitive teeth, and results usually occur within 4 to 8 weeks.[121] These results are encouraging, but far from perfect. The ideal desensitizing agent would possess the following properties: It would (1) cause no pain or irritation to the pulp, (2) be easy to use, (3) act rapidly, (4) have long-lasting effects, (5) be consistently effective, and (6) not stain the teeth.[117]

PLAQUE CONTROL

A simple, important, but often overlooked method to reduce hypersensitivity is improving

TABLE 15-12. Chemical and Physical Agents Used to Treat Dentin Sensitivity	
Mode of Action	**Agents**
	Chemical
Anti-inflammatory	Corticosteroids
Protein precipitating	Silver nitrate, zinc chloride, strontium chloride, formaldehyde
Tubule occluding	Calcium hydroxide, potassium nitrate, fluorides, sodium citrate, iontophoresis with 2 percent sodium fluoride, potassium oxalate
	Physical
Tubule sealing	Composites, resins, varnishes, sealants, glass ionomer cements, laser sealing of the tubules
Physical protection	Soft tissue grafts

Modified from Scherman A, Jacobsen PL. Managing dentin hypersensitivity: what treatment to recommend to patients. J Am Dent Assoc 1992;123:59. Reprinted by permission of ADA Publishing Co., Inc. Copyright © 1992 American Dental Association.

patient plaque control. Bacterial plaque is commonly observed in areas that are hypersensitive because of periodontal surgery.[118] Patients with poor plaque control experience more hypersensitivity[120] and are often reluctant to thoroughly clean hypersensitive areas. The dental hygienist can educate the patient about bacterial plaque acids and their contribution to hypersensitivity and reinforce the importance of meticulous daily oral hygiene.

CHEMICAL DESENSITIZING AGENTS

The common therapeutic measures for treating hypersensitive dentin are the use of specific toothpastes, gels, or rinses at home and the application of chemical agents in the dental office. Recommendations for home remedies and use of office treatments can provide effective combination therapy to relieve or reduce the condition. Based on their mode of action, chemical agents are classified into four categories: (1) anti-inflammatory agents; (2) protein-precipitating agents; (3) tubule-occluding agents; and (4) tubule sealants (see Table 15–12).

Home Use Agents. The use of a desensitizing dentifrice is the easiest first step in managing dentin hypersensitivity at home. Several toothpaste products are available that are simple to use and noninvasive. These agents promote compliance because almost everyone brushes his or her teeth. Potassium nitrate, strontium chloride, and sodium citrate are the active ingredients in desensitizing dentifrice formulations. The low concentration of these desensitizing agents allows for dispensing these dentifrices without a prescription. Data show that potassium nitrate is effective in reducing the pain of dentin hypersensitivity within 4 to 6 weeks.[117] The agents that combine desensitizing agents with fluoride are preferred because they provide both desensitizing action and caries control.

Fluoride preparations are also used for home treatment of dentin hypersensitivity. Unfortunately, they do not seem to have long-term effects.[113, 123, 124] In addition to their caries prevention benefits, sodium fluoride toothpaste or rinse, stannous fluoride gel, and sodium monofluorophosphate toothpaste can reduce hypersensitivity in 3 to 4 weeks.[125-127] Highly fluoridated (5,000 ppm) prescription dentifrices can reduce hypersensitivity and also provide a highly effective anti-caries benefit.[116]

No clinical studies have compared the fluoride compounds, so the best therapeutic agent for the treatment of dentin hypersensitivity is largely a matter of personal preference.[104] It is important to recommend home use of fluoride agents and desensitizing toothpastes to provide patients with both pain relief and caries prevention.[128]

Office Therapies. Professional application of high-concentration fluoride products is a common remedy for dentin hypersensitivity in the dental office. Agents are applied directly or by iontophoresis to the tooth surfaces. After the sensitive tooth is isolated, a 2 percent sodium fluoride paste can be massaged into the exposed surface with a wood point inserted into a porte polisher.[128] A kaolin- and glycerin-based 33.3 percent fluoride paste has also been used in this manner.[79] Alternatively, iontophoresis of a 2 percent sodium fluoride solution occludes the dentinal tubules.[124] This technique uses an electric current to create a positively charged tooth surface, which then attracts and embeds the negatively charged fluoride ions into the dentinal tubules.[117, 129] Although this technique reportedly provides immediate relief of pain,[124] it requires special equipment and multiple applications. It is also expensive and has not been shown to be superior to other methods.

Additional in-office chemical agents for reduction of hypersensitivity include monopotas-

TABLE 15–13. Treatment Recommendations for Dentin Hypersensitivity

Step	Rationale
1. Perform a thorough assessment and evaluate the cause	Other sources of pain should be eliminated.
2. Explain the problem and causes.	Informing the patient of the causes of hypersensitivity provides reassurance that the problem usually improves.
3. Reinforce proper and effective oral hygiene techniques to eliminate bacterial plaque.	Correction of easily preventable causes may eliminate the discomfort as well as prevent root caries and periodontal disease progression.
4. Provide dietary advice and counseling.	Diet modification may decrease the onset of hypersensitivity.
5. Recommend daily use of a desensitizing toothpaste (2- to 6-week trial).	A simple and generally effective form of therapy.
6. Provide in-office application of oxalate or fluoride products (2- to 10-week trial).	In-office therapy may provide immediate pain relief to be complemented by home therapy.
7. Recommend physical therapeutic agents and refer the patient to the dentist for treatment.	Sealing or covering dentinal tubules can be useful if other therapies do not relieve the pain.

Modified from Scherman A, Jacobsen PL. Managing dentin hypersensitivity: what treatment to recommend to patients. J Am Dent Assoc 1992;123:60. Reprinted by permission of ADA Publishing Co., Inc. Copyright © 1992 American Dental Association.

sium oxalate (Protect, John O. Butler, Chicago, IL) and ferric oxalate (Sensodyne Sealant, Block Drug, Jersey City, NJ). Both of these products are effective for pain relief,[130] but monopotassium oxalate is preferred by some.[117] Application is simple; the area is dried with cotton swabs and the compound is applied for 2 minutes.

PHYSICAL DESENSITIZING AGENTS

If chemical desensitizing agents do not provide relief, physical techniques, such as application of dentin bonding agents, including composite resins, varnishes, sealants, glass ionomer cements, and soft tissue grafts, can be employed (see Table 15–12).[117] These procedures seal or cover the dentinal tubules and require tooth preparation or periodontal surgery. These techniques can be useful if more conservative therapies are not effective. Composite resin with a glass ionomer liner is the preferred tooth preparation technique because it works well and lasts.

Treatment Recommendations

The management of dentin hypersensitivity can seem daunting because of the many desensitizing treatments available and their variable efficacy. In addition, the condition often improves with the passage of time. A recommended treatment plan to reduce dentin hypersensitivity is described in Table 15–13. Treatment begins with a complete examination to exclude other possible sources of pain.[117] Patient education and plaque control are major steps in the control of hypersensitivity because bacterial plaque is a known cause.[118] Dietary counseling may be helpful if patients consume large quantities of acidic or sugary foods and beverages. Foods to be avoided or used in moderation include citrus fruit juices, apple juice, wine, and yogurt.[120]

Treatment begins with a conservative approach to pain relief. The dental hygienist must recognize that a favorite desensitizing agent may not work on everyone, so trying different agents is helpful. Daily use of a desensitizing toothpaste by the patient and in-office treatment with potassium oxalate or fluoride are the first steps in treatment. If the discomfort persists after 2 to 6 weeks, other products should be tried. If these are not effective after several weeks, physical agents, such as a composite resin with a glass ionomer base, can be placed by the dentist.

Patient education is an important part of the successful treatment of dentin hypersensitivity. At the beginning of periodontal therapy, the patient should be advised of the risk of hypersensitivity and the availability of treatments. Patients who are warned about this problem will not be surprised if hypersensitivity develops and may be more willing to accept treatment alternatives.

THE ROLE OF THE DENTAL HYGIENIST IN PERIODONTAL MAINTENANCE

The prevalence of periodontal disease is well documented in epidemiologic studies of the United States dentate population.[131] With the recent decline in dental caries, treatment of periodontal disease has become increasingly important to dental hygienists, dentists, and the general public. Periodontal health is greatly dependent on routine professional care, so the demand for preventive and therapeutic periodontal services is likely to increase.[132-134] The dental hygienist is the primary provider of periodontal maintenance care to the public. This role is critical in the long-term success of therapy.

Dental hygienists are sometimes described as preventive oral health professionals, primary preventive therapists, periodontal therapists, co-therapists, or primary care providers of preventive and therapeutic procedures to manage periodontal disease.[35, 135-138] Whatever term is used, because of their skills, dental hygienists are valuable providers of long-term preventive and maintenance care after active periodontal therapy.[136, 137]

The contemporary role of the dental hygienist in periodontal and maintenance therapy has been described as a periodontal co-therapist[131] with both the dentist and the patient. This interrelationship is depicted in Figure 15-8. In collaboration with the dentist, the dental hygienist has the goal of providing the highest quality oral health care. The dental hygienist and dentist must integrate care into a single collaborative approach to quality patient care.[139] The dental hygienist also functions as a co-therapist with the patient, providing the knowledge and skills necessary to achieve successful long-term oral health for the individual.[136]

The patient must be an active partner with the dental hygienist to achieve and maintain periodontal health. The dental hygienist must be an effective communicator and an attentive and careful listener. The patient will then recognize the dental hygienist's commitment to provide the highest quality care and build trust and confidence in the partnership. Patients can then take responsibility for their own oral health. The role of the dental hygienist is a broad one that combines outstanding clinical skills in collaboration with other dental health professionals and a role as a partner in periodontal health.

SIGNIFICANCE OF PERIODONTAL MAINTENANCE

The vital role of periodontal maintenance in preserving periodontal health and the preven-

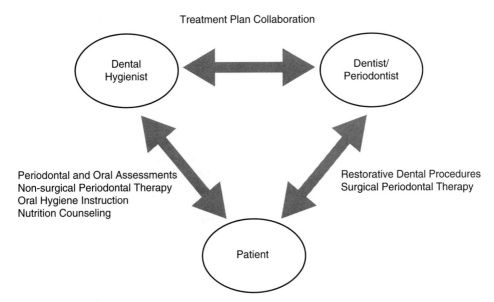

Treatment Plan Collaboration

Dental Hygienist

Dentist/ Periodontist

Periodontal and Oral Assessments
Non-surgical Periodontal Therapy
Oral Hygiene Instruction
Nutrition Counseling

Restorative Dental Procedures
Surgical Periodontal Therapy

Patient

FIGURE 15–8. The dental hygienist serves as a periodontal co-therapist in collaboration with both the dentist and periodontist. The patient is an active partner in achieving and maintaining periodontal health.

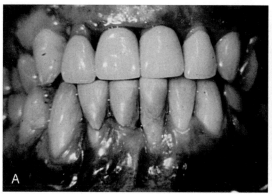
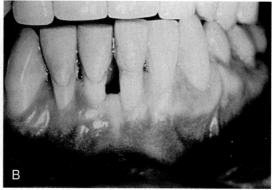

FIGURE 15-9. A. Patient presented with moderate periodontitis with recession and heavy accumulation of plaque and calculus. Following periodontal debridement, the patient was maintained on 3-month recalls. **B.** Patient's appearance following 2 years of periodontal maintenance. Note healthy appearance of the gingiva.

tion of new or recurrent disease after active therapy is indisputable. A wealth of clinical evidence confirms the efficacy of frequent monitoring and supportive care to achieve the goal of a healthy dentition for a lifetime. This goal is the ultimate measure of success for the periodontal maintenance population. To achieve this success, a collaborative effort between patient, dental hygienist, dentist, and periodontist is mandatory. Without a firm commitment from each, maintenance of optimal oral health is far more difficult. An example of successful periodontal maintenance care is presented in Figure 15-9.

The effectiveness of maintenance therapy is dependent on patient compliance. Adherence to both professional and personal plaque control recommendations is essential for a successful outcome. If the importance of continued maintenance therapy and daily home care is recognized and reinforced, patients are more likely to accept their crucial role in maintaining their own periodontal health.

A well-defined and well-executed maintenance protocol is the foundation of an effective long-term periodontal maintenance program.[36, 140] The components are compliance, assessment, prevention, and treatment. Patients must comply with recommended visit schedules. In gen-

eral, most patients benefit from a 3-month maintenance interval, although more frequent visits are sometimes necessary.[141] Regular periodontal assessment is imperative to evaluate clinical parameters, such as the physical characteristics of the tissues, probing pocket depths, clinical attachment levels, bleeding on probing, and radiographic alveolar bone changes. An indispensable component is reinforcement of the patient's oral hygiene practices because bacterial plaque is well established as the cause of periodontal disease. Periodic supervised care is important to permit early detection and treatment of new or recurrent disease in collaboration with the dentist and periodontist. Each periodontal maintenance visit also provides the opportunity to prevent and treat complications such as dentin hypersensitivity and root caries. Professional application of desensitizing and anti-caries agents is an important preventive and therapeutic procedure that is well within the scope of dental hygiene practice. Finally, thorough debridement of the entire dentition is necessary to eliminate all bacterial accumulations and calculus deposits, creating a plaque-free environment. These elements, as part of a periodontal maintenance program, lead to good oral health for the patient and provide a sense of satisfaction and reward for the dental hygienist.

STUDY QUESTIONS

MULTIPLE CHOICE

1. What evidence supports the effectiveness of periodontal therapy?

   a. untreated periodontal disease progresses, with a continual loss of periodontal attachment over time
   b. prevention of periodontal disease and retardation of disease progression, but prevention of tooth loss is more uncertain
   c. a regular maintenance program is not needed to assure long-term success
   d. supragingival plaque control alone can improve probing depths and clinical attachment in patients with periodontitis

2. As defined by the American Academy of Periodontology, what is nonsurgical periodontal therapy?

   a. plaque control, supragingival and subgingival scaling, root planing, and the use of chemical adjuncts
   b. plaque control, plaque removal, supragingival scaling, and the use of chemical adjuncts
   c. plaque control, plaque removal, supragingival and subgingival scaling, and the use of chemical adjuncts
   d. supragingival and subgingival scaling, root planing, and the use of chemical adjuncts
   e. plaque control, plaque removal, and supragingival and subgingival scaling

3. The most predictable measurement indicating further loss of clinical attachment levels in maintenance patients is:

   a. bleeding on probing
   b. increased amounts of suppuration
   c. higher plaque scores
   d. increased probing depths
   e. decreased alveolar bone height

4. A common reason for poor patient compliance to recommended oral hygiene regimens is:

   a. procedure too cumbersome
   b. physical or mental handicap
   c. procedure too time consuming
   d. recommendation of too many plaque control aids
   e. all of the above

5. The recommended periodontal maintenance interval after periodontal treatment is based on:

   a. degree of inflammation
   b. effectiveness of plaque control
   c. patient age
   d. record of compliance
   e. all of the above

6. The most common appearance of root caries is:

   a. a single tan to brown discoloration on the enamel surface at or near the cementoenamel junction
   b. a single tan to brown discoloration on the cemental surface at or near the cementoenamel junction
   c. multiple tan to brown discolorations on the enamel surface at or near the cementoenamel junction
   d. multiple tan to brown discolorations on the cemental surface at or near the cementoenamel junction

7. Daily application of topical fluoride gel is an effective method of root caries prevention.
   The most effective fluoride gel preparation for root caries control has not been determined.

   a. Both statements are TRUE.
   b. Both statements are FALSE.
   c. The first statement is TRUE, the second is FALSE.
   d. The first statement is FALSE, the second is TRUE.

8. Root hypersensitivity occurs in many patients with root surfaces exposed from periodontal therapy, malpositioned teeth, and improper tooth brushing techniques.
   Normal aging does not contribute to exposure of root surfaces or result in root hypersensitivity.

   a. Both statements are TRUE.
   b. Both statements are FALSE.
   c. The first statement is TRUE, the second is FALSE.
   d. The first statement is FALSE, the second is TRUE.

9. Management of dentinal sensitivity begins with recommending the use of fluoride toothpaste BECAUSE the sensitivity is more often related to root caries than exposure of root surfaces.

   a. Both the statement and reason are correct and related.
   b. Both the statement and reason are correct but NOT related.
   c. The statement is correct, but the reason is NOT.
   d. The statement is NOT correct, but the reason is correct.
   e. NEITHER the statement NOR the reason is correct.

10. 1.1% neutral sodium fluoride is effective in treating dentinal hypersensitivity BECAUSE it reduces the patient's susceptibility to root caries.

a. Both the statement and reason are correct and related.
b. Both the statement and reason are correct but NOT related.
c. The statement is correct, but the reason is NOT.
d. The statement is NOT correct, but the reason is correct.
e. NEITHER the statement NOR the reason is correct.

SHORT ANSWER

11. The success of periodontal maintenance greatly depends on the integration of several key elements. List the four major determinants of successful supportive periodontal therapy and explain the significance of each factor.

12. During the maintenance appointment, a periodontal evaluation is mandatory to assess the current periodontal status of the patient. What are the six components of the periodontal evaluation?

13. A 55-year-old woman has just completed nonsurgical periodontal therapy and is reluctant to return for a maintenance visit in 3 months. List strategies to encourage her compliance with the recommended supportive periodontal therapy interval.

14. A healthy 70-year-old man with a history of moderate to advanced periodontitis and an extensive restorative dental treatment reports to the dental hygienist for a 6-month dental checkup. During the clinical assessment, the dental hygienist notices moderate plaque accumulation and the patient reports having a "dry mouth" frequently. Devise a therapeutic treatment plan for this patient.

15. The dental hygienist is often described as a periodontal co-therapist. Describe the role of the dental hygienist as a co-therapist in periodontal maintenance therapy.

REFERENCES

1. American Academy of Periodontology. Glossary of periodontic terms. J Periodontol. 1986;(supplement):17.
2. American Academy of Periodontology. Current Procedural Terminology for Periodontics, 5th ed. Chicago: American Academy of Periodontology, 1988:14.
3. McGuire MK. Prognosis versus actual outcome: a long-term survey of 100 treated periodontal patients under maintenance care. J Periodontal 1991; 62:51-58.
4. Löe H, Morrison E. Epidemiology of periodontal disease. In Genco RJ, Goldman HM, Cohen DW, eds. Contemporary Periodontics. St. Louis: CV Mosby, 1990:106-116.
5. Greene JC. Periodontal disease in India: report of an epidemiological study. J Dent Res 1960;39:302-312.
6. Greville TNE. United States Life Tables by Dentulous or Edentulous Condition, 1971, and 1957-58. Bethesda, MD:US Department of Health, Education and Welfare, 1974; publication no. (HRA) 75-1338.
7. Löe H, Theilade E, Jensen SB. Experimental gingivitis in man. J Periodontol 1965:36:177-187.
8. Theilade E, Wright WH, Jensen SB, Löe H. Experimental gingivitis in man: II. A longitudinal clinical and bacterial investigation. J Periodontal Res 1966; 1:1-13.
9. Greenstein G. Periodontal response to mechanical non-surgical therapy: a review. J Periodontal 1992; 63:118-130.
10. Listgarten MA, Lindhe J, Hellden L. Effect of tetracycline and/or scaling on human periodontal disease: clinical, microbiological and histological observations. J Clin Periodontol 1978;5:246-271.
11. Slots J, Mashimo P, Levine MJ, Genco RJ. Periodontal therapy in humans: I. Microbiological and clinical effects of a single course of periodontal scaling and root planing, and of adjunctive tetracycline therapy. J Periodontol 1979;50:495-509.
12. Morrison EC, Ramfjord SP, Hill RW. Short-term effects of initial, non-surgical periodontal treatment (hygienic phase). J Periodontol 1980;7:199-211.
13. Badersten A, Nilveus R, Egelberg J. Effect of non-surgical periodontal therapy: I. Moderately advanced periodontitis. J Clin Periodontol 1981;8:57-72.
14. Badersten A, Nilveus R, Egelberg J. Effect of non-surgical periodontal therapy: II. Severely advanced periodontitis. J Clin Periodontol 1984;11:63-76.
15. Renvert S, Wikström M., Dahlén G, Slots J, Egelberg J. Effect of root debridement on the elimination of *Actinobacillus actinomycetemcomitans* and *Bacteroides gingivalis* from periodontal pockets. J Clin Periodontol 1990;17:345-350.
16. Hammerle CHF, Joss A, Lang NP. Short-term effects of initial periodontal therapy (hygienic phase). J Clin Periodontal 1991;18:233-239.
17. Kalkwarf KL, Kaldahl WB, Paul KD, Molvar MP. Evaluation of gingival bleeding following 4 types of periodontal therapy. J Clin Periodontol 1989;16:601-608.
18. Kaldahl WB, Kalkwarf KL, Patil KD, Molvar MP. Evaluation of gingival suppuration and supragingival plaque following 4 modalities of periodontal therapy. J Clin Periodontal 1990;17:642-649.
19. American Academy of Periodontology: Proceedings of the World Workshop in Clinical Periodontics. Chicago: American Academy of Periodontology, 1989:1-11,21.
20. Bragger U, Hakanson D, Lang NP. Progression of periodontal disease in patients with mild to moderate adult periodontitis. J Clin Periodontol 1992;19:659-666.
21. Axelsson P, Lindhe J. Effect of controlled oral hygiene procedures on caries and periodontal disease in adults. J Clin Periodontol 1978;5:133-151.

22. Axelsson P, Lindhe J. Effect of controlled oral hygiene procedures on caries and periodontal disease in adults: results after 6 years. J Clin Periodontol 1981;8:239-248.

23. Axelsson P, Lindhe J, Nystrom B. On the prevention of caries and periodontal disease: results of a 15-year longitudinal study in adults. J Clin Periodontol 1991;18:182-189.

24. Wood WR, Greco GW, McFall WT. Tooth loss in patients with moderate periodontitis after treatment and long-term maintenance care. J Periodontol 1989;60:516-520.

25. Merin RL. Results of periodontal treatment. In Carranza FA, ed. Glickman's Clinical Periodontology, 7th ed. Philadelphia: WB Saunders, 1990:977-987.

26. Wilson TG, Glover ME, Malik AK, Schoen JA, Dorsett D. Tooth loss in maintenance patients in a private periodontal practice. J Periodontol 1987;58:231-235.

27. Becker W, Becker BE, Berg LE. Periodontal treatment without maintenance: a retrospective study in 44 patients. J Periodontol 1984;55:505-509.

28. Becker W, Berg LE, Becker BE. Untreated periodontal disease: a longitudinal study. J Periodontol 1979;50:234-244.

29. Löe H, Anerud A, Boysen H, Morrison EC. The natural history of periodontal disease in man: rapid, moderate and no loss of attachment in Sri Lankan laborers 15 to 45 years of age. J Clin Periodontol 1986;13:431-440.

30. Bower RC. Current concepts of periodontal maintenance. Aust Dent J 1989;34:507-516.

31. Becker W, Becker BE, Berg LE. Long-term evaluation of periodontal treatment and maintenance in 95 patients. Int J Periodontics Restorative Dent 1984;4:54-71.

32. Caffesse RG. Maintenance therapy: preventing recurrence of periodontal diseases. In Genco RJ, Goldman HM, Cohen DW, eds. Contemporary Periodontics. St Louis: CV Mosby, 1990:483-492.

33. Proye M, Caton J, Polson A. Initial healing of periodontal pockets after a single episode of root planing monitored by controlled probing force. J Periodontol 1982;53:296-301.

34. Badersten A, Nilveus R, Egelberg J. Scores of plaque, bleeding, suppuration and probing depth to predict probing attachment loss: 5 years of observation following nonsurgical periodontal therapy. J Clin Periodontol 1990;17:102-107.

35. Hicks MJ, Uldricks JM, Whitacre HL, Anderson J, Moeschberger ML. A national study of periodontal assessment by dental hygienists. J Dent Hyg 1993;67:82-92.

36. DeVore CH, Hicks MJ, Claman L. A system for insuring success of long-term supportive periodontal therapy. J Dent Hyg 1989;63:214-220.

37. Dahlén G, Lindhe J, Sato K, Hanamura H, Okamoto H. The effect of supragingival plaque control on the subgingival microbiota in subjects with periodontal disease. J Clin Periodontol 1992;19:802-809.

38. Lindhe J, Socransky S, Nyman S, Haffajee A, Westfelt E. Critical probing depths in periodontal therapy. J Clin Periodontol 1982;9:323-336.

39. Greenwell H, Bissada NF, Wittwer JW. Periodontics in general practice: professional plaque control. J Am Dent Assoc 1990;121:642-646.

40. Mendoza AR, Newcomb GM, Nixon KC. Compliance with supportive periodontal therapy. J Periodontol 1991;62:731-736.

41. Wilson TG. Maintaining periodontal treatment. J Am Dent Assoc 1990;121:491-494.

42. Axelsson P, Lindhe J. The significance of maintenance care in the treatment of periodontal disease. J Clin Periodontol 1981;8:281-294.

43. Schmidt J, Morrison E, Kerry G, Caffesse R. Patient compliance with suggested maintenance recall in a private periodontal practice. J Periodontol 1990;61:316-317.

44. Wilson T, Glover M, Schoen J, Bans C, Jacobs T. Compliance with maintenance therapy in a private periodontal practice. J Periodontol 1984;55:468-473.

45. Hill RW, Ramfjord SP, Morrison EC, Appleberry EA, Caffesse RG, Kerry GJ, Nissle RR. Four types of periodontal treatment compared over two years. J Periodontol 1981;52:655-662.

46. Pihlstrom BL, McHugh RB, Oliphant TH. Molar and nonmolar teeth compared over 6½ years following two methods of periodontal therapy. J Periodontol 1984;55:499-504.

47. Knowles JW, Burgett FG, Nissle RR, Schnick RA, Morrison EC, Ramfjord SP. Results of periodontal treatment related to pocket depth and attachment level: eight years. J Periodontol 1979;50:225-233.

48. Wilson TG. Compliance: a review of the literature with possible applications to periodontics. J Periodontol 1987;58:706-714.

49. Becker BE, Karp CL, Becker W, Berg L. Personality differences and stressful life events: differences between treated periodontal patients with and without maintenance. J Clin Periodontol 1988;15:49-52.

50. Spolsky V. The epidemiology of gingival and periodontal disease. In Carranza FA, ed. Glickman's Clinical Periodontology, 7th ed. Philadelphia: WB Saunders, 1990:302-329.

51. Suomi JD, Greene JC, Vermillion JR, Doyle J, Chang JJ, Leatherwood EC. The effect of controlled oral hygiene procedures on the progression of periodontal disease in adults: results after the third and final year. J Periodontol 1971;42:152-160.

52. Boyer EM, Nikias MK. Self-reported compliance with a preventive dental regimen. Clin Preventive Dent 1983;5:3-7.

53. Strack BB, McCullough MA, Conine TA. Compliance with oral hygiene instructions. Dent Hyg 1980;54:181-184.

54. Johansson L, Oster B, Hamp S. Evaluation of cause-related periodontal therapy and compliance with maintenance care recommendations. J Clin Periodontol 1984;11:689-699.

55. Hellstadius K, Asman B, Gustafsson A. Improved maintenance of plaque control by electrical toothbrushing in periodontitis patients with low compliance. J Clin Periodontol 1993;20:235-237.

56. Heasman PA, Jacobs DJ, Chapple IL. An evaluation of the effectiveness and patient compliance with plaque control methods in the prevention of periodontal disease. Clin Preventive Dent 1989;11:24-28.

57. Kuhner MK, Raetzke PB. The effect of health beliefs on the compliance of periodontal patients with oral hygiene instructions. J Periodontol 1989;60:51-56.

58. Perry DA, Beemsterboer P, Carranza FA. Periodontal probing. In Techniques and Theory of Periodontal Instrumentation, 1st ed. Philadelphia: WB Saunders, 1990:29-61.

59. Ramfjord SP. Indices for prevalence and incidence of periodontal disease. J Periodontol 1959;30:51-59.

60. Gibbs CH, Hirschfeld JW, Lee JG, Low SB, Magnusson I, Thousand RR, Yerneni P, Clark WB. Description and clinical evaluation of a new computerized periodontal probe—the Florida probe. J Clin Periodontol 1988;15:137-144.

61. Consensus Report Section 1 Periodontal diseases:

Epidemiology and diagnosis, J Am Dent Assoc 1998; 129:9S-14S.

62. Lang NP, Joss A, Orsanic T, Gusberti FA, Siegrist BE. Bleeding on probing: a predictor for the progression of periodontal disease? J Clin Periodontol 1986; 13:590-596.

63. Van der Velden U. Influence of periodontal health on probing depth and bleeding tendency. J Clin Periodontol 1980;7:129.

64. Chaves ES, Caffesse RG, Morrison EC, Scutts DL. Diagnostic discrimination of bleeding on probing during maintenance periodontal therapy. Am J Dent 1990;3:167-170.

65. Wilkins EM. Examination procedures. In Clinical Practice of the Dental Hygienist, 6th ed. Philadelphia: Lea & Febiger, 1989:191-211.

66. Manson JD, Eley BM. Management of bone defects and furcation involvement. In Derrick DD, ed. Outline of Periodontics, 2nd ed. Cornwall: Butterworth, 1989:191.

67. Wilkins EM. The gingiva. In Clinical Practice of the Dental Hygienist, 6th ed. Philadelphia: Lea & Febiger: 1989:166-178.

68. Kennedy JE, Bird WC, Palcanis KG, Dorfman HS. A longitudinal evaluation of varying widths of attached gingiva. J Clin Periodontol 1985;12:667-675.

69. American Dental Association. Frequently asked questions. Patients and Consumers. ADA Website www.ada.org. March 1998.

70. American Academy of Periodontology: Supportive periodontal treatment. In Proceedings of the World Workshop in Clinical Periodontics. Chicago: American Academy of Periodontology, 1989.

71. Merin RL. Maintenance Care. In Carranza FA, ed. Glickman's Clinical Periodontology, 7th ed. Philadelphia: WB Saunders, 1990:964-977.

72. Fedi PF. Periodontal maintenance therapy. In The Periodontic Syllabus, 2nd ed. Philadelphia: Lea & Febiger, 1985:176-180.

73. Grossman E, Reiter G, Sturzenberger OP, de la Rosa M, Dickinson TD, Ferretti GA, Ludlam GE, Meckel AH. Six-month study of the effects of a chlorhexidine mouthrinse on gingivitis in adults. J Periodont Res 1986;21(suppl):33-43.

74. Siegrist BE, Gusberti FA, Brecx MC, Weber HP, Lang NP. Efficacy of supervised rinsing with chlorhexidine digluconate in comparison to phenolic and plant alkaloid compounds. J Periodont Res 1986;21(suppl):60-73.

75. Low SB, Ciancio SG. Reviewing nonsurgical periodontal therapy. J Am Dent Assoc 1990;121:467-470.

76. Wilkins EM. Clinical Practice of the Dental Hygienist, 3rd ed. Philadelphia: Lea & Febiger, 1971.

77. Wilkins EM. Bacterial plaque and other soft deposits. In Clinical Practice of the Dental Hygienist, 6th ed. Philadelphia: Lea & Febiger, 1989:235-246.

78. Nunn PF. "Selective polishing"—Time for a change? Access 1997;11:38-42.

79. Carranza FA. General principles of periodontal surgery. In Carranza FA, ed. Glickman's Clinical Periodontology, 7th ed. Philadelphia: WB Saunders, 1990:765-776.

80. Genco RJ. Classification and clinical and radiographic features of periodontal disease. In Genco RJ, Goldman HM, Cohen DW, eds. Contemporary Periodontics. St. Louis: CV Mosby, 1990:63-81.

81. Williams DM, Hughes FJ, Odell EW, Farthing PM. Clinical management of periodontal disease. In Pathology of Periodontal Disease, 1st ed. New York: Oxford University Press, 1992:125-143.

82. Hazen SP, Chilton NW, Mumma RD. The problem of root caries: I. Literature review and clinical description. J Am Dent Assoc 1973;86:137-144.

83. Schupbach P, Guggenheim B, Lutz F. Histopathology of root surface caries. J Dent Res 1990;69:1195-1204.

84. Syed SA, Loesche WJ, Pape HL, Grenier E. Predominant cultivable flora isolated from human root surface caries plaque. Infect Immun 1975;11:727-731.

85. Newbrun E. Microflora. In Cariology, 3rd ed. Carol Stream, IL: Quintessence, 1989:63-97.

86. Katz RV, Hazen SP, Chilton NW, Mumma RD. Prevalence and intraoral distribution of root caries in an adult population. Caries Res 1982;16:265-271.

87. Miller AJ, Brunelle JA, Carlos JP, Brown L, Löe H. Oral health of United States adults: national findings. Bethesda, MD: National Institute of Dental Research, 1987; NIH publication no. 87-2868.

88. Winn DM, Brunelle JA, Selwitz RH, Kaste LM, Oldakowski RJ, Kingman A, Brown LJ. Coronal and root caries in the dentition of adults in the United States, 1988-91. J Dent Res 1996;75(special issue):642-651.

89. Hix JO, O'Leary TJ. The relationship between cemental caries, oral hygiene status and fermentable carbohydrate intake. J Periodontol 1976;47:398-404.

90. Ravald N, Hamp SE. Prediction of root surface caries in patients reated for advanced periodontal disease. J Clin Periodontol 1981;8:400-414.

91. Beck JD, Kohout F, Hunt RJ. Identification of high caries risk adults: attitudes, social factors and diseases. Int Dent J 1988;38:231-238.

92. Regezi JA, Sciubba JJ. Salivary gland diseases. In Oral Pathology: Clinical-Pathologic Correlations, 1st ed. Philadelphia: WB Saunders, 1989:225-283.

93. Greenspan D. Xerostomia: diagnosis and management. Oncology 1996, 10:7-11.

94. Katz RV. Clinical signs of root caries: measurement issues from an epidemiologic perspective. J Dent Res 1990;69:1211-1215.

95. Newbrun E. Current concepts of caries etiology. In Cariology, 3rd ed. Carol Stream, IL: Quintessence, 1989:29-61.

96. Featherstone JDB. Prevention and reversal of dental caries: role of low level fluoride. Community Dent Oral Epidemiol 1999;27:31-40.

97. Stookey GK. Critical evaluation of the composition and use of topical fluorides. J Dent Res 1990;69(special issue):805-812.

98. Stamm JW, Banting DW. Comparison of root caries prevalence in adults with life-long residence in fluoridated and non-fluoridated communities. J Dent Res 1980;59(special issue A):405, abstract 552.

99. Burt BA, Ismail AI, Eklund SA. Root caries in an optimally fluoridated and a high-fluoride community. J Dent Res 1986;65:1154-1158.

100. Hunt RJ, Eldredge JB, Beck JD. Effect of residence in a fluoridated community on the incidence of coronal and root caries in an older adult population. J Public Health Dent 1989;49:138-141.

101. Leske G, Ripa L, Forte F, Varma A. Clinical trial of the effect of daily sodium fluoride mouthrinsing on root caries. J Dent Res 1988;67(special issue):171, abstract 469.

102. Paine ML, Slots J, Rich SK. Fluoride use in periodontal therapy: a review of the literature. J Am Dent Assoc 1998;129:69-77.

103. Stookey GK, Rodlun CA, Warrick JM, Miller CH. Professional topical fluoride systems vs. root caries in hamsters. J Dent Res 1989;68:372, abstract 1521.

104. Hastreiter RJ. Is 0.4 percent stannous fluoride gel an effective agent for the prevention of oral diseases? J Am Dent Assoc 1989;118:205-208.

105. Stookey GK, Rodlun CA, Warrick JM, Miller CH. Effect of fluoride dentifrices on root caries in hamsters. Caries Res 1989;23:429, abstract 84.
106. Wilkins EM. Fluorides. In Clinical Practice of the Dental Hygienist, 6th ed. Philadelphia: Lea & Febiger, 1989:394-418.
107. Jensen ME, Kohout F. The effect of a fluoridated dentifrice on root and coronal caries in an older adult population. J Am Dent Assoc 1988;117:829-832.
108. Horowitz HS. The prevention of oral disease: established methods of prevention. Br Dent J 1980;149:311-318.
109. Newbrun E. Control and prevention of dental caries. In Cariology, 3rd ed. Carol Stream, IL: Quintessence, 1989:357-375.
110. Sutcliffe P. A longitudinal clinical study of oral cleanliness and dental caries in schoolchildren. Arch Oral Biol 1973;18:765-770.
111. Wilkins EM. Diet and Dietary Analysis. In Clinical Practice of the Dental Hygienist, 6th ed. Philadelphia: Lea & Febiger, 1989:379-393.
112. Graf H, Galasse R. Morbidity, prevalence and intraoral distribution of hypersensitive teeth. J Dent Res 1977;56(suppl):A162.
113. Krauser JT. Hypersensitive teeth: Part I: Etiology. J Prosthet Dent 1986;56:153-156.
114. Brännstrom M. A hydrodynamic mechanism in the transmission of pain producing stimuli through dentin. In Andersson DJ, ed. Sensory Mechanisms in Dentine, vol. 1. London: Pergamon Press, 1963:73-79.
115. Kerns DG, Scheidt MJ, Pashley DH, Horner JA, Strong SL, Van Dyke TE. Dentinal tubule occlusion and root hypersensitivity. J Periodontol 1991;62:421-428.
116. Christensen GJ. Desensitization of cervical tooth structure. JADA 1998;129:765-766.
117. Scherman A, Jacobsen PL. Managing dentin hypersensitivity: what treatment to recommend to patients. J Am Dent Assoc 1992;123:57-61.
118. Wallace JA, Bissada NF. Pulpal and root sensitivity rated to periodontal therapy. Oral Surg Oral Med Oral Pathol 1990;69:743-747.
119. Fischer C, Wennberg A, Fischer RG, Attström R. Clinical evaluation of pulp and dentine sensitivity after supragingival and subgingival scaling. Endodontic Dent Traumatol 1991;7:259-265.
120. Trowbridge HO, Silver DR. A review of current approaches to in-office management of tooth hypersensitivity. Dent Clin North Am 1990;34:561-581.
121. Pashley DH. Dentin permeability, dentin sensitivity, and treatment through tubule occlusion. J Endodontics 1986;12:465-474.
122. Mjor I. Human coronal dentine: structure and reactions. Oral Surg Oral Med Oral Pathol 1972;33:810-823.
123. Ong G. Desensitizing agents: a review. Clin Preventive Dent 1986;8:14-18.
124. Kern DA, McQuade MJ, Scheidt MJ, Hanson B, Van Dyke TE. Effectiveness of sodium fluoride on tooth hypersensitivity with and without iontophoresis. J Periodontol 1989;60:386-389.
125. Krauser JT. Hypersensitive teeth: Part II. Treatment. J Prosthet Dent 1986;56:307-311.
126. McFall WT. A review of the active agents available for treatment of dentinal hypersensitivity. Endodontic Dent Traumatol 1986;2:141-149.
127. Kandelman D, Gagnon G, Ruel D, Peters D, Trepanier J. The effect of two fluoride toothpastes on dentinal sensitivity: a clinical evaluation. Oral Health 1988;78:63-65.
128. Wilkins EM. Hypersensitive teeth. In Clinical Practice of the Dental Hygienist, 6th ed. Philadelphia: Lea & Febiger, 1989:498-502.
129. Ciancio S. Delivery systems and clinical significance of available agents for dentinal hypersensitivity. Endodontic Dent Traumatol 1986;2:150-152.
130. Johnson R, Muzzin KB. Effects of potassium oxalate on dentin hypersensitivity in vivo. J Periodontol 1989;60:151-158.
131. Uldricks JM, Hicks MJ, Whitacre HL, Anderson J, Moeschberger ML. Dental hygienists' utilization of periodontal assessment skills and perceived collaboration with dentist-employer. J Dent Hyg 1993;67:22-29.
132. Douglass CW. The periodontal health status of the U.S. population. AADS Annual Session, March 1987.
133. Schallhorn R, Snider LS. Periodontal maintenance therapy. Dent Hyg 1981;103:227-231.
134. Löe H. Dental science and dental health: now and a century hence. J Dent Res 1988;67:797-798.
135. American Dental Hygienists' Association, Washington Office. Capitol Agenda. Access 1993;7:49-51.
136. McCullough C. Perio trends: the dental hygienist as periodontal cotherapist. Access 1993;7:36-37.
137. McCullough C. Perio trends: the critical role of the dental hygienist in periodontal therapy. Access 1993;7:27-29.
138. Walsh M. Trends and potentials for dental hygiene. J Public Health Dent 1985;45:60-64.
139. Darby M. Collaborative practice model: the future of dental hygiene. J Dent Educ 1983;47:589-593.
140. Wilkins EM. Evaluation and maintenance. In Clinical Practice of the Dental Hygienist, 6th ed. Philadelphia: Lea & Febiger, 1989:537-542.
141. Ramfjord SP. Maintenance care for treated periodontitis patients. J Clin Periodontol 1987;14:433-437.

Dorothy A. Perry / Phyllis L. Beemsterboer

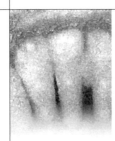

16

Periodontal Emergencies

Chapter Objectives

1. Define the role of the dental hygienist in the recognition and treatment of periodontal emergencies.
2. Describe the etiology of abscesses in periodontal tissues.
3. Compare and contrast the signs, symptoms, and treatment considerations in patients with gingival, periodontal, and periapical abscesses.
4. Describe the history of acute necrotizing ulcerative gingivitis and distinguish its clinical characteristics from those of other forms of acute oral infection.
5. Identify the lesions of acute herpetic gingivostomatitis and the recommended supportive treatment.

Key Terms

Acute herpetic gingivostomatitis
Acute necrotizing ulcerative gingivitis
Combination abscess
Endodontic abscess
Gingival abscess
Necrotizing ulcerative periodontitis

Periapical abscess
Pericoronitis
Periodontal abscess
Purulence
Suppuration

The ability to identify emergency periodontal conditions is an important skill for the dental hygienist. Knowledge of emergency situations and treatment priorities helps patients to receive the most timely and appropriate care. The dental hygienist must recognize conditions that do not represent variations of normal clinical presentation. In the case of periodontal emergency situations, delayed therapy can result in additional discomfort for the patient, with possible consequences of increased bone loss and damage to other periodontal tissues. Treatment of all periodontal emergency conditions requires co-therapy with the dentist or periodontist. Before any dental or dental hygiene procedure, a careful medical and dental history must be taken.

PERIODONTAL ABSCESSES

A **periodontal abscess** is an inflammation of bacterial origin that is associated with accumulations of **suppuration** or **purulence** (pus) in the periodontal tissues. The pus is often referred to as exudate, or purulent exudate. Such infections have rapid onset and are usually characterized by pain, swelling, and discomfort. The periodontal abscess is caused by bacteria that have become established in the tissue as a result of trauma, advancing disease process, or incomplete scaling and root planing. The response of the tissue to this infectious process is dependent on the patient's resistance. Individual factors, such as systemic disease, can affect the clinical situation. There are three basic types of abscesses: periodontal, gingival, and periapical. Each type may be acute or chronic, and there are **combination abscesses**.

Acute Periodontal Abscesses

Acute periodontal abscesses are associated with pre-existing periodontal disease. They may occur around any tooth in the mouth when the periodontal pocket becomes occluded, often as a result of a foreign object.[1] An exacerbated inflammatory reaction then occurs. If the pocket can drain through the sulcus or a fistula, the infection can stabilize. Stabilization rarely occurs if a foreign object, such as a peanut skin, popcorn hull, or berry seed, remains in the pocket.

Acute periodontal abscesses appear as shiny, red, raised, and rounded masses on the gingiva or mucosa. They can point and drain through the tissue or drain through the pocket opening. Suppuration (pus) is usually seen around the opening of the abscess and can often be expressed by finger pressure. Visual examination alone is not enough. Pus forms on the inner surface of the pocket wall and may not be seen on the exterior of the gingiva.[2] Symptoms include: (1) throbbing pain, (2) swelling, (3) deep red to blue discoloration of the affected tissue, (4) tooth sensitivity to pressure, and (5) tooth mobility (Figure 16–1) (see color figure).

The patient may also report that the tooth feels "high" because it may become slightly extruded.[1] Radiographs may be helpful in locating a pre-existing area of bone loss, which may be the origin of the abscess. However, the infection moves through the tissue in the direction of least resistance so that the external features may appear at some distance from the affected tooth. The opening of the fistula, or sinus orifice along the lateral aspect of the tooth in the adult dentition, is usually indicative of a periodontal abscess. However, it may be the result of a **periapical abscess**. In the primary dentition, the sinus orifice on the lateral aspect of the tooth is usually associated with periapical abscess.[2]

The microflora in the acute periodontal abscess is predominantly Gram-negative and anaerobic. In contrast, healthy gingival flora is predominantly Gram-positive and aerobic.[3]

TREATMENT CONSIDERATIONS

Treatment of acute periodontal abscesses consists mainly of drainage and the use of antibiotics or antimicrobial agents. The abscess must be treated immediately to alleviate pain and prevent spread of infection. It may be drained through the pocket opening or by access through an incision. Drainage through the pocket opening is usually possible. The teeth in the affected area are scaled and root planed with anesthesia, and curettage is performed to remove granulation tissue. Postoperative instructions call for rest, fluid intake, and warm salt water rinses to help reduce swelling. Follow-up treatment, often involving periodontal surgery, is required to eliminate the problem. After scaling, root planing, and curettage, local irrigation with 1 percent povidone or 3 percent hydrogen peroxide has been recommended to help kill the pathogenic bacteria and flush the abscess area.[1]

The initial treatment of the abscess through the pocket is often the responsibility of the dental hygienist. However, sometimes the procedure requires flap surgery at the initial appointment to obtain access to complete the debridement. This treatment is performed by the dentist or periodontist. Antibiotics and pain medications are not usually required.[4] If the patient has a fever or if lymphadenopathy is present, antibiotics should be prescribed. The antibiotic recommended can be an analog of tetracycline because these drugs have the ability to create high titers in the gingival sulcus and inhibit collagenase in the host.[5] Penicillin can also be prescribed.[4]

The repair potential for acute periodontal

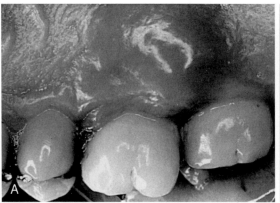
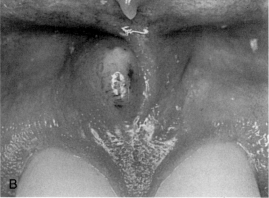

FIGURE 16–1. Acute Periodontal abscess. **A**. Clinical appearance of an acute periodontal abscess. There is marked swelling of the periodontal tissues. Clinically, the tissue appears shiny, reddened, and raised. The patient had severe pain. (Courtesy of Philip R. Melnick, DMD.) **B**. Acute periodontal abscess associated with a central incisor with a large fistulous track. The fistula drains periodically thus relieving the swelling and pain for a short time. The fistula then closes temporarily and the swelling and pain recur. (See Color figure.)

abscesses is excellent. Bone is lost rapidly during the acute phase, but with immediate recognition and treatment, the lost tissue can often be regained.[1]

Chronic Periodontal Abscess

Chronic periodontal abscesses resemble acute periodontal abscesses. There is an overgrowth of pathogenic organisms in suppurating periodontal abscess. However, chronic abscesses are usually painless because they drain into the oral cavity, either through the opening of the pocket or through a sinus tract. On careful questioning, patients often recount previous episodes of pain and swelling, probably caused by acute infection.[2]

The chronic periodontal abscess exhibits suppuration that exudes into the oral cavity on digital pressure through the pocket or sinus tract. The associated gingival tissue is red and swollen. As long as the chronic abscess is draining, it is rarely painful. The dental hygienist must understand that suppuration that exudes from the periodontium indicates chronic abscess and requires appropriate treatment (Figure 16-2).

TREATMENT CONSIDERATIONS

The treatment of chronic periodontal abscess is similar to the treatment of acute periodontal abscess. The lesion must be scaled and root planed, curettage performed, local antimicrobial therapy completed, and the patient seen for follow-up care to evaluate the need for further periodontal treatment, often including

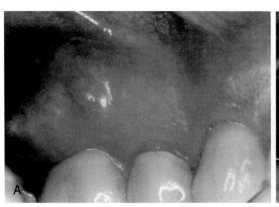
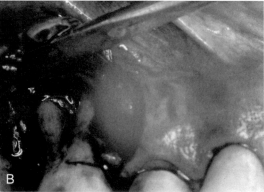

FIGURE 16–2. Chronic periodontal abscess. **A**. Inflammatory exudate drains through the opening of the pocket. **B**. On surgical opening of the defect, an extensive furcation involvement is seen. (Courtesy of Philip R. Melnick, DMD.)

periodontal surgery.[4] The patient must be made aware of the chronic condition, informed about possible acute episodes if no further treatment is performed, and encouraged to cooperate with meticulous supportive periodontal therapy. Patients often do not know that rapid bone loss occurs during acute episodes, placing the teeth in jeopardy. This knowledge must be communicated to the patient and may help convince the patient to seek further treatment to preserve the teeth.

Tooth Loss Associated with Periodontal Abscesses

It is important to understand that the presence of a periodontal abscess does not necessarily mean that the tooth must be extracted. A retrospective study of 114 patients treated and maintained at a university periodontology clinic, all having had moderate to severe periodontal disease, suggested that teeth that develop periodontal abscesses can be treated successfully and maintained for years. Symptoms of the infected teeth were pain, swelling, exudate and fistulous tracts. Of the subjects in the study, 109 periodontal abscesses occurred in a 13 year period, 45 percent were extracted, but 55 percent of the teeth were treated and maintained for an average of 12.5 years; the range was 5 to 29 years.[6] It is important for the dental hygienist to recognize periodontal abscesses and refer them for immediate treatment.

GINGIVAL ABSCESS

Gingival abscesses are primarily distinguished from acute periodontal abscesses by taking a good history. Gingival abscesses often occur in disease-free areas, and may be related to forceful inclusion of some foreign object into the area. Most frequently, gingival abscesses are found on the marginal gingiva and are not associated with any abnormality of the deeper tissues (Figure 16–3) (see color figure).[1]

A gingival abscess appears as a shiny, raised area of acute inflammation and may be painful. The swelling, although it may be quite large, is usually confined to the marginal gingiva.[2] A suppurative lesion is usually evident on the gingival tissues.

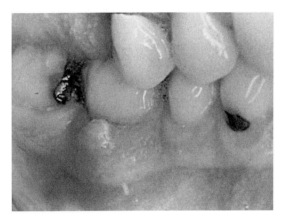

FIGURE 16–3. Gingival abscess. The gingival abscess appears as a localized area of swelling away from the pocket or sulcus. It is painful for the patient. (Courtesy of Philip R. Melnick, DMD.) (See Color figure.)

Treatment Considerations

The gingival abscess must be drained and irrigated. The treatment is usually performed by the dentist or periodontist. It is incised, drained, and irrigated with locally administered antimicrobials. Warm salt water rinses should be recommended for postoperative therapy. After the acute treatment of the abscess, the reduced lesion may require excision. Scaling and root planing of the teeth in the area is also recommended.[4]

ENDODONTIC ABSCESS

An **endodontic abscess** is sometimes difficult to distinguish from an acute periodontal abscess. The facial pain and tenderness to the tooth are similar in both cases. Endodontic abscesses result from infection through caries, traumatic fracture of the tooth, or the trauma of a dental procedure. In addition, pulpal infection to a tooth can be spread to the pulp from an adjacent infected tooth through the lateral canals.[7] Most commonly, microorganisms are spread from a carious lesion into the pulp through the dentinal tubules. The microorganisms colonize in the pulp and produce a variety of toxins that result in pulp cell death. Bacteria and their metabolic products then exit the apical foramen and can cause abscess formation.[8]

The endodontic abscess often appears on radiographs as a rounded radiolucency at the apex of the tooth. In this case it may be termed

TABLE 16–1. Characteristics of the Periodontal and Endodontic Abscess

Characteristic	Periodontal Abscess	Endodontic Abscess
Type of pain	Constant	Intermittent
	Localized	Hard to localize
	Severe, sharp	Extemely severe
Vitality	Vital	Usually nonvital
Radiographic image	Bone loss, but no apical radiolucency	Apical radiolucency common

a periapical abscess. However, early in abscess formation, the radiographic changes are much more subtle. Some abscesses drain through a sinus duct through the cortical bone, and some drain through the periodontal ligament, making them less identifiable on radiographs. Draining endodontic abscesses can resemble acute periodontal abscesses because their symptoms are similar.

In evaluating an abscess to determine its origin, it is helpful to know that 85 percent of tooth pain is pulpal and 15 percent is periodontal. In addition, many endodontically abscessed teeth test nonvital, which is a good distinguishing clue. However, some populations of patients, such as those being treated in the office of a periodontist, are much more likely to have periodontal abscesses than pulpal abscesses.[1] According to Killoy,[1] pain may be the feature that distinguishes periapical abscesses from periodontal abscesses. Periapical pain is characterized as sharp, severe, intermittent, and difficult to localize. In contrast, periodontal pain is usually constant, localized, and less severe. Ta-

ble 16-1 shows the characteristics of periodontal and endodontic abscesses.

Treatment Considerations

Treatment of endodontic abscesses requires endodontic therapy or extraction of the tooth. In addition to causing severe pain, untreated endodontic abscesses can lead to abscesses of the brain[9] or fasciitis of the neck or chest wall.[8] These extensions of infection into deeper tissues can be life threatening (Figure 16-4).

COMBINATION ABSCESSES

An abscess is an infectious process that can spread from the pulp to the periodontium, or from the periodontal pocket to the pulp. These circumstances lead to combination periapical and periodontal abscesses.

Combination abscesses have some combination of the signs and symptoms mentioned and may be difficult to diagnose. Periodontal and

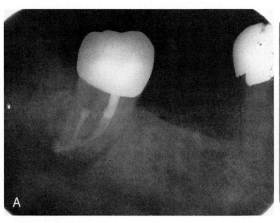
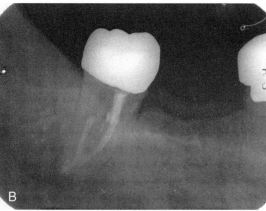

FIGURE 16–4. Periapical abscess. **A.** Radiographic appearance of an endodontic abscess. Radiolucency is seen at the apex of the root immediately after treatment. **B.** Radiographic appearance of the healed endodontic lesion 1 year after treatment. (Courtesy of Dr. Harold Goodis.)

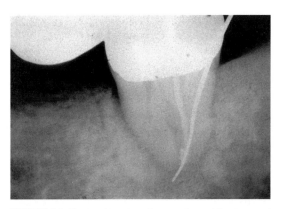

FIGURE 16–5. Combination abscess. A combination periodontal and periapical abscess. Gutta-percha points have been inserted through the opening to the oral cavity. They extend all the way to the apex of the roots. Widening of the periodontal ligament space can also be discerned. (Courtesy of Dr. Harold Goodis.)

periapical abscesses can cause extensive damage to the surrounding periodontium because symptoms can be intermittent, causing patients to delay treatment. These abscesses require extensive therapy, both periodontal and endodontic, and often result in tooth loss (Figure 16-5).

PERICORONITIS

Pericoronitis is an abscess associated with a partially or fully erupted tooth that is covered completely or partly by a flap of tissue called an operculum. The most commonly affected tooth is the mandibular third molar, but maxillary third molars and other teeth that are the most distal in the arch are also associated with the condition. As bacteria accumulate under the gingiva next to the tooth, the tissue responds by becoming inflamed and painful.[10] This condition is most commonly seen in young adults and has been a serious problem for military personnel, most of whom are 17 to 26 years old. Leone and Edenfield[11] reported that 20 percent of the military dental emergencies in World War II and 16 percent of those treated during the Vietnam conflict were pericoronitis. The population incidence was reported to be 1.9 cases of pericoronitis per 100 recruits.

The symptoms of acute pericoronitis are swelling of the operculum and other gingiva associated with the most distal tooth in the arch, redness, and pain. The tissue may be so swollen that it interferes with mastication because it may be compressed during chewing. Trismus (muscle spasm) may occur. (For a complete description of trismus, see Chapter 8.) The patient may also have a fever.[10] Purulent exudate occurs in about half of cases. Of 25 patients in a military population, few bled on palpation and none had a fever. However, pain, swelling, and redness were present in every instance. Pericoronitis may be a recurring situation. Two-thirds of the 25 patients reported a previous incidence of pericoronitis.[11]

Treatment Considerations

Treatment for pericoronitis varies according to the severity of the case, whether it is a recurrence, and if there are systemic complications. Treatment usually requires multiple visits.

Initial therapy is palliative and symptomatic to make the patient more comfortable. The infected area must be debrided, usually by flushing with warm water or dilute hydrogen peroxide, using a topical anesthetic. Much manipulation of the tissue may not be possible, and debridement with instruments may not be tolerable at the first visit. After this initial debridement, the patient should be instructed to rest at home, use warm salt water rinses, and drink fluids to avoid dehydration. Antibiotics should be prescribed if the patient has a fever.

The patient should return the next day. At that time, the tissue is usually considerably improved. At the second visit, the area should be flushed and instrumented if possible. More thorough patient education and plaque removal can be provided.[12]

After the acute condition has resolved, the patient should be evaluated by the dentist for further treatment. Extraction of the third molar, which is often only partially erupted, may be required. If the tooth is to be retained, the operculum can be surgically removed to obtain a more normal gingival contour. There is a relationship between pericoronitis and **acute necrotizing ulcerative gingivitis** (ANUG) to be discussed in the next section. Pericoronitis flaps are considered primary incubation sites for microbiota associated with ANUG, and the elimination of the flaps may reduce the likelihood of ANUG recurrences.[12]

NECROTIZING ULCERATIVE GINGIVITIS

NUG is an opportunistic infection of the gingiva that is associated with stress, lifestyle, and some chronic illnesses such as blood dyscrasias, human immunodeficiency virus (HIV) infection, and Down's syndrome. The disease was first described by Vincent[13] in the late 19th century. It was so common among troops fighting in the trenches in Europe during World War I that it was thought to be communicable and named "trench mouth." Now it is primarily seen in young adults under severe stress and individuals who are immunocompromised. It is no longer considered communicable.[13]

NUG is a recurring disease with complex bacteriology consisting of a large proportion of spirochetes and Gram-negative organisms. The bacteria invade the tissue and cause the characteristic appearance of the disease.[14] Recurrent NUG can result in attachment loss. When this occurs, the more appropriate name for the disease is **necrotizing ulcerative periodontitis** (NUP).

Characteristics of NUG

NUG has specific clinical characteristics that distinguish it from other forms of acute oral infections. The involved papillary gingiva becomes necrotic and appears cratered, or "punched out." The surface of the gingiva has a pseudomembranous coating made up of necrotic bacteria and tissue. The gingiva is reddened and painful. The lesions may be localized to specific areas or generalized throughout the mouth. Patients often have a strong and offensive breath odor, described as fetid, that can be detected anywhere in the room occupied by the patient. The three most reliable criteria for recognizing the disease were described by Stevens and co-workers[15]: (1) acute necrosis and ulceration of the interproximal papillae, (2) pain, and (3) bleeding.

Falker and co-workers[16] found that necrotic papillae, pain, and bleeding occurred 100 percent of the time in patients with ANUG who attended a dental school clinic. Fetid breath odor occurred in 97 percent of cases, pseudomembrane in 87 percent, lymphadenopathy in 61 percent, and fever in 39 percent. Smoking appeared to be a risk factor associated with NUG because 83 percent of patients who had symptoms smoked (Figure 16-6).

Treatment Considerations

Patients with NUG usually seek treatment for acute pain. Mechanical debridement to eliminate the bacterial organisms is recommended.[13] Treatment may need to progress over a few days during the acute phase of the disease because the pain prevents the patient and the dental hygienist from thoroughly cleaning the affected areas. The recommended treatment sequence requires several visits.[12, 13]

The first visit requires debridement to a limited extent. The use of ultrasonic instruments and topical or local anesthetics may be helpful in removing sloughing tissue, loose debris and supragingival plaque and calculus. Subgingival scaling and root planing should not be performed because of the possibility of extending the infection to deeper tissues and causing bacteremia.[12] Careful oral hygiene instruction should be provided. Systemic antibiotics may be prescribed by the dentist if the patient has a fever or lymphadenopathy.

The second treatment visit should occur 1 or 2 days later. In that short time, the condition usually improves enough to permit more thorough debridement and better home care. Subgingival scaling may be performed if the patient's sensitivity permits.[12] The third visit should occur 3 to 5 days after the first visit

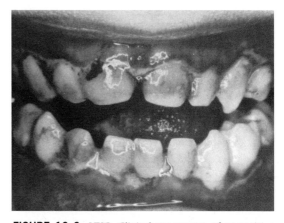

FIGURE 16-6. NUG. Clinical appearance of necrotizing ulcerative gingivitis in a 17-year-old male. Heavy plaque accumulation and pseudomembrane formation are seen. The condition was complicated by heavy plaque accumulation because it was too painful for the patient to brush properly. (Courtesy of Philip R. Melnick, DMD.)

so that debridement can be completed. Any defective amalgam margins should be smoothed or replaced to minimize plaque retention.

During the course of emergency management of ANUG, the patient should be given instructions to follow at home. Due to the nature of infection, the patient should rest, drink plenty of fluids, avoid spicy foods, and rinse with warm salt water as needed. If antibiotics have been prescribed, the patient should be strongly urged to fill the prescription and follow the treatment regimen.

After emergency treatment is completed, the patient should be evaluated by the dentist or periodontist. All factors related to plaque retention and control should be addressed. The disease often leaves cratered papillae that may require surgical correction. Supportive periodontal therapy should be provided at frequent intervals to minimize the risk of recurrence.

ACUTE HERPETIC GINGIVOSTOMATITIS

Acute herpetic gingivostomatitis is the oral manifestation of primary infection with the herpes virus, usually herpes simplex virus I (HSVI). Approximately 10 to 20 percent of patients with initial infection with HSVI are symptomatic.[17] Historically, acute herpetic gingivostomatitis has been seen primarily in infants and children. The disease is now more commonly found in young adults in their 20s and 30s, possibly as a result of primary infection with the genital herpes virus, herpes simplex virus II (HSVII). Primary herpetic gingivostomatitis in adolescents and older adults is usually HSVI, but may be the initial manifestation of HSVII. Many patients with primary herpetic infections become carriers of the disease through recurrent expressions of the virus as herpes labialis.[18]

The painful herpetic ulcers in the mouth that are associated with primary infection often cause reduction in food and fluid intake, which can be critical to health. This highly infectious disease requires education of patients, families, and office staff to prevent its spread. Dental and dental hygiene care should be postponed until the condition has subsided so that the clinician removes the risk of self-inoculation and does not spread the area of recurrence in the patient.

Acute herpetic gingivostomatitis is characterized by a set of systemic and intraoral symptoms. The disease is commonly associated with prodromal symptoms, such as fever, malaise, headache, irritability, and lymphadenopathy.[19] A good history and interview may be necessary to identify the prodromal symptoms when suspicious oral lesions are found.

Oral lesions begin as small, yellow vesicles. These vesicles coalesce to form larger, round ulcers with gray centers and bright red borders. The vesicles and ulcers may be present on any of the oral mucous membranes, including the lips, tongue, gingiva, and buccal mucosa, and appear generally throughout the oral cavity.[18] The patient may have serious, even extreme, pain. Recognition of the disease is based on knowledge of the appearance of the ulcers and on questioning regarding systemic manifestations. Diagnostic tests can be used to confirm the presence of the virus, but are not routinely performed (Figure 16–7).

Treatment Considerations

The treatment of acute herpetic gingivostomatitis is supportive because the disease runs its course in 7 to 10 days. Gingival inflammation can be reduced by patient plaque removal if the patient can tolerate the discomfort. Instrumentation should not be performed because of the possibility of transmission of the virus to the dental hygienist and other workers. Even if the hygienist has been previously exposed to

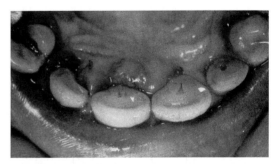

FIGURE 16–7. Acute herpetic gingivostomatitis. This disease appears as a generalized infection characterized by vesicle formation and reddened tissue. Tissue changes were seen around all of the anterior teeth. This patient had severe gingival pain which caused him to seek treatment. (Courtesy of Philip R. Melnick, DMD.)

herpes virus, the possibility of initiating herpetic whitlow from an inadvertent puncture. Whitlow is the term for the herpetic lesion that occurs most often on the fingers of the dental hygienist where the inoculation of herpes virus occurred.[12]

The patient should be encouraged to maintain an adequate diet, perform oral hygiene as much as possible, and, if necessary, use over-the-counter topical anesthetics to control the discomfort. Topical anesthetics should be used cautiously to avoid anesthetizing the throat. That feeling can be frightening, especially for children.[18] For more controlled delivery, topical anesthetics can be swabbed on the lesions rather than rinsed or sprayed.

CONCLUSION

Dental hygienists must be familiar with the identification and initial treatment of periodontal emergencies because it is part of professional responsibility. Recognizing emergency conditions as quickly as possible helps to limit the destructive processes, start timely care, and restore patients to comfort and function.

STUDY QUESTIONS

MULTIPLE CHOICE

1. The periodontal abscess is characterized by all of the following symptoms except one. Which is the exception?

   a. bleeding
   b. pain
   c. swelling
   d. tenderness

2. The microflora in the acute periodontal abscess is predominantly:

   a. Gram-negative and anaerobic
   b. Gram-positive and aerobic
   c. Gram-negative and aerobic
   d. Gram-positive and anaerobic

3. An acute periodontal abscess can occur as the result of all of the following except one. Which is the exception?

   a. dental procedures
   b. a popcorn hull or berry seed
   c. subgingival scaling
   d. antibiotic usage

4. What is the term for an abscess that is found on marginal gingiva and is not involved in the deeper periodontium?

   a. acute periodontal abscess
   b. chronic periodontal abscess
   c. gingival abscess
   d. periapical abscess
   e. pericoronitis

5. What is the term for an abscess that is the result of a pulpal infection from caries or trauma?

   a. acute periodontal abscess
   b. chronic periodontal abscess
   c. gingival abscess
   d. periapical abscess
   e. pericoronitis

6. A periapical abscess that is draining can resemble which of the following?

   a. acute periodontal abscess
   b. allergic reaction
   c. pericoronitis
   d. linear gingival erythema

7. A periapical abscess must be treated as soon as possible BECAUSE infection from this lesion could be life-threatening.

   a. both the statement and the reasons are correct.
   b. both the statement and the reason are correct but NOT related.
   c. The statement is correct, but the reason is NOT.
   d. The statement is NOT correct, but the reason is correct.
   e. NEITHER the statement NOR the reason is correct.

8. An abscess is an infectious process that can spread from the periodontal pocket to the pulp.
   An abscess is an infectious process that can spread from the pulp to the periodontal pocket.

   a. both statements are TRUE.
   b. both statements are FALSE.
   c. the first statement is TRUE, the second is FALSE.
   d. the first statement is FALSE, the second is TRUE.

9. Which disease is highly infectious?

   a. acute herpetic gingivostomatitis
   b. acute necrotizing ulcerative gingivitis
   c. acute periodontal abscess
   d. periapical abscess
   e. pericoronitis

10. What is the term for an abscess that is associated with partially or fully erupted teeth?

    a. acute periodontal abscess
    b. chronic periodontal abscess
    c. gingival abscess
    d. periapical abscess
    e. pericoronitis

SHORT ANSWER

11. What are the postoperative instructions for a patient after treatment of a periodontal abscess?

    _____

    _____

12. How does the clinician differentiate between acute and chronic periodontal abscess?

    _____

    _____

13. Describe the difference between pain from a periapical abscess and pain from a periodontal abscess.

_____

_____

14. Describe the clinical characteristics of necrotizing ulcerative gingivitis that distinguish it from other forms of acute oral infection.

_____

_____

15. Identify the oral lesions of acute herpetic gingivostomatitis, and describe the recommended treatment.

_____

_____

16. Identify the oral lesions of acute herpetic gingivostomatitis, and describe the recommended treatment.

_____

_____

REFERENCES

1. Killoy WJ. Treatment of periodontal abscesses. In Genco RJ, Goldman HM, Cohen DW, eds. Contemporary Periodontics, CV Mosby, St. Louis: 1990:475-482.
2. Carranza FA Jr. Clinical diagnosis. In Carranza FA and Newman MG, eds. Clinical Periodontology, 8th ed. Philadelphia: WB Saunders, 1996:344-362.
3. Newman MG, Sims TN. The predominant cultivable microbiota of the periodontal abscess. J Periodontol 1978;50:350.
4. Carranza FA Jr. Treatment of the periodontal abscess. In Carranza FA and Newman MG, eds. Clinical Periodontology, 8th ed. Philadelphia: WB Saunders, 1996:483-485.
5. Jolkovsky DL, Ciancio SC. Antimicrobial agents in periodontal therapy. In Carranza FA and Newman MG, eds. Clinical Periodontology, 8th ed. Philadelphia: WB Saunders, 1996:511-522.
6. McLeod DE, Lainson PA, Spivey JD. Tooth loss due to periodontal abscess: a retrospective study. J Periodontol 1997;68:963-966.
7. Kureishi A, Chow AW. The tender tooth dentoalveolar, pericoronal, and periodontal infections. Infect Dis Clin North Am 1988;2:163-182.
8. Macfarlane TW. Plaque-related infections. J Med Microbiol 1989;29:161-170.
9. Saal CJ, Mason JC, Cheuk SL, Hill MK. Brain abscess from chronic odontogenic cause: report of a case. J Am Dent Assoc 1988;117:453-455.
10. Genco RJ. Periodontal diagnosis, prognosis, and treatment planning. In Genco RJ, Goldman HM, Cohen DW, eds. Contemporary Periodontics. St. Louis: CV Mosby, 1990:348-359.
11. Leone SA, Edenfield MJ. Third molars and acute pericoronitis: a military problem. Mil Med 1987;152:146-149.
12. Carranza FA Jr. Treatment of acute gingival disease. In Carranza FA, ed. Glickman's Clinical Periodontology, 7th ed. Philadelphia: WB Saunders, 1990: 657-667.
13. Cogen RB. Acute necrotizing ulcerative gingivitis. In Genco RJ, Goldman HM, Cohen DW, eds. Contemporary Periodontics, St. Louis: CV Mosby, 1990:460-465.
14. Caton J. Periodontal diagnosis and diagnostic aids. In Nevins M, Becker W, Kornman K, eds. Proceedings of the World Workshop in Clinical Periodontics, Chicago: American Academy of Periodontology, 1989:I-2.
15. Stevens AW, Cogen RB, Cohen-Cole S, Freeman A. Demographic and clinical data associated with acute necrotizing ulcerative gingivitis in a dental school population. J Clin Periodontol 1984;11:487-493.
16. Falker WA, Martin SA, Vincent JW, Tall BD, Nauman RK, Suzuki JB. A clinical, demographic and microbiologic study of ANUG patients in an urban dental school. J Clin Periodontol 1987;14:307-314.
17. Rose F. Infective forms of gingivostomatitis. In Genco RJ, Goldman HM, Cohen DW, eds. Contemporary Periodontics. St. Louis: CV Mosby, 1990:243-250.
18. Balciunas BA, Overholser CD. Diagnosis and treatment of common oral lesions. Am Fam Physician 1987;35:206-220.
19. Balciunas BA, Kelly M, Siegel MA. Clinical management of common oral lesions. Cutis 1991;47:31-36.

17

Gary C. Armitage

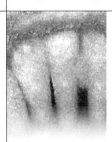

Systemic Factors Influencing Periodontal Diseases

*C*hapter *O*bjectives

1. Understand systemic factors that influence dental hygiene care.
2. Describe conditions that require consultation with a patient's physician.
3. Describe changes in oral tissues observed with systemic diseases and conditions.
4. List modifications needed to best treat patients with systemic conditions.

*K*ey *T*erms

Blood dyscrasias
Cardiovascular diseases
Dermatologic diseases
Endocrine disturbances and
   abnormalities

Infectious diseases
Joint diseases and disorders
Neurologic disorders
Oral cancer
Tobacco use

Systemic factors can have a profound effect on the diagnosis, pathogenesis, and treatment of periodontal infections. There are several ways in which systemic factors or diseases can influence the recognition and management of periodontal infections. Some systemic diseases have signs and symptoms that mimic those of plaque-induced gingivitis or periodontitis, thereby increasing the likelihood of a misdiagnosis. Systemic problems in some patients can (1) increase their susceptibility to infection, (2) interfere with wound healing, (3) require modification of standard approaches to treatment, and (4) complicate factors associated with patient cooperation. In many instances, medical treatment of systemic diseases affects the clinical presentation and course of periodontal infections.

People are now living longer than ever before. As a result, the patient population in a typical dental practice includes an increasing number of individuals with complex systemic problems, many of which are being treated with a wide variety of medications. To intelligently treat periodontal infections in such a population, the knowledgeable clinician must understand how the patient's systemic problems influence the selection of periodontal treatment and the anticipated response to treatment. This chapter provides an introduction to this subject and reviews some common systemic conditions that are encountered in a dental and dental hygiene practice.

CARDIOVASCULAR DISEASES

In the United States, more than 40 million people have some form of cardiovascular disease. In this group of diseases, the most common conditions include hypertension (high blood pressure), coronary artery disease, valvar heart disease, cardiac arrhythmias, and congestive heart failure. Because cardiovascular diseases are so prevalent in the population, many patients with these conditions will seek dental care. In general, dental and periodontal treatment is not contraindicated in most patients with cardiovascular disease. In many cases, it is advisable to obtain a medical consultation from the patient's physician before treatment is initiated. A request for a medical consultation usually involves preparing a written summary of the patient's cardiovascular problem and a statement of what type of dental or periodontal treatment is planned. This information is useful to the physician in deciding whether any special precautions are required for the anticipated dental treatment. When dental health care workers request medical consultations, it is their responsibility to have a reasonable idea of

what pretreatment precautions might be necessary.

Hypertension

High blood pressure is a major risk factor for cardiovascular disease, stroke, and kidney failure. Tens of millions of people in the United States have high blood pressure or are taking antihypertensive medications.[1] Hypertension has been called the "silent killer" because it is frequently asymptomatic and more than half of the patients with hypertension are unaware that they have it.[2] The prevalence of the disease increases dramatically with age.[2] Variations also occur with gender and race.[3] In general, patients with readings $\geq 140/90$ mm Hg are considered to be hypertensive.[4, 5] Table 17-1 shows the 1997 classification of hypertension published by the Joint National Committee on the detection, evaluation, and treatment of high blood pressure.[4]

Dental health care workers can play an important role in detecting previously undiagnosed and asymptomatic cases of hypertension. Adult dental patients should routinely have their blood pressure measured at each visit. When elevated blood pressure is detected, patients should be advised to see their physician. In individuals with uncontrolled hypertension,

TABLE 17-1. Classification of Adult Blood Pressure and Dental Treatment Modifications[4, 5]

Category	Systolic Pressure (mm Hg)	Diastolic Pressure (mm Hg)	Dental Treatment
Normal	< 130	< 85	No modification of dental care
High normal	130–139	85–89	No modification of dental care
Hypertension			
Stage I	140–159	90–99	No modification of dental care, medical referral, inform patient
Stage II	160–179	100–109	Selective dental care,* medical referral
Stage III	180–209	110–119	Emergent nonstressful procedures,† immediate medical referral/consultation
Stage IV	≥ 210	≥ 120	Emergent nonstressful procedures,† immediate medical referral

*Selective dental care may include, but is not limited to, dental prophylaxis, nonsurgical periodontal therapy, restorative procedures, and nonsurgical endodontic therapy.
†Emergent nonstressful procedures may include, but are not limited to, dental procedures that may help alleviate pain, infection or masticatory dysfunction. These procedures should have limited physiological and psychological effects. An example of an emergent nonstressful procedure might be a simple incision and drainage of an intraoral fluctuant dental abscess. The medical benefits achieved by performing emergent nonstressful procedures in stage III and IV hypertensive patients should outweigh the risk of complications secondary to the patient's hypertensive state.
Used with permission. From Muzyka BC, Glick M. The hypertensive dental patient. J Am Dent Assoc 1997;128:1109–1120. Copyright 1997, American Dental Association.

elective dental treatment should be deferred because stress associated with dental procedures can further elevate blood pressure and thereby increase the risk of stroke and assorted cardiovascular or renal problems. However, patients with medically well-controlled hypertension can safely receive nearly all forms of dental and periodontal therapy.

The use of epinephrine-containing local anesthetics is not contraindicated in patients with well-controlled hypertension. However, it is advisable to use minimal amounts of epinephrine, such as 0.04 mg per dental visit (approximately two cartridges containing 1:100,000 parts epinephrine). If pain is anticipated in association with the planned dental or periodontal treatment, complete local anesthesia is desirable to minimize the release of endogenous epinephrine.[6, 7] In addition, special care must be taken to use adequate aspiration before the anesthetic is administered to avoid intravascular injection.

Physicians prescribe many types of medications for hypertensive patients, including diuretics (e.g., thiazides), sympatholytics (e.g., beta-adrenergic blockers, such as propanolol), vasodilators (e.g., hydralazine HCl), and angiotensin-converting enzyme inhibitors (e.g., enalapril). As with all patients who are taking medication, it is important for the dental health care worker to review the list of drugs taken by the patient and become familiar with their mode of action and potential side effects. Some of the side effects of these medications are drowsiness, mental depression, confusion, and xerostomia (dry month). The *Physician's Desk Reference* or a drug reference text would be an excellent source of information about medications.

Coronary Artery (Ischemic Heart) Disease

Atherosclerosis is the deposition of cholesterol-containing material in the walls of arteries that results in a narrowing, and eventually the occlusion, of the affected blood vessels. Atherosclerotic changes in the coronary arteries that feed the heart can lead to ischemic heart disease, which is the leading cause of sudden death in the United States. The two most common clinical manifestations of ischemic heart disease are angina pectoris and myocardial infarction (heart attack).

Angina pectoris is a severe, recurring chest pain that frequently radiates into the left shoulder and arm. It is an intense, crushing pain that can also move across the chest and down each arm. Sometimes the pain involves the neck, lower jaw, and face. It is caused by the deprivation of oxygen to the cardiac muscle secondary to reduced blood flow, frequently as a consequence of atherosclerotic narrowing of the coronary arteries. However, it also can be caused by specific situations, such as strenuous physical exertion or extreme psychological stress, in which the oxygen demands of the heart muscle are not met.

A condition in which anginal pain is predictable and controlled by medication is called "stable angina."[8] Patients with stable angina frequently control their anginal pain by taking one or more of the following types of drugs: nitrates (e.g., nitroglycerin), beta-adrenergic blockers, and calcium channel blockers (e.g., nifedipine). Gingival enlargement is one of the common side effects of nifedipine (Procardia) and certain other calcium channel blockers.[9-13] The gingival enlargement can make oral hygiene difficult and thereby increase the risk of plaque-induced diseases, such as dental caries and periodontal disease (Figure 17–1).

Patients with stable angina can safely receive routine dental care, but it is advisable to minimize stress by scheduling relatively short morning appointments so that the patient is well rested. As with hypertensive patients, local anesthesia should be used for potentially painful procedures to minimize the release of endogenous epinephrine.[6, 7] If an anginal attack occurs during the delivery of dental care, treatment should be discontinued, the patient should be

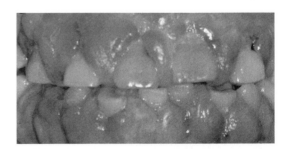

FIGURE 17–1. Drug-influenced gingival enlargement in a 53-year-old male who was taking verapamil for a cardiac arrhythmia, nifedipine to control anginal pain, and cyclosporine (an immunosuppressive agent) to combat rejection of a transplanted kidney. A reported side effect of all three drugs is gingival enlargement. (Courtesy of Dr. V. Godfrey.)

placed in a semisupine position, and standard emergency procedures should be performed.

Myocardial infarction (heart attack) is caused by sudden occlusion of the blood supply to a portion of the heart. Heart attacks are frequently caused by occlusion of a coronary artery by atherosclerotic deposits or a blood clot (thrombus). Patients who are recovering from a recent heart attack should not receive elective dental treatment until their condition is medically stabilized, usually for 6 months or until treatment is approved by their physician. Once their condition is stabilized, however, patients can receive almost any routine dental treatment.

Valvar Heart Disease

Any dental or periodontal procedure that introduces bacteria into the bloodstream of patients with valvar heart disease can increase their risk of a potentially fatal heart infection called *infective endocarditis*. In general, damaged heart valves are more susceptible to colonization by bacteria. In addition, the stasis of blood, frequently associated with defective heart valves, increases the likelihood that bacteria will be able to successfully attach to fibrin deposits that can form on the heart at sites where blood flow is impaired. To reduce the risk of infective endocarditis, these high-risk patients should take prescribed doses of antibiotics before undergoing any procedures in which gingival bleeding might be induced (e.g., periodontal examination, scaling of the teeth). It is important for dental health care workers to have a basic understanding of the general types of valvar heart disease so that they can more effectively consult with physicians about any pretreatment precautions that should be taken for high-risk patients.

The primary function of heart valves is to allow the unidirectional forward flow of blood through the heart. Diseases of the heart valves can be either acquired or congenital. Acquired diseases are far more common. Approximately half of all acquired heart valve lesions occur as isolated *stenosis*, or narrowing, of the orifice of either the aortic or the mitral valve. Stenosis leads to the failure of a valve to open completely, thereby retarding the forward flow of blood through the heart. Valvar insufficiency is the failure of a heart valve to close completely,

thereby leading to regurgitation, or flow of blood in a reverse direction. Stenosis and insufficiency often affect the same valve.

Many methods are employed by physicians to detect heart disease. One of them is to listen to heart sounds with a stethoscope to detect, among other things, the presence or absence of a heart murmur. Murmurs are simply the sounds that are produced by the turbulent flow of blood through the heart. Valvar disease is only one of many possible causes of a heart murmur. Some murmurs are caused by abnormalities of the heart (organic murmurs); others are termed "innocent" or "functional" murmurs. When patients report that they have a heart murmur, it is usually advisable to consult with their physician to determine whether any precautions are necessary before dental procedures are performed. Patients with organic murmurs may require preoperative coverage with antibiotics; those with innocent or functional murmurs usually do not. The final decision depends on the physician's analysis of the source and nature of the murmur.

Acquired valvar heart disease is often found in patients with a history of rheumatic fever,[14] ischemic heart disease,[15] systemic lupus erythematosus,[16] a variety of connective tissue disorders,[17] and several other systemic diseases.[18]

Rheumatic fever is an acute systemic inflammatory disease that sometimes follows throat infections with group A streptococci. In response to streptococcal antigens associated with the infection, antibodies are produced that cross-react with host tissues, especially those of the heart and kidneys. As a result, antistreptococcal antibodies can react with heart valve tissues and cause inflammation and damage to the valves. This damage may lead to scarring of the heart valves and thereby increase the risk that infective endocarditis will develop as a result of the transient bacteremias associated with many dental procedures. Before performing dental procedures (including oral examinations with periodontal probing or exploring) in a patient with a history of rheumatic fever, the clinician should consult with the patient's physician to determine whether preoperative coverage with antibiotics is necessary. In general, patients with a history of rheumatic fever with valvar dysfunction require antibiotic coverage. Those with functionally normal valves do not.[19]

A relatively common valvar abnormality is

mitral valve prolapse ("floppy" valve syndrome). Approximately 7 percent of the United States population between the ages of 20 and 40 years have this cardiac abnormality.[20] In patients with this condition, the leaflets of the mitral valve partially lose their elasticity and billow, or balloon back, into the left atrium during systole.[20] The underlying causes for this loss of valvar elasticity are unknown. In some cases, valvar damage occurs and causes incomplete closure of the valve, which leads to local regurgitation, or backward flow of blood. In patients with mitral valve prolapse, prophylactic antibiotic coverage for dental procedures is usually needed only if regurgitation or valvular insufficiency has been demonstrated.[21] Of course, the final decision as to whether antibiotic coverage is required is made by the patient's physician.

The American Heart Association has recommended that prophylactic antibiotic coverage be provided for some, but not all, patients with cardiac conditions as shown in Cardiac Conditions Associated with Endocarditis. In patients at high risk for infective endocarditis, the course of antibiotics to be administered depends on a variety of factors (Table 17–2), but for most adults, the standard recommended regimen is 2.0 g amoxicillin 1 hour before the dental procedure.[19]

Cardiac Arrhythmias

Irregular heartbeat can be associated with a variety of systemic conditions, such as high fevers from certain infectious diseases, ischemic heart disease, congestive heart failure, mitral valve prolapse, rheumatic heart disease, myocardial infarction, hypertension, certain allergic reactions (anaphylaxis), and hyperthyroidism. There are many forms of cardiac arrhythmia, some of which can be controlled by medications. Others require the insertion of electronic devices (e.g., pacemakers and defibrillators).

Dental procedures can be safely performed in most patients who are under medical treatment for cardiac arrhythmias. However, patients who are taking antiarrhythmic drugs can experience a variety of side effects that may complicate or worsen their dental and periodontal problems. For example, some antiar-

TABLE 17–2. American Heart Association Recommendations of Prophylactic Antibiotic Coverage for Dental Procedures in Patients with High- and Moderate-Risk for Infective Endocarditis[19]

Situation	Agent	Regimen*
Standard general prophylaxis	Amoxicillin	Adults: 2.0 g; children: 50 mg/kg orally 1 hour before procedure
Unable to take oral medications	Ampicillin	Adults: 2.0 g intramuscularly (IM) or intravenously (IV); children: 50 mg/kg IM or IV within 30 minutes before procedure
Allergic to penicillin	Clindamycin	Adults: 600 mg; children: 20 mg/kg orally 1 hour before procedure
	OR	
	Cephalexin† or cefadroxil†	Adults: 2.0 g; children: 50 mg/kg orally 1 hour before procedure
	OR	
	Azithromycin or clarithromycin	Adults: 500 mg; children: 15 mg/kg orally 1 hour before procedure
Allergic to penicillin and unable to take oral medications	Clindamycin	Adults: 600 mg; children: 20 mg/kg IV within 30 minutes before procedure
	OR	
	Cefazolin†	Adults: 1.0 g; children: 25 mg/kg IM or IV within 30 minutes before procedure

*Total children's dose should not exceed adult dose.

†Cephalosporins should not be used in individuals with immediate-type hypersensitivity reaction (urticaria, angioedema, or anaphylaxis) to penicillins.

Used with permission. From Dajani AS, Taubert KA, Wilson W, Bolger AF, Bayer A, Ferrieri P, Gewitz MH, Shulman ST, Nouri S, Newburger JW, Hutto C, Pallasch TJ, Gage TW, Levison ME, Peter G, Zuccaro G Jr. Prevention of bacterial endocarditis: Recommendations by the American Heart Association. J Am Dent Assoc 1997;128:1142–1151. Copyright 1997, American Dental Association.

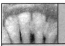

CARDIAC CONDITIONS ASSOCIATED WITH ENDOCARDITIS[19]

Endocarditis Prophylaxis Recommended

High-risk category

- Prosthetic cardiac valves, including bioprosthetic and homograft valves
- Previous bacterial endocarditis
- Complex cyanotic congenital heart disease (e.g., single ventricle states, transposition of the great arteries, tetralogy of Fallot)
- Surgically constructed systemic pulmonary shunts or conduits

Moderate-risk category

- Most other congenital cardiac malformations (other than above and below)
- Acquired valvar dysfunction (e.g., rheumatic heart disease)
- Hypertrophic cardiomyopathy
- Mitral valve prolapse with valvar regurgitation and/or thickened leaflets

Endocarditis Prophylaxis Not Recommended

Negligible-risk category (no greater risk than the general population)

- Isolated secundum atrial septal defect
- Surgical repair of atrial septal defect, ventricular septal defect or patent ductus arteriosus (without residua beyond 6 mo.)
- Previous coronary artery bypass graft surgery
- Mitral valve prolapse without valvar regurgitation
- Physiologic, functional, or innocent heart murmurs
- Previous Kawasaki disease without valvar dysfunction
- Previous rheumatic fever without valvar dysfunction
- Cardiac pacemakers (intravascular and epicardial) and implanted defibrillators

rhythmic drugs, such as disopyramide (Norpace), mexiletine (Mexitil), verapamil (Calan), and diltiazem (Cardizem), may lead to xerostomia (dry mouth), which can facilitate plaque retention and increase the patient's susceptibility to dental caries and periodontal disease. Drugs such as phenytoin (Dilantin), verapamil, and diltiazem may lead to severe gingival enlargement, which makes plaque control difficult (see Figure 17-1). In some patients, mexiletine and quinidine (Cardioquin) may cause neutropenia (i.e., a decrease in circulating neutrophils), which can increase their susceptibility to periodontal and other infections. It is important for dental health care workers to familiarize themselves with the actions and side effects of the medications that their patients are taking to determine whether the drugs might adversely influence or complicate dental and periodontal therapy.

Some cases of cardiac arrhythmia are best treated by surgical insertion of a battery-oper-

ated electronic device (i.e., pacemaker) under the skin of the upper chest wall. Wire leads connect the pacemaker to an electrode that is placed in contact with heart tissue. The pacemaker sends periodic electrical impulses to the heart, thereby regulating its rate of contraction. The American Heart Association guidelines do not recommend that patients with pacemakers be given antibiotics before dental procedures.[19] However, for certain patients, the physician or cardiologist will recommend antibiotic coverage.

In one type of arrhythmia, portions of the heart undergo rapid irregular twitching referred to as *fibrillation*. Devices called defibrillators are designed to send electrical impulses to the heart to shock it into a normal pattern of contraction. Defibrillators can be implanted subcutaneously in the abdomen with electrodes connected to the heart. The devices detect the onset of fibrillation and automatically send small electrical shocks to the heart to correct the situation. As with pacemakers, prophylactic antibiotic coverage is not usually required before dental procedures.[19]

Congestive Heart Failure

Elective dental procedures should not be performed in patients with congestive heart failure unless their condition has been stabilized by medical treatment. In cases of congestive heart failure, the heart is unable to supply the body with sufficient oxygenated blood. As a result, the patient has difficulty breathing after minimal exertion.

Patients whose condition is under good medical control can safely receive routine dental treatment. However, appointments should be short to minimize stress. When these patients are treated, the dental chair should be kept in an erect or partially reclining position. If these patients are placed in a fully reclining position, gravity promotes the return of peripheral blood to the central circulation, thereby placing an extra burden on the heart. For these patients, it is a good idea to have supplemental oxygen on hand in case some difficulty in breathing is encountered.

Patients Who Are Taking Anticoagulants

Many patients with a history of cardiovascular disease take medications called anticoagulants (blood thinners). These reduce the risk of the development of blood clots that can block the circulation to vital organs such as the brain, heart, and lungs. Patients who have prosthetic heart valves or have had a recent heart attack (myocardial infarction) or stroke (blockage of blood flow to the brain) frequently receive anticoagulant therapy. The medications that are usually administered are heparin or warfarin derivatives. Coumadin (warfarin) is the agent that is most often used on an outpatient basis. Subgingival instrumentation associated with routine dental hygiene procedures in anticoagulated patients can result in more gingival bleeding than is ordinarily encountered. However, the bleeding is usually easily controlled by applying pressure with a gauze sponge. When treating these patients, it is important to minimize the soft tissue trauma associated with subgingival instrumentation.

Many patients with a history of cardiovascular disease take small daily doses (80–325 mg/day) of aspirin, which retards the formation of blood clots by inhibiting platelet aggregation. At these doses, aspirin does not significantly alter the bleeding time,[22] and postoperative bleeding from dental hygiene procedures is usually not a problem.

JOINT DISEASES AND DISORDERS

Joint diseases and disorders that are frequently seen in dental patients and that can complicate or modify the approach to dental or periodontal treatment are (1) arthritis and (2) artificial or prosthetic joints.

Arthritis

Arthritis is a general term that means inflammation of a joint. It is a common condition that affects, in one form or another, as many as 85 percent of adults older than 45 years. It is associated with many systemic diseases, including rheumatoid arthritis (rheumatism), osteoarthritis, systemic lupus erythematosus, scleroderma, and gout. The primary dental problem that arthritis causes in some patients is difficulty in performing oral hygiene procedures. This problem is particularly common in patients with rheumatoid arthritis and osteoarthritis involving the hands. Arthritic involvement of the hands can result in the inability to grasp such items as a toothbrush and to manipulate dental floss or other interproximal cleaning devices. This inability may stem from actual loss of joint flexibility or from intense pain associated with inflamed joints of the hands and fingers. Dental hygienists must recognize this potential problem and determine whether special plaque control devices, such as a powered toothbrush, are needed. In addition, as with all patients who have difficulty cleaning their teeth, it is advisable to schedule more frequent professional care.

Patients with severe arthritis often take anti-inflammatory medications to reduce local inflammation and decrease the amount of joint pain. In some cases, relatively high doses of aspirin are prescribed by the patient's physician. Aspirin can retard the formation of blood clots, so some increased bleeding may occur

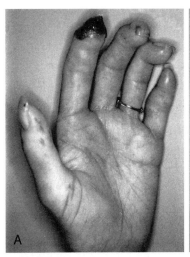
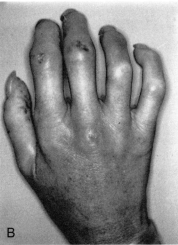

FIGURE 17–2. Hands of a 50-year-old woman with progressive systemic sclerosis exhibiting arthritic enlargement of the finger joints. Sores on the hands and tips of the fingers (Raynaud's disease) are secondary to inadequate circulation from blood vessel involvement. In addition to these changes, loss of skin flexibility made it impossible for the patient to grasp a toothbrush.

during routine scaling and root planing procedures. In most patients, this problem is not significant, and any localized gingival bleeding resulting from subgingival instrumentation can be controlled by pressure with a gauze sponge.

It is important to remember that arthritis can be the result of many systemic diseases and that arthritis is only one of several medical problems that may have dental implications. For example, patients with progressive systemic sclerosis (PSS), or scleroderma, experience multiple dental and periodontal problems that are directly attributable to their systemic disease.[23] PSS is a chronic connective tissue disease of unknown cause in which abnormal amounts of collagen are continuously deposited in a variety of organ systems, including the skin, lungs, and kidneys. Death as a result of PSS often occurs because of kidney or respiratory failure. As the disease progresses, the skin loses much of its elasticity and becomes almost leather-like. Severe arthritis and stiffening of the hands is common (Figure 17-2). It is difficult for these patients to hold or manipulate plaque control devices, and their firm, inflexible skin often prevents them from opening their mouths wide enough to allow the dentist or dental hygienist access to perform routine procedures. As a result, patients with PSS tend to experience high rates of dental caries and periodontal disease. Significant gingival recession is a common feature

(Figure 17-3). An unusual oral finding that is seen in some patients with PSS is the uniform widening of the periodontal ligament space as seen in radiographs (Figure 17-4)[24]. Although PSS is not a common disease, it is a dramatic example of a systemic disease that can present challenges to the dentist and dental hygienist in providing adequate oral health care.

Artificial Joints

In some patients with arthritis, the destruction of joint tissues can result in severe pain and loss of function. In such cases, it is often necessary to replace the affected joint with an artifi-

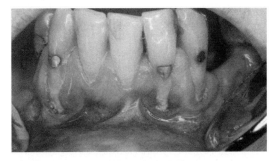

FIGURE 17–3. Marked gingival recession in a patient with progressive systemic sclerosis. Gingival recession is a common feature in patients with long-standing disease. Same patient as shown in Figure 17-2.

cial or prosthetic device. Through modern orthopedic surgery, it is possible to replace joints of the hip, knee, elbow, wrist, and shoulder. Complete replacement of the hip joint is the most common procedure. Because more than 450,000 joint prostheses are placed annually in the United States, patients with these devices are frequently seen in most dental practices.[25]

Infection, in one form or another, occurs in approximately 1 percent of joint prostheses and is a major cause of their failure.[26] The sources of "late" infections of joint prostheses (i.e., infections that occur more than 3 months after joint placement) are not known, but bacteremias originating from acute dental, respiratory tract, dermatologic, or urinary tract infections are prime suspects.[26-30] It appears that the highest risk of late infections of joint prostheses is up to 2 years after joint replacement.[31]

Most patients with total joint replacements, orthopedic pins, and plates do not routinely require antibiotic prophylaxis prior to dental treatment.[25] However, certain patients may be at increased risk of hematogenous joint infection and should be considered as candidates for antibiotic coverage prior to extensive bacteremia-producing dental procedures. Antibiotic prophylaxis regimens for patients at potential increased risk of hematogenous total joint infection, suggested by a panel of experts from the American Dental Association and the American Academy of Orthopaedic Surgeons, are shown next.

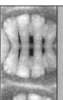

PATIENTS AT POTENTIAL INCREASED RISK OF HEMATOGENOUS TOTAL JOINT INFECTION[25]

Immunocompromised/Immunosuppressed Patients

- Inflammatory arthropathies: rheumatoid arthritis, lupus erythematosus
- Disease-, drug-, or radiation-induced immunosuppression

Other Patients

- Insulin-dependent (Type I) diabetes
- First 2 years following joint placement
- Previous prosthetic joint infections
- Malnourishment
- Hemophilia

Used with permission. Fitzgerald RH Jr, Jacobson JJ, Luck JV Jr, Nelson CL, Nelson JP, Osmon DR, Pallasch TJ, Whall CW Jr, Tipton WW Jr. Advisory statement: Antibiotic prophylaxis for dental patients with total hip joint replacements. J Am Dent Assoc 1997; 128:1004–1008. Copyright 1997, American Dental Association.

ENDOCRINE DISTURBANCES AND ABNORMALITIES

Diabetes Mellitus

It is estimated that more than 10 million people in the United States have diabetes mellitus (DM), but only half of them have been diagnosed.[32] DM is a group of disorders that share the common feature of elevated glucose level in the blood. The underlying problem in DM is an insufficient supply or impaired availability of insulin, a pancreatic hormone that is necessary for the regulation of carbohydrate metabolism. Insulin contains two polypeptide chains and is produced by the β-cells of the islets of Langerhans in the pancreas. There are two main types of DM: type I, or insulin-dependent diabetes mellitus (IDDM), and type II, or non–insulin-dependent diabetes mellitus (NIDDM). There is a genetic predisposition to the development of these two forms of diabetes.

Approximately 10 to 20 percent of all cases of diabetes mellitus are of the IDDM (type I) variety.[33] In this form of the disease, there is a severe deficiency of insulin secondary to the

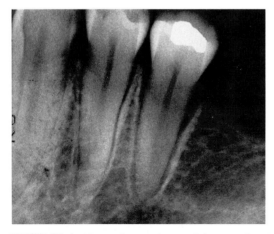

FIGURE 17–4. The uniform widening of the periodontal ligament space in a 28-year-old woman with progressive systemic sclerosis. The tooth was not mobile.

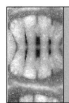

SUGGESTED ANTIBIOTIC PROPHYLAXIS REGIMENS FOR PATIENTS AT AN INCREASED RISK OF HEMATOGENOUS TOTAL JOINT INFECTION[25]

Patients not allergic to penicillin:

- Cephalexin, cephradine, or amoxicillin—2 g orally 1 hour prior to dental procedure

Patients not allergic to penicillin and unable to take oral medications:

- Cefazolin—1 g intramuscularly or intravenously 1 hour prior to procedure OR
- Ampicillin—2 g intramuscularly or intravenously 1 hour prior to procedure

Patients allergic to penicillin:

- Clindamycin—600 mg orally 1 hour prior to dental procedure

Patients allergic to penicillin and unable to take oral medications:

- Clindamycin—600 mg intravenously 1 hour prior to dental procedure

Used with permission. Fitzgerald RH Jr, Jacobson JJ, Luck JV Jr, Nelson CL, Nelson JP, Osmon DR, Pallasch TJ, Whall CW Jr, Tipton WW Jr. Advisory statement: Antibiotic prophylaxis for dental patients with total hip joint replacements. J Am Dent Assoc 1997; 128:1004–1008. Copyright 1997, American Dental Association.

destruction of pancreatic β-cells. Destruction occurs because of autoimmune reactions to β-cells that develop in response to environmental injury from some viruses.[34] In other instances, destruction of β-cells may be caused by tumors, surgery, and toxic reactions to drugs or chemicals.[34] Onset of the disease is usually rapid and occurs around the time of puberty. Medical control of IDDM requires periodic self-injection with one or more prescribed insulin preparations.

Patients with NIDDM (type II) account for 80 to 90 percent of all cases of DM.[33] In the early stages, the pancreatic β-cells are intact and capable of producing insulin. There are, however, two general metabolic defects associated with the development of NIDDM: (1) impaired secretion of insulin and (2) insulin resis-

tance.[35] Although the precise reasons for these abnormalities are unknown, defective cell receptors for insulin are believed to play a role in insulin resistance.[33] The onset of the disease is slow, and it usually affects individuals who are older than 30 years.[33] The incidence of the disease increases with age. Medical control of early forms of NIDDM can frequently be achieved by dietary modifications. If problems persist, oral hypoglycemic agents are used that stimulate insulin release from the pancreas and enhance insulin uptake by the tissues. In many patients with long-standing NIDDM, loss of pancreatic β-cells eventually occurs, and periodic insulin injections are required to achieve medical control of the disease.

Patients with either form of diabetes suffer a wide variety of cardiovascular, kidney, eye, and neurologic problems.[33] In addition, patients with uncontrolled or poorly controlled DM appear to be more susceptible to infections, including periodontal diseases.[36-44] The precise reasons for this increased susceptibility are unknown, but certain antibacterial functions of neutrophils appear to be abnormal.[45-48] Other common oral problems associated with diabetes include asymptomatic parotid gland enlargement[49] and dry mouth secondary to decreased salivary flow.[50]

There is a long-standing clinical impression that control of gingival inflammation through periodontal therapy and good daily oral hygiene reduces insulin requirements in patients with diabetes.[51] In other words, satisfactory metabolic control of diabetes is made easier if periodontal infections are arrested. Scientific evidence supporting this impression is minimal, but preliminary data suggest that it might be correct.[52-54] However, not all studies have found that treatment of periodontitis improves the metabolic control of diabetes.[55]

Patients with IDDM or NIDDM tolerate most routine dental procedures well, and no special precautions are usually necessary. However, because they are at greater risk for periodontal disease, it is advisable to schedule preventive dental care at more frequent intervals. Before dental visits, patients with diabetes should be instructed to continue their medication schedule as prescribed by their physician. For morning appointments, they should eat a normal breakfast to reduce the chances of becoming hypoglycemic during the visit.

Occasionally, before a dental visit, diabetic patients do not eat their normal diet and self-administer too much insulin. This practice can precipitate a dangerous emergency called insulin shock, in which the patient becomes severely hypoglycemic. The condition frequently develops rapidly and with little warning. The initial signs and symptoms of insulin shock include mental confusion, slurred speech, rapid heartbeat, nausea, and cold, clammy skin. If the condition is not promptly treated, the patient's blood pressure may drop precipitously. As a result, the patient may lose consciousness and have seizures. Death can occur if emergency measures are not taken. Fortunately, insulin shock is relatively easy to recognize, and the initial management of the emergency is simple. Because the underlying problem in cases of insulin shock is dangerously low levels of blood sugar (glucose), initial emergency care involves the prompt administration of a sugar-containing beverage, such as orange juice. Any easily administered sugar source will suffice (e.g., candy, honey, soft drinks). In addition, many patients will know what is happening and why they are being asked to consume a sugar-containing substance. Once the patient has consumed the sugar, recovery usually begins within a few minutes. If the patient does not respond, a medical emergency response team should be called to the scene.

Pregnancy

Increased gingival inflammation (gingivitis) is frequently associated with pregnancy.[56-60] The gingivitis can be severe, with the tissues becoming swollen and red (Figure 17–5). Patients often report bleeding gums because the tissues bleed on the slightest provocation. The gingivitis is most severe during the first and second trimesters. It decreases somewhat around the eighth month and after parturition.[57, 58] If left untreated, the severe gingivitis associated with pregnancy may lead to the development of periodontitis, with the loss of alveolar bone and even teeth.[56, 60]

It is not known precisely why gingivitis intensifies during pregnancy, but it has been clearly established that the inflammation is caused by plaque.[57, 58] It has been suggested that vascular alterations associated with the hormonal changes of pregnancy (i.e., elevated se-

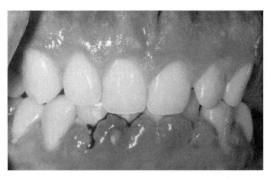

FIGURE 17–5. Severely inflamed and enlarged gingival tissues around the lower anterior teeth of a 28-year-old woman who was in the fifth month of an uncomplicated pregnancy. The patient's chief dental complaint was bleeding gums.

rum levels of estrogen and progesterone) make the gingiva more susceptible to plaque-induced inflammation.[60] For example, increased progesterone levels can result in dilation of the gingival capillaries, increased vascular permeability, and increased flow of gingival crevicular fluid.[60] These changes could facilitate the entry of irritating bacterial products from plaque into the gingival tissue, thereby promoting the inflammatory response. In addition, estrogen and progesterone can promote the growth of certain suspected periodontal pathogens such as *Prevotella intermedia*.[61, 62] In other words, hormonal changes associated with pregnancy can affect the composition of the subgingival flora, thereby promoting the development of gingivitis and, in some cases, even periodontitis.

The importance of these observations is that because pregnant women may be more susceptible to periodontal diseases, they should receive closely supervised oral health care and intensified preventive services during pregnancy. Pregnant patients should be informed that they are at increased risk for periodontal disease. They should then be shown how to perform daily oral hygiene procedures thoroughly. In addition, when a patient becomes pregnant, it is usually advisable to schedule professional teeth cleaning at more frequent intervals than before the pregnancy. For example, a patient who was being followed at 6-month intervals before her pregnancy might be seen at 3-month intervals during the pregnancy. Preventive oral health services should be a routine part of prenatal care.

Fluctuations in Female Sex Hormone Levels

Increased gingival inflammation associated with physiologic fluctuations in the levels of female sex hormones is observed during puberty[63] and the menstrual cycle.[64] Acquired fluctuations occur in some patients who are taking oral contraceptives.[65-70] The mechanisms responsible for this increased susceptibility to plaque-induced gingival inflammation are probably the same as those in pregnancy. In addition, the clinical features of the gingival changes that occur during puberty or the menstrual cycle and in patients who are taking oral contraceptives sometimes resemble those seen in pregnant women. When oral contraceptives were introduced, relatively high doses of hormones were used and the gingival effects were significant.[71, 72] Gingival changes associated with modern low-dose contraceptives are not as severe.[70] The gingival inflammation in patients with physiologic or acquired fluctuations in female sex hormones is caused by plaque. Therefore, the oral hygiene practices in these patients must be carefully monitored to reduce the likelihood of periodontal problems.

Psychological Stress

Many patients are under psychological stress because of pressures associated with daily life. The effect of stress on the general systemic well-being of patients is a complex and often controversial subject. However, there is a long-standing clinical impression that patients who are under emotional tension have an increased susceptibility to certain periodontal infections.[73, 74] The truth of this assumption has not been determined. Subtle endocrine disturbances associated with stress, including the secretion of adrenal hormones, such as corticosteroids and catecholamines (e.g., norepinephrine), affect the periodontal tissues and make them more susceptible to the damaging effects of the products of plaque bacteria.[75, 76] The hypothesis has also been advanced that corticosteroids released in response to stressful situations act as growth factors for certain suspected periodontopathogens.[76] It has been firmly established that in some patients, immunosuppression can occur during periods of stressful life events.[77-82]

The clinical impression that stress is an important factor in the pathogenesis of certain periodontal diseases is strongest in the case of necrotizing ulcerative gingivitis (NUG).[83-85] This periodontal infection, also known as "trench mouth" or Vincent's infection, is characterized by the rapid onset of gingival pain and the presence of interproximal necrosis and ulceration (Figure 17–6). Most patients with NUG exhibit one or more of the following predisposing factors: (1) recent emotional stress, (2) heavy cigarette smoking, (3) lack of sleep, and (4) poor dietary habits.[86]

A growing body of evidence is emerging that certain psychosocial factors, including emotional stress, are associated with an increased risk of developing periodontitis.[87-95] Nevertheless, the evidence supporting a connection is still preliminary and any association remains to be scientifically validated. A significant problem in trying to show a relationship between stress and any disease is that it is difficult to objectively determine the presence and magnitude of stress. In addition, people who are under stress frequently have a number of lifestyle variables that could negatively influence the course of periodontal infections, such as poor oral hygiene and cigarette smoking. Nevertheless, when patients with certain periodontal diseases (especially NUG) state that they have recently been under considerable stress, it is possible that their emotional status may be contributing to their disease. Depending on a variety of circumstances, it may be advisable to inform some patients of the possible relationship between

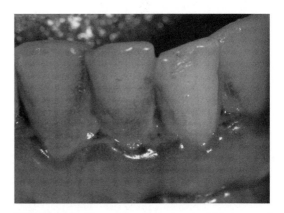

FIGURE 17–6. Necrotizing ulcerative gingivitis in a medically healthy 21-year-old male who was under severe emotional stress. Note the interproximal necrosis and ulceration.

stress and periodontal infections. For some patients, merely knowing that stress might negatively affect the course of their periodontal disease encourages them to modify their lifestyle or to seek psychological counseling. However, even in patients who make no effort to change their stress level, local treatment of the periodontal infection through plaque control instruction and scaling and root planing is the most significant step toward arresting the disease. At best, stress may be a modifying factor, not the cause of the periodontal infection.

INFECTIOUS DISEASES

The presence of certain **infectious diseases** in patients is a source of concern to oral health care providers. Some infections may have one or more of the following effects: (1) modify or increase the patient's susceptibility to oral diseases, (2) create diagnostic challenges because of their oral manifestations, and (3) cause infection-control problems that increase the risk of transmitting the disease to other patients and health care workers.

Viral Hepatitis

The liver is a multifunctional vital organ that plays a major role in metabolizing lipids and carbohydrates, producing serum proteins, and detoxifying drugs (e.g., alcohol). Hepatitis, or inflammation of the liver, can be caused by a variety of factors. The two most common factors are certain viral infections and ingestion of drugs or toxic chemicals. Viral hepatitis is a general term that refers to a group of liver infections caused by at least five distinct deoxyribonucleic acid (DNA)-containing viruses designated as types A, B, C (non-A, non-B), D, and E (non-A, non-B). Hepatitis A virus (HAV) is primarily transmitted in food that has been contaminated with sewage. The liver disease caused by HAV is sometimes called infectious hepatitis. The hepatitis E virus (HEV) is an enteric form of non-A and non-B which is primarily found in the water supply after catastrophic seasonal flooding in third-world countries throughout Central and South America, Asia, India, and Africa. All of the other hepatitis viruses (B, C, and D) are primarily transmitted by the inadvertent introduction of infected blood

or blood products into the circulation. Liver infections caused by this group of viruses are often collectively referred to as serum hepatitis. Infection with the hepatitis B virus (HBV) is the most common cause of this form of hepatitis.

Serum hepatitis (Types B, C, and D) is of particular concern to oral health care workers because they are at increased risk for the disease if they come in contact with saliva or blood from infected patients. In addition, hepatitis viruses survive on inadequately sterilized dental instruments and therefore can be transmitted to other patients. Approximately 90 percent of all patients infected with HBV completely recover from the infection, and 60 to 70 percent never have any symptoms (i.e., subclinical infection). However, the disease is fatal 0.2 to 0.5 percent of the time.[96] Once infected with HBV, approximately 2 to 10 percent of patients remain chronically infected and become carriers of the virus.[96] Chronic infection with the virus often leads to further liver damage, and in many patients, a fatal liver malignancy develops (i.e., hepato-cellular carcinoma). Therefore, all health care providers who are exposed to the blood and saliva of potential carriers of HBV must be immunized against the disease, and appropriate infection control procedures must be used at all times. It is not possible to determine from a self-reported medical history whether a patient is a carrier of HBV because many infected patients may be asymptomatic. Therefore, it is necessary to assume that all patients are potential carriers of HBV. For this reason, rigorous infection control procedures must be followed for every patient.

Acquired Immune Deficiency Syndrome

Acquired immune deficiency syndrome (AIDS) is caused by infection with the human immunodeficiency virus (HIV), which is a ribonucleic acid (RNA)-containing retrovirus. It is transmitted primarily through sexual activities that result in the transfer of certain body fluids, such as blood or semen, from one individual to another. Other major routes of transmission include the sharing of contaminated needles by intravenous drug users (i.e., parenteral route) and transmission from infected mothers to their newborns. In comparison to many other viruses, HIV is relatively difficult to transmit. It is not passed from person to person through food, clothing, sneezing, shaking hands, or casual contact.

HIV infects and eventually kills a wide range of cells, but it has a particular predilection for subpopulations of CD4-positive helper T-cells (i.e., thymus-derived lymphocytes that promote certain immunologic reactions and carry a cell surface receptor designated as CD4). The depletion of CD4-positive helper T-cells can result in severe immunosuppression that makes the patient susceptible to many life-threatening fungal, bacterial, and viral infections. Infection with one or more of these opportunistic pathogens is the major cause of AIDS-related death.[97] Some other common cellular targets of the virus are monocytes, endothelial cells, and certain cells of the central nervous system. HIV infection of the brain can result in severe neurologic dysfunction, including paralysis and dementia.[97]

After exposure to the virus, the usual way to determine whether an individual has become infected with HIV is the finding of antibody against HIV in the bloodstream. If this antibody is detected, the patient is said to have "seroconverted," or become seropositive for the HIV antibody. Seroconversion usually occurs within 3 to 6 months after exposure to HIV. Soon after individuals become infected with HIV, they frequently have influenza-like symptoms, including sore throat, fever, muscle and joint pain, diarrhea, headache, and rashes. These symptoms usually last for only a few weeks. Patients then may remain asymptomatic for many years. The estimated median time from infection to the development of AIDS is 8 to 11 years.[98] Each year, in the group of asymptomatic HIV-positive individuals, approximately 6 to 10 percent have symptoms and go on to develop AIDS.[99] The vast majority of patients with AIDS die of opportunistic fungal, bacterial, or viral infections of the lungs or brain. A smaller, but significant, percentage of patients die of malignancies, such as Kaposi's sarcoma or lymphomas.[97]

Depending on the population examined and the diagnostic criteria used, epidemiologic surveys indicate that 15 to 74 percent of HIV-infected individuals have oral manifestations of the disease.[97] The most frequently reported oral lesion in patients with AIDS is a fungal infection called candidiasis.[100-104] This infection is caused by the overgrowth of *Candida albicans*, a yeast commonly found in the normal oral flora. Approximately half of patients with AIDS have oral candidiasis.[100-104] Lesions can develop on virtually any mucosal surface in the mouth and perioral tissues. The clinical features of candidiasis are variable. However, in one common form (i.e., "thrush," or acute pseudomembranous candidiasis), the palate and buccal mucosa are covered with white patches that can be wiped off, leaving a reddened, ulcerated, and tender mucosal surface (Figure 17–7). Treatment usually involves the administration of topical or systemic antifungal agents. Because the condition is frequently uncomfortable, elective dental and periodontal procedures should be delayed until the infection is controlled. Candidiasis can also occur in HIV-negative patients. This infection usually occurs in patients who take an antibiotic, such as tetracycline, which suppresses the oral flora and allows *Candida* to overgrow as an opportunistic pathogen. It also can occur under ill-fitting artificial dentures and partial dentures in elderly patients who are not infected with HIV.

HIV-infected patients, especially those who already have AIDS or are on the verge of manifesting it, often contract several viral infections of the oral cavity. According to most epidemiologic reports, the most common of these is caused by a herpesvirus called the Epstein-Barr virus (EBV).[100-104] Before the era of AIDS, EBV was primarily associated with two types of ma-

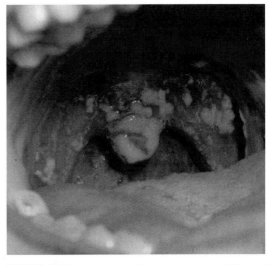

FIGURE 17–7. Acute pseudomembranous candidiasis of the soft palate in a 36-year-old man with acquired immune deficiency syndrome. (Courtesy of Dr. D. Greenspan.)

lignancies: Burkitt's lymphoma (a neoplasm of B-lymphocytes) and certain nasopharyngeal carcinomas. In HIV-positive patients, EBV has been strongly linked to a generally asymptomatic oral lesion called "hairy leukoplakia."[97] This corrugated white lesion usually occurs on the lateral border of the tongue (Figure 17-8). In some patients, hairy leukoplakia is the first sign of HIV infection. Many HIV-positive individuals with the lesion have full-blown AIDS within 36 months.[105] In addition to EBV, other DNA-containing viruses cause oral lesions at a higher rate in HIV-positive compared with HIV-negative patients. These include human papilloma viruses, which cause "oral warts"; herpes simplex, which is the cause of herpetic ulcerations; and herpes zoster, which causes chickenpox and shingles.

Some HIV-positive patients also have severe and aggressive forms of periodontal disease, such as necrotizing ulcerative gingivitis/periodontitis (NUG/NUP) and rapidly progressive periodontitis.[101, 104, 106-108] The amount and rapidity of tissue destruction in patients with NUP can be particularly striking (Figure 17-9). These diseases of bacterial origin are not unique to immunosuppressed HIV-positive individuals, but most studies show that they occur with some regularity in this population of patients.[101-108] The types of bacteria that have been associated with severe cases of periodontitis appear to be similar in both HIV-positive and HIV-negative patients.[109] These bacteria include *Actinobacillus actinomycetemcomitans, Porphyromonas gingivalis, Campylobacter rectus, Prevotella intermedia, Peptostreptococ-*

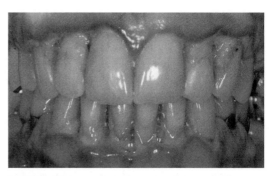

FIGURE 17–9. Necrotizing ulcerative periodontitis in a 42-year-old man with acquired immune deficiency syndrome. The periodontal tissues were sore and tender. Other oral manifestations of human immunodeficiency virus infection in this patient included candidiasis and hairy leukoplakia. (Courtesy of Dr. R. Fujitaki.)

cus micros, Eikenella corrodens, and various *Treponema* species (spirochetes).

The initial treatment of NUG, NUP, and severe periodontitis in all patients, regardless of their HIV serostatus, involves oral hygiene instructions and thorough scaling and root planing. In immunosuppressed patients, it is particularly advisable to recommend the use of an antimicrobial mouth rinse containing chlorhexidine to assist in the reduction of the plaque bacteria.[110] Because patients with NUG or NUP frequently have tender gingival tissues, multiple visits and local anesthesia are usually required.

The risk to a dentist or dental hygienist of contracting AIDS from an HIV-infected patient during dental and periodontal procedures is small.[97] The primary danger to health care providers is through the accidental introduction of the patient's blood into the care provider's bloodstream (i.e., parenteral exposure). In a dental setting in which proper infection control procedures are used, practically the only way that this type of accident can occur is through needle sticks or cuts from sharp instruments. Even if this type of accident occurs, the risk of becoming infected with HIV is still small. For example, in one study of 860 medical personnel who had parenteral exposure to HIV-infected blood, only 4 (0.5 percent) sero-converted.[111]

For infection control purposes, dentists and dental hygienists must assume that all of their patients carry multiple infectious diseases. This assumption must be made because some people are asymptomatic carriers of infectious diseases, such as hepatitis B, HIV, and tuberculosis. When any dental or periodontal procedures are

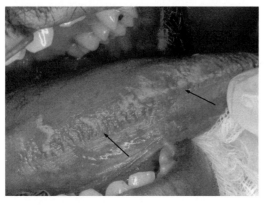

FIGURE 17–8. Hairy leukoplakia on the lateral border of the tongue in a 48-year-old man with acquired immune deficiency syndrome. (Courtesy of Dr. D. Greenspan.)

performed, precautions must be taken to mini-mize the risk of contracting or transmitting in-fectious diseases. These precautions include the routine use of gloves, face masks and shields, safety glasses, and protective clothing or gowns. All instruments and handpieces should be sterilized, and the dental unit and chair should be properly prepared with rigorous in-fection control procedures. If these precautions are followed, the risk of contracting or transmit-ting a serious infectious disease in the dental office is small.

Herpes Simplex Infections

Herpes viruses are a group of DNA-containing viruses. One member of this group, known as herpes simplex virus-1 (HSV-1) primarily binds to nerve terminals within the epithelial tissues of the mouth and skin.[112] A second virus, her-pes simplex-2 (HSV-2) primarily affects the geni-tals. In a few instances, HSV-1 affects the geni-tals and HSV-2 can affect the oral tissues. Previous exposure and infection with HSV-1 is common, with approximately 90 percent of the population demonstrating antibody to the vi-rus.[113] Most of the time, infection with HSV-1 occurs during childhood. Patients usually have some symptoms of the common cold, such as low-grade fever and a runny nose. HSV-1 has an unusual natural cycle. After initial infection of an epithelial surface, the virus migrates along branches of the main sensory nerve of the face (i.e., trigeminal nerve) to the trigeminal gan-glion, where it becomes latent, or inactive. Later in life, the virus can be reactivated by a variety of stimuli, migrate to the original site of infection, and cause mucosal or dermal ulcer-ations.[112] This condition is called secondary, or recurrent, HSV infection. It occurs in approxi-mately 40 percent of the population at some point.[113]

Intraoral herpetic ulcerations may appear on the tongue, buccal mucosa, and gingiva (Fig-ures 17–10 and 17–11). The lesions are of rapid onset and painful. The patient usually has a fever and does not feel well. Herpetic gingival lesions are sometimes confused with gingival changes associated with NUG because both dis-eases have rapid onset and are painful. It is important to clinically distinguish between the two diseases because bacterial infections, such as NUG, can be treated by removal and control

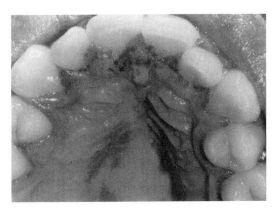

FIGURE 17–10. Herpetic gingival infection in an other-wise healthy 18-year-old male. Note the interproximal le-sions. As is the case with acute necrotizing ulcerative gingi-vitis, the disease is of sudden onset and painful. However, unlike acute necrotizing ulcerative gingivitis, there is no cratering of the interproximal papillae (compare with Fig-ure 17-6).

of dental plaque, whereas viral infections do not respond to such treatment. It is usually easy to eliminate NUG as the problem because patients with this bacterial infection rarely do not have ulcerations of the buccal mucosa or tongue. In addition, the gingival lesions of NUG are usually confined to interproximal gingival tissues that have a cratered, or "punched-out," appearance (see Figure 17-6).

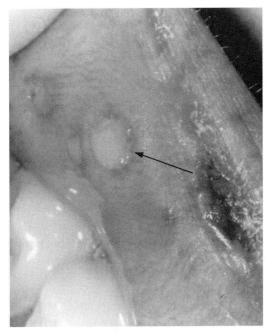

FIGURE 17–11. Herpetic ulcerations of the buccal mu-cosa of the same patient shown in Figure 17-10.

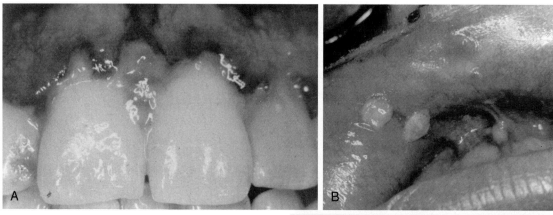

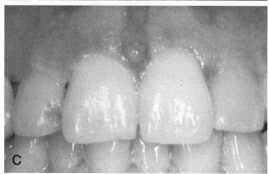

FIGURE 17–12. **A.** Herpetic gingival infection in an otherwise healthy 25-year-old male. **B.** Ulcerations of the adjacent oral mucosa of the upper lip were also present. **C.** The same patient 11 days later. There has been spontaneous resolution of the gingival lesions. No periodontal therapy was administered because herpetic lesions are usually self-limiting and run their course in 10 to 14 days. (Courtesy of Dr. R. E. Robinson.)

In medically healthy individuals, herpetic lesions are usually self-limiting and resolve without therapy within 10 to 14 days (Figure 17–12). Supportive measures, such as adequate bed rest and ingestion of fluids, are usually all that is necessary. However, it is sometimes advisable to have patients see their physician to determine whether there is a serious underlying medical problem that has precipitated the recurrent herpetic infection.

Human Papillomavirus Infections

The cellular targets for these DNA-containing viruses are epithelial cells. Certain subtypes of human papillomavirus (HPV) cause the widely familiar skin (cutaneous) wart. They have a high degree of host and target-cell specificity. There are more than 65 known subtypes of HPV, of which at least 11 affect the oral epithelium.[114] The HPV subtypes that cause cutaneous warts are usually different from those that cause oral lesions, but there are some exceptions. The most common oral lesion associated with HPV is a benign epithelial tumor called an oral squamous cell papilloma. As many as 80 percent of these lesions are caused by HPV subtypes 6 and

11.[114] They can appear on any soft tissue surface in the mouth, but they have a predilection for the soft palate. Gingival lesions occasionally occur (Figures 17–13 and 17–14). They have a characteristic cauliflower-like appearance and a white or pink exterior. They can usually be successfully treated by surgical removal.

Transmission is believed to occur by direct contact with a lesion that is actively shedding virus particles. The risk to a dental health care worker of contracting the virus from an infected patient is virtually nonexistent if appropriate barrier techniques are used, such as

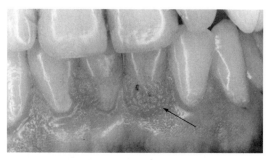

FIGURE 17–13. Multiple gingival papillomas (arrow) in the lower anterior area of a medically healthy 32-year-old male. The lesions had been present for 3 years.

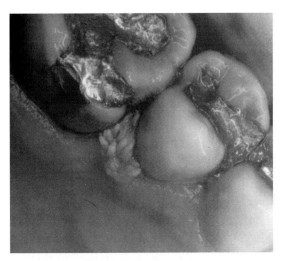

FIGURE 17–14. Solitary gingival papilloma with a hyperkeratotic surface between an upper first molar and a second bicuspid in a medically healthy 15-year-old female. The patient was unaware of the lesion.

wearing gloves, a face mask or shield, and protective eyewear.

Some HPV (primarily subtype 16), in conjunction with other risk factors, such as tobacco and alcohol use, are believed to have an association with a type of **oral cancer** called squamous cell carcinoma.[115, 116] However, most papilloma-like lesions do not lead to oral cancer. As with all soft tissue lesions or abnormalities, their presence should be pointed out to the patient and the dentist should be notified so that the lesions can be appropriately treated.

DERMATOLOGIC DISEASES

Many diseases that involve the skin can also affect the soft tissues of the mouth. This observation is not surprising because the skin and oral mucous membranes share many histologic characteristics. The list of diseases with skin involvement that may have an oral counterpart is long, but a few of the more notable diseases are malignant melanoma, squamous cell carcinoma, Kaposi's sarcoma, candidiasis, HPV infection, psoriasis, and vesiculobullous diseases, such as erythema multiforme, pemphigus vulgaris, pemphigoid, and lichen planus.

The dental hygienist is sometimes the first member of the oral health care team to detect soft tissue lesions of the mouth. If such a lesion is observed, it may be impossible to determine immediately whether the lesion is an infection, an innocent oral manifestation of a skin condition, or a potentially lethal oral cancer. Dental hygienists should be able to distinguish between normal and abnormal hard and soft oral tissues. The dental hygienist is expected to detect oral lesions, not to diagnose them. The importance of detecting abnormalities cannot be overemphasized. For example, prompt detection of a white lesion of the oral mucosa, which is later found to be an early squamous cell carcinoma, can be lifesaving. Detection of oral cancers at an early stage in their growth, when they are small and easy to treat, is the single most important factor in the successful treatment or cure of cancer.

In addition to their role in the detection of abnormalities, dental hygienists frequently treat patients who have painful oral lesions associated with certain dermatologic diseases. Uncomfortable oral lesions can complicate routine approaches to periodontal therapy by preventing the patient from performing adequate oral hygiene procedures or by making subgingival instrumentation more difficult. There are many examples of systemic conditions in which this problem occurs, but lichen planus is probably the most common dermatologic disease that may cause painful oral lesions.

Lichen Planus

Lichen planus is a chronic inflammatory skin and mucosal disease that affects approximately 1 percent of the general population.[117] Although the causes of lichen planus are unknown, cell-mediated autoimmune reactions against basal epithelial cells are involved. Lesions of the oral mucosa appear in approximately 75 percent of patients with lichen planus, and 30 percent have only oral lesions.[117] It affects men and women more or less equally.

The most common type of lichen planus is the reticular form, which is characterized by the presence of lace-like white lesions on the buccal mucosa (Figure 17–15). The tongue and gingiva are also frequently involved.[118] The lesions usually produce no symptoms, but in one prospective study of 181 patients with reticular lichen planus, 55 percent reported some oral discomfort because of the lesions.[118] Two other, less common types of lichen planus are the atrophic and erosive forms. Both types fre-

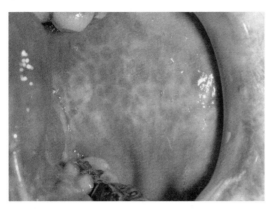

FIGURE 17–15. Reticular form of lichen planus on the left buccal mucosa of a 43-year-old female. The lace-like white lesions (striae of Wickham) are characteristic of lichen planus. (Courtesy of Dr. D. Greenspan.)

quently cause painful gingival lesions. Gingival lesions in the atrophic form usually consist of fiery red tissues that are sore and tender (Figure 17-16). Erosive forms of lichen planus are also uncomfortable because of the development of mucosal ulcerations. Approximately 85 percent of patients with the atrophic or erosive forms of lichen planus report pain and soreness.[118]

The pain associated with oral lichen planus lesions can often be reduced by the topical or systemic administration of steroids.[119] Some success has also been reported in reducing the gingival discomfort by instituting a professionally supervised intensive program of oral hygiene instruction in which an antimicrobial mouth rinse (0.2 percent chlorhexidine) was used.[120] Even though dental plaque is not the

cause of lichen planus, it appears that plaque-induced inflammation superimposed on sites affected by lichen planus can contribute to the patient's discomfort.[120]

ORAL CANCER

Cancer is a general term for a large group of potentially fatal diseases in which there is an uncontrolled growth of genetically altered abnormal cells. Such cells are generally referred to as malignant because, if not eliminated, they can lead to death. Death is usually the result of the destruction or replacement of tissues of one or more vital organs by cancer cells. Certain cancers are sometimes referred to as malignant neoplasms (new growths) or malignant tumors (swellings). Some neoplasms and tumors are composed of morphologically and genetically normal cells. Such growths are usually not life-threatening and are called benign neoplasms or tumors.

There are many causes of cancer. Frequently, more than one factor leads to the formation of cancer cells. Important risk factors that predispose to the development of oral cancer include smoking or other **tobacco use,** excessive alcohol intake, exposure to ionizing radiation, ingestion of environmental toxins and chemicals, and infection with certain viruses. Cancers can affect essentially all organ systems and types of tissues. An oral cancer is any malignant growth that originates from tissues of the mouth. There are two basic ways in which cancer cells can

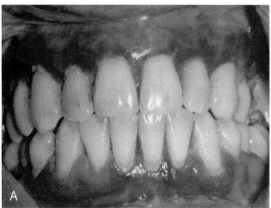

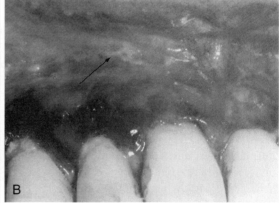

FIGURE 17–16. **A**. Atrophic form of lichen planus in a 52-year-old man affecting gingival tissues around the upper and lower teeth. In this form of lichen planus, the gingival tissues are usually bright red and tender. The tenderness interfered with the patient's ability to perform plaque control procedures. **B**. Lace-like white lesions of the alveolar mucosa, apical to the mucogingival junction of the upper right lateral and central incisors (arrow).

spread: (1) by local invasion of adjacent tissues and (2) by a process called metastasis, in which malignant cells are carried away from the site of origin to another part of the body. Metastasis occurs when malignant cells are shed by the tumor, enter the blood-stream or lymphatic system, and are carried to other tissues.

It has already been mentioned in the discussion of dermatologic diseases that the dental hygienist plays an important role in detecting oral cancers by determining whether the oral tissues are normal. Oral cancers can cause a variety of signs and symptoms. For example, white or red lesions of the oral mucosa could be cancerous. Long-standing ulcerations or un-healed sores of the mouth or lips should be particularly suspected of being cancerous (Figure 17–17). Unexplained lumps or swellings of the mouth or face could be the first sign of certain cancers. In rare instances, even common signs of periodontitis, such as loose teeth and radiographically visible bone loss, can be signs of a malignant lesion (Figure 17–18).

The most frequent type of oral cancer is squamous cell carcinoma, a malignancy that develops from epithelial cells. In the United States, approximately 30,000 new cases of oral squamous cell carcinoma are diagnosed each year. The formation of oral squamous cell carcinoma is strongly linked to pipe and cigarette smoking.[121] Heavy smokers frequently have visible changes in their palatal tissues (Figure 17–

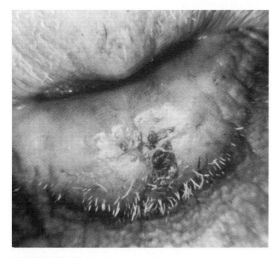

FIGURE 17–17. Squamous cell carcinoma on the lower lip of a 68-year-old man. The patient had noticed the lesion for 18 months and wanted to know, "Why hasn't the sore healed?" Long-standing unhealed sores can be a sign of cancer.

19). The chronic use of smokeless tobacco (snuff) has also been linked to the development of this type of oral cancer.[122] Most snuff users habitually place the tobacco between the gingiva and cheek and leave it there for prolonged periods. In almost all cases, the oral mucosa has dramatic and clinically obvious changes (Figure 17–20).

Treatment of cancer usually involves a combination of approaches, all of which are aimed at eradicating the malignancy. Basic cancer therapy techniques involve (1) surgical excision of the lesion, (2) administration of anticancer drugs (chemotherapy), and (3) irradiation of the malignancy. In addition, with some types of hematologic malignancies (e.g., certain leukemias), the diseased bone marrow is purposely destroyed by lethal doses of radiation and high doses of bone marrow–killing drugs. This treatment is followed by the insertion of healthy bone marrow from an immunologically compatible donor. This form of therapy is referred to as bone marrow transplantation.

Oral health care practitioners are frequently called on to provide important dental and periodontal services before or during cancer treatment. In some forms of cancer therapy, such as bone marrow transplantation and chemotherapy, patients may become susceptible to infections because of the severe immunosuppression induced by the cancer treatment. In such cases, it is important to eliminate all ongoing oral infections before the cancer treatment.

Most chemotherapeutic approaches to the treatment of cancer use toxic drugs that are capable of killing malignant cells. Unfortunately, when such drugs are systemically administered, they also kill normal cells, thereby creating a variety of severe side effects. Some cancer-fighting drugs cause painful oral ulcerations that make routine plaque control procedures impossible (Figures 17–21 and 17–22). Therefore, it is important to bring the patient's oral diseases under control before toxic anti-cancer drugs are administered.

Radiation therapy is sometimes used to treat some cancers of the head and neck. Although during modern radiation therapy, attempts are made to shield nondiseased tissues from the lethal doses of radiation, some damage to the salivary glands can occur. In such cases, the patient may experience a temporary, but sometimes permanent, reduction in salivary flow.

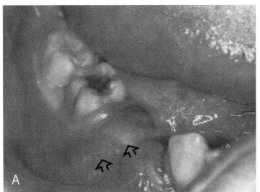

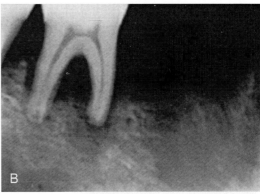

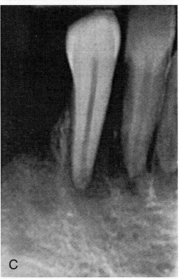

FIGURE 17–18. **A**. Painless swelling in the lower right jaw of a 19-year-old male with Burkitt's lymphoma. Several teeth in the quadrant were loose. **B** and **C**. Radiographs of the lower right quadrant. The diffuse radiolucencies around the teeth and in the surrounding alveolar bone show sites where the malignancy has destroyed bone.

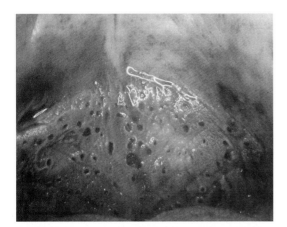

FIGURE 17–19. Soft tissue changes on the soft palate of a 41-year-old man who was a heavy drinker and cigarette smoker (3 packs/day). The lesions were not yet malignant, but extensive use of alcohol and tobacco products increases the risk of oral cancer (squamous cell carcinoma).

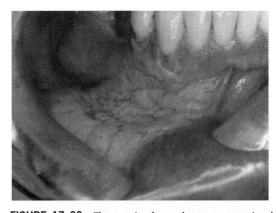

FIGURE 17–20. Changes in the oral mucosa associated with the use of smokeless tobacco (snuff) in a 42-year-old male. For 20 years (approximately 10 times/day), the patient had placed snuff between the buccal mucosa and gingiva. Use of smokeless tobacco can lead to the development of squamous cell carcinomas. Note the gingival recession on the facial surface of the lower cuspid. Such recession is a common finding at sites where the snuff is placed.

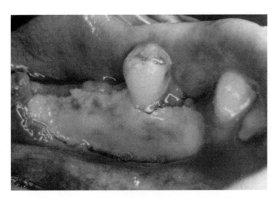

FIGURE 17–21. Severe gingival ulcerations in a 27-year-old female who was treated for cancer (lymphosarcoma) with a systemically administered toxic anticancer drug (methotrexate). Oral ulcerations can be a side effect of some drugs used for cancer treatment (see Figure 17–22).

The resulting xerostomia (dry mouth) can promote plaque retention and increase the patient's risk of severe dental caries. Dental hygienists play an important role in preventing this complication by helping affected patients to improve their oral hygiene practices. Another possible side effect of radiation treatment of head and neck tumors is temporary damage to the oral mucosa. In such cases, mucosal tissues lining the oral cavity receive "radiation burns." These burns make the mouth tender.

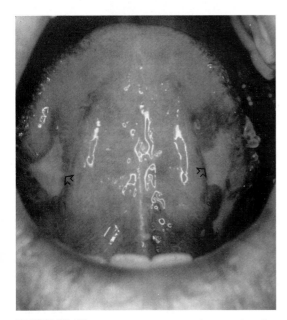

FIGURE 17–22. Severe ulcerations on the ventral surface of the tongue in a 20-year-old male who was being treated for testicular cancer (choriocarcinoma) with a toxic anticancer drug (dactinomycin).

This condition is sometimes called "radiation-induced mucositis." Because routine oral hygiene procedures are difficult in such situations, it is often advisable to see patients at frequent intervals for prophylaxis during the course of the radiation treatment. Frequent treatment may minimize the chances of plaque-induced diseases.

BLOOD DYSCRASIAS

The term "**blood dyscrasias**" refers to a large group of disorders that affect cellular elements of the blood (i.e., red or white blood cells). Patients with blood dyscrasias are occasionally encountered in most dental practices. In some of these disorders, there is impaired function of infection-fighting white blood cells, such as polymorphonuclear neutrophilic leukocytes (PMN or neutrophils). As a result, periodontal diseases and other oral infections can worsen in patients who have either impaired PMN function or a significant decrease in normal numbers of PMNs (i.e., leukopenia). Commonly encountered blood disorders that affect white blood cell populations include aplastic anemia, agranulocytosis, cyclic neutropenia, and several forms of leukemia.

Aplastic Anemia, Agranulocytosis, and Cyclic Neutropenia

The term "aplastic anemia" refers to a dramatic reduction in the ability of bone marrow to produce most of the cellular components of blood. It can be caused by a variety of factors, but environmental exposure to toxic chemicals (e.g., benzene) or certain drugs (e.g., chloramphenicol) has been implicated as the cause in some patients. In some cases, no cause can be identified (i.e., idiopathic aplastic anemia). Patients with this disease experience a rapidly progressive form of periodontitis (Figure 17–23), probably because of the significant decline in the numbers of neutrophils, which are necessary to fight infection.[123, 124]

Agranulocytosis is the depletion of the granulocyte precursors in the bone marrow. Because PMNs are one type of granulocyte, severe periodontal infections are frequently a feature of this disease.[125, 126] In addition, oral ulcerations occur with some regularity. As with aplastic

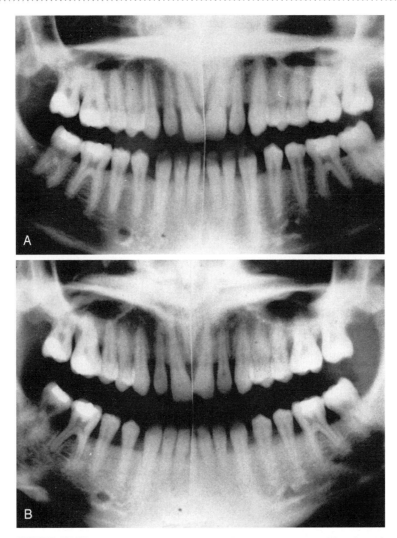

FIGURE 17–23. A. Rapidly progressive periodontitis in a 19-year-old male with aplastic anemia. Radiograph in **B** was taken 12 months after the one shown in **A**. Note the marked loss of alveolar bone that had occurred in this young patient in only 1 year. Patients with aplastic anemia and some other blood dyscrasias are highly susceptible to periodontal infections.

anemia, this disorder can be caused by a reaction to certain medications (e.g., chloramphenicol, methimazole).

Cyclic neutropenia is a blood dyscrasia of unknown etiology in which there are periodic reductions in neutrophil populations in the blood and bone marrow. As might be expected, patients with this disease experience flare-ups of any existing periodontal infections during the period of PMN depletion.[127]

The dental hygienist can play an important role in the management of the oral problems experienced by patients with these blood dyscrasias. Periodontal diseases in affected patients are all caused by dental plaque. Therefore, be-

cause these patients are at increased risk for periodontal infections, they should be given a rigorous program designed to prevent gingivitis and periodontitis. Even in these high-risk patients, periodontal damage will not occur if dental plaque is adequately controlled.

Leukemias

Leukemias are a group of cell malignancies of the bone marrow. Although the precise causes of leukemia are unknown, some forms have been strongly linked to certain viruses or exposure to ionizing radiation.[128] In these diseases, abnormal white blood cells replace and actively suppress the differentiation of normal bone marrow tissue. As the normal marrow is replaced, a significant depletion of infection-fighting normal white blood cells occurs. In addition, there is a drastic reduction in the production of platelets, which are necessary for the normal clotting of blood. As a result, patients with leukemia (particularly those with acute forms) are at increased risk for infections and bleeding problems. Overwhelming infection and uncontrollable bleeding are the two primary causes of death in patients with leukemia.

There are several forms of leukemia. The major types are acute lymphoblastic leukemia, acute myeloblastic leukemia, chronic myeloid leukemia, and chronic lymphocytic leukemia.[128] The acute forms have a sudden onset and lead to death within a few months unless treated. Chronic forms develop slowly and usually have a relatively long clinical course. In general, 80 percent of patients with acute lymphoblastic leukemia are younger than 15 years, whereas most patients with acute myeloblastic leukemia are between the ages of 15 and 39 years. The chronic forms of leukemia usually affect adults. In all types of leukemia, increased susceptibility to infection (including periodontal diseases) can be a problem because of the immunosuppression associated with the disease or its treatment. Of all patients with leukemia, those with the chronic forms are most likely to be seen in a dental practice because they are often being medically managed on an outpatient basis. Because of their increased susceptibility to periodontal infections, patients with leukemia should have their teeth professionally cleaned at frequent intervals and should be given rigorous plaque control programs.

In some forms of leukemia (particularly acute myeloblastic leukemia), gingival enlargement occurs as a result of the accumulation of leukemic cells in the gingival tissues and swelling caused by plaque-induced inflammation.[129] This oral manifestation of leukemia is relatively rare and is usually seen only in very sick, hospitalized patients.

Some patients with acute leukemia are treated with bone marrow transplantation. This treatment involves the intentional destruction of the abnormal marrow before the insertion of normal marrow cells. Because severe immunosuppression occurs with this treatment, it is advisable to eliminate all sources of oral infection before the patient's malignant bone marrow is destroyed.[129] This step is important because uncontrolled oral infections can be fatal in severely immunosuppressed patients. For this reason, dentists and dental hygienists are an important part of the medical teams that perform bone marrow transplantation procedures.

NEUROLOGIC DISORDERS

Patients with a variety of **neurologic disorders** are frequently encountered in dental practices. Many diseases affect the nervous system, and an equally large number of conditions have neurologic manifestations.[130] For the oral health care practitioner, patients with diseases of the nervous and neuromuscular systems present three basic problems: (1) physical inability to perform adequate oral hygiene procedures because of difficulties associated with hand and movement coordination; (2) mental or physical inability to cooperate with the practitioner; and (3) changes in oral tissues that increase the risk for dental diseases.

The first two present an obvious set of patient-management difficulties. Because these patients often have low levels of cooperation and poorly executed personal oral hygiene procedures, they should be seen regularly for professionally administered oral care. Dental hygienists can play a particularly important role in teaching the patient's daily caregiver how to perform oral hygiene procedures for the patient.

Phenytoin-Influenced Gingival Enlargement

Gingival enlargement associated with the administration of anticonvulsant drugs, such as phenytoin, is probably the most common change in the oral tissues of patients with neurologic problems. Phenytoin is often prescribed by the patient's neurologist to control cerebral seizures (epilepsy), which are disorders in which the brain undergoes an involuntary burst of chaotic electrical activity. Most patients with cerebral seizures are of normal intelligence and can lead productive lives if their seizures are controlled. A troublesome side effect of phenytoin is the development of gingival enlargement, which can cause esthetic and plaque control problems for the patient (Figure 17-24). Approximately 50 percent of patients who take phenytoin for a long time experience this side effect, although its reported incidence varies from 0 to 84.5 percent, depending on the criteria used for enlargement.[131] Plaque control problems associated with gingival enlargement can lead to periodontitis and tooth loss. In cases of severe enlargement, surgical excision of the gingival tissue is required.

Although the mechanisms associated with phenytoin-influenced gingival enlargement are not completely understood, evidence shows that plaque-induced inflammation plays an important role in the process.[131, 132] Therefore, patients who have this side effect should be urged to practice meticulous oral hygiene procedures. In addition, frequent visits for professionally administered cleaning of the teeth is advisable. Patients who have undergone periodontal surgery to remove the enlarged gingiva are likely to experience a recurrence unless rigorous daily plaque control procedures are practiced.[132] Recurrence is also likely for patients who experience drug-influenced gingival enlargement as a side effect of certain immunosuppressive drugs (e.g., cyclosporine) that are used to combat rejection of transplanted organs or some medications (e.g., verapamil, nifedipine) that are used to treat cardiovascular problems.

Gingival enlargement also occurs in some patients who are not taking any medications.

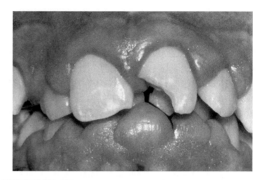

FIGURE 17–25. Hereditary gingival fibromatosis in a medically healthy 15-year-old male. Although the gingival enlargement resembles that associated with the ingestion of phenytoin (see Figure 17-24), the patient was not taking any medications. The chipped front tooth was caused by a sports accident.

Such patients have a rare condition known as hereditary gingival fibromatosis (Figure 17-25).[133, 134] The disease is transmitted as an autosomal dominant trait that is not fully expressed in every case.[135]

TOBACCO USE AND PERIODONTAL DISEASES

In addition to the catastrophic consequences of cigarette smoking, such as emphysema, lung cancer, heart disease, and oral cancer, evidence is mounting that tobacco use is an important risk factor for periodontal diseases.[136-140] The mechanisms by which smoking increases susceptibility to periodontal infections are not completely known, but it is likely that smoking suppresses certain components of the immune system.[141, 142] Impaired neutrophil function induced by products of tobacco smoke appear to be particularly important.[143-145]

Oral health care professionals can play an important role in smoking cessation programs. However, understanding and tact are needed. Patients with periodontitis frequently ask the dentist or dental hygienist, "Does cigarette smoking play a role in my gum disease?" When such questions are asked, it is advisable to inform the patient that periodontal diseases are infections and that smoking appears to reduce the resistance to infections. However, even in smokers, it is possible to treat periodontitis if the plaque bacteria are well controlled. Because smokers are addicted to their habit, it is not wise to tell them that their gum disease will

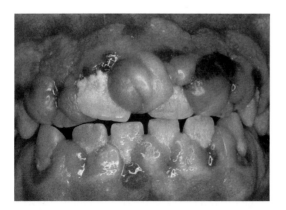

FIGURE 17–24. Phenytoin-influenced gingival enlargement in a 23-year-old male who was taking phenytoin, an anticonvulsant agent, to help control cerebral seizures (epilepsy). He had been taking the drug for 5 years.

worsen unless they stop smoking. This statement only discourages the patient. Addictions are difficult to break, and patients should be given hope that their periodontal disease can be controlled without cessation of smoking. However, controlling periodontal disease is more difficult if the patient continues to smoke.

CONCLUSION

This chapter has outlined some of the ways in which systemic factors affect the diagnosis, pathogenesis, and treatment of dental diseases. Systemic conditions that are most often encountered in a typical dental practice have been emphasized. As a key member of the oral health care team, the dental hygienist will be called on to treat patients with medical problems. The dental hygienist must realize how a patient's systemic condition influences the development and progression of dental or periodontal diseases. The presence of some systemic diseases or conditions may require modification of standard approaches to the treatment of plaque-induced oral diseases. For example, patients with diabetes mellitus should undergo more frequent supportive periodontal therapy than nondiabetics because diabetic patients are at increased risk for periodontitis. Certain systemic conditions require pretreatment precautions to avoid harming the patient. In patients with certain forms of valvar heart disease, prophylactic antibiotic coverage is usually required before dental procedures are performed to reduce the risk of infective endocarditis.

To provide optimal prevention and treatment of dental and periodontal diseases, it is necessary to consider the entire patient. Plaque-induced oral diseases in most patients with medical problems can be safely and effectively treated in a dental setting. Even in very ill patients, treatment of plaque-induced infections is important because a comfortable disease-free mouth can greatly improve the patient's quality of life. Treatment of dental diseases in patients with medical problems is helpful and causes no harm as long as the oral health care provider understands the importance of taking appropriate precautions and modifying therapeutic approaches as dictated by the systemic history and condition of the patient.

STUDY QUESTIONS

MULTIPLE CHOICE

1. When should adult dental patients have their blood pressure measured?

    a. at the initial visit
    b. at every visit
    c. when symptoms are present
    d. when the physician advises

2. What drug is often associated with gingival tissue enlargement?

    a. nifedipine
    b. amoxicillin
    c. hydralazine
    d. nitroglycerin

3. Preoperative coverage with antibiotics is usually recommended for patients with mitral valve prolapse with regurgitation BECAUSE the potential for vegetative infection of the heart valves is increased in these patients.

    a. Both the statement and reason are correct and related.
    b. Both the statement and reason are correct but NOT related.
    c. The statement is correct, but the reason is NOT.
    d. The statement is NOT correct, but the reason is correct.
    e. NEITHER the statement NOR the reason is correct.

4. Why is the presence of valvar heart disease in a patient a source of concern during dental and periodontal procedures?

    a. bacteria can increase the risk of infection
    b. damaged heart valves are susceptible to bacterial infection
    c. stasis of blood increases bacterial attachment sites
    d. all of the above

5. Patients with total hip or knee replacements who are at increased risk for prosthetic joint infection after scaling and root planing include those with:

    a. systemic sclerosis
    b. stage III hypertension
    c. insulin-dependent (Type 1) diabetes
    d. prosthetic joints in service for more than 3 years

6. Increased gingival inflammation in females has been observed in which of the following conditions:

    a. menstruation
    b. pregnancy
    c. puberty
    d. all of the above

7. Which type of hepatitis virus is primarily transmitted through contaminated food?

    a. Hepatitis A virus
    b. Hepatitis B virus
    c. Hepatitis C virus (non-A, non-B)
    d. Hepatitis D virus

8. After becoming infected with the human immunodeficiency virus, patients remain asymptomatic for an estimated median time of:

    a. 2 to 5 years
    b. 8 to 11 years
    c. 12 to 15 years

9. Which statement describes oral lichen planus?

    a. it affects approximately 10 percent of the population
    b. it affects men and women equally
    c. the common form is erosive
    d. the lesions are never painful

10. A dramatic reduction in the ability of bone marrow to produce cellular blood components occurs in which of the following conditions:

    a. agranulocytosis
    b. aplastic anemia
    c. cyclic neutropenia
    d. all of the above

SHORT ANSWER

11. Why has high blood pressure been called the "silent killer"?

    _____

    _____

    _____

12. What are the two most common clinical manifestations of coronary heart disease?

    _____

    _____

    _____

13. What is the main concern for patients receiving anticoagulant therapy during scaling procedures?

_____

_____

_____

14. What is the major cause of failure in most joint prosthesis replacements?

_____

_____

_____

15. What are the signs and symptoms of insulin shock?

_____

_____

_____

16. Describe the difference between infectious hepatitis and serum hepatitis, and explain why these diseases are of concern to dental health care workers.

_____

_____

_____

17. The most frequently reported oral lesion in patients with acquired immune deficiency syndrome is symptomatic of an infection called:

_____

_____

_____

18. What is the most important initial treatment for patients with acute necrotizing ulcerative gingivitis, acute necrotizing ulcerative periodontitis, or rapidly progressive forms of periodontitis?

_____

_____

_____

19. What is the most frequent type of oral cancer diagnosed in the United States?

_____

_____

_____

20. Why does smoking increase a patient's susceptibility to periodontal infection?

_____

_____

_____

REFERENCES

1. Council on Community Health, Hospital, Institutional and Medical Affairs. Hypertension update: a survey of the literature of interest to dentists. J Am Dent Assoc 1989;118:645–646.
2. Council on Dental Health and Health Planning, Bureau of Health Education and Audiovisual Services. Breaking the silence on hypertension: a dental perspective. J Am Dent Assoc 1985;110:781–782.
3. Fay JT, O'Neal R. Dental responsibility for the medically compromised patient. J Oral Med 1984;39:148–156.
4. Joint National Committee on Detection, Evaluation and Treatment of High Blood Pressure. The fifth report of the Joint National Committee on Detection, Evaluation and Treatment of High Blood Pressure (JNC V). Arch Intern Med 1993;153:154–183.
5. Muzyka BC, Glick M. The hypertensive dental patient. J Am Dent Assoc 1997;128:1109–1120.
6. Hasse AL, Heng MK, Garrett NR. Blood pressure and electrocardiographic response to dental treatment with use of local anesthesia. J Am Dent Assoc 1986;113:639–642.
7. Abraham-Inpijn L, Borgmeijer-Hoelen A, Gortzak RAT. Changes in blood pressure, heart rate, and electrocardiogram during dental treatment with use of local anesthesia. J Am Dent Assoc 1988;116:531–536.
8. Farkas JA, Goebel WM. Assessing the risk of angina for dental therapy. Oral Surg Oral Med Oral Pathol 1984;58:253–256.
9. Barclay S, Thomason JM, Idle JR, Seymour RA. The incidence and severity of nifedipine-induced gingival overgrowth. J Clin Periodontol 1992;19:311–314.
10. Nery EB, Edson RG, Lee KK, Pruthi VK, Watson J. Prevalence of nifedipine-induced gingival hyperplasia. J Periodontol 1995;66:572–578.
11. Katz J, Givol N, Chaushu G, Taicher S, Shemer J. Vigabatrin-induced gingival overgrowth. J Clin Periodontol 1997;24:180–182.
12. Jorgensen MG. Prevalence of amlodipine-related gingival hyperplasia. J Periodontol 1997;68:676–678.
13. Bullon P, Machuca G, Martinez-Sahuquillo A, Rojas J, Lacalle JR, Rios JV, Velasco E. Clinical assessment of gingival size among patients treated with diltiazem. Oral Surg Oral Med Oral Pathol 1995;79:300–304.
14. Little JW, Falace DA. Rheumatic fever, rheumatic heart disease, and murmurs. In Dental Management of the Medically Compromised Patient, 3rd ed. St. Louis: CV Mosby, 1988:100–110.
15. Friedlander AH, Yoshikawa TT. Pathogenesis, management, and prevention of infective endocarditis in the elderly dental patient. Oral Surg Oral Med Oral Pathol 1990;69:177–181.
16. Zysset MK, Montgomery MT, Redding SW, Dell'Italia LJ. Systemic lupus erythematosus: a consideration for antimicrobial prophylaxis. Oral Surg Oral Med Oral Pathol 1987;64:30–34.
17. Perloff JK. Evolving concepts of mitral-valve prolapse. N Engl J Med 1982;307:369–370.

18. Devereux RB, Kramer-Fox R, Kligfield P. Mitral valve prolapse: causes, clinical manifestations, and management. Ann Intern Med 1989;111:305–317.

19. Dajani AS, Taubert KA, Wilson W, Bolger AF, Bayer A, Ferrieri P, Gewitz MH, Shulman ST, Nouri S, Newburger JW, Hutto C, Pallasch TJ, Gage TW, Levison ME, Peter G, Zuccaro G Jr. Prevention of bacterial endocarditis: Recommendations by the American Heart Association. J Am Dent Assoc 1997;128:1142–1151.

20. MacMahon SW, Roberts JK, Kramer-Fox R, Zucker DM, Roberts RB. Mitral valve prolapse and infective endocarditis. Am Heart J 1987;113:1291–1298.

21. McKinsey DS, Ratts TE, Bisno AL. Underlying cardiac lesions in adults with infective endocarditis: the changing spectrum. Am J Med 1987;82:681–688.

22. Hancock EW. Coronary artery disease: epidemiology and prevention. In Rubenstein E, Federman DD, eds. Scientific American Medicine. New York: Scientific American, 1991:1 (section VIII):1–10.

23. Nagy G, Kovács J, Zeher M, Czirják L. Analysis of the oral manifestations of systemic sclerosis. Oral Surg Oral Med Oral Pathol 1994;77:141–146.

24. Alexandridis C, White SC. Periodontal ligament changes in patients with progressive systemic sclerosis. Oral Surg Oral Med Oral Pathol 1984;58:113–118.

25. Fitzgerald RH Jr, Jacobson JJ, Luck JV Jr, Nelson CL, Nelson JP, Osmon DR, Pallasch TJ, Whall CW Jr, Tipton WW Jr. Advisory statement: Antibiotic prophylaxis for dental patients with total hip joint replacements. J Am Dent Assoc 1997;128:1004–1008.

26. Little JW. The need for antibiotic coverage for dental treatment of patients with joint replacements. Oral Surg Oral Med Oral Pathol 1983;55:20–23.

27. Ahlberg Å, Carlsson ÅS, Lindberg L. Hematogenous infection in total joint replacement. Clin Orthop Rel Res 1978;137:69–75.

28. Thyne GM, Ferguson JW. Antibiotic prophylaxis during dental treatment in patients with prosthetic joints. J Bone Joint Surg 1991;73B:191–194.

29. Ching DWT, Gould IM, Rennie JAN, Gibson PH. Prevention of late haematogenous infection in major prosthetic joints. J Antimicrob Chemother 1989; 23:676–680.

30. Bartzokas CA, Johnson R, Jane M, Martin MV, Pearce PK, Saw Y. Relation between mouth and haematogenous infection in total joint replacements. Br Med J 1994;309:506–508.

31. Hanssen AD, Osmon DR, Nelson CL. Prevention of deep periprosthetic joint infection. J Bone Joint Surg [Am] 1996;78-A:458–471.

32. National Diabetes Data Group. Diabetes in America: diabetes data compiled 1984. Bethesda, MD: National Institutes of Health, 1985;NIH publication no. 85–1268.

33. Cotran RS, Kumar V, Robbins SL. The pancreas. In Robbins Pathologic Basis of Disease, 4th ed. Philadelphia: WB Saunders, 1989:981–1010.

34. Lernmark Å, Nerup J. Etiology, pathogenesis, and natural history of insulin-dependent (type 1) diabetes. In DeGroot LJ, ed. Endocrinology, vol. 2. Philadelphia: WB Saunders, 1989:1357–1368.

35. Cahill GF. Beta-cell deficiency, insulin resistance, or both? N Engl J Med 1988;318:1268–1270.

36. Bartolucci EG, Parkes RB. Accelerated periodontal breakdown in uncontrolled diabetes. Oral Surg Oral Med Oral Pathol 1981;52:387–390.

37. Löe H. Periodontal disease: the sixth complication of diabetes mellitus. Diabetes Care 1993;16:329–334.

38. Safkan-Seppälä B, Ainamo J. Periodontal conditions in insulin-dependent diabetes mellitus. J Clin Periodontol 1992;19:24–29.

39. Gusberti FA, Syed SA, Bacon G, Grossman N, Loesche WJ. Puberty gingivitis in insulin-dependent diabetic children: I. Cross-sectional observations. J Periodontol 1983;54:714–720.

40. Hugoson A, Thorstensson H, Falk H, Kuylenstierna J. Periodontal conditions in insulin-dependent diabetics. J Clin Periodontol 1989;16:215–223.

41. Cianciola LJ, Park BH, Bruck E, Mosovich L, Genco RJ. Prevalence of periodontal disease in insulin-dependent diabetes mellitus (juvenile diabetes). J Am Dent Assoc 1982;104:653–660.

42. Shlossman M, Knowler WC, Pettit DJ, Genco RJ. Type 2 diabetes mellitus and periodontal disease. J Am Dent Assoc 1990;121:532–536.

43. Emrich LJ, Shlossman M, Genco RJ. Periodontal disease in non-insulin-dependent (type II) diabetes mellitus. J Periodontol 1991;62:123–130.

44. Nelson RG, Shlossman M, Budding LM, Pettit DJ, Saad MF, Genco RJ, Knowler WC. Periodontal disease and NIDDM in Pima Indians. Diabetes Care 1990;13:836–840.

45. Kjersem H, Hilsted J, Madsbad S, Wandall JH, Johansen KS, Borregaard N. Polymorphonuclear leucocyte dysfunction during short term metabolic changes from normo- to hyperglycemia in type 1 (insulin dependent) diabetic patients. Infection 1988;16:215–221.

46. Wilson RM, Reeves WG. Neutrophil phagocytosis and killing in insulin-dependent diabetes. Clin Exp Immunol 1986;63:478–484.

47. Marhoffer W, Stein M, Maeser E, Federlin K. Impairment of polymorphonuclear leukocyte function and metabolic control of diabetes. Diabetes Care 1992; 15:256–260.

48. McMullen JA, Van Dyke TE, Horosweicz HU, Genco RJ. Neutrophil chemotaxis in individuals with advanced periodontal disease and a genetic predisposition to diabetes mellitus. J Periodontol 1981;52:167–173.

49. Russotto SB. Asymptomatic parotid gland enlargement in diabetes mellitus. Oral Surg Oral Med Oral Pathol 1981;52:594–598.

50. Conner S, Iranpour B, Mills J. Alteration in parotid salivary flow in diabetes mellitus. Oral Surg Oral Med Oral Pathol 1970;30:55–59.

51. Williams RC, Mahan CJ. Periodontal disease and diabetes in young adults. JAMA 1960;172:776–778.

52. Miller LS, Manwell MA, Newbold D, Reding ME, Rasheed A, Blodgett J, Kornman KS. The relationship between reduction in periodontal inflammation and diabetes control: a report of 9 cases. J Periodontol 1992;63:843–848.

53. Taylor GW, Burt BA, Becker MP, Genco RJ, Shlossman M, Knowler WC, Pettitt DJ. Severe periodontitis and risk for poor glycemic control in patients with non-insulin-dependent diabetes mellitus. J Periodontol 1996;67:1085–1093.

54. Grossi SG, Skrepcinski FB, DeCaro T, Robertson DC, Ho AW, Dunford RG, Genco RJ. Treatment of periodontal disease in diabetics reduces glycated hemoglobin. J Periodontol 1997;68:713–719.

55. Aldridge JP, Lester V, Watts TLP, Collins A, Viberti G, Wilson RF. Single-blind studies of the effects of improved periodontal health on metabolic control in type 1 diabetes mellitus. J Clin Periodontol 1995; 22:271–275.

56. Maier AW, Orban B. Gingivitis and pregnancy. Oral Surg Oral Med Oral Pathol 1949;2:334–373.

57. Löe H, Silness J. Periodontal disease in pregnancy: I.

Prevalence and severity. Acta Odontol Scand 1963;21:533-551.

58. Silness J, Löe H. Periodontal disease in pregnancy: II. Correlation between oral hygiene and periodontal condition. Acta Odontol Scand 1964;22:121-135.

59. Löe H. Periodontal changes in pregnancy. J Periodontol 1965;36:209-217.

60. Sooriyamoorthy M, Gower DB. Hormonal influences on gingival tissue: relationship to periodontal disease. J Clin Periodontol 1989;16:201-208.

61. Kornman KS, Loesche WJ. The subgingival microbial flora during pregnancy. J Periodontal Res 1980; 15:111-122.

62. Korman KS, Loesche WJ. Direct interaction between estradiol and progesterone with *Bacteroides asaccharolyticus* and *Bacteroides melaninogenicus*. Infect Immun 1982;35:256-263.

63. Sutcliffe P. A longitudinal study of gingivitis and puberty. J Periodontal Res 1972;7:52-58.

64. Holm-Pedersen P, Löe H. Flow of gingival exudate as related to menstruation and pregnancy. J Periodontal Res 1967;2:13-20.

65. Lindhe J, Björn A-L. Influence of hormonal contraceptives on the gingiva of women. J Periodontal Res 1967;2:1-6.

66. El-Ashiry GM, El-Kafrawy AH, Nasr MF, Younis N. Comparative study of the influence of pregnancy and oral contraceptives on the gingivae. Oral Surg Oral Med Oral Pathol 1970;30:472-475.

67. Knight GM, Wade AB. The effects of hormonal contraceptives on the human periodontium. J Periodontal Res 1974;9:18-22.

68. Kalkwarf KL. Effect of oral contraceptive therapy on gingival inflammation in humans. J Periodontol 1978;49:560-563.

69. Pankhurst CL, Waite IM, Hicks KA, Allen Y, Harkness RD. The influence of oral contraceptive therapy on the periodontium: duration of drug therapy. J Periodontol 1981;52:617-620.

70. Perry DA. Oral contraceptives and periodontal health. J West Soc Periodontol 1981;29:72-80.

71. Lynn BD. "The pill" as an etiologic agent in hypertrophic gingivitis. Oral Surg Oral Med Oral Pathol 1967;24:333-334.

72. Kaufman AY. An oral contraceptive as an etiologic factor in producing hyperplastic gingivitis and a neoplasm of the pregnancy tumor type. Oral Surg Oral Med Oral Pathol 1969;28:666-670.

73. Burstone MS. The psychosomatic aspects of dental problems. J Am Dent Assoc 1946;33:862-871.

74. Moulton R, Ewen S, Thieman W. Emotional factors in periodontal disease. Oral Surg Oral Med Oral Pathol 1952;5:833-860.

75. Kardachi BJR, Clarke NG. Aetiology of acute necrotizing ulcerative gingivitis: a hypothetical explanation. J Periodontol 1974;45:830-832.

76. Loesche WJ, Syed SA, Laughon BE, Stoll J. The bacteriology of acute necrotizing ulcerative gingivitis. J Periodontol 1982;53:223-230.

77. Ader R, Cohen N, Felten D. Psychoneuroimmunology: conditioning and stress. Lancet 1995;345:99-103.

78. Kiecolt-Glaser JK, Dura JR, Speicher CE, Trask OJ, Glaser R. Spousal caregivers of dementia victims: Longitudinal changes in immunity and health. Psychosom Med 1991;53:345-362.

79. Herbert TB, Cohen S. Stress and immunity in humans: A meta-analytic review. Psychosom Med 1993;55:364-379.

80. Kort WJ. The effect of chronic stress on the immune response. Adv Neuroimmunol 1994;4:1-11.

81. Sheridan JF, Dobbs C, Brown D, Zwilling B. Psychoneuroimmunology: Stress effects on pathogenesis and immunity during infection. Clin Microbiol Rev 1994;7:200-212.

82. Stone AA, Bovbjerg DH. Stress and humoral immunity: a review of the human studies. Adv Neuroimmunol 1994;4:49-56.

83. Shannon IL, Kilgore WG, O'Leary TJ. Stress as a predisposing factor in necrotizing ulcerative gingivitis. J Periodontol Periodontics 1969;40:240-242.

84. Formicola AJ, Witte ET, Curran PM. A study of personality traits and acute necrotizing ulcerative gingivitis. J Periodontol 1970;41:36-38.

85. Shields WD. Acute necrotizing ulcerative gingivitis: a study of some of the contributing factors and their validity in an Army population. J Periodontol 1977;48:346-349.

86. Armitage GC. Biologic Basis of Periodontal Maintenance Therapy. Berkeley: Praxis, 1980:146-154.

87. Marcenes WS, Croucher R, Sheiham A, Marmot MG. The relationship between self-reported oral symptoms and life-events. Psychol Health 1993;8:123-134.

88. Marcenes W, Sheiham A. The relationship between marital quality and oral health status. Psychol Health 1996;11:357-369.

89. Monteiro da Silva AM, Oakley DA, Newman HN, Nohl FS, Lloyd HM. Psychosocial factors and adult onset rapidly progressive periodontitis. J Clin Periodontol 1996;23:789-794.

90. Monteiro da Silva AM, Newman HN, Oakley DA, O'Leary R. Psychosocial factors, dental plaque levels and smoking in periodontitis patients. J Clin Periodontol 1998;25:517-523.

91. Moss ME, Beck JD, Kaplan BH, Offenbacher S, Weintraub JA, Koch GG, Genco RJ, Machtei EE, Tedesco LA. Exploratory case-control analysis of psychosocial factors and adult periodontitis. J Periodontol 1996;67:1060-1069.

92. Linden GJ, Mullally BH, Freeman R. Stress and the progression of periodontal disease. J Clin Periodontol 1996;23:675-680.

93. Croucher R, Marcenes WS, Torres MCMB, Hughes WS, Sheiham A. The relationship between life-events and periodontitis. A case-control study. J Clin Periodontol 1997;24:39-43.

94. Deinzer R, Rüttermann S, Möbes O, Herforth A. Increase in gingival inflammation under academic stress. J Clin Periodontol 1998;25:431-433.

95. Axtelius B, Söderfeldt B, Nilsson A, Edwardsson S, Attström R. Therapy-resistant periodontitis. Psychosocial characteristics. J Clin Periodontol 1998;25:482-491.

96. Hollinger FB. Hepatitis B virus. In Fields BN, Knipe DM, eds. Fields Virology, 2nd ed. New York: Raven Press, 1990:2171-2236.

97. Greenspan D, Schiødt M, Greenspan JS, Pindborg JJ. Aids and the Mouth. Copenhagen: Munksgaard, 1990:15-198.

98. Ward JW, Drotman DP. Epidemiology of HIV and AIDS. In Wormser GP, ed. AIDS and Other Manifestations of HIV Infection, 2nd ed. New York: Raven Press, 1992:1-15.

99. Tindall B, Cooper DA, Donovan B, Penny R. Primary human immunodeficiency virus infection: clinical and serologic aspects. In Sande MA, Volberding PA, eds. The Medical Management of AIDS. Philadelphia: WB Saunders, 1988:75-89.

100. Silverman S, Migliorati CA, Lozada-Nur F, Greenspan D, Conant MA. Oral findings in people with or at risk for AIDS: a study of 375 homosexual males. J Am Dent Assoc 1986;112:187-192.

101. Reichart PA, Gelderblom HR, Becker J, Kuntz A. AIDS and the oral cavity. The HIV-infection: virology, etiology, origin, immunology, precautions and clinical observations in 110 patients. Int J Oral Maxillofac Surg 1987;16:129-153.

102. Barone R, Ficarra G, Gaglioti D, Orsi A, Mazzotta F. Prevalence of oral lesions among HIV-infected intravenous drug abusers and other risk groups. Oral Surg Oral Med Oral Pathol 1990;69:169-173.

103. Ramirez V, Gonzalez A, de la Rosa E, Gonzalez M, Rivera I, Hernandez C, Ponce de Leon S. Oral lesions in Mexican HIV-infected patients. J Oral Pathol Med 1990;19:482-485.

104. Laskaris G, Hadjivassiliou M, Stratigos J. Oral signs and symptoms in 160 Greek HIV-infected patients. J Oral Pathol Med 1992;21:120-123.

105. Greenspan D, Greenspan JS, Hearst NG, Pan L-Z, Conant MA, Abram DI, Hollander H, Levy JA. Relation of oral hairy leukoplakia to infection with the human immunodeficiency virus and the risk of developing AIDS. J Infect Dis 1987;155:475-481.

106. Shulten EAJM, ten Kate RW, van der Waal I. Oral manifestations of HIV infection in 75 Dutch patients. J Oral Pathol Med 1989;18:42-46.

107. Porter SR, Luker J, Scully C, Glover S, Griffiths MJ. Orofacial manifestations of a group of British patients infected with HIV-1. J Oral Pathol Med 1989;18:47-48.

108. Winkler JR, Robertson PB. Periodontal disease associated with HIV infection. Oral Surg Oral Med Oral Pathol 1992;73:145-150.

109. Moore LVH, Moore WEC, Riley C, Brooks CN, Burmeister JA, Smibert RM. Periodontal microflora of HIV positive subjects with gingivitis or adult periodontitis. J Periodontol 1993;64:48-56.

110. Winkler JR, Murray PA, Grassi M, Hammerle C. Diagnosis and management of HIV-associated periodontal lesions. J Am Dent Assoc 1989;119(suppl):25S-34S.

111. Marcus R, CDC Cooperative Needlestick Surveillance Group. Surveillance of health care workers exposed to blood from patients infected with human immunodeficiency virus. N Engl J Med 1988;319:1118-1123.

112. Scully C. Orofacial herpes simplex virus infections: current concepts in the epidemiology, pathogenesis, and treatment, and disorders in which the virus may be implicated. Oral Surg Oral Med Oral Pathol 1989;68:701-710.

113. Regezi JA, Sciubba J. Vesiculo-bullous diseases. In Oral Pathology: Clinical-Pathological Correlations, 2nd ed. Philadelphia: WB Saunders, 1993:1-9.

114. Chang F, Syrjanen S, Kellokoski J, Syrjänen K. Human papillomavirus (HPV) infections and their associations with oral disease. J Oral Pathol Med 1991;20:305-317.

115. Woods KV, Shillitoe EJ, Spitz MR, Schantz AP, Adler-Storthz K. Analysis of human papillomavirus DNA in oral squamous cell carcinomas. J Oral Pathol Med 1993;22:101-108.

116. Ostwald C, Müller P, Barten M, Rutsatz K, Sonnenburg M, Milde-Langosch K, Löning T. Human papillomavirus DNA in oral squamous cell carcinomas and normal mucosa. J Oral Pathol Med 1994;23:220-225.

117. Scully C, El-Kom M. Lichen planus: review and update on pathogenesis. J Oral Pathol 1985;14:431-458.

118. Silverman S, Gorsky M, Lozada-Nur F. A prospective follow-up study of 570 patients with oral lichen planus: persistence, remission, and malignant association. Oral Surg Oral Med Oral Pathol 1985;60:30-34.

119. Vincent SD, Fotos PG, Baker KA, Williams TP. Oral lichen planus: the clinical, historical, and therapeutic features of 100 cases. Oral Surg Oral Med Oral Pathol 1990;70:165-171.

120. Holmstrup P, Schiøtz A, Westergaard J. Effect of dental plaque control on gingival lichen planus. Oral Surg Oral Med Oral Pathol 1990;69:585-590.

121. Silverman S, Gorsky M. Epidemiologic and demographic update in oral cancer: California and national data—1973 to 1985. J Am Dent Assoc 1990;120:495-499.

122. Winn DM, Blot WJ, Shy CM, Pickle LW, Toledo A, Fraumeni JF. Snuff dipping and oral cancer among women in the southern United States. N Engl J Med 1981;304:745-749.

123. Opinya GN, Kaimenyi JT, Meme JS. Oral findings in Franconi's anemia: a case report. J Periodontol 1988;59:461-463.

124. Stamps JT. The role of oral hygiene in a patient with idiopathic aplastic anemia. J Am Dent Assoc 1974;88:1025-1027.

125. Awbrey JJ, Hibbard ED. Congenital agranulocytosis. Oral Surg Oral Med Oral Pathol 1973;35:526-530.

126. Hou G-L, Tsai C-C. Oral manifestations of agranulocytosis associated with methimazole therapy. J Periodontol 1988;59:244-248.

127. Smith JF. Cyclic neutropenia. Oral Surg Oral Med Oral Pathol 1964;18:312-320.

128. Scheinberg DA, Golde DW. The leukemias. In Isselbacher KJ, Braunwald E, Wilson JD, Martin JB, Fauci AS, Kasper DL, eds. Harrison's Principles of Internal Medicine, 13th ed. New York: McGraw-Hill, 1994: 1764-1771.

129. Barrett AP. Gingival lesions in leukemia: a classification. J Periodontol 1984;55:585-588.

130. Haerer AF. DeJong's The Neurologic Examination, 5th ed. Philadelphia: JB Lippincott, 1992:1-844.

131. Angelopoulos AP, Goaz PW. Incidence of diphenylhydantoin gingival hyperplasia. Oral Surg Oral Med Oral Pathol 1972;34:898-906.

132. Donnenfeld OW, Stanley HR, Bagdonoff L. A nine month clinical and histological study of patients on diphenylhydantoin following gingivectomy. J Periodontol 1974;45:547-557.

133. Becker W, Collings CK, Zimmerman ER, De La Rosa M, Singdahlsen D. Hereditary gingival fibromatosis. Oral Surg Oral Med Oral Pathol 1967;24:313-318.

134. Kilpinen E, Raeste A-M, Collan Y. Hereditary gingival hyperplasia and physical maturation. Scand J Dent Res 1978;86:118-123.

135. Jorgenson RJ, Cocker ME. Variation in the inheritance and expression of gingival fibromatosis. J Periodontol 1974;45:472-477.

136. Haber J, Wattles J, Crowley M, Mandell R, Joshipura K, Kent RL. Evidence for cigarette smoking as a major risk factor for periodontitis. J Periodontol 1993;64:16-23.

137. Ahlquist M, Bengtsson C, Hollender L, Lapidus L, Österberg T. Smoking habits and tooth loss in Swedish women. Community Dent Oral Epidemiol 1989; 17:144-147.

138. Österberg T, Mellström D. Tobacco smoking: a major risk factor for loss of teeth in three 70-year-old cohorts. Community Dent Oral Epidemiol 1986;14:367-370.

139. Grossi SG, Zambon JJ, Ho AW, Koch G, Dunford RG, Machtei EE, Norderyd OM, Genco RJ. Assessment of risk for periodontal disease: I. Risk indicators for attachment loss. J Periodontol 1994;65:260-267.

140. Bergström J, Preber H. Tobacco use as a risk factor. J Periodontol 1994;65:545-550.

141. Bennet KR, Read PC. Salivary immunoglobulin A levels in normal subjects, tobacco smokers, and patients with minor aphthous ulcerations. Oral Surg Oral Med Oral Pathol 1982;53:461-465.

142. Costabel U, Bross KJ, Reuter C, Rühle K-H, Matthys H. Alterations in immunoregulatory T-cell subsets in cigarette smokers: a phenotypic analysis of bronchoalveolar and blood lymphocytes. Chest 1986; 90:39-44.

143. Kenney EB, Kraal JH, Saxe SR, Jones J. The effect of cigarette smoke on human oral polymorphonuclear leukocytes. J Periodontal Res 1977;12:227-234.

144. Lannan S, McLean A, Drost E, Gillooly M, Donaldson K, Lamb D, MacNee W. Changes in neutrophil morphology and morphometry following exposure to cigarette smoke. Int J Exp Pathol 1992;73:183-191.

145. Selby C, Drost E, Brown D, Howie S, MacNee W. Inhibition of neutrophil adherence and movement by acute cigarette smoke exposure. Exp Lung Res 1992;18:813-827.

Appendix I: Answers to Study Questions

CHAPTER 1

1. a	6. d
2. a	7. a
3. a	8. c
4. b	9. d
5. c	10. e

11. Provides historical perspective and encourages learners to direct, modify, and expand their professional actions.
12. Recognition that dental diseases were caused by factors outside the teeth. Slowly until the twentieth century.
13. Historical perspective permits the learner to evaluate new findings and knowledge with an understanding of what has been known and tried in the past.
14. Home tooth cleaning devices, dentifrices, and mouth rinses have been recommended since ancient times. From chew sticks to electric toothbrushes, toothpicks to chlorhexidine rinse, people have always been concerned about oral cleanliness.

CHAPTER 2

1. c	7. c
2. b	8. b
3. a	9. a
4. a	10. c
5. c	11. a
6. d	

12. The sulcus depth is a histologic term. It may differ from probe depth because of a number of variables, such as insertion pressure and tissue penetration.
13. Tooth anchorage, tissue development and maintenance, metabolic transport, and sensory functions.
14. Coral pink, with or without melanin pigmentation, knife-edged, with stippling and a firm consistency.
15. Contains PMNs, enzymes, and other elements that are presumed to protect against the extension of plaque into the sulcus.
16. Contains elements that damage and inactivate bacteria, and enzymes to inhibit tissue destruction.

CHAPTER 3

1. c	6. a
2. d	7. c
3. a	8. b
4. c	9. c
5. a	10. a

11. To provide a picture of the prevalence and severity of dental disease.
12. Gingivitis characterized by bleeding does not always progress to periodontal disease.
13. Place metal instruments on both sides of the tooth and move it back and forth.
14. Improved oral hygiene, greater education levels, more dental care, less smoking, increased use of fluorides and systemic antibiotics.
15. The role of the dental hygienist will increase based on epidemiologic data.

CHAPTER 4

1. d	6. a
2. e	7. b
3. a	8. b
4. b	9. c
5. d	10. e

11. Increase in numbers of (a) rods and spirochetes, (b) Gram-negative organisms, (c) obligate anaerobes, (d) bacteria utilizing proteins as energy source.
12. Corncob formation–filamentous bacteria surrounded by cocci; or test-tube brush formation–filamentous bacteria surrounded by Gram-negative rods; or one organism acting as a bridge between two others that do not interact.
13. (a) Gram-negative anaerobic rods, particularly *Porphyromonas gingivalis*.
    (b) The Gram-negative anaerobic *Actinobacillus actinomycetemcomitans*.
    (c) Intermediate-sized spirochetes and the Gram-negative anaerobic rod *Prevotella intermedia*.
14. Endotoxin or lipopolysaccharide, a component of the cell wall, which is released when the integrity of the cell wall is disrupted.

15. The enzyme glucosyltransferase cleaves sucrose and transfers the glucose moiety to the growing polymer.

CHAPTER 5

1. c	6. a
2. a	7. b
3. a	8. c
4. a	9. a
5. d	10. d

11. It was associated with the inflammation process, and its removal resulted in gingival improvement.
12. Calcium and phosphate.
13. The importance of calculus removal to long-term gingival health.
14. The pyrophosphate in the toothpaste inhibits the growth of hydroxyapatite crystal in supragingival calculus.
15. Faulty restorations, poorly contoured crowns, the presence of orthodontic appliances or partial dentures, and smoking.

CHAPTER 6

1. d	6. b
2. b	7. c
3. b	8. d
4. a	9. b
5. a	10. c

11. Chronic plaque-associated gingivitis, gingival hypertrophy, medication-induced gingival hyperplasia, steroid hormone-influenced gingivitis, and other gingival diseases.
12. No specific type of organism has been identified as the etiologic agent.
13. Gingival inflammation, dark red appearance, swelling, and bleeding on probing.
14. Good plaque control performed daily by the patient.

CHAPTER 7

1. b	6. c
2. c	7. d
3. b	8. a
4. c	9. c
5. d	10. d

11. Refractory periodontitis continues to progress despite appropriate periodontal therapy. Recurrent periodontitis occurs after periodontitis has been treated, but the etiology (plaque or calculus) returns.
12. Specific microorganisms, early age of onset, rapid rate of tissue reduction, possible defects in the immune system.
13. *Actinobacillus actinomycetemcomitans.*
14. Tetracyclines concentrate in the gingival fluid and many pathogenic organisms are susceptible to their antibiotic effect.

15. The dental hygienist may be the first to recognize periodontitis, suggest treatment, perform treatment, and suggest referral to a specialist when the disease is unusual, advanced, or may be related to systemic disease.

CHAPTER 8

1. d	6. a
2. c	7. c
3. d	8. a
4. c	9. d
5. c	10. c

11. Recognize, record, and refer.
12. Orthofunction or physiologic occlusion.
13. Adaptive capability of the oral system.
14. Size and shape of the roots, quantity and quality of the bone, microbiology of the plaque, and oral habits.
15. Traumatic.
16. No.
17. 5 to 60 percent.
18. Tooth wear, tooth fracture, restoration fracture, myalgia, damage to the periodontium, hypertrophy of muscles, and headache.
19. Muscle palpation, mandibular movement, joint function, joint sounds, intercuspal position, excursive movement, tooth mobility and wear, radiographic evaluation.
20. Muscle and fascial disorders.

CHAPTER 9

1. a	6. a
2. b	7. c
3. b	8. b
4. d	9. c
5. d	10. b

11. By evaluating the systemic conditions that can affect dental treatment.
12. Add up the number of surfaces with plaque and compute the percentage of this figure against the total number of tooth surfaces measured.
13. Bone loss, occlusal forces, trauma, endodontic therapy, hormonal changes, or disease.
14. Evaluation for caries, restoration status, contact relationship, anomalies of tooth form, parafunctional habits, tooth wear, and sensitivity.
15. Fuzziness and breaks in the continuity of the lamina dura.

CHAPTER 10

1. b	6. d
2. d	7. c
3. a	8. a
4. c	9. a
5. c	10. b

11. To eliminate and control etiologic and predisposing factors, maintain health, and prevent the occurrence of disease.

12. Case type, amount of experience, practice setting, dentist philosophy, and state practice act.
13. Age, systemic health, type of periodontal disease, oral condition, and attitude of the patient.
14. Good, fair, guarded, poor.
15. Number of teeth, amount of calculus, condition of periodontium and restorations, developmental anomalies, patient sensitivity, and patient attitude.

CHAPTER 11

1. c	6. b
2. a	7. a
3. a	8. d
4. b	9. c
5. d	10. c

11. Maintenance of gingival and periodontal health, caries control, managing complex plaque control problems, patient responsibility, and patient motivation.
12. Personal preference and ease of use.
13. Alters the bacterial cell wall and interferes with adsorption of the bacteria to the teeth.
14. Motivating and changing patient behavior.
15. Attachment loss and recession expose root surfaces to the oral environment.

CHAPTER 12

1. c	6. a
2. a	7. c
3. c	8. b
4. d	9. c
5. e	10. b

11. Scaling removes calculus, whereas root planing removes a portion of the root surfaces.
12. Short-term goals are plaque control and smooth tooth surfaces; the long-term goal is gingival health.
13. Exposed dentinal tubules are stimulated, causing the flow of tubule contents outward, affecting the odontoblastic process and resulting in pain.
14. Fluoride, calcium hydroxide, varnish, potassium oxalate, ferric oxalate, potassium nitrate toothpaste, and strontium chloride toothpaste.
15. Yes, it has been proven with in vitro investigations.

CHAPTER 13

1. c	6. a
2. e	7. a
3. c	8. d
4. c	9. c
5. d	10. b

11. Gain access to the root surfaces for treatment.
12. Pocket depth, bone loss, tooth value, patient's plaque control, patient's age and health, patient's preference.
13. Healing by selected cell repopulation; a barrier membrane is placed that excludes epithelial cells, allowing only cells from the periodontal ligament and bone to grow.

14. A flap that is sutured at a more apical location on the tooth root to reduce the pocket depth.
15. Patient advocate, plaque control educator, and provider of postoperative care.

CHAPTER 14

1. d	6. b
2. c	7. a
3. c	8. a
4. b	9. d
5. b	10. d

11. Direct contact of bone to the dental implant.
12. Acceptability and compliance of the patient, surgical technique, and quality of the restorative dentistry.
13. Steel curettes can roughen surfaces, enhancing plaque accumulation.
14. Bleeding on probing, exudate, progression of bone loss, mobility, a dull percussion sound, and peri-implant radiolucency.
15. Complying with daily oral hygiene care and regular attendance at supportive periodontal therapy appointments.

CHAPTER 15

1. a	6. d
2. c	7. a
3. d	8. c
4. e	9. e
5. e	10. b

11. Collaboration between dental hygienist, patient, dentist, and periodontist; partnership between patient and oral health care team; patient acceptance of responsibility; understanding of many factors that effect periodontal disease.
12. Probing pocket depths, gingival recession, bleeding on probing and suppuration, mobility, furcations, mucogingival involvement.
13. Simplify, accommodate, remind of appointments, keep records of compliance, inform, provide positive reinforcement.
14. Medication review, oral hygiene instruction, diet modification, fluoride therapy.
15. Collaborate with dentists to provide the highest quality oral health care, and have the knowledge and skills to achieve successful long-term oral health in partnership with the patient.

CHAPTER 16

1. a	6. a
2. a	7. a
3. d	8. c
4. c	9. a
5. d	10. e

11. Warm saltwater rinses, rest, and fluid intake.
12. Acute abscesses are usually painful.
13. Periapical pain is sharp, severe, intermittent, and hard to localize, whereas periodontal pain is constant, localized, and less severe.

14. Necrotizing ulcerative gingivitis causes papillary gingiva that is necrotic, cratered, red, painful, and bleeding. It also causes a fetid oral odor.
15. Oral lesions start as small, yellow vesicles that become larger, round ulcers, with gray centers and red borders. Treatment is supportive and includes the use of topical anesthetics, oral hygiene, and adequate diet.

CHAPTER 17

1. b	6. d
2. a	7. a
3. a	8. b
4. d	9. b
5. c	10. d

11. May be asymptomatic and increases with age. Patients may be unaware that they have it.
12. Angina pectoris and myocardial infarction.
13. Controlling gingival bleeding.
14. Infection.
15. Mental confusion, slurred speech, rapid heartbeat, nausea, and cold, clammy skin.
16. Infectious hepatitis is transmitted in contaminated food. Serum hepatitis is transmitted in blood. Health care workers are at risk because infection with hepatitis viruses can lead to liver damage and death.
17. Candidiasis.
18. Oral hygiene instruction and scaling of the teeth.
19. Squamous cell carcinoma.
20. It is thought to suppress certain components of the immune system.

Appendix II: Case Studies

PERIODONTAL CHARTING RECORD

NAME **CASE 1**   Medical Alert **ALLERGIC TO PENICILLIN**

Date

Mobility												1		1		
Probe 3																
Probe 2																
Probe 1	757	647	946	535	535	435	636	735	536	634	436	735	537	777	545	545

Buccal

Lingual (teeth 1–16)

Date

Probe 1	746	657	736	434	434	478	567	855	545	636	637	747	756	757	779	547
Probe 2																
Probe 3																

LEGENDS:
- ▤ IMPLANT
- ● BLEEDING
- ⊙ EXUDATE
- FURCATIONS:
  - ∧ CLASS I
  - △ CLASS II
  - ▲ CLASS III
- **OH** OVERHANG
- ∿ MARGINAL RIDGE DISCREPANCY
- ↑↓ EXTRUSION
- ‖ OPEN CONTACT
- ↻↺ ROTATION
- → DRIFTING OR
- ↙↖ TILTING

Date

Probe 3																
Probe 2																
Probe 1	534	444	555	545	544	546	646	656	635	536	734	435	545	446	544	447

Lingual (teeth 32–17)

Buccal

Date

Probe 1	649	955	644	434	434	535	666	666	666	655	735	536	536	466	544	436
Probe 2																
Probe 3																
Mobility																

PLAQUE CONTROL RECORD

Date _____
Teeth: 1 2 3 4 5 6 7 8 9 10 11 12 13 14 15 16 / 32 31 30 29 28 27 26 25 24 23 22 21 20 19 18 17
Plaque score **100%**

Date _____
Teeth: 1 2 3 4 5 6 7 8 9 10 11 12 13 14 15 16 / 32 31 30 29 28 27 26 25 24 23 22 21 20 19 18 17
Plaque score _____

Date _____
Teeth: 1 2 3 4 5 6 7 8 9 10 11 12 13 14 15 16 / 32 31 30 29 28 27 26 25 24 23 22 21 20 19 18 17
Plaque score _____

CASE 1

See the patient chart, radiographs, and clinical photographs. Refer to the color insert.

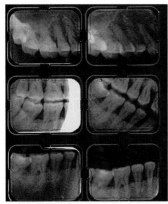
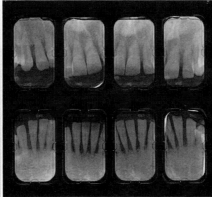
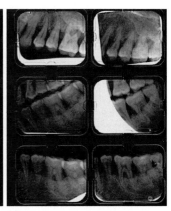

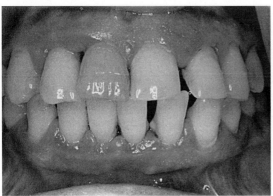
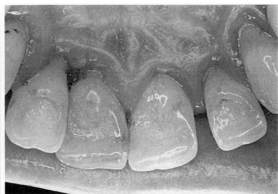

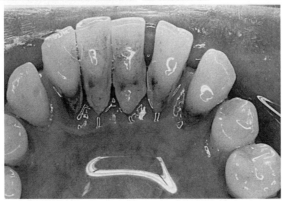

DESCRIPTION: MTA is a 62-year-old male who recently emigrated from the Middle East. He has a college education and is interested in keeping his teeth. He was surprised to learn that he had "gum problems", because he had "never had any trouble with my teeth." You are the dental hygienist working in a periodontist's office. MTA has brought the full mouth series of radiographs taken at the referring dentist's office and is reluctant to have further radiographs taken. MTA is in good general health, is 5'11" in height, weighs 185 pounds, his blood pressure is 140/85 RAS, and his pulse is 82. He has a history of myocardial infarction two years ago and takes the following medications:

Nifedipine (Procardia), 20 mg TID
Warfarin sodium (Coumadin), 7.5 mg/5 mg on alternate days
Furosemide (Lasix), 40 mg daily
Lovistatin (Mevacor), 40 mg daily.

MTA reports a reaction of swelling of the feet and hands following treatment with procaine penicillin given to him as a child.

Based on the description, charting, three intraoral photographs and radiographs, answer the following questions:

1. The most likely diagnosis for this case is which of the following?

    a. Gingivitis
    b. Localized moderate periodontitis
    c. Generalized moderate periodontitis
    d. Localized severe periodontitis
    e. Generalized severe periodontitis

2. The periodontal disease case type designation for MTA is which of the following?

    a. Case Type I
    b. Case Type II
    c. Case Type III
    d. Case Type IV
    e. Case Type V

3. The molar bitewing radiographs have large white areas. The most probable cause of this artifact is:

    a. Improper development
    b. Patient moved during exposure
    c. Improper x-ray tube alignment
    d. Film slipped in holder

4. What premedication should be given to MTA prior to his treatment?

    a. Amoxicillin (oral)
    b. Clindamycin (oral)
    c. Erythromycin (oral)
    d. None required

5. MTA has extremely poor plaque control. The oral hygiene regimen you prescribe should include all of the following EXCEPT one. Which one is the EXCEPTION?

    a. Electric and/or manual toothbrush
    b. Antimicrobial rinses
    c. Toothpicks used on a handle
    d. Fluoride rinses

6. In order to avoid the risk of excessive bleeding

during dental hygiene appointments, the most appropriate treatment plan is:

    a. Half-mouth debridement per treatment visit
    b. Full-mouth debridement
    c. ½ to 1 quadrant debridement per treatment visit
    d. Gross scaling followed by quadrant debridement

7. This patient will require local anesthesia during treatment. The best choice among available local anesthetics is:

    a. Lidocaine with 1:100,000 epinephrine (Xylocaine)
    b. Procaine hydrochloride (Novocaine)
    c. Mepivacaine 3% (Carbocaine)
    d. Lidocaine with 1:50,000 epinephrine (Xylocaine)

8. MTA is concerned about the maxillary right quadrant because "the teeth are loose." He asks you if you think he can keep all of his teeth. After reviewing the oral findings and the radiographs, you consider the prognosis of tooth #14 to be:

    a. Good
    b. Fair
    c. Poor
    d. Guarded
    e. Not treatable

9. The shape of the gingiva in the mandibular incisors suggests some hyperplastic gingiva may have developed. This condition was most likely caused by:

    a. Plaque and calculus
    b. Medications
    c. Drifting of teeth
    d. Genetic predisposition
    e. Trauma from occlusion

10. Teeth numbers 23, 24, 25, and 26 have been scheduled for extraction. The most likely reason for this course of action is:

    a. Heavy calculus
    b. Lack of bone support
    c. Poor plaque control
    d. Advanced mobility

11. At the one-month evaluation of MTA after dental hygiene treatment, how much resolution in probing depths would you expect to see?

    a. less than 1 mm
    b. 1 mm to 2 mms
    c. more than 2 mms
    d. Varies with age

PERIODONTAL CHARTING RECORD

NAME _____ CASE 2 _____ Medical Alert _____

Date

Mobility															
Probe 3															
Probe 2															
Probe 1	434	434	434	423	323	323	323	323	423	423	434	434	434	444	

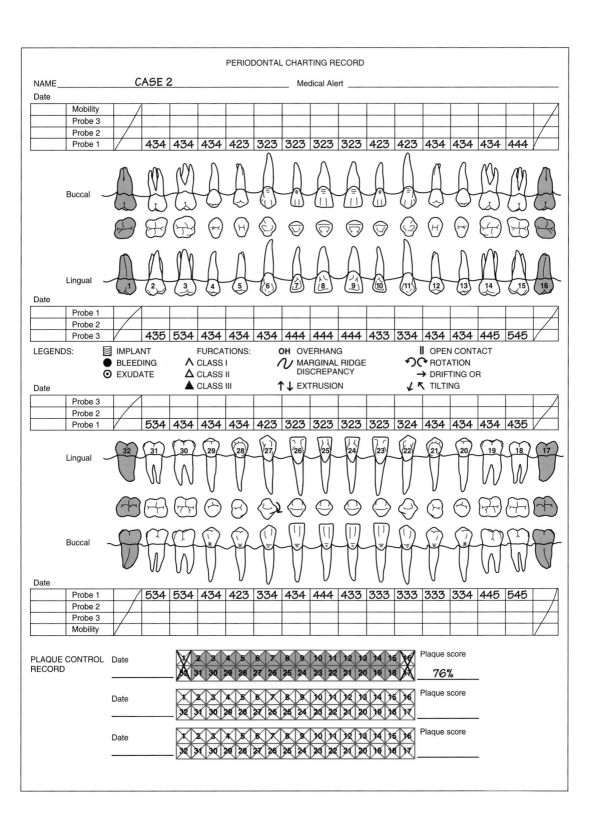

Buccal

Lingual (teeth 1–16)

Date

Probe 1															
Probe 2															
Probe 3	435	534	434	434	434	444	444	444	433	334	434	434	445	545	

LEGENDS:
- IMPLANT
- ● BLEEDING
- ◉ EXUDATE

FURCATIONS:
- ∧ CLASS I
- △ CLASS II
- ▲ CLASS III

OH OVERHANG
- ∿ MARGINAL RIDGE DISCREPANCY
- ↑↓ EXTRUSION

- ‖ OPEN CONTACT
- ↻ ROTATION
- → DRIFTING OR
- ↙ ↖ TILTING

Date

Probe 3															
Probe 2															
Probe 1	534	434	434	434	423	323	323	323	323	324	434	434	434	435	

Lingual (teeth 32–17)

Buccal

Date

Probe 1	534	534	434	423	334	434	444	433	333	333	333	334	445	545	
Probe 2															
Probe 3															
Mobility															

PLAQUE CONTROL RECORD

Date _____ Plaque score **76%**

Date _____ Plaque score _____

Date _____ Plaque score _____

CASE 2

See patient chart and clinical photographs. Refer to color insert.

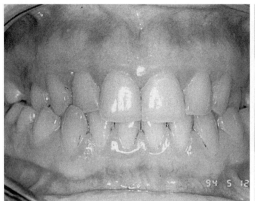
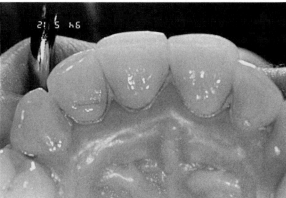

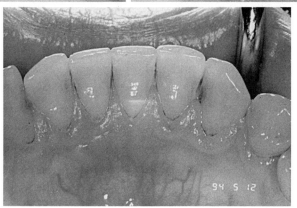

DESCRIPTION: EBC is a 24-year-old Caucasian female in the second trimester of her first pregnancy. She came to see your employer, a general dentist, because her "gums hurt and bleed when I eat and try to brush." EBC is in good general health. She is taking over-the-counter multivitamin tablets and no prescription medications. EBC is 5'4" tall, weighs 143 pounds, her blood pressure is 110/72 RAS, pulse 79. She has no history of chronic illness or hospitalization, no drug allergies, and is not under the care of a physician for anything other than prenatal care. EBC does not smoke or drink alcoholic or caffeinated beverages. EBC recently moved into the area and has not been seen in this office before. No dental radiographs have been taken. The patient is referred to you for care.

Based on the description, charting, and three intraoral photographs, answer the following questions:

1. The most likely diagnosis for this case is which of the following?

   a. Gingivitis
   b. Localized moderate periodontitis
   c. Generalized moderate periodontitis
   d. Localized severe periodontitis
   e. Generalized severe periodontitis

2. The periodontal disease case type designation for EBC is which of the following?

   a. Case Type I
   b. Case Type II
   c. Case Type III
   d. Case Type IV
   e. Case Type V

3. All of the following could contribute to the swollen edematous gingival margins EXCEPT one. Which one of the following is the EXCEPTION?

   a. Poor plaque control
   b. Subgingival calculus
   c. Hormonal changes due to the pregnancy
   d. Tooth positioning including crossbite and rotated teeth
   e. Age of the patient

4. The dental hygiene treatment plan for EBC most likely will include which of the following?

   a. Multiple short scaling sessions with home care instruction
   b. Full-mouth debridement in one long session
   c. Site-specific antibiotic therapy
   d. Systemic tetracycline therapy

5. Based on the case history, the best time to begin scaling and root planing is:

   a. Immediately
   b. During the third trimester
   c. After the baby is born
   d. After the baby is weaned

6. Following improvement in plaque control, how much change in probing depths would be expected?

   a. Complete resolution
   b. Partial resolution
   c. No resolution
   d. Gradual deepening

7. EBC relates that she cannot brush and floss because the tissue is tender. What is the most appropriate advice to provide this patient?

   a. "Do the best you can."
   b. "Don't be such a baby."
   c. "Don't bother until after the baby comes, then it won't hurt."
   d. "Let's find a method that will work."

8. The pattern of plaque present in the patient's mouth suggests plaque control instruction that focuses on which of the following?

   a. Electric and/or manual toothbrush
   b. Interproximal brushing
   c. Flossing
   d. Oral antimicrobial rinses
   e. Fluoride rinses

9. Dark staining appears at the gingival margin throughout the patient's mouth. The stain is most likely caused by what mechanism?

   a. Tobacco use
   b. Red wine consumption
   c. Coffee or tea consumption
   d. Chromogenic bacteria in plaque

10. The most appropriate form of pain control to be used during scaling and root planing for EBC is which of the following?

    a. No local anesthesia is indicated
    b. Topical anesthesia only
    c. Infiltration and block anesthesia with vasoconstrictor
    d. Infiltration and block anesthesia without vasoconstrictor

11. Reevaluation following dental hygiene treatment should occur:

    a. 4 to 6 weeks after treatment
    b. 3 months after treatment
    c. 6 months after treatment
    d. 12 months after treatment

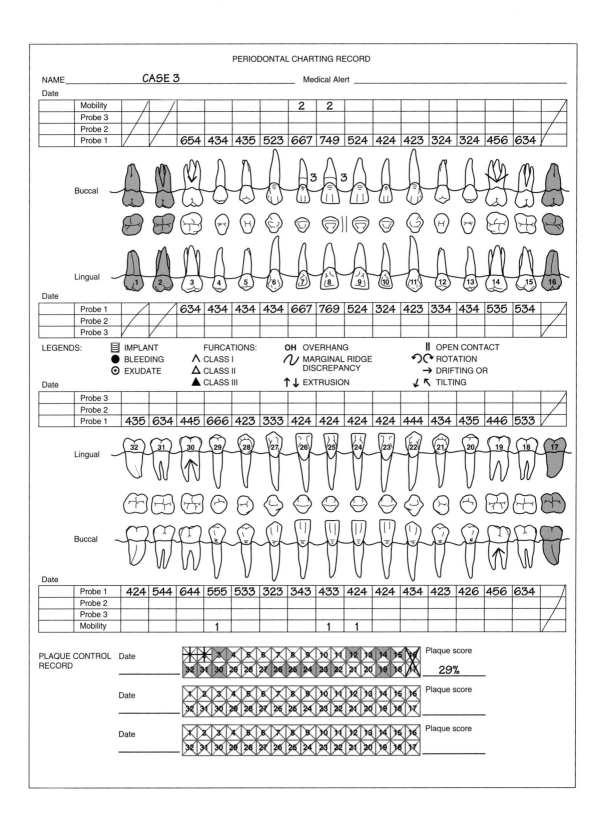

PERIODONTAL CHARTING RECORD

NAME _____ CASE 3 _____   Medical Alert _____

Date

Mobility						2	2									
Probe 3																
Probe 2																
Probe 1		654	434	435	523	667	749	524	424	423	324	324	456	634	

Buccal

(3 3 markings shown)

Lingual — teeth 1 2 3 4 5 6 7 8 9 10 11 12 13 14 15 16

Date

Probe 1		634	434	434	434	667	769	524	324	423	334	434	535	534	
Probe 2																
Probe 3																

LEGENDS: ▤ IMPLANT   FURCATIONS: **OH** OVERHANG   ‖ OPEN CONTACT
● BLEEDING   ∧ CLASS I   ∿ MARGINAL RIDGE   ↻↺ ROTATION
⊙ EXUDATE   △ CLASS II   DISCREPANCY   → DRIFTING OR
▲ CLASS III   ↑↓ EXTRUSION   ↙↖ TILTING

Date

Probe 3																
Probe 2																
Probe 1	435	634	445	666	423	333	424	424	424	424	444	434	435	446	533	

Lingual — teeth 32 31 30 29 28 27 26 25 24 23 22 21 20 19 18 17

Buccal

Date

Probe 1	424	544	644	555	533	323	343	433	424	424	434	423	426	456	634	
Probe 2																
Probe 3																
Mobility				1				1	1							

PLAQUE CONTROL RECORD

Date _____   Plaque score **29%**
(upper row teeth: 1 2 3 4 5 6 7 8 9 10 11 12 13 14 15 16)
(lower row teeth: 32 31 30 29 28 27 26 25 24 23 22 21 20 19 18 17)

Date _____   Plaque score _____

Date _____   Plaque score _____

CASE 3

See patient chart, radiographs, and clinical photographs. Refer to color insert.

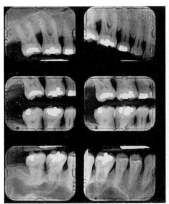
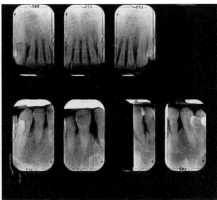
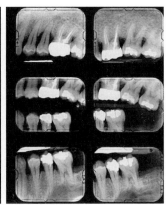

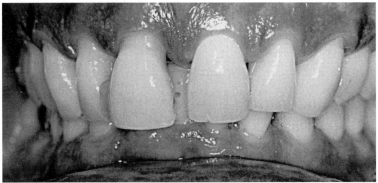

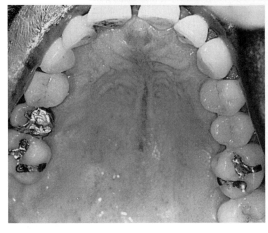
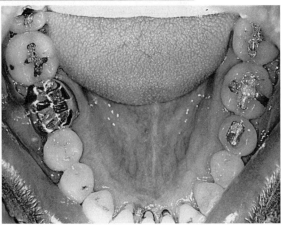

DESCRIPTION: DEN is a 55-year-old African American male. Although he has received fairly regular dental care in the past, it has been several years since he has been seen for treatment. DEN has come to your general dentist employer because he noticed that there are spaces between his front teeth that were not there before. He is worried about losing more teeth. DEN has a history of atrial fibrillation and has been wearing a pacemaker for five years. He is also under the care of a physician for high blood pressure. DEN is 5′8″, weighs

210 pounds, his blood pressure is 138/88 RAS, and his pulse is 80. His medications are:

Atenolol (Tenormin), 50 mg daily
Hydrochlorothiazide (Esidrix), 75 mg daily
Over-the-counter multivitamin, one per day.

DEN smokes ½ pack of cigarettes per day and is a social drinker. He presents with moderate subgingival calculus, and moderate amounts of plaque and stain.

Based on the description, charting, three intraoral photographs, and radiographs, answer the following questions:

1. The most likely diagnosis for this case is which of the following?

   a. Gingivitis
   b. Localized moderate periodontitis
   c. Generalized moderate periodontitis
   d. Localized severe periodontitis
   e. Generalized severe periodontitis

2. The periodontal disease case type designation for DEN is which of the following?

   a. Case Type I
   b. Case Type II
   c. Case Type III
   d. Case Type IV
   e. Case Type V

3. DEN's chief complaint is drifting of the anterior teeth. Which of the following most likely causes this condition?

   a. Tongue thrust
   b. Bone loss
   c. Brushing habits
   d. Traumatic occlusion

4. The long-term prognosis is most likely very poor for which of the following teeth?

   a. 2
   b. 6
   c. 8
   d. 19
   e. 31

5. Treatment planning options for dental hygiene care would include all of the following EXCEPT one. Which one is the EXCEPTION?

   a. Full mouth debridement
   b. Gross scaling
   c. Quadrant scaling and root planing
   d. Half-mouth-scaling and root planing

6. Instrumentation during dental hygiene treatment may be complicated by all of the following EXCEPT one. Which one is the EXCEPTION?

   a. Deep pockets
   b. Heavy subgingival calculus
   c. Cervical caries
   d. Margins of restorations
   e. Hypertensive medications

7. Ultrasonic instrumentation is contraindicated in this patient because:

   a. The calculus is not very heavy
   b. The patient is on antihypertensive medications
   c. The patient has a pacemaker
   d. The teeth are too mobile

8. Which of the following oral hygiene devices would be most efficient for DEN to use for plaque removal in the class I furcation areas?

   a. Electric toothbrush
   b. Single-tufted toothbrush
   c. Floss
   d. Toothpick on a handle

9. The heavy stain observed on the lingual surfaces of the maxillary and mandibular anterior teeth is most likely related to:

   a. Tobacco use
   b. Red wine consumption
   c. Coffee or tea consumption
   d. Chromogenic bacteria in plaque

10. Tobacco and alcohol use are related to more severe periodontal diseases.
    The plaque control regimen should include devices for cleaning interproximal surfaces as well as buccal and lingual surfaces.

    a. Both statements are TRUE.
    b. Both statements are FALSE.
    c. The first statement is TRUE and the second is FALSE.
    d. The first statement is FALSE and the second is TRUE.

11. After reevaluation. DEN will most likely need to be referred to a periodontist for management of the remaining deep pockets.
    It is appropriate to begin periodontal maintenance after treatment is completed by the periodontist.

    a. Both statements are TRUE.
    b. Both statements are FALSE.
    c. The first statement is TRUE and the second is FALSE.
    d. The first statement is FALSE and the second is TRUE.

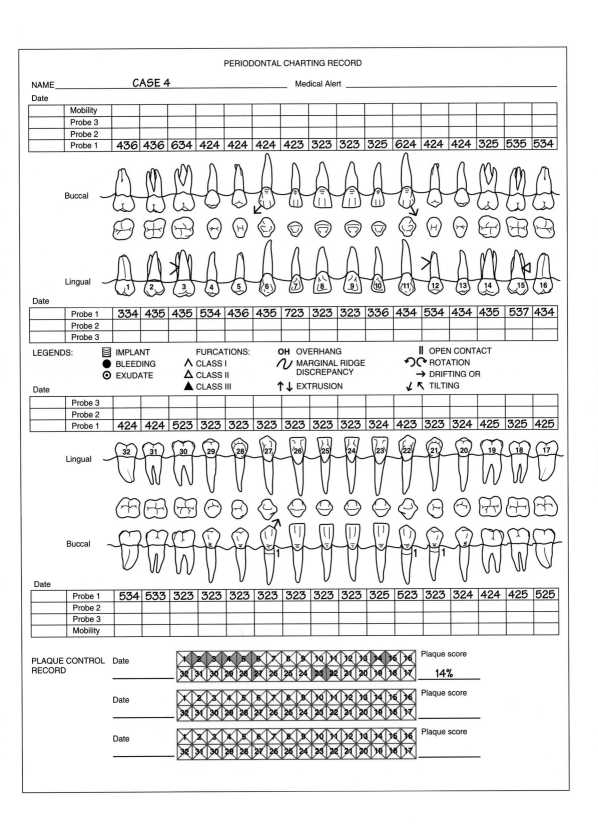

PERIODONTAL CHARTING RECORD

NAME **CASE 4**   Medical Alert

Date

Mobility																	
Probe 3																	
Probe 2																	
Probe 1	436	436	634	424	424	424	423	323	323	325	624	424	424	325	535	534

Buccal

Lingual

Teeth: 1 2 3 4 5 6 7 8 9 10 11 12 13 14 15 16

Date

Probe 1	334	435	435	534	436	435	723	323	323	336	434	534	434	435	537	434
Probe 2																	
Probe 3																	

LEGENDS:

▤ IMPLANT	FURCATIONS:	OH OVERHANG ‖ OPEN CONTACT
● BLEEDING	∧ CLASS I	∿ MARGINAL RIDGE ↻↺ ROTATION
⊙ EXUDATE	△ CLASS II	DISCREPANCY → DRIFTING OR
	▲ CLASS III	↑↓ EXTRUSION ↙↖ TILTING

Date

Probe 3																	
Probe 2																	
Probe 1	424	424	523	323	323	323	323	323	323	324	423	323	324	425	325	425

Lingual

Teeth: 32 31 30 29 28 27 26 25 24 23 22 21 20 19 18 17

Buccal

Date

Probe 1	534	533	323	323	323	323	323	323	323	325	523	323	324	424	425	525
Probe 2																	
Probe 3																	
Mobility																	

PLAQUE CONTROL RECORD Date _____

Plaque score **14%**

Date _____

Plaque score

Date _____

Plaque score

CASE 4

See patient chart, radiographs, and clinical
photographs. Refer to color insert.

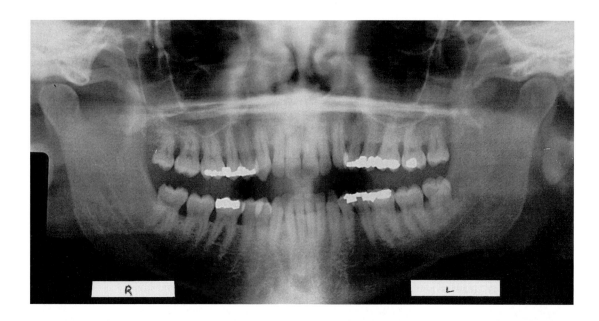

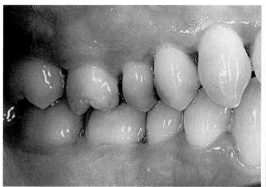

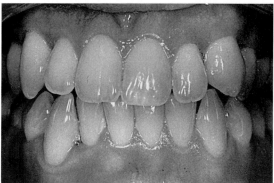

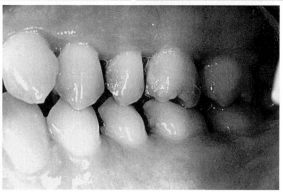

DESCRIPTION: JEP is a 35-year-old Hispanic female. She is in good health and has come to your general dentist employer for routine dental care. JEP is very cooperative and interested in maintaining her dental health. JEP has no history of diseases other than childhood chickenpox. She is not currently under the care of a physician, but has annual physical examinations. JEP is 5′7″ tall, weighs 150 pounds, her blood pressure is 126/82 RAS, and her pulse is 76. JEP had restorative dental treatment ten years ago and has had no new caries experience since then. She brushes and flosses her teeth twice per day and reports that one tooth (she points to #21, buccal surface) is sensitive to cold.

Based on the description, charting, three intraoral photographs, and radiographs, answer the following questions:

1. The most likely diagnosis for this case is which of the following?

   a. Gingivitis
   b. Localized moderate periodontitis
   c. Generalized moderate periodontitis
   d. Localized severe periodontitis
   e. Generalized severe periodontitis

2. The periodontal disease case type designation for JEP is which of the following?

   a. Case Type I
   b. Case Type II
   c. Case Type III
   d. Case Type IV
   e. Case Type V

3. The 5-mm probing depth on #32 distal is best described as:

   a. Normal anatomy
   b. Recession
   c. Moderate bone loss
   d. Gingival pocket

4. The 5-mm probing depth on #31 distal is best described as:

   a. Normal anatomy
   b. Recession
   c. Moderate bone loss
   d. Gingival pocket

5. The plaque control program for JEP should emphasize:

   a. Sulcular brushing technique
   b. Triangular tooth picks
   c. Cone-shaped interproximal brushes
   d. Flossing technique

6. Plaque accumulation on tooth #27 mesial is most likely related to:

   a. Frenum pull
   b. Tooth position
   c. Traumatic brushing technique
   d. Gingival recession

7. The dental hygiene treatment plan is for quadrant scaling and root planing. The most likely quadrant to begin treatment is which of the following?

   a. Upper right
   b. Lower right
   c. Upper left
   d. Lower left

8. The sensitivity on tooth #21 buccal was most likely caused by:

   a. Tooth position
   b. Traumatic brushing technique
   c. Stiff-bristled tooth brushes
   d. Traumatic occlusion

9. In order to complete the preventive program for JEP, the home care regimen should include morning and evening use of which product?

   a. Fluoride toothpaste
   b. Fluoride mouthrinse
   c. Chlorhexidine gluconate mouthrinse
   d. Essential oil mouthrinse

10. Following scaling and root planing therapy, you should expect resolution of the probing depths in which of the following areas?

    a. Maxillary right molars
    b. Maxillary left molars
    c. Mandibular right molars
    d. Mandibular left molars

11. The recommended recall interval for JEP would be which of the following?

    a. 1 to 2 months
    b. 3 to 4 months
    c. 6 to 9 months
    d. 9 to 12 months

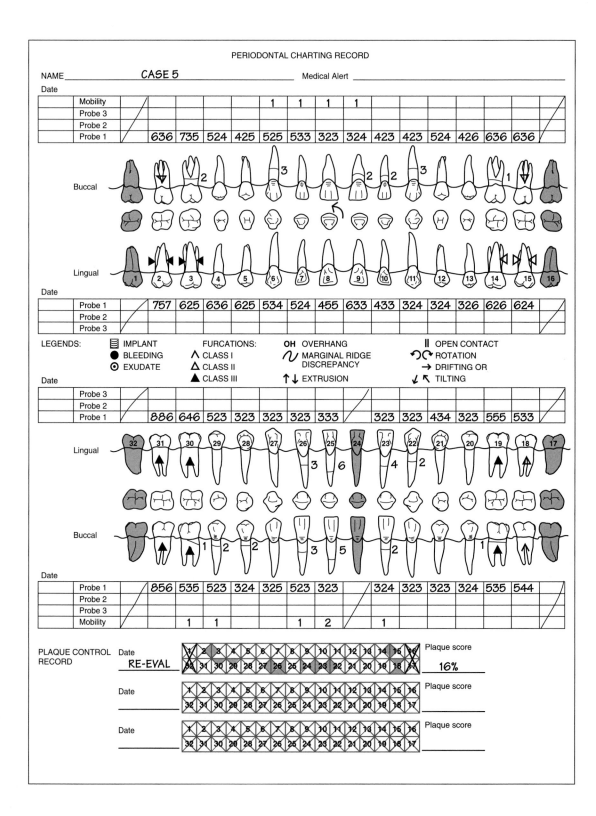

PERIODONTAL CHARTING RECORD

NAME _____ CASE 5 _____   Medical Alert _____

Date

Mobility						1	1	1	1							
Probe 3																
Probe 2																
Probe 1		636	735	524	425	525	533	323	324	423	423	524	426	636	636	

Buccal

Lingual

Date

Probe 1		757	625	636	625	534	524	455	633	433	324	324	326	626	624	
Probe 2																
Probe 3																

LEGENDS:

▤ IMPLANT	FURCATIONS:	**OH** OVERHANG	‖ OPEN CONTACT
● BLEEDING	∧ CLASS I	∿ MARGINAL RIDGE DISCREPANCY	↺↻ ROTATION
⊙ EXUDATE	△ CLASS II		→ DRIFTING OR
	▲ CLASS III	↑↓ EXTRUSION	↙↖ TILTING

Date

Probe 3																
Probe 2																
Probe 1		886	646	523	323	323	323	333		323	323	434	323	555	533	

Lingual

Buccal

Date

Probe 1		856	535	523	324	325	523	323		324	323	323	324	535	544	
Probe 2																
Probe 3																
Mobility			1	1			1	2		1						

PLAQUE CONTROL RECORD

Date		Plaque score
RE-EVAL		16%
Date		Plaque score
Date		Plaque score

CASE 5

See patient chart, radiographs, and clinical photographs. Refer to color insert.

Set 1

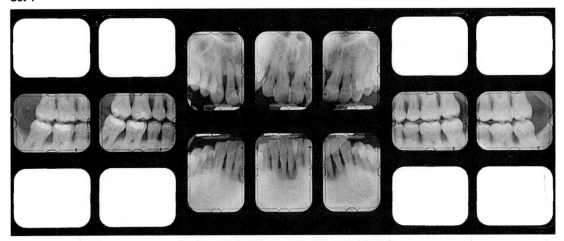

Set 2

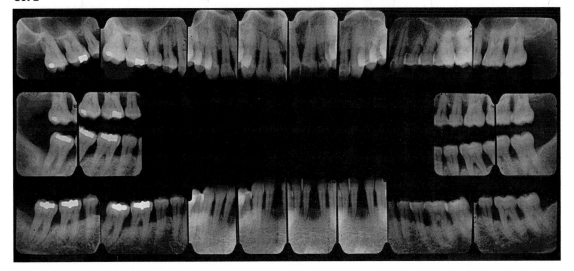

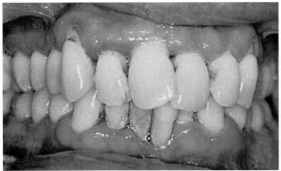
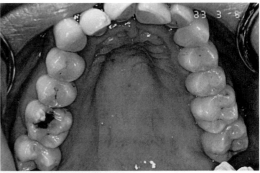
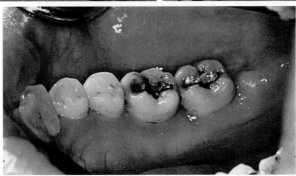

DESCRIPTION: EJT is a 41-year-old Caucasian male. He is in excellent health, is not under the care of a physician, and takes no medications. EJT was provided initial therapy at his general dentist's office but became unhappy when he was told he might lose all his teeth. EJT was then referred to the periodontist for whom you work. He brought his old x-rays with him (Set 1), and you took the new full mouth set (Set 2). He told you, "I know I have serious gum problems. I was not treated right by my dentist. All he did was pull my front tooth! I want to keep all my teeth; don't even talk to me about false teeth!" EJT brushes his teeth three times per day, and he uses floss and an interproximal brush once per day. He smokes one pack of cigarettes a day, and does not drink. You encounter considerable residual calculus, burnished on the root surfaces.

Based on the description, charting, three intraoral photographs, and two sets of radiographs, answer the following questions:

1. The most likely diagnosis for this case is which of the following?

   a. Gingivitis
   b. Localized moderate periodontitis
   c. Generalized moderate periodontitis
   d. Localized severe periodontitis
   e. Generalized severe periodontitis

2. The periodontal disease case type designation for EJT is which of the following?

   a. Case Type I
   b. Case Type II
   c. Case Type III
   d. Case Type IV
   e. Case Type V

3. The prognosis for EJT's teeth is generally:

   a. Guarded
   b. Poor
   c. Fair
   d. Good

4. You would expect healing of the gingiva to be delayed in this patient for which of the following reasons?

   a. Age
   b. Smoking
   c. Medications
   d. Rotated teeth
   e. Traumatic occlusion

5. Plaque control in the lower anterior teeth is complicated by all of the following circumstances EXCEPT one. Which one is the EXCEPTION?

   a. Smoking
   b. Root proximity
   c. Compliance
   d. Age

6. You recorded the probe depths in the chart one month after scaling and root planing was

completed at the general dentist's office. What was the likely probe depth on tooth #30 mesial and distal prior to the initial therapy?

a. 3 mm
b. 5 mm
c. 7 mm
d. 9 mm

7. The teeth with the poorest prognosis are those with:

a. No furcations
b. Class I furcations
c. Class II furcations
d. Class III furcations

8. Based on the patient history and clinical presentation, you would expect the periodontal infection to be:

a. Aggressive
b. Refractory
c. Recurrent
d. Chronic

9. Based on your probing depths made one month after initial therapy at the general dentist's office, further periodontal treatment would include all of the following EXCEPT one. Which one is the EXCEPTION?

a. Repeat scaling and root planing
b. 6-month recall
c. Periodontal surgery
d. Locally delivered antibiotic therapy

10. Systemic antibiotic therapy may be appropriate for EJT for which of the following reasons?

a. Poor plaque control
b. Medical contraindication
c. Virulent subgingival plaque
d. Expected extraction of multiple teeth

11. It is important to wait at least one week after scaling and root planing to reprobe the treated areas.
Probe depths improve after scaling and root planing due to reduction in edematous gingiva and healed connective tissue that resists penetration by the probe tip.

a. Both statements are TRUE.
b. Both statements are FALSE.
c. The first statement is TRUE and the second is FALSE.
d. The first statement is FALSE and the second is TRUE.

PERIODONTAL CHARTING RECORD

NAME _____ CASE 6 _____ Medical Alert _____

Date

Mobility																	
Probe 3																	
Probe 2																	
Probe 1					334	433	333	333	333	333							

Buccal

Lingual

1 2 3 4 5 6 7 8 9 10 11 12 13 14 15 16

Date

Probe 1					434	433	333	333	333	333							
Probe 2																	
Probe 3																	

LEGENDS:

IMPLANT	FURCATIONS:	OH OVERHANG	‖ OPEN CONTACT
● BLEEDING	∧ CLASS I	∿ MARGINAL RIDGE DISCREPANCY	↺↻ ROTATION
⊙ EXUDATE	△ CLASS II		→ DRIFTING OR
	▲ CLASS III	↑↓ EXTRUSION	↙↖ TILTING

Date

Probe 3																	
Probe 2																	
Probe 1					424	424	424	424	424	424							

Lingual

32 31 30 29 28 27 26 25 24 23 22 21 20 19 18 17

Buccal

Date

Probe 1					424	424	424	424	424	424							
Probe 2																	
Probe 3																	
Mobility																	

PLAQUE CONTROL RECORD

Date _____ 1 2 3 4 5 6 7 8 9 10 11 12 13 14 15 16 / 32 31 30 29 28 27 26 25 24 23 22 21 20 19 18 17   Plaque score _____

Date _____ 1 2 3 4 5 6 7 8 9 10 11 12 13 14 15 16 / 32 31 30 29 28 27 26 25 24 23 22 21 20 19 18 17   Plaque score _____

Date _____ 1 2 3 4 5 6 7 8 9 10 11 12 13 14 15 16 / 32 31 30 29 28 27 26 25 24 23 22 21 20 19 18 17   Plaque score _____

CASE 6

See patient chart and clinical photographs. Refer to color insert.

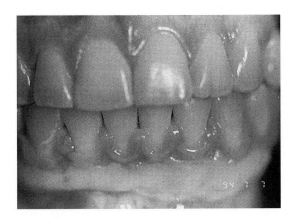

DESCRIPTION: PLB is a 25-year-old Caucasian female. Her medical history is unremarkable, no history of disease and no hospitalizations. The only medication she is taking is oral contraceptives. She is a graduate student completing her doctorate at the local university and is under a great deal of stress. PLB does not smoke and consumes an occasional glass of wine. PLB is 5'8" tall, weighs 130 pounds, her blood pressure is 100/70 RAS, pulse 72. Upon examination you find she has moderate to heavy subgingival calculus and minimal attachment loss. She is concerned about the appearance of the gingiva on the mandibular anterior area. It has been several years since PLB had her teeth cleaned, and she reports being treated by a periodontist. She had some periodontal surgery as a teenager.

Based on the case description, the charting of the anterior teeth, and one photograph answer the following questions:

1. The extremely rolled gingival margin evident on the mandibular anterior is most likely the result of which of the following?

   a. Oral contraceptives
   b. Parafunctional habit
   c. Familial predisposition
   d. Plaque and calculus

2. The light band of keratinized gingival tissue apical to the gingival margin on the mandible is most likely indicative of which of the following?

   a. Racial pigmentation
   b. *Candida albicans* infection
   c. Healed gingival graft
   d. Normal attached gingiva

3. After thorough debridement and improved patient plaque control, the tissue on the mandibular anterior is most likely to do which of the following?

   a. Shrink but retain some rolled characteristics
   b. Shrink, leaving no rolled appearance
   c. Remain unchanged
   d. Continue to enlarge over time

Answers to Case-based questions plus brief explanation:

CASE 1

1. e (extensive bone loss throughout the dentition)
2. d (advanced periodontitis)
3. c (cone cuts)
4. d (history of MI does not require premedication)
5. d (no history of caries)
6. c (shorter appointments treating fewer teeth)
7. a (vasoconstrictor of 1:100 epinephrine is advised)
8. d (probably will not respond to therapy)
9. b (Nifedipine is associated with gingival enlargement)
10. b (untreatable due to lack of bone)
11. b (deep, inflamed pockets are reduced 1 to 2 mm)

CASE 2

1. a (no bone loss)
2. a (gingival involvement only)
3. e (age is unrelated)
4. a (less fatiguing and permits oral hygiene reinforcement)
5. a (resolve infection as soon as possible)
6. b (due to hormone changes in pregnancy)
7. d (positive and encouraging)
8. c (interproximal plaque present throughout)
9. d (indicated by history)
10. c (local anesthesia needed for pain control)
11. a (reprobe in 4 to 6 weeks to permit connective tissue healing)

CASE 3

1. d (not severe in all areas)
2. d (determine type by most severe area)
3. b (normal masticatory pressures exceed bone support)
4. c (severe bone loss)
5. b (does not adequately debride pockets)

6. e (no effects on gingiva or patient management)
7. c (electromagnetic field created in ultrasonic handpiece)
8. d (best access)
9. a (smoker)
10. d (alcohol use is not related to severity of periodontal diseases)
11. c (maintenance begins immediately after initial therapy)

CASE 4

1. c (generalized bone loss)
2. c (severe bone loss)
3. a (relationship to external oblique ridge)
4. c (bone loss on radiographs)
5. d (interproximal plaque present)
6. b (rotated buccally)
7. c (most severe involvement)
8. b (excessive brushing pressure)
9. a (adequate for caries prevention)
10. c and d (no furcation involvement)
11. b (to maintain furcation areas)

CASE 5

1. e (most severe bone loss)
2. d (based on bone loss)
3. b (may respond to therapy)
4. b (nicotine effects on vascularization)
5. d (age is not a disease or symptom)
6. c (1 to 2 mm deeper prior to treatment)
7. d (bone loss and plaque control)
8. d (no history of adequate treatment)
9. b (recall is not sufficient treatment)
10. c (helps control infection)
11. d (4 to 6 weeks required for connective tissue healing)

CASE 6

1. d (response to local irritants)
2. c (large healed gingival graft)
3. a (severe rolling rarely resolves completely after scaling and root planing)

Appendix III: Color Supplement

CASE 1

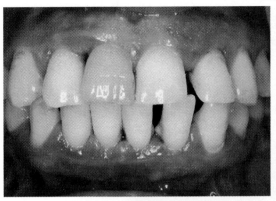
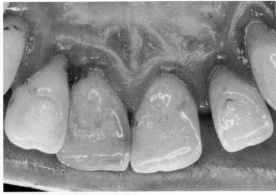

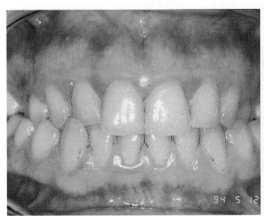

CASE 2

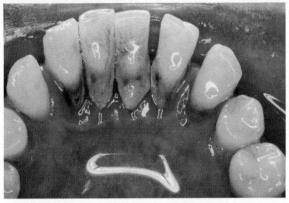
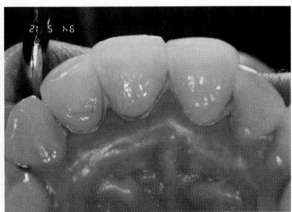

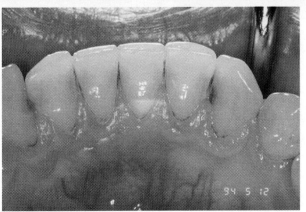

CASE 3

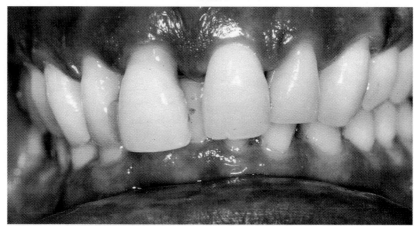

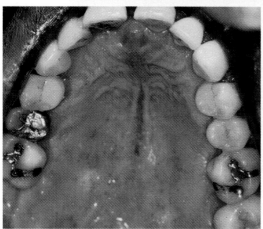
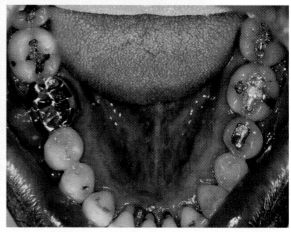

CASE 4

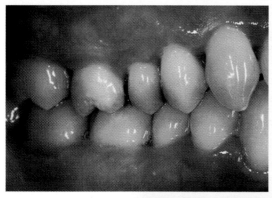
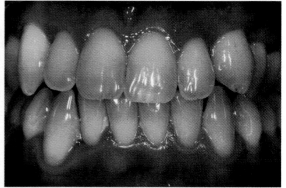

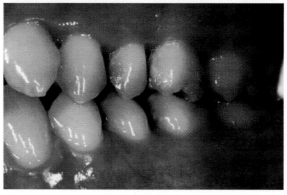

CASE 5

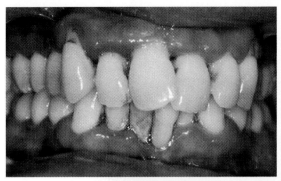
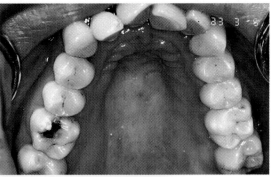

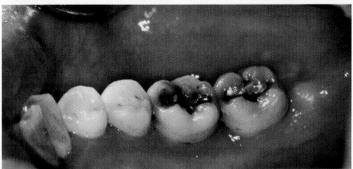

CASE 6

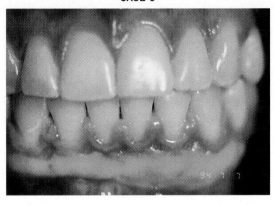

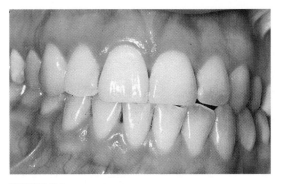

FIGURE 6-1. Normal gingiva.

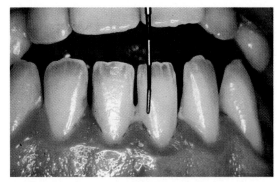

FIGURE 6-2. Plaque-associated gingivitis.

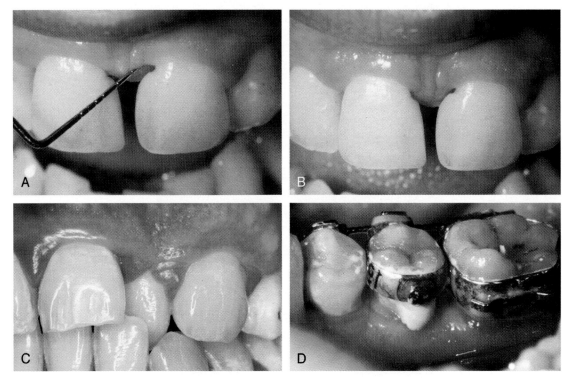

FIGURE 6-4. **A** and **B.** Overcontoured restoration. **C.** Malposition of tooth. **D.** Orthodontic bands and excess cement.

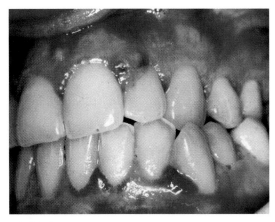

FIGURE 6-5. Pregnancy gingivitis.

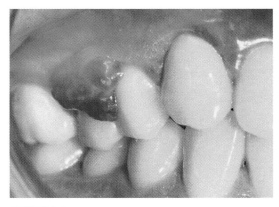

FIGURE 6-6. Pyogenic granuloma.

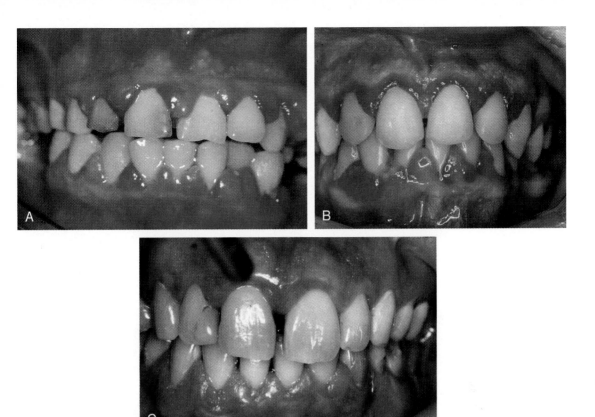

FIGURE 6-7. **A** to **C.** Medication-induced gingival enlargement.

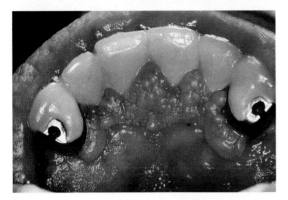

FIGURE 6-8. Medication-induced enlargement.

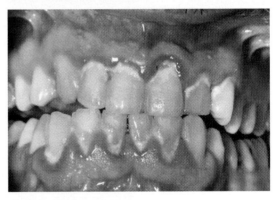

FIGURE 6-9. Gingivitis modified by malnutrition.

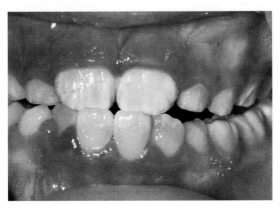

FIGURE 6-10. Streptococcal-associated gingival lesions.

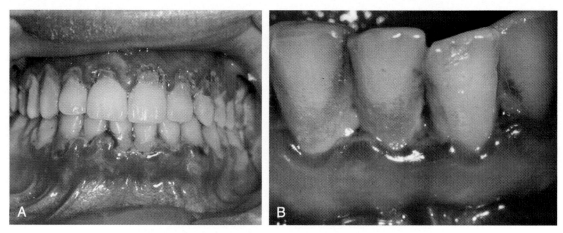

FIGURE 6-11. **A** and **B.** ANUG, generalized.

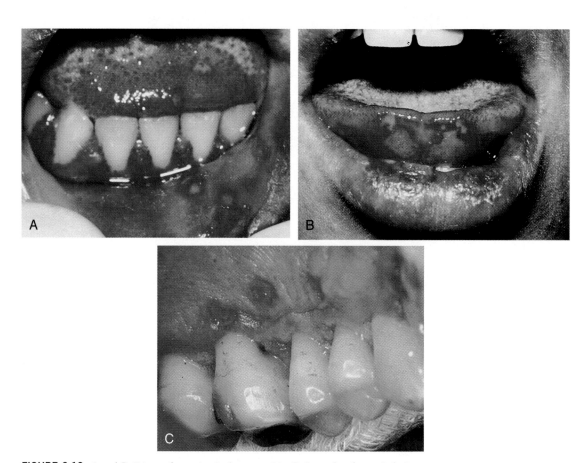

FIGURE 6-12. **A** and **B.** Primary herpetic gingivostomatitis. **C.** Secondary herpetic lesions.

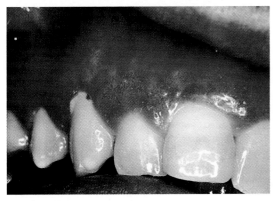

FIGURE 6-13. Gingival candidiasis.

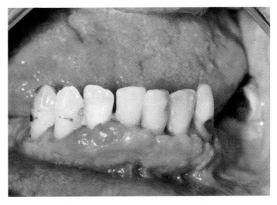

FIGURE 6-14. Idiopathic gingival enlargement.

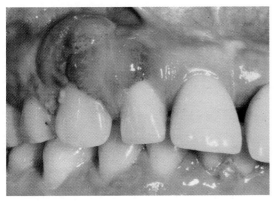

FIGURE 6-15. Acute leukemia–associated gingival lesions.

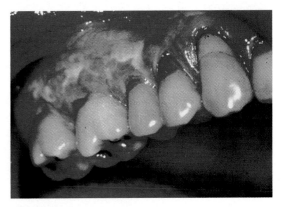

FIGURE 6-16. Lichen planus.

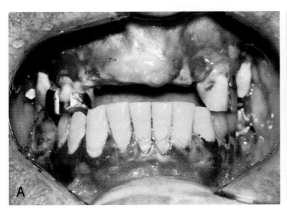

FIGURE 6-17. A and **B.** Pemphigoid.

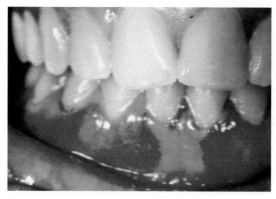

FIGURE 6-18. Desquamative gingivitis.

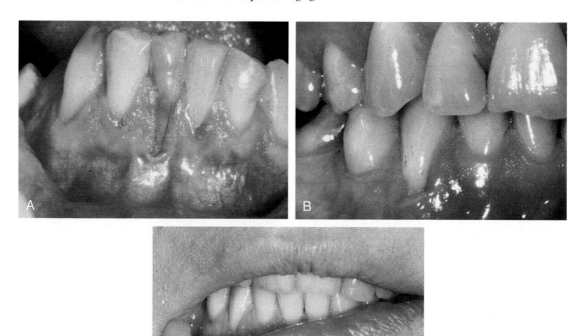

FIGURE 6-19. **A.** Gingival trauma. **B.** Factitious injury. **C.** Cause of injury.

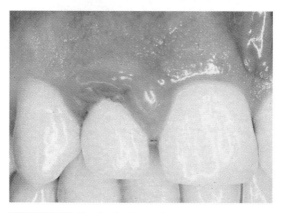

FIGURE 6-20. Foreign-body reaction.

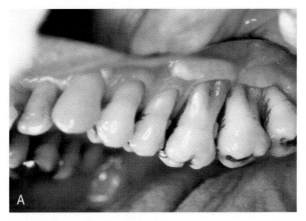

FIGURE 7-1. Clinical attachment loss.

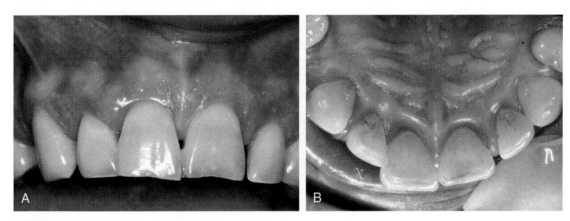

FIGURE 7-2. **A** and **B.** Slight periodontitis.

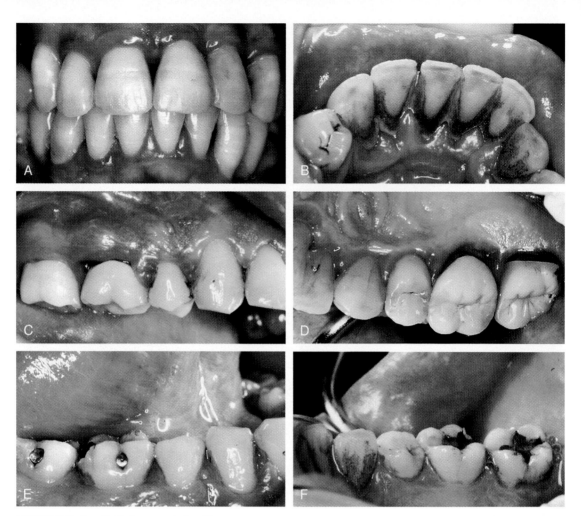

FIGURE 7-3. A to **F.** Moderate periodontitis.

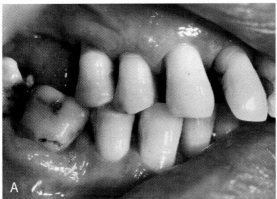

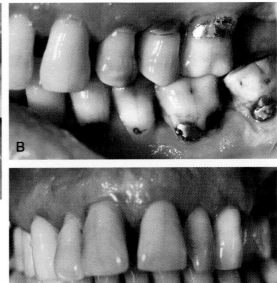

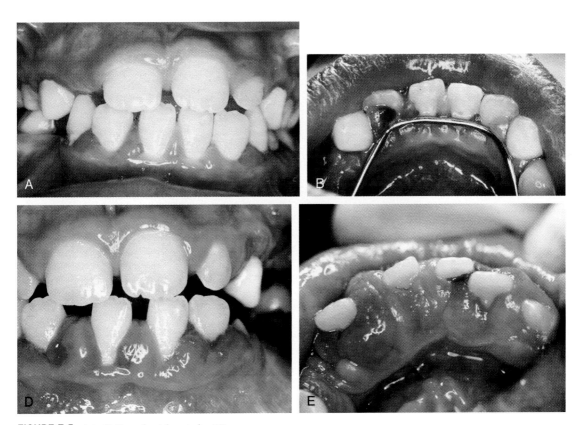

FIGURE 7-4. **A** to **C.** Advanced periodontitis.

FIGURE 7-5. **A** to **E.** Prepubertal periodontitis.

409

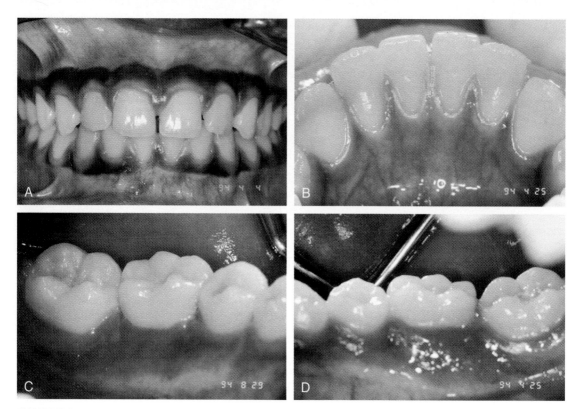

FIGURE 7-6. A to **D.** Localized juvenile periodontitis.

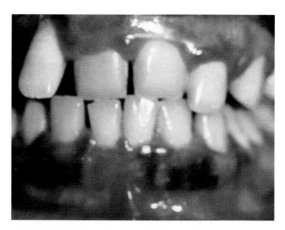

FIGURE 7-7. Generalized juvenile periodontitis.

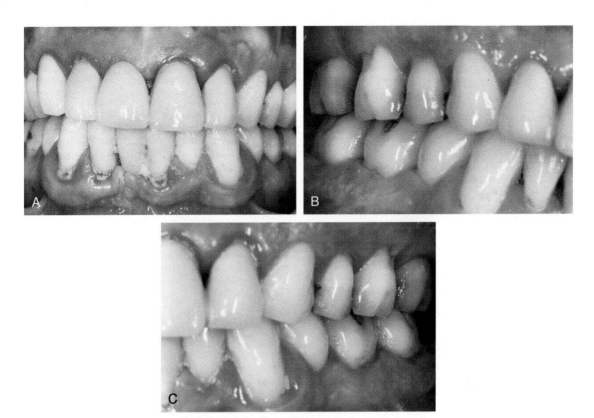

FIGURE 7-8. A to C. Rapidly progressive periodontitis.

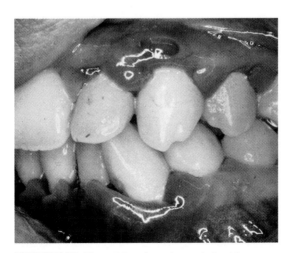

FIGURE 7-10. Necrotizing ulcerative periodontitis.

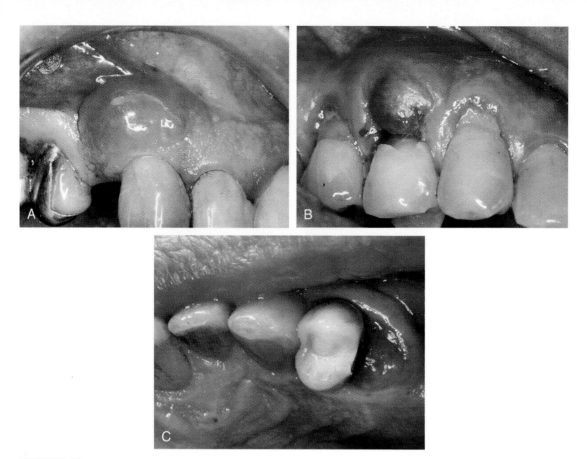

FIGURE 7-11. A to **C.** Acute periodontal abscess.

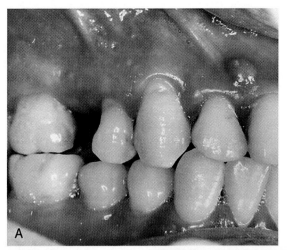

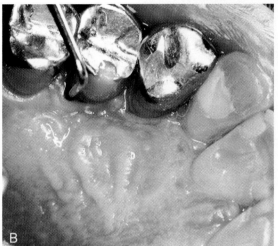

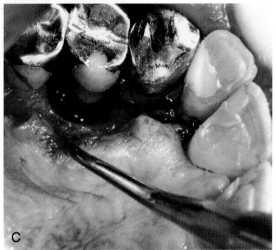

FIGURE 7-12. A to **C.** Acute periodontal abscess.

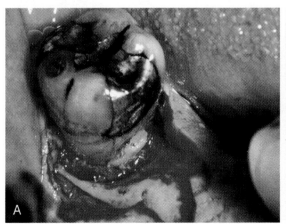

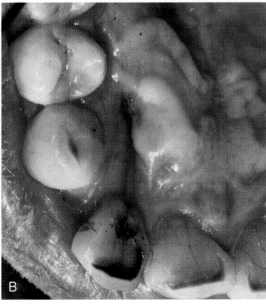

FIGURE 7-13. A. Cementicle (cementum spur). **B.** Developmental groove.

413

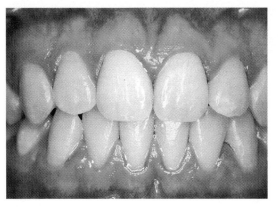

FIGURE 9-5. Inflamed gingiva.

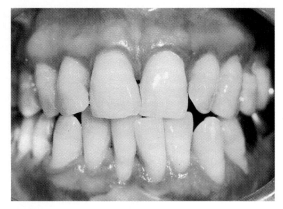

FIGURE 9-6. Inflamed gingiva.

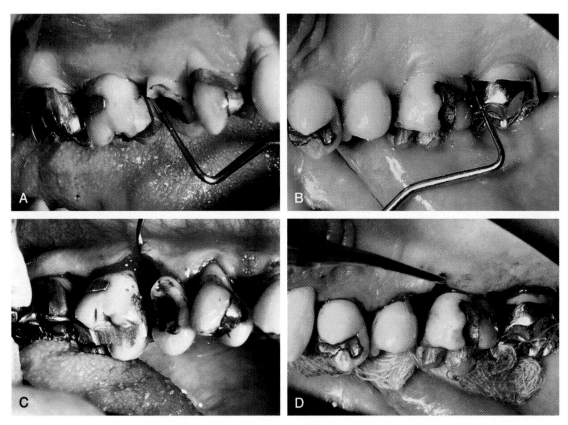

FIGURE 13-10. **A** and **B.** Modified Widman flap—presurgical. **C** and **D.** Modified Widman flap—flap reflected.

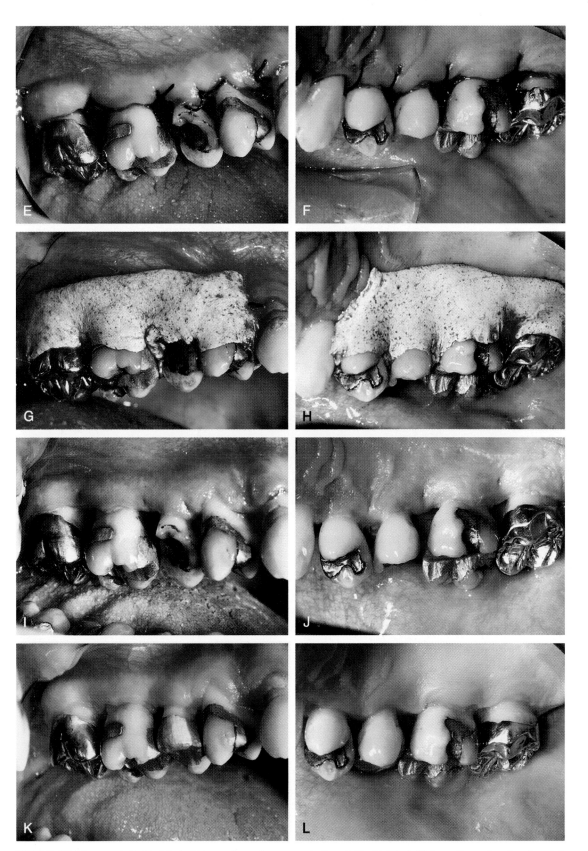

FIGURE 13-10. **E** and **F.** Modified Widman flap—flap sutured. **G** and **H.** Modified Widman flap—dressing. **I** and **J.** Modified Widman flap—1-week healing. **K** and **L.** Modified Widman flap—3-month healing.

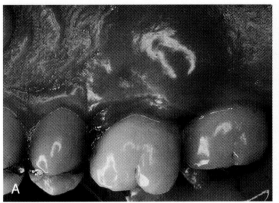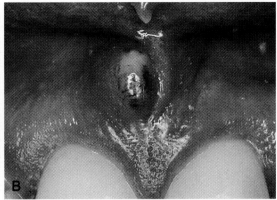

FIGURE 16-1. **A** and **B.** Acute periodontal abscess.

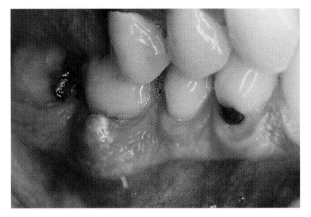

FIGURE 16-3. Gingival abscess.

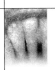

Index

Note: Page numbers in *italics* refer to illustrations. Page numbers followed by the letter b refer to boxed material; those followed by t refer to tables.

A

AAP. See *American Academy of Periodontology (AAP)* entries.

Abfraction, 173-174, 175t

Abrasion, causing tooth wear, 173, *173,* 175t

Abscess(es), associated with partially or fully erupted tooth, 334
  combination, 333-334, *334*
  endodontic, 332-333, *333*
    characteristics of, 333t
  gingival, 332, *332*
  periapical, 330
  periodontal, 122-124, *123-124,* 330-332
    acute, 330-331, *331*
      treatment of, 330-331
    characteristics of, 333t
    chronic, 331, *331*
      treatment of, 331-332
    tooth loss associated with, 332
    treatment of, 124
  stitch, 263

Abutments, implants as, 274, *274*

Acquired immunodeficiency syndrome (AIDS), 352-355, *353-354*
  periodontal disease associated with, epidemiology of, 49-50

ADA (American Dental Association) approval, of implants, 280

Adhesins, in bacterial colonization of pellicle, 57-58

Aerobes, 56

Aerosols, 238

Age, patient, as indication for periodontal surgery, 248-249

Agranulocytosis, 361-362

AHA (American Heart Association) recommendations, for prophylactic antibiotics for patients at risk for infective endocarditis, 344t

AIDS (acquired immunodeficiency syndrome), 352-355, *353-354*
  periodontal disease associated with, epidemiology of, 49-50

Allergic (hypersensitivity) reactions, 31-32

Allograft(s), from cadaver bone, 259

Alloplastic graft(s), 259-260

Aluminum oxide–coated titanium implant, 277. See also *Implant(s).*

Alveolar bone, 24, *25*
  dehiscence and fenestration in, 26, *26*
  preservation of, as objective of periodontal maintenance, 296-297

Alveolar mucosa, assessment of, 157, *157*

Alveolar process, 24-26, *25*
  components of, 24-25
  remodeling of, 25-26

Amalgam overhang, affecting plaque retention, 78-79, *78-79*
  removal of, tools used in, 79, *79*

American Academy of Periodontology (AAP) case types, 188b
  treatment planning for, 190-191, 190b

American Academy of Periodontology (AAP) classification, of disease, 109, 109b, 180b

American Academy of Periodontology (AAP) definition, of scaling, 221

American Dental Association (ADA) approval, of implants, 280

American Heart Association (AHA) recommendations, for prophylactic antibiotics for patients at risk for infective endocarditis, 344t

Ammonium compounds, plaque control with, 211

Anaerobes, 56

Anemia, aplastic, periodontitis associated with, 361, *362*

Angina pectoris, *342,* 342-343

Antibiotics, for periodontal disease, 128-132
  controlled-release, local delivery of, 130-131, *131*
  enzyme suppression effect of, 131-132
  systemic, 129
  treatment considerations in, 129-130
  prophylactic, 344t, 349b

Antibody(ies), 30

Anticalculus agents, 76
  plaque control with, 213-214

Anticoagulants, for cardiovascular disease, 346

Aplastic anemia, periodontitis associated with, 361, *362*

Arrhythmias, 344-346

Arthralgia, 141

Arthritis, 346-347, *347*

Arthrocentesis surgery, for temporomandibular disorders, 149

Arthroscopic surgery, for temporomandibular disorders, 149

Arthus (immune complex) reactions, in hypersensitivity Type III, 32

2621